Crosstalk Between Autophagy and Oxidative Stress

Crosstalk Between Autophagy and Oxidative Stress

Guest Editors

Marina Garcia-Macia
Álvaro F. Fernández

MDPI

Basel • Beijing • Wuhan • Barcelona • Belgrade • Novi Sad • Cluj • Manchester

Guest Editors

Marina Garcia-Macia
Institute of Functional Biology and Genomics (IBFG)
University of Salamanca
Salamanca
Spain

Álvaro F. Fernández
Departamento de Bioquímica y Biología Molecular
Universidad de Oviedo
Oviedo
Spain

Editorial Office
MDPI AG
Grosspeteranlage 5
4052 Basel, Switzerland

This is a reprint of the Special Issue, published open access by the journal *Antioxidants* (ISSN 2076-3921), freely accessible at: https://www.mdpi.com/journal/antioxidants/special_issues/78WOUJ8YQ6.

For citation purposes, cite each article independently as indicated on the article page online and as indicated below:

Lastname, A.A.; Lastname, B.B. Article Title. *Journal Name* **Year**, *Volume Number*, Page Range.

ISBN 978-3-7258-5823-1 (Hbk)
ISBN 978-3-7258-5824-8 (PDF)
https://doi.org/10.3390/books978-3-7258-5824-8

Contents

About the Editors

Marina Garcia-Macia

Marina Garcia-Macia is a Ramón y Cajal researcher at the University of Salamanca, where she leads the MacPhagy research group. She completed her B.Sc., M.Sc. and PhD in Biology at the University of Oviedo. Then, she completed a postdoc at the Albert Einstein College of Medicine (NY, USA) and another at the University of Newcastle (UK). In 2019, she joined the Neuroenergetics and Metabolism group, in Salamanca, to continue her research career by directing her line of research in Batten Disease and becoming a young leader. She is part of various scientific networks, including Women in Autophagy (WIA), SEBBM and SEFAGIA. Her scientific career has always been linked to the study of autophagy. In her study of cellular recycling, she has used different models, from beef to mice, including zebrafish, hamsters, and cell cultures, to understand everything from aging to obesity, including neurodegenerative or liver diseases.

Álvaro F. Fernández

Álvaro F. Fernández is an Associate Professor at the University of Oviedo (Spain), where he leads the AU·SIS (Autophagy & Autosis) group. He obtained his Ph.D. in Cancer Research at the University of Oviedo, studying the functional and pathological roles of the mammalian orthologues of autophagy protease Atg4 (called autophagins) in Prof. Carlos López-Otín's lab. After that, he was a postdoctoral fellow in Dr. Beth Levine's group in the Center for Autophagy Research at the University of Texas Southwestern Medical Center in Dallas (USA), focusing his research on understanding the link between autophagy, aging, and cell death.

Preface

Our knowledge of the role of autophagy in pathophysiology is increasing year by year, as we seek to comprehend how this protective pathway is activated upon different stressors, including the presence of free radicals. Thus, we invited contributions from experts across disciplines to explore the latest advancements in understanding how autophagy and oxidative stress communicate within cellular environments. By fostering collaborative discussions, this reprint seeks to deepen our insights into these interconnected processes, paving the way for innovative therapeutic strategies and unveiling novel targets for intervention.

Marina Garcia-Macia and Álvaro F. Fernández
Guest Editors

antioxidants

MDPI

Editorial

Autophagy: The Last Antioxidant to Unravel

Álvaro F. Fernández [1,2,3,*,†] and Marina García-Macia [4,5,*,†]

1 Departamento de Bioquímica y Biología Molecular, Universidad de Oviedo, 33006 Oviedo, Spain
2 Instituto Universitario de Oncología del Principado de Asturias (IUOPA), 33007 Oviedo, Spain
3 Instituto de Investigación Sanitaria del Principado de Asturias (ISPA), 33011 Oviedo, Spain
4 Institute of Functional Biology and Genomics (IBFG), Universidad de Salamanca-CSIC, 37007 Salamanca, Spain
5 Department of Biochemistry and Molecular Biology, Universidad de Salamanca, 37007 Salamanca, Spain
* Correspondence: fernandezferalvaro@uniovi.es (Á.F.F.); marinagarciamacia@usal.es (M.G.-M.)
† These authors contributed equally to this work.

Christian de Duve used the term "Autophagy" for the first time during a conference focused on lysosomes in 1963, but the scientific revolution caused by this cellular recycling system could not be foreseen at that moment. More than fifty years later, Yoshinori Oshumi was awarded the Nobel Prize for the description of the autophagy-related (ATG) genes, and to this very date, key aspects of this cellular process have been reported by hundreds of groups all over the world. Autophagy is a fundamental cellular process that maintains homeostasis, as it eliminates undesirable cytoplasmic components. It can be activated in response to various stresses, such as nutrient deprivation, hypoxia, drugs, and infections. Recent strong evidence indicates that autophagy is a crucial mediator in the regulation of the oxidative stress response. The more obvious role, when encountering oxidative stress, is removing oxidized proteins or organelles, including damaged mitochondria that generate excessive ROS. However, the knowledge about the interplay between autophagy and the antioxidant transcriptional factor Nrf2 opened the door to a myriad of new roles of autophagy as an antioxidant process. Exploring when and how autophagy modulates antioxidant defenses seems completely necessary. For this reason, we set up this Special Issue, aiming to provide a comprehensive platform for researchers to delve into the cross-regulation between autophagy and oxidative stress.

In this regard, we have included interesting reviews about the mechanistic aspects of the autophagy and oxidative stress interplay (Contributions 1 and 2), a crosstalk that could lead to new forms of cellular death (Contribution 3). Unraveling the basic mechanisms that control this interplay is the cornerstone for further understanding its role in different diseases. Additionally, this Special Issue also displays manuscripts focusing on how the antioxidant stimulation of autophagy is triggered upon certain pathological conditions (Contributions 4 to 9). We did not only focus on human health; very interesting articles about how autophagy can be a tool to improve animal welfare were also included in this Special Issue (Contributions 10 and 11).

Cells try to maintain homeostasis through different pathways that can be activated at the same time or in a sequential order. One of these signaling pathways is the route of the mitogen-activated protein kinases (MAPKs), so it is not a surprise that MAPKs, activated by ROS, are able to modulate autophagy, as it is deeply explained in Contribution 1. The source of ROS is also discussed in this Special Issue. While the main origin of ROS is mitochondria, we often neglect to acknowledge the importance of peroxisomes. Strikingly, peroxisomes also have antioxidant enzymes, so they can be central to the regulation of oxidative stress. When peroxisomes are not functional, they are recycled by a specific type of autophagy: pexophagy. This nexus between peroxisome-dependent oxidative stress regulation and the role of pexophagy is reviewed in Contribution 2. Moreover, these authors go further, addressing the relevance of pexophagy for neurodegenerative diseases too. Interestingly, even though autophagy is mostly considered a pro-survival mechanism, it can be aberrantly activated and lead to cellular death. Autosis is one of these types of death, and it is described thoroughly in Contribution 3. Defects in redox balance and accumulation of oxidative damage led to cellular death too, but the actual role of ROS in autosis is not well understood. The authors of this contribution review what is known about the interplay of ROS in autosis and suggest some audacious hypotheses to test in the future.

Aging is a complex process where both autophagy and oxidative stress participate. Autophagy generally declines with age while oxidative stress builds up. Also, senescent cells accumulate with aging, which can be established as a mark of a more detrimental decay. The use of different types of antioxidants is one of the recent strategies to improve aging and prolong lifespan (Contributions 4 and 5). These authors used flavonoid-related molecules that can be found in grapes, such as procyanidin A1 from peanut skin extract (PSE) and delphinidin, which impact the upstream steps of the autophagic pathway. In these articles, authors blocked autophagy at different levels and found that the antioxidant effect was eliminated. A different strategy, a probiotic yeast (Milmed), was used in Contribution 6. In this case, the beneficial effects of this antioxidant were also tested in vivo, and Milmed increased lifespan in C. elegans.

Aging is the most important risk factor for many diseases, such as cancer. Autophagy and oxidative stress also play a crucial role during the development of this pathology. Tumoral hypoxia or nutrient deprivation fosters oxidative stress that, in turn, activates autophagy to promote tumor cell survival. This is studied deeply in Contribution 7. Additionally, neurodegeneration and alcohol-related brain damage were addressed in Contribution 8. The authors establish the activation of CYP2E1 as the difference between both disorders, while autophagy and oxidative stress aspects are very similar in both diseases. In terms of therapies, stem cells and regenerative medicine are the focus of Contribution 9. Stem cell biology requires both autophagy and oxidative stress in fine balance since they contribute to cell survival, self-renewal, and differentiation. The fate of stem cells is critical to address age-related decline and enhance the potential of regenerative therapies.

Several reasons justify animal welfare research, but the economic value outweighs many of them. In this Special Issue, we learn how pollution affects chicken kidneys and produces nephrotoxicity, increasing oxidative stress and reducing autophagy. This problem severely impacts egg and meat production. Here, authors from contribution 10 tackle the problem with a strategy that is similar to the one previously mentioned in papers focusing on aging. This time, using another flavonoid, luteolin, in the diseased chickens. This treatment reduced oxidative stress and increased autophagy via SIRT1 activation, which resulted in the alleviation of the kidney damage. Apart from poultry, beef cattle are central to the livestock economy, mainly for milk production. Mastitis is a common illness in cows that reduces dairy production. Last but not least, Contribution 11 evaluates how *Streptococcus* infects mammary glands to produce mastitis. They discovered that mammary cells stimulated the antioxidant defenses through Nfr2 and Sirt1, and both activated autophagy.

In summary, this Special Issue provides new knowledge about the role of autophagy as a defense against oxidative stress. The numerous manuscripts cover everything from basic mechanisms to pathophysiology, not only related to human diseases but also considering animal welfare. But still, autophagy will for sure keep surprising the field with unexpected, new roles, as an antioxidant response, and more.

Author Contributions: Conceptualization, Á.F.F. and M.G.-M.; writing—original draft preparation, review and editing, Á.F.F. and M.G.-M. All authors have read and agreed to the published version of the manuscript.

Funding: This research received no external funding.

Conflicts of Interest: The authors declare no conflicts of interest.

List of Contributions:

1. Desideri, E.; Castelli, S.; Ciriolo, M.R. MAPK Signaling in the Interplay Between Oxidative Stress and Autophagy. *Antioxidants* **2025**, *14*, 662. https://doi.org/10.3390/antiox14060662.
2. Wei, X.; Manandhar, L.; Kim, H.; Chhetri, A.; Hwang, J.; Jang, G.; Park, C.; Park, R. Pexophagy and Oxidative Stress: Focus on Peroxisomal Proteins and Reactive Oxygen Species (ROS) Signaling Pathways. *Antioxidants* **2025**, *14*, 126. https://doi.org/10.3390/antiox14020126.
3. Guerra-Andrés, M.; Martínez-Rojo, I.; Piedra-Macías, A.; Lavado-Fernández, E.; García-Macia, M.F.; Fernández, Á. Oxidative Stress in the Regulation of Autosis-Related Proteins. *Antioxidants* **2025**, *14*, 958. https://doi.org/10.3390/antiox14080958.
4. Li, Y.; Xiang, L.; Qi, J. Procyanidin A1 from Peanut Skin Exerts Anti-Aging Effects and Attenuates Senescence via Antioxidative Stress and Autophagy Induction. *Antioxidants* **2025**, *14*, 322. https://doi.org/10.3390/antiox14030322.
5. Bahar, M.E.; Hwang, J.S.; Lai, T.H.; Byun, J.-H.; Kim, D.-H.; Kim, D.R. The Survival of Human Intervertebral Disc Nucleus Pulposus Cells under Oxidative Stress Relies on the Autophagy Triggered by Delphinidin. *Antioxidants* **2024**, *13*, 759. https://doi.org/10.3390/antiox13070759.
6. Armeli, F.; Mengoni, B.; Schifano, E.; Lenz, T.; Archer, T.; Uccelletti, D.; Businaro, R. The Probiotic Yeast, Milmed, Promotes Autophagy and Antioxidant Pathways in BV-2 Microglia Cells and *C. elegans*. *Antioxidants* **2025**, *14*, 393. https://doi.org/10.3390/antiox14040393.
7. Cabrera-Serrano, A.J.; Sánchez-Maldonado, J.M.; González-Olmedo, C.; Carretero-Fernández, M.; Díaz-Beltrán, L.; Gutiérrez-Bautista, J.F.; García-Verdejo, F.J.; Gálvez-Montosa, F.; López-López, J.A.; García-Martín, P.; et al. Crosstalk Between Autophagy and Oxidative Stress in Hematological Malignancies: Mechanisms, Implications, and Therapeutic Potential. *Antioxidants* **2025**, *14*, 264. https://doi.org/10.3390/antiox14030264.
8. Ruiter-Lopez, L.; Khan, M.A.S.; Wang, X.; Song, B.-J. Roles of Oxidative Stress and Autophagy in Alcohol-Mediated Brain Damage. *Antioxidants* **2025**, *14*, 302. https://doi.org/10.3390/antiox14030302.
9. Rossin, D.; Perrelli, M.-G.; Lo Iacono, M.; Rastaldo, R.; Giachino, C. Dynamic Interplay Between Autophagy and Oxidative Stress in Stem Cells: Implications for Regenerative Medicine. *Antioxidants* **2025**, *14*, 691. https://doi.org/10.3390/antiox14060691.
10. Zhang, K.; Li, J.; Dong, W.; Huang, Q.; Wang, X.; Deng, K.; Ali, W.; Song, R.; Zou, H.; Ran, D.; et al. Luteolin Alleviates Cadmium-Induced Kidney Injury by Inhibiting Oxidative DNA Damage and Repairing Autophagic Flux Blockade in Chickens. *Antioxidants* **2024**, *13*, 525. https://doi.org/10.3390/antiox13050525.
11. Khan, S.; Wang, T.; Cobo, E.R.; Liang, B.; Khan, M.A.; Xu, M.; Qu, W.; Gao, J.; Barkema, H.W.; Kastelic, J.P.; et al. Antioxidative Sirt1 and the Keap1-Nrf2 Signaling Pathway Impair Inflammation and Positively Regulate Autophagy in Murine Mammary Epithelial Cells or Mammary Glands Infected with *Streptococcus uberis*. *Antioxidants* **2024**, *13*, 171. https://doi.org/10.3390/antiox13020171.

antioxidants

MDPI

Review

MAPK Signaling in the Interplay Between Oxidative Stress and Autophagy

Enrico Desideri [1,†], Serena Castelli [2,3,†] and Maria Rosa Ciriolo [3,4,*]

1 Department of Life Sciences, Health and Health Professions, Link Campus University, Via del Casale di San Pio V, 44, 00165 Rome, Italy; e.desideri@unilink.it
2 Department of Human Sciences and Promotion of the Quality of Life, San Raffaele Roma Open University, Via di Val Cannuta, 247, 00166 Rome, Italy; serena.castelli@uniroma5.it
3 IRCCS San Raffaele Roma, Via di Val Cannuta, 247, 00166 Rome, Italy
4 Department of Biology, University of Rome "Tor Vergata", Via Della Ricerca Scientifica, 00133 Rome, Italy
* Correspondence: ciriolo@bio.uniroma2.it
† These authors are co-first authorship.

Abstract: The term autophagy identifies several mechanisms that mediate the degradation of intracellular and extracellular components via the lysosomal pathway. Three main forms of autophagy exist, namely macroautophagy, chaperone-mediated autophagy, and endosomal microautophagy, which have distinct mechanisms but share lysosomes as the final destination of their cargo. A basal autophagic flux is crucial for the maintenance of cellular homeostasis, being involved in the physiological turnover of proteins and organelles. Several stressors, including nutrient shortage and genotoxic and oxidative stress, increase the autophagic rate, which prevents the accumulation of damaged and potentially harmful cell components, thus preserving cell viability. In this context, several studies have highlighted the role of MAPKs, serine–threonine kinases activated by several stimuli, in linking oxidative stress and autophagy. Indeed, several oxidative stressors activate autophagy by converging on MAPKs, directly or indirectly. In this regard, the different transcription factors that bridge MAPKs and autophagic activation are here described. In this review, we summarize the current knowledge regarding the regulation of autophagy by MAPK, including the atypical ones, with a particular focus on the regulation of autophagy by oxidative stress.

Keywords: autophagy; MAPK; oxidative stress; CMA; eMI; atypical MAPK

1. Introduction

Autophagy is a collective term that identifies different evolutionary conserved mechanisms involved in the elimination of intracellular and extracellular material via the lysosomes. It plays a pivotal role in maintaining cellular homeostasis, as it can degrade damaged or aggregated proteins, organelles, as well as intracellular pathogens, preventing negative consequences [1]. According to the specificity of substrates degraded by autophagy, autophagy can be divided into non-selective and selective autophagy; the latter refers to the degradation of specific organelles (e.g., mitophagy, ribophagy, pexophagy, and so on) or proteins. Selective autophagy usually requires adaptor proteins that recognize the protein/organelle to be degraded and direct the assembly of the autophagic machinery. Selective autophagy is important during cell differentiation, development, and aging [2]. While autophagy is always active at low rates in physiological conditions, its activity is boosted when cells face stress conditions, such as nutrient deprivation or oxidative stress. In this condition, autophagy acts as a survival mechanism that degrades non-essential or damaged molecules to limit cell damage and/or use their building blocks to sustain the fundamental functions of the cell [3].

In this review, we describe the current knowledge about the regulation of the different types of autophagy by mitogen-activated protein kinases (MAPKs), a family of kinases that responds to both intrinsic and extrinsic stimuli and acts as a key determinant of cell fate upon stress conditions, being involved in the regulation of both death and survival mechanisms. In particular, we will highlight how the different MAPKs influence autophagy in conditions of oxidative stress and the underlying molecular mechanism.

2. Mechanism and Functions of Autophagy

2.1. Mechanism of Autophagy

Among the many variants of autophagy so far cited, the three main types are: macroautophagy; endosomal microautophagy (eMI); and chaperone-mediated autophagy (CMA) (Figure 1). They differ in the way the substrates are recognized and transported to the lysosomes for degradation [2]. In macroautophagy, portions of the cytoplasm or single organelles are engulfed into double-membraned structures, while in eMI and CMA, the cargo is captured by the endosomes and the lysosomes, respectively.

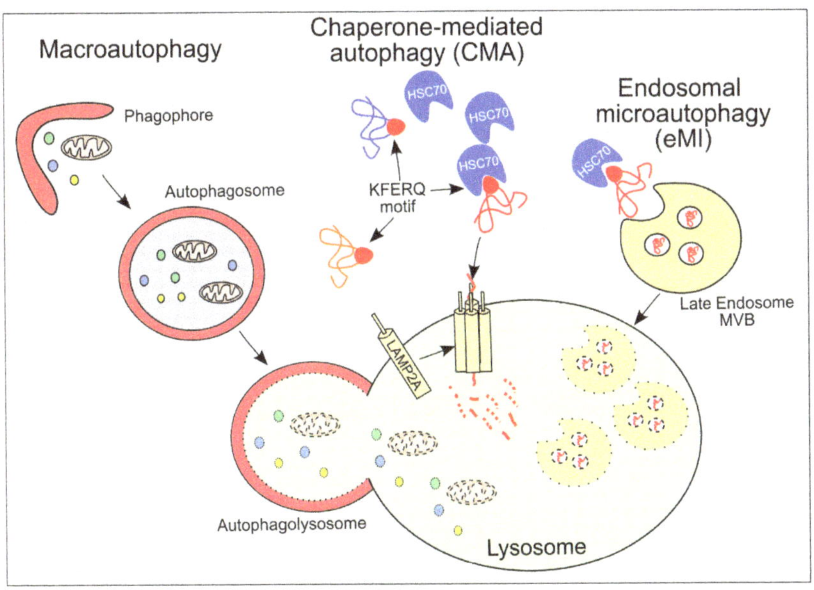

Figure 1. Mechanisms of the different types of autophagy, namely macroautophagy, chaperone-mediated autophagy (CMA), and endosomal microautophagy (eMI), all converging into lysosomal degradation.

2.1.1. Macroautophagy

In macroautophagy (hereinafter called autophagy) cytoplasmic cargoes are sequestered into double-walled membranes called autophagosomes, which originate from the expansion of crescent-shaped structures, the phagophore, and then fuse with the lysosomes to allow the degradation of their content. Thus, the process includes several steps, including phagophore formation, elongation, and autophagosome–lysosome fusion, each regulated by one or more regulatory complexes. The initiation of autophagosome formation is governed by the unc-51-like kinase (ULK) complex, a multiprotein complex composed of FIP200, ATG13, ATG101, and ULK1/ULK2 [3]. ATG13 forms a heterodimer with ATG101, representing a subcomplex binding ULK1 and FIP200, which contains the catalytic domain [4].

Under normal conditions, the ULK1 complex is ubiquitously localized in the cell and inhibited by the mammalian target of rapamycin complex 1 (mTORC1). After a stimulus that induces autophagy, mTORC1 is inactivated, allowing the activation of the ULK complex, which forms visible dots in proximity to the endoplasmic reticulum (ER) membrane, co-localizing specifically with omegasomes, ER structures supporting autophagosome formation [5]. After ULK1/ULK2 is activated, phosphorylation of ATG13 and FIP200 and autophosphorylation of ULK proteins occur. The active ATG13-ULK-FIP200 complex recruits other autophagy-related (ATG) proteins determining the initiation of autophagosome formation and culminating in nucleation, with the activation of class III phosphatidylinositol 3-kinase (PIK3C3) complex, composed of BECN1, AMBRA1, ATG14L, VPS15, and VPS34 and that produce phosphatidylinositol 3-phosphate (PIP3) on the ER membrane, leading to the recruitment of WD-repeat protein interacting with phosphoinositides (WIPI) proteins [4]. There are four WIPI proteins, but WIPI2 is the most abundant and its depletion profoundly impacts autophagy [5]. WIPI2 interacts with ATG16L1, included in the ATG5–ATG12–ATG16L1 (E3-like) complex, and recovers ATG9-positive vesicles allowing the autophagosome nucleation [4]. The E3 Complex promotes the lipidation of different ATG8 proteins, which include LC3 and GABARAP, allowing the binding of ATG2 through its LC3-interacting region (LIR). ATG2 is considered a lipid transfer unit from the ER to the de novo synthesized organelle by supplying phospholipids for autophagosome formation [6,7].

The lipidation of LC3 is a multi-step process similar to ubiquitination that starts with the cleavage of newly synthesized LC3 (pro-LC3) by ATG4 to form LC3-I, which localizes to the cytosol. LC3-I has a C-terminal glycine residue that is susceptible to conjugation. The conjugation requires the adenylation by the ATG7 (E1-like), forming a thioester intermediate. Then, LC3-I binds ATG3 (E2-like) and is finally conjugated with the amine group of phosphatidylethanolamine (PE) localized to the nascent autophagosomes. The amount of lipidated LC3 (LC3-II) is widely used as an indicator of the number of autophagosomes in the cells [8]. The presence of LC3-II on both the inner and outer membrane of autophagosomes allows not only autophagosome formation but also cargo selection via the interaction with several adaptor proteins harboring an LIR motif (e.g., p62, BNIP3) [9]. Recently, human ATG4 has been also described as capable of autophagosome formation independently of its protease activity and able to traffic ATG9-vesicles, with its proximity network. This non-canonical function is carried out specifically during PINK1/Parkin-dependent mitophagy. Indeed, the disruption of the four ATG4s genes using the CRISPRCas9 technique elegantly highlighted that ATG4A and ATG4D, together with proximal proteins involved in the transport process and lipid modification (including LPS responsive beige-like anchor protein, LRBA), play a role in ATG9 recruitment during mitophagy [10]. ATG4 also contributes to LC3-II deconjugation, which allows the release and recycling of LC3. ATG4B has been proposed as the main responsible for LC3 delipidation. Its regulation occurs through ULK1-mediated phosphorylation on serine 316 of ATG4B, which inhibits its catalytic activity. On the contrary, phosphatase PP2A-PP2R3B can dephosphorylate ATG4B. These opposite activities of ULK1 and PP2A proteins regulate the cellular activity of ATG4B and, consequently, LC3 processing [9].

The specificity of the autophagic system is given by proteins known as autophagic receptors that facilitate the engulfment of specific cargoes into autophagosomes. The main feature of autophagic receptors is the presence of both a LIR sequence in their structure, which mediates the binding with LC3-II, and a ubiquitin-binding domain (UBD), which allows them to act as a bridge between cargo to be degraded and the forming autophagosome.

In the majority of cases, autophagic receptors bind poly-ubiquitin chains, but they can also have a direct interaction with the cargo. In this latter case, the expression of cargo-localizing receptors is directly regulated by stress conditions, including starvation and hypoxia [11]. A crucial example of a cargo-localizing receptor is the nuclear receptor coactivator 4 (NCOA4), which has been recently identified as an autophagic receptor specifically recognizing ferritin heavy-chains (FTH1). Excessive intracellular iron is sequestered by ferritin, to prevent harmful consequences. In case of low iron levels, NCOA4 conveys ferritin-iron complexes into the lysosome, where ferritin is degraded, and free iron is released into the cytosol. This process is referred to as ferritinophagy [12–14].

In the case of autophagic receptors binding poly-ubiquitin chains, ubiquitination of substrates by ubiquitin ligases is the major regulatory mechanism. This process allows proteins or organelles that cannot be repaired to be specifically marked and represents a particular advantage in recognizing damaged organelles contained in a network, such as that of mitochondria and ER. In the former, autophagic degradation must be preceded by an isolation process. The selective degradation of mitochondria by autophagy (mitophagy) is preceded by mitochondria fragmentation (fission) due to the activity of dynamin-related protein 1 (DRP1), mitochondrial fission factor (MFF), and mitochondrial fission protein 1 (FIS1) proteins. On the contrary, the activity of proteins involved in mitochondrial fusion, such as mitofusin 1 and 2 (MFN1 and MFN2) is inhibited [15].

For ER (ER-phagy), the mechanism is widely unclear; FAM134B has been identified as a receptor involved in the selectiveness of autophagy but it is not the only player [16].

Virtually all organelles can be degraded by selective macroautophagy. In addition to the above-mentioned mitophagy and ER-phagy, also lipid droplets (lipophagy), protein aggregates (aggrephagy), lysosomes (lysophagy) and pathogens (xenophagy) can be degraded by autophagy [17].

The removal of ubiquitin from the substrate is mediated by deubiquitinating enzymes (DUBs), which cleave single or poly-ubiquitin chains from proteins, releasing free ubiquitin. The deubiquitination process impacts biological processes, such as DNA damage response and DNA repair pathways, and it is involved in the regulation of cancer metabolism [18,19].

The best-studied autophagy receptor is sequestosome-1 (SQSTM-1/p62) [20]. Ubiquitin chains are recognized and bound by p62 monomers with low affinity, but following the homo-oligomerization, p62 oligomers show high avidity to bind poly-ubiquitin chains [13]. The affinity between the ubiquitin-associated domain (UBA) of p62 and the cargoes to be degraded is regulated by S403 phosphorylation, which can stabilize the sequestosome structure. The S403 phosphorylation of the UBA domain of p62 is mediated by Casein kinase 2 (CK2). Interestingly, it has been demonstrated that CK2 over-expression reduces mutant Huntingtin aggregation, consistent with the knowledge that toxic protein aggregations are cleared through autophagy [21].

Other autophagic receptors binding poly-ubiquitin chains in mammalian cells are neighbors of BRCA1 (NBR1), Tax1 binding protein 1 (TAX1BP1), nuclear dot protein 52 (NDP52), and optineurin. Together with p62, they all are soluble proteins having domains capable of binding ubiquitin marks. Considering the similarity to p62, they are all defined as sequestosome-like cargo receptors (SLRs) [22].

Autophagosomes containing their cargo are transported to the lysosomes using dynein motor proteins. The mature autophagosomes acquire SNARE proteins, which are also present on the lysosome membrane. When these two organelles are close enough, SNARE proteins form trans-SNARE complexes, namely an α-helical bundle that forces the fusion of the lysosomal membrane with the autophagosome outer membrane. Two SNARE complexes are involved in autophagosome and lysosome membrane fusion, classified based on the presence of a conserved glutamine (Q) (Q-SNARE) or arginine (R) (R-SNARE) residue in the SNARE motif [23].

The organelle deriving from the fusion between autophagosome and lysosome is called the autophagolysosome. After the autophagosome fusion with the lysosome, the acidic lysosomal hydrolases initially break down the autophagosome inner membrane and finally the autophagosome cargo [24]. Lysosomes contain more than 60 hydrolases, which include proteases, sulfatases, nucleases, lipases, phosphatases, glycosidases, and nucleases. They allow the cells to degrade many types of cargo, including nucleic acids and bacteria. Among lysosomal hydrolases, cathepsins are the most abundant. They are proteases classified into serine cathepsins (A and G), aspartic cathepsins (D and E), and cysteine cathepsins.

These enzymes optimally work in the lysosomal acidic conditions (pH 4.5–5.5), maintained by an H^+-ATPase, or V-ATPase, present at the lysosomal membrane and that translocates two protons into the lysosome by consuming one ATP. The requirement of an acidic pH prevents cell auto-digestion in case of lysosomal damage and the release of lysosomal enzymes into the cytosol.

When the degradation is complete, macromolecule building blocks are transported out of the lysosomes via exporters or vesicular trafficking to be used for ATP production or as precursors of anabolic pathways [25].

2.1.2. Chaperone-Mediated Autophagy

Chaperone-mediated autophagy (CMA) is a selective type of autophagy that degrades proteins bearing a recognition motif (KFERQ-like motif), biochemically related to the KFERQ sequence present in the first CMA substrate identified, RNAse A. The KFERQ motif is recognized by the chaperone HSPA8/HSC70 (heat shock protein family A (Hsp70) member 8) [26]. The KFERQ-like motif is present in a good percentage (up to 30%) of cytosolic proteins and is sufficient to allow their degradation by CMA, but it is often not accessible to HSC70 unless the protein is at least partially unfolded and/or modified by PTM. The HSC70-protein complex promotes the interaction with LAMP2A, the CMA receptor located on the lysosome membrane. The interaction of the CMA substrate with the cytosolic tail of LAMP2A promotes LAMP2A oligomerization and the formation of a multiprotein complex that facilitates substrate unfolding and internalization. Once the LAMP2A complex completes this role, it returns to the monomeric form, ready for a new translocation cycle. This assembly/disassembly dynamic of LAMP2A is regulated by glial fibrillary acidic protein (GFAP) and elongation factor 1α (EF1α). GFAP is responsible for the stabilization of the LAMP2A multimeric complex, responsible for the internalization of the substrate. The phosphorylated form of GFAP, instead, has a higher affinity for EF1α, forming with it a complex on the lysosomal membrane. When the substrate is translocated, EF1α is released and pGFAP becomes available to be bound. The affinity of GFAP for pGFAP is higher than that for LAMP2A; for this reason, GFAP/pGFAP dimer forms and GFAP/LAMP2A complex disassembles [27].

Another regulatory mechanism of CMA is mTORC2, which negatively impacts CMA by phosphorylating and activating AKT. Active AKT, indeed, can phosphorylate GFAP releasing it from LAMP2A, disassembling the translocation complex of CMA. On the contrary, a positive regulation depends on the Pleckstrin homology (PH) domain and leucine-rich repeat protein phosphatase 1 (PHLPP1) since it can remove the phosphorylation of Akt induced by mTORC2. In the same way, Torin-1 inhibits the function of mTORC2, by blocking the activation of AKT and inducing CMA [26–28].

The regulation can also occur at the level of chaperones responsible for substrate translocation, such as HSPA8 and heat shock protein 90 (Hsp90). These chaperones bind LAMP2A, regulating its recycling [29].

The levels of LAMP2A are crucial in the regulation of the CMA pathway. The transcription factor NFAT-1 can regulate the expression of LAMP2A based on intracellular ROS levels. Indeed, an increase in ROS leads to the recruitment of NFAT-1 on the LAMP2 promoter, upregulating its expression. In light of this, modulation of ROS is used as a suitable approach to regulate CMA. For instance, 6-Aminonicotinamide (6-AN), a ROS inducer, promotes CMA, as well as, vitamin E, as an antioxidant, reduces CMA levels [30].

2.1.3. Endosomal Microautophagy (eMI)

In endosomal microautophagy (eMI), the cytoplasmic cargo is engulfed by late endosome/multi-vesicular bodies. The initial step, shared with CMA, is the recognition of a pentapeptide amino acid KFERQ-like targeting motif in the substrate protein by the HSC70 chaperone. This chaperone, through interaction with the chaperone Bag6, interacts with phosphatidylserine residues of late endosomes, instead of lysosomes as it occurs in CMA. The internalization inside the vesicles is mediated by the endosomal sorting complexes required for transport (ESCRT) machinery (Tsg101 and Alix) and the ATPase Vps4, which is responsible for the invagination of the membrane [31]. In the formed multivesicular bodies, the KFERQ-containing protein can be degraded after fusion with lysosomes or secreted after the fusion with the plasma membrane [32]. Extracellular release of eMI cargoes could represent an alternative way for cells to remove molecules particularly when degradation is impaired, and to execute immune signaling and pathogen surveillance. The fusion between the late endosome body and the plasma membrane is responsible for the formation of exosomes, a subset of extracellular vesicles enriched in endosomal proteins [33].

On the other hand, the fusion between late endosomes and lysosomes contributes to proteostasis and organelle turnover; moreover, it takes part in the autophagic response to aminoacid starvation. Indeed, it has been demonstrated that eMI activation can contribute in the case of prolonged starvation, acting as a regulatory pathway. Among its substrates, there are also some selective autophagy receptors (including p62 and LC3-II), probably degraded through the eMI pathway to avoid the activation of bulk macroautophagy [29]. Recent studies showed that eMI is preferentially activated by some selective stressors. They include high glucose conditions, H_2O_2 treatment, and genotoxic insults such as etoposide. On the contrary, serum starvation and short-time serum and aminoacid depletion treatment do not alter eMI activation. Notably, during oxidative stress, MAPK/JNK signaling is involved in eMI induction [32,34]. It has also been demonstrated a cross-talk between eMI and CMA as a compensatory mechanism. Indeed, when lysosomal-associated membrane protein 2A (LAMP2A) is knocked down and CMA blocked, eMI activity is increased; conversely, Vps4A/B knock-down blocked eMI and induced higher CMA activity [35].

2.2. Functions of Autophagy

The role of autophagy in cellular physiology is extensive, including adaptation to metabolic stress, degradation of potentially dangerous cargoes, and prevention of genomic modifications.

Glucose represents the major energy source for several cell types. In the case of low glucose levels, autophagy mediates the response aimed at meeting the intracellular energy requirements for cell survival through the catabolism of reserves and the recycling of intracellular macromolecules. A crucial hub responsible for glucose sensing is the highly conserved mTOR complex, composed of mTORC1 and mTORC2. Upon glucose availability, mTORC1 is activated to stimulate the anabolic process and promote proliferation [36]. Glucose scarcity inhibits mTORC1 both blocking cell growth and proliferation and inducing autophagy. Being the synthesis of macromolecules, mainly protein synthesis, the most expensive process in terms of energy, mTORC1-driven response blocks anabolism and promotes the usage of reserves.

However, beyond emphasizing the energy provided by autophagy, the energy required by autophagy itself has also to be highlighted. Thus, autophagy activation may depend on the ability of the cell to carry out the process spending the minimum amount of energy. Whether this ability is restricted, other vital processes are prioritized [37].

On the other hand, energy stresses responsible for autophagy induction also include nutrient excess, especially high glucose concentrations, resulting in an autophagy-mediated cell death, also known as "autosis". Autosis is a programmed cell death, beyond apoptosis and necrosis, that is recognized by a large number of autolysosomes present in the cytoplasm and the fact that no proteins, aside from those belonging to the autophagic core, are required to mediate this type of death [38]. Indeed, autophagic cell death can be blocked by the depletion of ATG proteins [39]. In this condition, reactive oxygen species (ROS) have been identified as the major players in the overwhelmed induction of autophagy by activating the Mitogen-activated protein kinase (MAPK) signaling pathway [40]. Moreover, upon an overload of nutrients, ER stress can also occur following the increased protein entry in ER and the consequent augment of unfolded proteins. The unfolded protein response (UPR) is in turn responsible for activating autophagy [41]. Indeed, autophagy has an active role in protein turnover, orchestrating protein degradation together with the proteasome. The ubiquitin–proteasome system (UPS) is responsible for the degradation of about one-third of newly synthesized proteins. Even though UPS and autophagy are mechanistically different, an important common feature is the presence of ubiquitin sequence marking targets [42]. Generally, the majority of short-lived proteins are degraded by UPS, whereas long-lived proteins are preferentially degraded via autophagy, but this division is not strictly enforced. In addition, the relative contribution of autophagy depends on the cell type and the environment; indeed, this process contributes to cellular remodeling and adaptations to changes in the availability of different nutrients [43]. For instance, autophagy plays a pivotal role in physiological bone remodeling, which is crucial for the formation and maintenance of bone morphology and the repair of damaged bones. The differentiation of bone marrow mesenchymal stem cells requires AMP-activated protein kinase (AMPK)/mTOR signaling axis-mediated autophagy during the early stage. In contrast, protein kinase B (AKT)/mTOR signaling axis activation is needed in the late stage. The key role of autophagy in this differentiation process is also demonstrated by the loss of autophagic capability in fully differentiated osteoblasts. In this context, ROS are responsible for autophagy activation through MAPK induction [44]. Beyond bone marrow mesenchymal stem cells, it has also been demonstrated that autophagy is involved in the differentiation of several cell types, including immune cells [45], hematopoietic cells [46], neurons [47], by removing proteins that should not be present in each specific stage of differentiation.

The above-mentioned functions define autophagy as a crucial process to maintain homeostasis; consequently, perturbations of this degradation process are associated with numerous diseases, such as infections, cancer, and neurodegeneration [48].

Autophagy acts as an innate immune mechanism aimed at removing pathogens invading cells. This type of selective autophagy is known as xenophagy [49]. After the permeabilization of the phagosome through which the bacterium enters the cell, it will be promptly ubiquitinated and recognized by ubiquitin-binding autophagic receptors. Consistently, the deletion of genes codifying for key autophagic players determines an uncontrolled replication of bacteria in mammalian cells, making cells extremely susceptible to infection. For instance, murine myeloid-derived cells knock-out in the ATG5 gene show a higher vulnerability to *Mycobacterium tuberculosis* infection [50]. Knockdown of p62 or inactivation of ATG5 has been shown to increase viral capsid accumulation and accelerate cell death induced by the Sindbis virus [51].

Based on this, bacteria and viruses have developed mechanisms to elude autophagy degradation. In several cases, bacteria inhibit autophagy activation at different levels to carry on the infection or mask their surface to avoid ubiquitination [52]. For instance, *Francisella tularensis* escapes from autophagic destruction by coating its surface with polysaccharidic O-antigens that protect it against polyubiquitination [53].

Being autophagy a self-clearance pathway, among its functions there is also the removal of oxidized cellular components and, consequently, the regulation of intracellular ROS content. ROS are small molecules, including one-electron reduction products such as superoxide anions ($O^{\bullet 2-}$), hydroxyl radicals ($^{\bullet}OH$), peroxyl ($RO_2^{\bullet}$), and alkoxy ($RO^{\bullet}$), two-electron reduction products such as hydrogen peroxide (H_2O_2). ROS and RNS (reactive nitrogen species) are mainly produced in mitochondria by the electron transport chain, thus their production is strictly associated with the metabolic status of the cells. Basal levels of ROS have a physiological function of signaling, acting as second messengers, and activating transcriptional factors. At high concentrations, ROS/RNS can react with organelle and macromolecules resulting in their oxidation. The net content of ROS depends on the balance between ROS production and elimination, thanks to the action of antioxidant mechanisms [54]. Autophagy is part of the adaptive antioxidant response of cells, and it is responsible for the different capacities of cells to cope with ROS originating from different insults based also on a different ROS threshold required to activate autophagy [55].

3. Regulation of Autophagy

Autophagy is a homeostatic mechanism, and it is not surprising that autophagic levels can significantly fluctuate when cellular homeostasis is perturbed, regardless of whether it is the consequence of nutrient shortage, pathogen infections, or exposure to pro-oxidant agents. In all these cases, the autophagy rate is enhanced to cope with stress conditions and to preserve cell integrity and viability [56]. At the same time, it should also be considered that an excessive degradation of cell components can be detrimental to the cells and eventually lead to cell death [57]. The term autophagic cell death was introduced to identify a type of cell death that can be blocked by genetic inhibition of autophagy [58]. As high autophagic activity was reported in many dying cells and no specific morphological features of autophagic cell death have ever been identified, it is not trivial to discriminate between a cell death "by autophagy" and one that is only dependent or triggered by autophagy, like autosis [59]. Regardless of this difference, cells must fine-tune autophagy activity and duration to make sure that it is always proportional to the intensity of the stimulus to prevent undesired detrimental effects. A common trait of all types of autophagy is that they all require lysosomes to complete the process. Therefore, changes in lysosomal activity, positioning, and expression of lysosomal membrane proteins impact autophagy activity [60,61]. The regulation of the specific forms of autophagy, namely CMA and eMI, is still poorly studied but it generally occurs at either substrate recognition or at the lysosomal level [26,62]. On the contrary, the regulation of macroautophagy is well characterized and all steps of the autophagy pathway, from autophagosome formation and maturation to autophagosome fusion with lysosomes, are subject to regulation [3]. Regulation of macroautophagy can occur at multiple levels: transcriptional, post-transcriptional, and post-translational.

3.1. Transcriptional Regulation

The transcriptional regulation depends on the expression of autophagic genes; the increase of even a few of them is sufficient to stimulate autophagy. Several transcription factors have been shown to regulate autophagy, either activating or inhibiting it.

3.1.1. TFEB

The transcription factor TFEB is considered the master regulator of autophagy and lysosomal biogenesis, and many genes involved in different steps of the autophagic pathway, including Beclin-1, LC3, and p62, are TFEB targets [63]. Consequently, the increase of TFEB expression causes activation of autophagy. Various transcriptional factors, in turn, can regulate TFEB expression, including CREB, which also regulates ATG7 and ULK1, by recruiting its coactivator CRTC2 [64]. TFEB can be also regulated through phosphorylation that sequesters it into the cytosol and prevents its nuclear activity. The main kinase responsible for TFEB phosphorylation in the presence of aminoacids is mTOR [65]. In particular, mTORC1 directly phosphorylates TFEB at Ser142 and Ser211 sites, inactivating it. 14-3-3 proteins also bind phosphorylated TFEB and prevent its nuclear translocation [63]. Moreover, AKT directly phosphorylates TFEB at Ser467 and represses its nuclear translocation independently of mTORC1 [66].

3.1.2. FoxO

Beyond TFEB, members of the Forkhead Box O (FoxO) family can also regulate autophagic genes. FoxO3 induces a bulk induction of autophagy, determining atrophy in myotubes by promoting genes such as LC3 and GABARAPl1 [67]. Moreover, FoxO3 can induce autophagy in a FoxO1-dependent manner. Specifically, FoxO3 promotes the phosphorylation of FoxO1 by AKT1, causing translocation of FoxO1 to the cytoplasm, leading to the induction of autophagy [68].

3.1.3. Peroxisome Proliferator–Activated Receptors (PPARs)

The transcription factors of the PPARs family, such as PPARα and PPARγ, regulate gene expression upon metabolic variations and have opposite roles in the regulation of autophagy. PPARα is activated by free fatty acids and it can bind promoters of autophagic-related genes, regulating the expression of LC3, BNIP3, ATG7, and Beclin1. Pharmacological activation of PPARα is sufficient to release autophagy inhibition in the fed state, inducing lipophagy, and PPARα knockout mice are partially defective in activating autophagy during fasting [69]. During adipogenesis, it has been demonstrated that PPARγ induces LC3, Beclin1, and ATG4b, directly regulating autophagy, and indirectly promotes the expression of TFEB and FoxO1 inducing autophagy to remove proteins not useful in the differentiation step ongoing [70].

3.1.4. p53

The transcription factor and tumor suppressor p53 has a dual role in modulating autophagy, depending on its subcellular localization. Nuclear p53 activates ATG genes, among which ATG4A, ATG5, and WIPI1, and genes inhibiting mTOR, such as AMPK and TSC2. Another p53 target is DRAM1, which promotes the acidification of lysosomes and, consequently, autophagy. On the contrary, cytosolic p53 inhibits autophagy through different pathways, such as the inhibition of AMPK, mTOR activation, and the ubiquitination and degradation of Beclin1 [71].

3.1.5. AMPK

A crucial stress sensor responsible for maintaining energy balance is AMPK, which also acts as an epigenetic regulator. Indeed, it can modulate the activity of histone acetyltransferases (HATs) and histone deacetylases (HDACs). Among HDACs influenced by AMPK, there is SIRT1, which induces autophagy by promoting the deacetylation of ATGs and FOXO1 genes. Under nutrient-deprived conditions, AMPK can phosphorylate GAPDH, which, in turn, translocates into the nucleus where it interacts with SIRT1 and activates its histone deacetylation function. This mechanism allows the release of epigenetic acetylation readers, such as bromodomain-containing protein 4 (BRD4), and the expression of autophagic and lysosomal genes. When nutrients are available, autophagy and lysosomal gene expression are repressed by the binding of BRD4 to the promoter and, consequently, the recruitment of a methyltransferase that induces histone demethylation [72]. Another target of AMPK is Acetyl-CoA synthetase short-chain family member 2 (ACSS2), whose function is to convert acetate into acetyl-CoA. When phosphorylated by AMPK, ACSS2 can translocate into the nucleus to interact with TFEB and to locally produce acetyl-CoA necessary for histone acetylation, inducing the expression of autophagic genes [73].

3.1.6. HATs

The activity of acetyltransferase, including p300, can also be modulated by mTOR [72]. In particular, when activated, mTORC1 phosphorylates p300 and prevents the binding to the RING domain, inhibiting the catalytic function. As a consequence, autophagy induced by starvation is suppressed and lipogenesis is activated [74].

Regarding the epigenetic regulation of autophagy, DNA methyltransferases (DNMTs) and ten-eleven translocation (TET) proteins are responsible for methylation levels of several autophagic genes and, consequently, they can activate or suppress autophagy. For instance, TET1 can regulate the expression of ATG13 and DNA damage-regulated autophagy modulator protein 1 [75]; DNMT3 is responsible for methylating the DNA of the LC3 gene, resulting in a reduction of basal autophagy [76].

3.2. *Post-Transcriptional Regulation*

In addition to transcription factors, a significant number of non-coding RNAs (microRNA, circRNA, and lncRNA) participate in autophagy modulation. Among them, miR-101 inhibits RAB5A, ATG4C and, together with miR-376b, ATG4D; miR-103a-3p inhibits ATG5 [77].

3.3. *Post-Translational Regulation*

Post-translational modifications are widely present in autophagy regulation, comprehending ubiquitination, phosphorylation, glycosylation, methylation, acetylation, and protein lipidation (N-myristoylation, S-palmitoylation, S-prenylation, glycosylphosphatidylinositol (GPI) anchoring, and cholesterylation) [78]. Several of the abovementioned transcriptional factors are also responsible for directly regulating post-translational modifications of autophagic proteins, such as AKT, that phosphorylates Beclin1 at Ser295 and inhibits autophagy [79], whereas the phosphorylation at Ser91/94 by AMPK induces autophagy [80].

A crucial point of post-translational regulation of autophagy is the regulation of LC3 protein levels and function. The ubiquitin-activating enzyme UBA6 and the ubiquitin ligase BIRC6 cooperate and suppress autophagy by promoting LC3 monoubiquitination and proteasomal degradation [81]. LC3 phosphorylation at Ser12 by PKA suppresses its activity and inhibits autophagy. Metabolic and pathological inducers of autophagy caused dephosphorylation of endogenous LC3 [82].

4. Regulation of Autophagy by ROS

Oxidative stress is a major modulator of autophagy, as many stimuli that activate autophagy cause an increase in ROS. ROS can regulate autophagy both directly and indirectly. For instance, nutrient deprivation, the archetypal autophagy inducer, increases mitochondrial ROS levels, possibly due to an increased electron leakage [83].

A rapid accumulation of ROS during nutrient starvation promotes autophagy activation. Nutrient starvation stimulates the production of mitochondrial ROS, mainly H_2O_2, that can oxidize the cysteine protease ATG4, responsible for regulating LC3 interaction with autophagosomes. Oxidation inhibits ATG4 and promotes the lipidation of LC3 and autophagosome formation [84]. Since mitochondria are the main responsible for ROS production, ROS can promote mitophagy to avoid excessive oxidative stress. One of the mechanisms responsible for mitophagy activation by ROS is the induction of Parkin translocation to mitochondria, mainly driven by superoxide [85]. Additionally, the non-canonical mitophagic pathway regulated by BNIP3 can be modulated by ROS [86,87].

The regulation of autophagy by ROS can also be indirect, via modulation of autophagic gene expression; it is the case of Beclin1 and NF-kB expression prompted by ROS and that consequently activates autophagy [88]. Moreover, ROS can activate AMPK and stimulate autophagy to allow the cells to counteract oxidative stress and preserve cell viability. Several AMPK cysteine residues, like Cys299, Cys304, and Cys312, can be oxidized and modified, for instance by S-glutathionylation, causing a conformational change in AMPK that facilitates protein phosphorylation at Thr172. This event anticipates the activation of AMPK mediated by a high AMP:ATP ratio. [89].

ROS-mediated autophagy activation can also play a propaedeutic role in cell death by autosis. ROS-mediated loss of cardiolipin in neurons causes autosis [90], and high LPS-mediated activation induces ROS-mediated autophagic cell death in macrophages [91].

The ability of ROS to induce autophagic cell death can also be exploited as an anti-cancer strategy, as was shown in glioma [92], colon [93], and chronic myeloid leukemia [94]. ROS-mediated activation of autophagy can also trigger ferroptosis, an iron-dependent cell death mechanism, since autophagy regulates intracellular iron levels through ferritin degradation and transferrin receptor induction [95].

5. Mitogen-Activated Protein Kinases (MAPKs)

Mitogen-activated protein kinases (MAPKs) are a family of serine/threonine kinases that transduce extracellular and intracellular stimuli into a variety of cellular responses. The best-characterized members are the four conventional MAPKs: the extracellular signal-regulated kinases 1/2 (ERK1/2), c-Jun amino (N)-terminal kinases 1/2/3 (JNK1/2/3), p38 (p38α, β, γ, and δ), and ERK5 [96]. Other MAPKs have been described and classified as atypical MAPKs, because they are activated via different, often unclear mechanisms and their functions differ from those of conventional MAPK. Atypical MAPKs are ERK3/4/7/8 and Nemo-like kinase (NLK) [97,98].

Each conventional MAPK is the endpoint of a three-tier cascade starting with a MAP kinase kinase kinase (MAP3K) that is activated by upstream signals like cytokines or growth factors, often through G-protein-coupled or tyrosine kinase receptors [96].

Active MAP3Ks phosphorylate and activate one or more MAP kinase kinases (MAP2Ks), which, in turn, phosphorylate-specific MAPKs on threonine and/or tyrosine residue located within a Thr-Xxx-Tyr motif [96]. MAPKs, in particular JNK and p38, can also be activated in response to several stressors originating from either outside or inside the cell, such as oxidative and genotoxic stress. An overview of the MAPK cascades and their output is shown in Figure 2. The activation mechanism of MAPK by oxidative stress is often not completely understood but it involves the activation of protein tyrosine kinase [99], inhibition of protein phosphatases [100], or direct activation of upstream kinases. One well-known example is represented by the MAP3K apoptosis signal-regulating kinase 1 (ASK1). ASK1 is usually inhibited by the binding of thioredoxin 1 (TRX1), a small antioxidant protein. Upon ROS production, TRX1 cysteine residues are oxidized, causing the release of ASK1 and its activation. Active ASK1 phosphorylates the MAP2Ks MKK3/4/6, which, in turn, activate JNK and p38 and induce the cell death pathway [101].

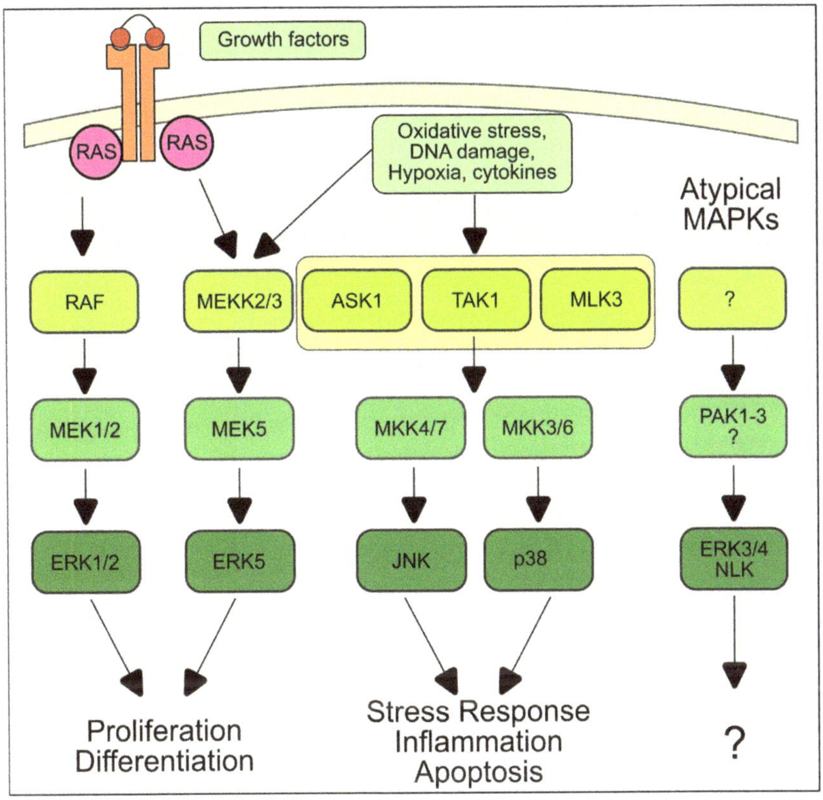

Figure 2. Cascades of conventional and atypical MAPKs. Conventional MARKs activate responses as proliferation, differentiation, and apoptosis whereas atypical MAPKs are involved in the autophagy response, but their roles are still unclear (?).

Once activated, MAPKs phosphorylate a considerable number of targets, either in the cytosol or in the nucleus, resulting in the modulation of a wide range of processes, such as cell survival, proliferation, differentiation, migration, and death [102]. In an over-simplistic view, the ERK pathway was traditionally considered associated with cell proliferation and differentiation, while JNK and p38 are involved in stress response and activation of cell death pathways. The presence of several isoforms of each MAPK with tissue specificity, the presence of scaffolding proteins and phosphatases that operate a spatiotemporal regulation of MAPK activation, and the connectivity among components of the MAPK pathway, add additional layers of complexity in the MAPK network and make the result of MAPK activation highly dependent on the type and duration of the stimulus and the cellular context [103].

6. Role of MAPK in the Regulation of Autophagy

As downstream effectors of ROS, multiple reports have shown that MAPKs regulate autophagy, either activating or inhibiting it, depending on the stimulus and the cell type (Figure 3). However, the identity of the downstream effectors is not always known.

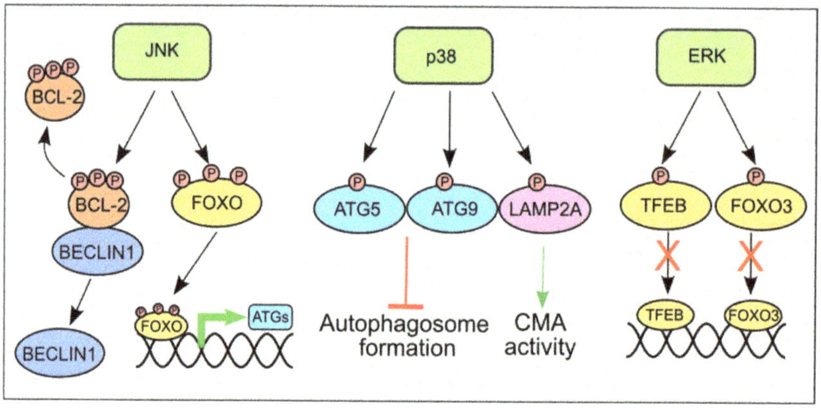

Figure 3. Regulation of autophagy by MAPKs. As downstream effectors of ROS, MAPKs can either activate (green arrows) or inhibit (red arrow with blunted end) autophagy by phosphorylating several downstream targets, promoting (black arrow), or inhibiting (black arrow with red crosses) their functions.

6.1. JNK

Several reports in the last decades have highlighted the role of JNK in the regulation of autophagy, specifically macroautophagy, and there is a consensus in defining JNK as a positive regulator. Mechanistically, JNK-dependent regulation of autophagy can be either transcriptional-independent or transcriptional-dependent. In 2006, Wei and colleagues demonstrated that JNK1, but not JNK2, phosphorylates the anti-apoptotic protein Bcl-2 upon nutrient deprivation [104]. The magnitude and/or the kinetic Bcl-2 phosphorylation by JNK1 determines whether Bcl-2 phosphorylation triggers a pro-survival (autophagy) or pro-death (apoptosis) response. Upon short-term nutrient deprivation, the phosphorylation by JNK1 at residues Thr69, Ser70, and Ser87 of Bcl-2 disrupts the binding with Beclin1, promoting autophagosome formation. In this condition, the interaction of Bcl-2 with the pro-apoptotic protein Bax is not affected, so the anti-antiapoptotic functions of Bcl-2 are preserved. If nutrient deprivation is prolonged, maximal Bcl-2 phosphorylation disrupts the binding with Bax, promoting apoptosis [105]. Thus far, this is the sole example of a direct involvement of JNK in the regulation of autophagy through direct phosphorylation of a protein linked to autophagy. The literature regarding the transcriptional-dependent regulation of autophagy by JNK is, on the contrary, quite rich. This is not surprising as many JNK downstream targets are transcription factors. JNK is a positive regulator of the FoxO transcription factors. Active JNK phosphorylates FoxO at several residues, promoting nuclear translocation and expression of its targets [106]. Several ATG genes, including LC3 and BNIP3, are among FoxO targets [107], and constitutive activation of FoxO3A was shown to be sufficient to induce autophagy [67]. In addition, FoxO can regulate autophagy through epigenetic mechanisms involving histone modifications that promote the expression of the autophagy and lysosomal biogenesis regulator TFEB [108]. Among the other JNK targets c-Jun, one of the subunits of the AP-1 transcription factor, upregulates Beclin1 expression to induce autophagy [109]. To date, nothing is known about the possible regulation of CMA by the JNK pathway, while a role in eMI has been reported in Drosophila. Here, the authors showed that JNK signaling mediates ROS-induced activation of eMI in the fly fat body, although the JNK targets are not yet identified [34].

6.2. p38

Similar to JNK, numerous reports are linking p38 activation to autophagy modulation. However, unlike JNK, there is conflicting data on whether p38 is a positive or negative regulator of autophagy. Regardless of the effect of p38 activation, regulation of autophagy seems to predominantly take place via phosphorylation of protein involved in autophagy. For example, ATG5, a protein involved in autophagosome formation, can be phosphorylated at Thr75 in a p38-dependent manner [110]. Phosphorylation of ATG5 by p38 blocks autophagy by inhibiting autophagosome maturation, highlighting a negative role of p38 on autophagy. In a similar paper, p38 was shown to inhibit autophagy in glial cells by phosphorylating ULK1 [111]. Additional reports demonstrated that p38 can inhibit autophagy also via indirect mechanisms. In 2010, the group of Sharon Tooze demonstrated that p38 inhibits autophagy by controlling the interaction of p38IP with ATG9, a member of autophagy core machinery [112]. Similarly, we showed that ROS-dependent activation of p38 indirectly limits starvation-induced autophagy via a feedback loop that decreases ROS levels by redirecting glucose metabolism from glycolysis to the pentose phosphate pathway (PPP), thus increasing NADPH production to preserve cell viability under conditions of nutrient deprivation [113].

While many papers indicate that p38 activation inhibits autophagy, others go in the opposite direction. Activation of p38 was shown to regulate autophagy through the phosphorylation of glycogen synthase kinase 3b (GSK3b) on Ser9 [114]. Whether p38 directly phosphorylates GSK3b was not clarified. More recently, p38 was shown to phosphorylate TFEB at Ser401, leading to TFEB activation to promote monocyte-to-macrophage differentiation [115]. In the paper, the effect on autophagy was not analyzed; however, being many autophagy and lysosomal genes among TFEB targets, it is reasonable to speculate that this activation would increase autophagy. The knowledge regarding the other types of autophagy is extremely limited. Only one paper highlighted the direct role of p38 in the regulation of CMA. The authors demonstrated that in response to ER stress p38 can localize to the lysosome and directly phosphorylate the CMA lysosomal receptor LAMP2A at Thr211 and Thr213, inducing LAMP2A oligomerization and CMA activation [116]. Another paper showed that p38 phosphorylates TFEB by inhibiting its activity. TFEB is a transcription factor promoting LAMP2 expression and, consequently, increasing activation of CMA. For this reason, several p38 inhibitors are used as CMA promoters since they induce TFEB translocation into the nucleus [117]. To date, nothing is known about whether p38 also influences eMI.

6.3. ERK1/2

The number of reports regarding the regulation of autophagy by ERK in conditions of oxidative stress is not huge, as it is more often studied in the context of the RAS/RAF/MEK/ERK pathway in tumors in which this pathway is altered. For instance, RAS or ERK blockade was shown to increase autophagy in pancreatic cancer [118]. Along the same line, ERK was shown to inhibit FoxO3, a positive regulator of autophagy [119], and to phosphorylate TFEB at Ser142 when sufficient nutrients are present, sequestering TFEB in the cytosol. In starvation conditions, ERK does not bind TFEB, leaving it to translocate into the nucleus [120].

Both lines of evidence agree on the inhibitory function of ERK on autophagy. Interestingly, ERK was shown to localize to the cytoplasmic face of autophagosomes and to interact with some ATG proteins. In this case, autophagosomes act as a scaffold in the spatio-temporal regulation of ERK phosphorylation in response to growth factors [121]. Whether active ERK localized at the autophagosome has any effect on ATG proteins and autophagy is not known. As for CMA and eMI, there are currently no reports on the regulation by ERK.

6.4. ERK5

A limited number of papers described the involvement of ERK5 signaling in autophagy, without an agreement on the output of its activation. The MEKK2/3-MEK5-ERK5 pathway was shown to promote basal mitophagy in cultured cells [122], while in neuronal cells MEK5 inhibition was shown to activate autophagy in a mTOR-independent and ERK5-independent manner [123]. Another paper indicated that ERK5 inhibition activates autophagy, but in this case, the effect was attributed to ER stress caused by ERK5 inhibition, rather than a direct modulation of ERK5 on autophagy [124].

6.5. Atypical MAPK

Very few reports investigated the influence of atypical MAPKs, in particular NLK, on autophagy. NLK was shown to be activated by stress conditions such as hyperosmotic and oxidative stress in HEK293 cells and to phosphorylate Raptor and inhibit mTORC1 [125], suggesting that NLK stimulates autophagy, although this possibility was not tested. A more recent paper by Tejwani and colleagues suggests an opposite effect of NLK. They show that in neuronal cells NLK inhibits lysosomal biogenesis and autophagy by promoting the destabilization of nuclear TFEB [126].

7. Conclusions

In detailing the fundamentals of the interplay between redox regulation and autophagy, this review is structured to provide an outline of the underlying principles of how MAPKs are contributing. For autophagy functioning cells use an orchestrated system, which includes multifaceted input cues that cause a signal to be generated. The general set-up is completed by appropriate feedback systems, the detailed mechanisms of which still need to be uncovered. Autophagy and MAPK are both modulated by several stimuli, and it is therefore not surprising that there is plenty of literature showing their interconnection, at least for what regards macroautophagy. The biochemistry of gene activation through redox-sensitive transcription factors has largely been elucidated. However, several key questions remain to be answered. One major question concerns the hierarchy of redox regulation. In this context, ROS are among the main stimuli responsible for the activation of autophagy through MAPKs. This makes cellular antioxidant defenses crucial because they regulate the amount of ROS imposing the threshold for autophagic activation [83]. As mentioned in the published literature and in several instances in the present review, there are the so-called master regulators, but the question arises: who regulates the regulator? Therefore, cell fate is regulated by cellular antioxidant capacity; in fact, cells with prominent antioxidant defenses, such as the aforementioned liver cells [127], cardiac cells [40], and bone marrow mesenchymal cells [44] exploit ROS to activate autophagy avoiding cell death. A better understanding will require network analysis in terms of feedback and feedforward loops at spatiotemporal patterns. It is not surprising that the final effect of MAPK activation is strongly cell-dependent and stimulus-dependent, reflecting the complex regulation of the MAPK pathways that determine their outputs. This depends on a better understanding of the molecular mechanisms linking MAPK and autophagy, as many papers are more focused on the final effects of MAPK modulation than on how the regulation takes place. Another important consideration concerns the duration of the stimulus, which determines whether the cellular response will be pro-survival or pro-death. In fact, the activation of autophagy is directly associated with the cell's ability to survive under stress conditions, either by utilizing alternative energy sources or by engaging the autophagic pathway to eliminate the source of stress itself (e.g., misfolded proteins, bacteria, viruses). However, if the stimulus is prolonged, apoptosis tends to become the predominant outcome. This aspect further complicates the relationship between oxidative stress and the autophagic response, also introducing limitations in the potential therapeutic exploitation of this interplay. Similarly, a major research challenge exists in further elucidating the molecular details linking MAPK and other types of autophagy, whose regulatory mechanisms remain poorly understood.

Author Contributions: E.D. and S.C. conceptualized the review, performed the literature search for articles, and wrote the manuscript; M.R.C. supervised the study and revised the manuscript. All authors have read and agreed to the published version of the manuscript.

Funding: This work was supported by European Union—Next Generation EU and Italian Ministry of University and Research (MUR-PRIN_2022_PNRR No. P2022XZKBM, MUR-PNRR M4C2I1.3 PE6 project PE00000019 Heal Italia No. E83C22004670001); Italian Association for Cancer Research (AIRC) No. IG 2023 ID 29207.

Conflicts of Interest: The authors declare no conflicts of interest.

References

1. Aguilera, M.O.; Delgui, L.R.; Reggiori, F.; Romano, P.S.; Colombo, M.I. Autophagy as an Innate Immunity Response against Pathogens: A Tango Dance. *FEBS Lett.* **2024**, *598*, 140–166. [CrossRef] [PubMed]
2. Gómez-Virgilio, L.; Silva-Lucero, M.-D.-C.; Flores-Morelos, D.-S.; Gallardo-Nieto, J.; Lopez-Toledo, G.; Abarca-Fernandez, A.-M.; Zacapala-Gómez, A.-E.; Luna-Muñoz, J.; Montiel-Sosa, F.; Soto-Rojas, L.O.; et al. Autophagy: A Key Regulator of Homeostasis and Disease: An Overview of Molecular Mechanisms and Modulators. *Cells* **2022**, *11*, 2262. [CrossRef] [PubMed]
3. Yamamoto, H.; Zhang, S.; Mizushima, N. Autophagy Genes in Biology and Disease. *Nat. Rev. Genet.* **2023**, *24*, 382–400. [CrossRef]
4. Qi, S.; Kim, D.J.; Stjepanovic, G.; Hurley, J.H. Structure of the Human Atg13-Atg101 HORMA Heterodimer: An Interaction Hub within the ULK1 Complex. *Structure* **2015**, *23*, 1848–1857. [CrossRef] [PubMed]
5. Zachari, M.; Ganley, I.G. The Mammalian ULK1 Complex and Autophagy Initiation. *Essays Biochem.* **2017**, *61*, 585–596. [CrossRef]
6. Bozic, M.; van den Bekerom, L.; Milne, B.A.; Goodman, N.; Roberston, L.; Prescott, A.R.; Macartney, T.J.; Dawe, N.; McEwan, D.G. A Conserved ATG2-GABARAP Family Interaction Is Critical for Phagophore Formation. *EMBO Rep.* **2020**, *21*, e48412. [CrossRef]
7. Osawa, T.; Noda, N.N. Atg2: A Novel Phospholipid Transfer Protein That Mediates de Novo Autophagosome Biogenesis. *Protein Sci.* **2019**, *28*, 1005–1012. [CrossRef]
8. Maruyama, T.; Noda, N.N. Autophagy-Regulating Protease Atg4: Structure, Function, Regulation and Inhibition. *J. Antibiot.* **2017**, *71*, 72–78. [CrossRef]
9. Pengo, N.; Agrotis, A.; Prak, K.; Jones, J.; Ketteler, R. A Reversible Phospho-Switch Mediated by ULK1 Regulates the Activity of Autophagy Protease ATG4B. *Nat. Commun.* **2017**, *8*, 294. [CrossRef]
10. Nguyen, T.N.; Padman, B.S.; Zellner, S.; Khuu, G.; Uoselis, L.; Lam, W.K.; Skulsuppaisarn, M.; Lindblom, R.S.J.; Watts, E.M.; Behrends, C.; et al. ATG4 Family Proteins Drive Phagophore Growth Independently of the LC3/GABARAP Lipidation System. *Mol. Cell* **2021**, *81*, 2013–2030.e9. [CrossRef]
11. Faruk, M.O.; Ichimura, Y.; Komatsu, M. Selective Autophagy. *Cancer Sci.* **2021**, *112*, 3972–3978. [CrossRef] [PubMed]
12. Le, Y.; Liu, Q.; Yang, Y.; Wu, J. The Emerging Role of Nuclear Receptor Coactivator 4 in Health and Disease: A Novel Bridge between Iron Metabolism and Immunity. *Cell Death Discov.* **2024**, *10*, 312. [CrossRef]
13. Zaffagnini, G.; Martens, S. Mechanisms of Selective Autophagy. *J. Mol. Biol.* **2016**, *428*, 1714–1724. [CrossRef] [PubMed]
14. Mancias, J.D.; Wang, X.; Gygi, S.P.; Harper, J.W.; Kimmelman, A.C. Quantitative Proteomics Identifies NCOA4 as the Cargo Receptor Mediating Ferritinophagy. *Nature* **2014**, *509*, 105–109. [CrossRef]
15. Chen, W.; Zhao, H.; Li, Y. Mitochondrial Dynamics in Health and Disease: Mechanisms and Potential Targets. *Signal Transduct. Target. Ther.* **2023**, *8*, 333. [CrossRef]
16. Gubas, A.; Dikic, I. ER Remodeling via ER-Phagy. *Mol. Cell* **2022**, *82*, 1492–1500. [CrossRef]
17. Wu, M.-Y.; Li, Z.-W.; Lu, J.-H. Molecular Modulators and Receptors of Selective Autophagy: Disease Implication and Identification Strategies. *Int. J. Biol. Sci.* **2024**, *20*, 751–764. [CrossRef]
18. Snyder, N.A.; Silva, G.M. Deubiquitinating Enzymes (DUBs): Regulation, Homeostasis, and Oxidative Stress Response. *J. Biol. Chem.* **2021**, *297*, 101077. [CrossRef] [PubMed]
19. Han, S.; Wang, R.; Zhang, Y.; Li, X.; Gan, Y.; Gao, F.; Rong, P.; Wang, W.; Li, W. The Role of Ubiquitination and Deubiquitination in Tumor Invasion and Metastasis. *Int. J. Biol. Sci.* **2022**, *18*, 2292–2303. [CrossRef]

20. Runwal, G.; Stamatakou, E.; Siddiqi, F.H.; Puri, C.; Zhu, Y.; Rubinsztein, D.C. LC3-Positive Structures Are Prominent in Autophagy-Deficient Cells. *Sci. Rep.* **2019**, *9*, 10147. [CrossRef]
21. Matsumoto, G.; Wada, K.; Okuno, M.; Kurosawa, M.; Nukina, N. Serine 403 Phosphorylation of P62/SQSTM1 Regulates Selective Autophagic Clearance of Ubiquitinated Proteins. *Mol. Cell* **2011**, *44*, 279–289. [CrossRef] [PubMed]
22. Adriaenssens, E.; Ferrari, L.; Martens, S. Orchestration of Selective Autophagy by Cargo Receptors. *Curr. Biol.* **2022**, *32*, R1357–R1371. [CrossRef] [PubMed]
23. Wang, Y.; Li, L.; Hou, C.; Lai, Y.; Long, J.; Liu, J.; Zhong, Q.; Diao, J. SNARE-Mediated Membrane Fusion in Autophagy. *Semin. Cell Dev. Biol.* **2016**, *60*, 97–104. [CrossRef]
24. Saha, S.; Panigrahi, D.P.; Patil, S.; Bhutia, S.K. Autophagy in Health and Disease: A Comprehensive Review. *Biomed. Pharmacother.* **2018**, *104*, 485–495. [CrossRef]
25. Xiong, J.; Zhu, M.X. Regulation of Lysosomal Ion Homeostasis by Channels and Transporters. *Sci. China Life Sci.* **2016**, *59*, 777–791. [CrossRef]
26. Jafari, M.; McCabe, M.; Cuervo, A.M. Chaperone-Mediated Autophagy: Mechanisms and Physiological Relevance. *Curr. Opin. Physiol.* **2022**, *30*, 100597. [CrossRef]
27. Bandyopadhyay, U.; Sridhar, S.; Kaushik, S.; Kiffin, R.; Cuervo, A.M. Identification of Regulators of Chaperone-Mediated Autophagy. *Mol. Cell* **2010**, *39*, 535–547. [CrossRef] [PubMed]
28. Arias, E.; Koga, H.; Diaz, A.; Mocholi, E.; Patel, B.; Cuervo, A.M. Lysosomal mTORC2/PHLPP1/Akt Regulate Chaperone-Mediated Autophagy. *Mol. Cell* **2015**, *59*, 270–284. [CrossRef]
29. Alfaro, I.E.; Albornoz, A.; Molina, A.; Moreno, J.; Cordero, K.; Criollo, A.; Budini, M. Chaperone Mediated Autophagy in the Crosstalk of Neurodegenerative Diseases and Metabolic Disorders. *Front. Endocrinol.* **2019**, *9*, 778. [CrossRef]
30. Hubert, V.; Weiss, S.; Rees, A.J.; Kain, R. Modulating Chaperone-Mediated Autophagy and Its Clinical Applications in Cancer. *Cells* **2022**, *11*, 2562. [CrossRef]
31. Krause, G.J.; Cuervo, A.M. Assessment of Mammalian Endosomal Microautophagy. *Methods Cell Biol.* **2021**, *164*, 167–185. [CrossRef] [PubMed]
32. Vélez, E.J.; Véron, V.; Gouis, J.; Reji, S.; Dias, K.; Herpin, A.; Beaumatin, F.; Seiliez, I. Endosomal Microautophagy Is Activated by Specific Cellular Stresses in Trout Hepatocytes. *bioRxiv* **2024**. bioRxiv:2024.09.26.615173.
33. Buratta, S.; Tancini, B.; Sagini, K.; Delo, F.; Chiaradia, E.; Urbanelli, L.; Emiliani, C. Lysosomal Exocytosis, Exosome Release and Secretory Autophagy: The Autophagic- and Endo-Lysosomal Systems Go Extracellular. *Int. J. Mol. Sci.* **2020**, *21*, 2576. [CrossRef]
34. Mesquita, A.; Glenn, J.; Jenny, A. Differential Activation of eMI by Distinct Forms of Cellular Stress. *Autophagy* **2021**, *17*, 1828–1840. [CrossRef]
35. Krause, G.J.; Kirchner, P.; Stiller, B.; Morozova, K.; Diaz, A.; Chen, K.-H.; Krogan, N.J.; Agullo-Pascual, E.; Clement, C.C.; Lindenau, K.; et al. Molecular Determinants of the Crosstalk between Endosomal Microautophagy and Chaperone-Mediated Autophagy. *Cell Rep.* **2023**, *42*, 113529. [CrossRef]
36. Ben-Sahra, I.; Manning, B.D. mTORC1 Signaling and the Metabolic Control of Cell Growth. *Curr. Opin. Cell. Biol.* **2017**, *45*, 72–82. [CrossRef]
37. Park, J.-M.; Lee, D.-H.; Kim, D.-H. Redefining the Role of AMPK in Autophagy and the Energy Stress Response. *Nat. Commun.* **2023**, *14*, 2994. [CrossRef] [PubMed]
38. Liu, Y.; Shoji-Kawata, S.; Sumpter, R.M.; Wei, Y.; Ginet, V.; Zhang, L.; Posner, B.; Tran, K.A.; Green, D.R.; Xavier, R.J.; et al. Autosis Is a Na+,K+-ATPase-Regulated Form of Cell Death Triggered by Autophagy-Inducing Peptides, Starvation, and Hypoxia-Ischemia. *Proc. Natl. Acad. Sci. USA* **2013**, *110*, 20364–20371. [CrossRef]
39. Chen, Y.; McMillan-Ward, E.; Kong, J.; Israels, S.J.; Gibson, S.B. Oxidative Stress Induces Autophagic Cell Death Independent of Apoptosis in Transformed and Cancer Cells. *Cell Death Differ.* **2008**, *15*, 171–182. [CrossRef]
40. Chen, J.; Guo, R.; Yan, H.; Tian, L.; You, Q.; Li, S.; Huang, R.; Wu, K. Naringin Inhibits ROS-Activated MAPK Pathway in High Glucose-Induced Injuries in H9c2 Cardiac Cells. *Basic Clin. Pharmacol. Toxicol.* **2014**, *114*, 293–304. [CrossRef]
41. Kwon, J.; Kim, J.; Kim, K.I. Crosstalk between Endoplasmic Reticulum Stress Response and Autophagy in Human Diseases. *Anim. Cells Syst.* **2023**, *27*, 29–37. [CrossRef] [PubMed]
42. Li, Y.; Li, S.; Wu, H. Ubiquitination-Proteasome System (UPS) and Autophagy Two Main Protein Degradation Machineries in Response to Cell Stress. *Cells* **2022**, *11*, 851. [CrossRef]
43. Mizushima, N.; Klionsky, D.J. Protein Turnover via Autophagy: Implications for Metabolism. *Annu. Rev. Nutr.* **2007**, *27*, 19–40. [CrossRef] [PubMed]
44. Zhu, C.; Shen, S.; Zhang, S.; Huang, M.; Zhang, L.; Chen, X. Autophagy in Bone Remodeling: A Regulator of Oxidative Stress. *Front. Endocrinol.* **2022**, *13*, 898634. [CrossRef] [PubMed]
45. Clarke, A.J.; Simon, A.K. Autophagy in the Renewal, Differentiation and Homeostasis of Immune Cells. *Nat. Rev. Immunol.* **2019**, *19*, 170–183. [CrossRef]

46. Riffelmacher, T.; Simon, A.-K. Mechanistic Roles of Autophagy in Hematopoietic Differentiation. *FEBS J.* **2017**, *284*, 1008–1020. [CrossRef]
47. Stavoe, A.K.H.; Holzbaur, E.L.F. Autophagy in Neurons. *Annu. Rev. Cell Dev. Biol.* **2019**, *35*, 477–500. [CrossRef]
48. Levine, B.; Kroemer, G. Biological Functions of Autophagy Genes: A Disease Perspective. *Cell* **2019**, *176*, 11–42. [CrossRef]
49. Reggio, A.; Buonomo, V.; Grumati, P. Eating the Unknown: Xenophagy and ER-Phagy Are Cytoprotective Defenses against Pathogens. *Exp. Cell Res.* **2020**, *396*, 112276. [CrossRef]
50. Castillo, E.F.; Dekonenko, A.; Arko-Mensah, J.; Mandell, M.A.; Dupont, N.; Jiang, S.; Delgado-Vargas, M.; Timmins, G.S.; Bhattacharya, D.; Yang, H.; et al. Autophagy Protects against Active Tuberculosis by Suppressing Bacterial Burden and Inflammation. *Proc. Natl. Acad. Sci. USA* **2012**, *109*, E3168–E3176. [CrossRef]
51. Orvedahl, A.; MacPherson, S.; Sumpter, R.; Tallóczy, Z.; Zou, Z.; Levine, B. Autophagy Protects against Sindbis Virus Infection of the Central Nervous System. *Cell Host Microbe.* **2010**, *7*, 115–127. [CrossRef] [PubMed]
52. Lei, Y.; Klionsky, D.J. The Emerging Roles of Autophagy in Human Diseases. *Biomedicines* **2021**, *9*, 1651. [CrossRef] [PubMed]
53. Case, E.D.R.; Chong, A.; Wehrly, T.D.; Hansen, B.; Child, R.; Hwang, S.; Virgin, H.W.; Celli, J. The Francisella O-Antigen Mediates Survival in the Macrophage Cytosol via Autophagy Avoidance. *Cell Microbiol.* **2014**, *16*, 862–877. [CrossRef]
54. Castelli, S.; De Falco, P.; Ciccarone, F.; Desideri, E.; Ciriolo, M.R. Lipid Catabolism and ROS in Cancer: A Bidirectional Liaison. *Cancers* **2021**, *13*, 5484. [CrossRef] [PubMed]
55. Castelli, S.; Ciccarone, F.; De Falco, P.; Ciriolo, M.R. Adaptive Antioxidant Response to Mitochondrial Fatty Acid Oxidation Determines the Proliferative Outcome of Cancer Cells. *Cancer Lett.* **2023**, *554*, 216010. [CrossRef]
56. Li, J.; Liu, R. Autophagy in Cellular Stress Responses. In *Oxidative Stress: Human Diseases and Medicine*; Huang, C., Zhang, Y., Eds.; Springer: Singapore, 2021; pp. 133–154; ISBN 978-981-16-0522-2.
57. Liu, S.; Yao, S.; Yang, H.; Liu, S.; Wang, Y. Autophagy: Regulator of Cell Death. *Cell Death Dis.* **2023**, *14*, 648. [CrossRef]
58. Galluzzi, L.; Vitale, I.; Abrams, J.M.; Alnemri, E.S.; Baehrecke, E.H.; Blagosklonny, M.V.; Dawson, T.M.; Dawson, V.L.; El-Deiry, W.S.; Fulda, S.; et al. Molecular Definitions of Cell Death Subroutines: Recommendations of the Nomenclature Committee on Cell Death 2012. *Cell Death Differ.* **2012**, *19*, 107–120. [CrossRef]
59. Liu, Y.; Levine, B. Autosis and Autophagic Cell Death: The Dark Side of Autophagy. *Cell Death Differ.* **2015**, *22*, 367–376. [CrossRef]
60. Yim, W.W.-Y.; Mizushima, N. Lysosome Biology in Autophagy. *Cell Discov.* **2020**, *6*, 6. [CrossRef]
61. Korolchuk, V.I.; Saiki, S.; Lichtenberg, M.; Siddiqi, F.H.; Roberts, E.A.; Imarisio, S.; Jahreiss, L.; Sarkar, S.; Futter, M.; Menzies, F.M.; et al. Lysosomal Positioning Coordinates Cellular Nutrient Responses. *Nat. Cell Biol.* **2011**, *13*, 453–460. [CrossRef]
62. Wang, L.; Klionsky, D.J.; Shen, H.-M. The Emerging Mechanisms and Functions of Microautophagy. *Nat. Rev. Mol. Cell Biol.* **2023**, *24*, 186–203. [CrossRef] [PubMed]
63. Song, T.-T.; Cai, R.-S.; Hu, R.; Xu, Y.-S.; Qi, B.-N.; Xiong, Y.-A. The Important Role of TFEB in Autophagy-Lysosomal Pathway and Autophagy-Related Diseases: A Systematic Review. *Eur. Rev. Med. Pharmacol. Sci.* **2021**, *25*, 1641–1649. [CrossRef] [PubMed]
64. Seok, S.; Fu, T.; Choi, S.-E.; Li, Y.; Zhu, R.; Kumar, S.; Sun, X.; Yoon, G.; Kang, Y.; Zhong, W.; et al. Transcriptional Regulation of Autophagy by an FXR-CREB Axis. *Nature* **2014**, *516*, 108–111. [CrossRef] [PubMed]
65. Napolitano, G.; Esposito, A.; Choi, H.; Matarese, M.; Benedetti, V.; Di Malta, C.; Monfregola, J.; Medina, D.L.; Lippincott-Schwartz, J.; Ballabio, A. mTOR-Dependent Phosphorylation Controls TFEB Nuclear Export. *Nat. Commun.* **2018**, *9*, 3312. [CrossRef]
66. Palmieri, M.; Pal, R.; Sardiello, M. AKT Modulates the Autophagy-Lysosome Pathway via TFEB. *Cell Cycle* **2017**, *16*, 1237–1238. [CrossRef]
67. Zhao, J.; Brault, J.J.; Schild, A.; Cao, P.; Sandri, M.; Schiaffino, S.; Lecker, S.H.; Goldberg, A.L. FoxO3 Coordinately Activates Protein Degradation by the Autophagic/Lysosomal and Proteasomal Pathways in Atrophying Muscle Cells. *Cell Metab.* **2007**, *6*, 472–483. [CrossRef]
68. Zhou, J.; Liao, W.; Yang, J.; Ma, K.; Li, X.; Wang, Y.; Wang, D.; Wang, L.; Zhang, Y.; Yin, Y.; et al. FOXO3 Induces FOXO1-Dependent Autophagy by Activating the AKT1 Signaling Pathway. *Autophagy* **2012**, *8*, 1712–1723. [CrossRef]
69. Lee, J.M.; Wagner, M.; Xiao, R.; Kim, K.H.; Feng, D.; Lazar, M.A.; Moore, D.D. Nutrient-Sensing Nuclear Receptors Coordinate Autophagy. *Nature* **2014**, *516*, 112–115. [CrossRef]
70. Ahmed, M.; Lai, T.H.; Hwang, J.S.; Zada, S.; Pham, T.M.; Kim, D.R. Transcriptional Regulation of Autophagy Genes via Stage-Specific Activation of CEBPB and PPARG during Adipogenesis: A Systematic Study Using Public Gene Expression and Transcription Factor Binding Datasets. *Cells* **2019**, *8*, 1321. [CrossRef]
71. Lei, Y.; Klionsky, D.J. Transcriptional Regulation of Autophagy and Its Implications in Human Disease. *Cell Death Differ.* **2023**, *30*, 1416–1429. [CrossRef]
72. Shi, Y.; Shen, H.-M.; Gopalakrishnan, V.; Gordon, N. Epigenetic Regulation of Autophagy Beyond the Cytoplasm: A Review. *Front. Cell Dev. Biol.* **2021**, *9*, 675599. [CrossRef] [PubMed]
73. Bulusu, V.; Tumanov, S.; Michalopoulou, E.; van den Broek, N.J.; MacKay, G.; Nixon, C.; Dhayade, S.; Schug, Z.T.; Vande Voorde, J.; Blyth, K.; et al. Acetate Recapturing by Nuclear Acetyl-CoA Synthetase 2 Prevents Loss of Histone Acetylation during Oxygen and Serum Limitation. *Cell Rep.* **2017**, *18*, 647–658. [CrossRef] [PubMed]

74. Wan, W.; You, Z.; Xu, Y.; Zhou, L.; Guan, Z.; Peng, C.; Wong, C.C.L.; Su, H.; Zhou, T.; Xia, H.; et al. mTORC1 Phosphorylates Acetyltransferase P300 to Regulate Autophagy and Lipogenesis. *Mol. Cell* **2017**, *68*, 323–335.e6. [CrossRef] [PubMed]
75. Fu, R.; Ding, Y.; Luo, J.; Huang, K.M.; Tang, X.J.; Li, D.S.; Guo, S.W. Ten-Eleven Translocation 1 Regulates Methylation of Autophagy-Related Genes in Human Glioma. *Neuroreport* **2018**, *29*, 731–738. [CrossRef]
76. González-Rodríguez, P.; Cheray, M.; Füllgrabe, J.; Salli, M.; Engskog-Vlachos, P.; Keane, L.; Cunha, V.; Lupa, A.; Li, W.; Ma, Q.; et al. The DNA Methyltransferase DNMT3A Contributes to Autophagy Long-Term Memory. *Autophagy* **2021**, *17*, 1259–1277. [CrossRef]
77. Ma, Q.; Long, S.; Gan, Z.; Tettamanti, G.; Li, K.; Tian, L. Transcriptional and Post-Transcriptional Regulation of Autophagy. *Cells* **2022**, *11*, 441. [CrossRef]
78. Shao, Y.; Hu, J.; Li, H.; Lu, K. Regulation of Autophagy by Protein Lipidation. *Adv. Biotechnol.* **2024**, *2*, 33. [CrossRef]
79. Wang, R.C.; Wei, Y.; An, Z.; Zou, Z.; Xiao, G.; Bhagat, G.; White, M.; Reichelt, J.; Levine, B. Akt-Mediated Regulation of Autophagy and Tumorigenesis through Beclin 1 Phosphorylation. *Science* **2012**, *338*, 956–959. [CrossRef]
80. Kim, J.; Kim, Y.C.; Fang, C.; Russell, R.C.; Kim, J.H.; Fan, W.; Liu, R.; Zhong, Q.; Guan, K.-L. Differential Regulation of Distinct Vps34 Complexes by AMPK in Nutrient Stress and Autophagy. *Cell* **2013**, *152*, 290–303. [CrossRef]
81. Jia, R.; Bonifacino, J.S. Negative Regulation of Autophagy by UBA6-BIRC6-Mediated Ubiquitination of LC3. *Elife* **2019**, *8*, e50034. [CrossRef]
82. Cherra, S.J.; Kulich, S.M.; Uechi, G.; Balasubramani, M.; Mountzouris, J.; Day, B.W.; Chu, C.T. Regulation of the Autophagy Protein LC3 by Phosphorylation. *J. Cell Biol.* **2010**, *190*, 533–539. [CrossRef]
83. Marchi, S.; Giorgi, C.; Suski, J.M.; Agnoletto, C.; Bononi, A.; Bonora, M.; De Marchi, E.; Missiroli, S.; Patergnani, S.; Poletti, F.; et al. Mitochondria-Ros Crosstalk in the Control of Cell Death and Aging. *J. Signal. Transduct.* **2012**, *2012*, 329635. [CrossRef] [PubMed]
84. Scherz-Shouval, R.; Shvets, E.; Fass, E.; Shorer, H.; Gil, L.; Elazar, Z. Reactive Oxygen Species Are Essential for Autophagy and Specifically Regulate the Activity of Atg4. *EMBO J.* **2007**, *26*, 1749–1760. [CrossRef] [PubMed]
85. Xiao, B.; Deng, X.; Lim, G.G.Y.; Xie, S.; Zhou, Z.D.; Lim, K.-L.; Tan, E.-K. Superoxide Drives Progression of Parkin/PINK1-Dependent Mitophagy Following Translocation of Parkin to Mitochondria. *Cell Death Dis.* **2017**, *8*, e3097. [CrossRef]
86. Ney, P.A. Mitochondrial Autophagy: Origins, Significance, and Role of BNIP3 and NIX. *Biochim. Biophys. Acta* **2015**, *1853*, 2775–2783. [CrossRef]
87. Castelli, S.; Ciccarone, F.; Tavian, D.; Ciriolo, M.R. ROS-Dependent HIF1α Activation under Forced Lipid Catabolism Entails Glycolysis and Mitophagy as Mediators of Higher Proliferation Rate in Cervical Cancer Cells. *J. Exp. Clin. Cancer Res.* **2021**, *40*, 94. [CrossRef] [PubMed]
88. Azad, M.B.; Chen, Y.; Gibson, S.B. Regulation of Autophagy by Reactive Oxygen Species (ROS): Implications for Cancer Progression and Treatment. *Antioxid. Redox Signal* **2009**, *11*, 777–790. [CrossRef]
89. Agostini, F.; Bisaglia, M.; Plotegher, N. Linking ROS Levels to Autophagy: The Key Role of AMPK. *Antioxidants* **2023**, *12*, 1406. [CrossRef]
90. Kirkland, R.A.; Adibhatla, R.M.; Hatcher, J.F.; Franklin, J.L. Loss of Cardiolipin and Mitochondria during Programmed Neuronal Death: Evidence of a Role for Lipid Peroxidation and Autophagy. *Neuroscience* **2002**, *115*, 587–602. [CrossRef]
91. Xu, Y.; Kim, S.O.; Li, Y.; Han, J. Autophagy Contributes to Caspase-Independent Macrophage Cell Death. *J. Biol. Chem.* **2006**, *281*, 19179–19187. [CrossRef]
92. Li, L.; Ishdorj, G.; Gibson, S.B. Reactive Oxygen Species Regulation of Autophagy in Cancer: Implications for Cancer Treatment. *Free. Radic. Biol. Med.* **2012**, *53*, 1399–1410. [CrossRef] [PubMed]
93. Lee, Y.J.; Kim, N.-Y.; Suh, Y.-A.; Lee, C. Involvement of ROS in Curcumin-Induced Autophagic Cell Death. *Korean J. Physiol. Pharmacol.* **2011**, *15*, 1–7. [CrossRef]
94. Jiang, S.; Fan, J.; Wang, Q.; Ju, D.; Feng, M.; Li, J.; Guan, Z.-B.; An, D.; Wang, X.; Ye, L. Diosgenin Induces ROS-Dependent Autophagy and Cytotoxicity via mTOR Signaling Pathway in Chronic Myeloid Leukemia Cells. *Phytomedicine* **2016**, *23*, 243–252. [CrossRef] [PubMed]
95. Park, E.; Chung, S.W. ROS-Mediated Autophagy Increases Intracellular Iron Levels and Ferroptosis by Ferritin and Transferrin Receptor Regulation. *Cell Death Dis.* **2019**, *10*, 822. [CrossRef]
96. Braicu, C.; Buse, M.; Busuioc, C.; Drula, R.; Gulei, D.; Raduly, L.; Rusu, A.; Irimie, A.; Atanasov, A.G.; Slaby, O.; et al. A Comprehensive Review on MAPK: A Promising Therapeutic Target in Cancer. *Cancers* **2019**, *11*, 1618. [CrossRef]
97. Hadwiger, J.A.; Aranda, R.G.; Fatima, S. Atypical MAP Kinases—New Insights and Directions from Amoeba. *J. Cell Sci.* **2023**, *136*, jcs261447. [CrossRef]
98. Daams, R.; Massoumi, R. Nemo-Like Kinase in Development and Diseases: Insights from Mouse Studies. *Int. J. Mol. Sci.* **2020**, *21*, 9203. [CrossRef]

99. Lin, Y.-J.; Yang, C.-C.; Lee, I.-T.; Wu, W.-B.; Lin, C.-C.; Hsiao, L.-D.; Yang, C.-M. Reactive Oxygen Species-Dependent Activation of EGFR/Akt/P38 Mitogen-Activated Protein Kinase and JNK1/2/FoxO1 and AP-1 Pathways in Human Pulmonary Alveolar Epithelial Cells Leads to Up-Regulation of COX-2/PGE2 Induced by Silica Nanoparticles. *Biomedicines* **2023**, *11*, 2628. [CrossRef] [PubMed]
100. Ravindran, J.; Gupta, N.; Agrawal, M.; Bala Bhaskar, A.S.; Lakshmana Rao, P.V. Modulation of ROS/MAPK Signaling Pathways by Okadaic Acid Leads to Cell Death via, Mitochondrial Mediated Caspase-Dependent Mechanism. *Apoptosis* **2011**, *16*, 145–161. [CrossRef]
101. Sakauchi, C.; Wakatsuki, H.; Ichijo, H.; Hattori, K. Pleiotropic Properties of ASK1. *Biochim. Biophys. Acta Gen. Subj.* **2017**, *1861*, 3030–3038. [CrossRef]
102. Gehart, H.; Kumpf, S.; Ittner, A.; Ricci, R. MAPK Signalling in Cellular Metabolism: Stress or Wellness? *EMBO Rep.* **2010**, *11*, 834–840. [CrossRef] [PubMed]
103. Fey, D.; Croucher, D.R.; Kolch, W.; Kholodenko, B.N. Crosstalk and Signaling Switches in Mitogen-Activated Protein Kinase Cascades. *Front. Physiol.* **2012**, *3*, 355. [CrossRef]
104. Wei, Y.; Pattingre, S.; Sinha, S.; Bassik, M.; Levine, B. JNK1-Mediated Phosphorylation of Bcl-2 Regulates Starvation-Induced Autophagy. *Mol. Cell* **2008**, *30*, 678–688. [CrossRef]
105. Wei, Y.; Sinha, S.; Levine, B. Dual Role of JNK1-Mediated Phosphorylation of Bcl-2 in Autophagy and Apoptosis Regulation. *Autophagy* **2008**, *4*, 949–951. [CrossRef] [PubMed]
106. Essers, M.A.G.; Weijzen, S.; de Vries-Smits, A.M.M.; Saarloos, I.; de Ruiter, N.D.; Bos, J.L.; Burgering, B.M.T. FOXO Transcription Factor Activation by Oxidative Stress Mediated by the Small GTPase Ral and JNK. *EMBO J.* **2004**, *23*, 4802–4812. [CrossRef]
107. Mammucari, C.; Milan, G.; Romanello, V.; Masiero, E.; Rudolf, R.; Del Piccolo, P.; Burden, S.J.; Di Lisi, R.; Sandri, C.; Zhao, J.; et al. FoxO3 Controls Autophagy in Skeletal Muscle in Vivo. *Cell Metab.* **2007**, *6*, 458–471. [CrossRef]
108. Shin, H.-J.R.; Kim, H.; Oh, S.; Lee, J.-G.; Kee, M.; Ko, H.-J.; Kweon, M.-N.; Won, K.-J.; Baek, S.H. AMPK-SKP2-CARM1 Signalling Cascade in Transcriptional Regulation of Autophagy. *Nature* **2016**, *534*, 553–557. [CrossRef]
109. Li, D.-D.; Wang, L.-L.; Deng, R.; Tang, J.; Shen, Y.; Guo, J.-F.; Wang, Y.; Xia, L.-P.; Feng, G.-K.; Liu, Q.Q.; et al. The Pivotal Role of C-Jun NH2-Terminal Kinase-Mediated Beclin 1 Expression during Anticancer Agents-Induced Autophagy in Cancer Cells. *Oncogene* **2009**, *28*, 886–898. [CrossRef] [PubMed]
110. Keil, E.; Höcker, R.; Schuster, M.; Essmann, F.; Ueffing, N.; Hoffman, B.; Liebermann, D.A.; Pfeffer, K.; Schulze-Osthoff, K.; Schmitz, I. Phosphorylation of Atg5 by the Gadd45β-MEKK4-P38 Pathway Inhibits Autophagy. *Cell Death Differ.* **2013**, *20*, 321–332. [CrossRef]
111. He, Y.; She, H.; Zhang, T.; Xu, H.; Cheng, L.; Yepes, M.; Zhao, Y.; Mao, Z. P38 MAPK Inhibits Autophagy and Promotes Microglial Inflammatory Responses by Phosphorylating ULK1. *J. Cell Biol.* **2018**, *217*, 315–328. [CrossRef]
112. Webber, J.L.; Tooze, S.A. Coordinated Regulation of Autophagy by P38alpha MAPK through mAtg9 and p38IP. *EMBO J.* **2010**, *29*, 27–40. [CrossRef]
113. Desideri, E.; Vegliante, R.; Cardaci, S.; Nepravishta, R.; Paci, M.; Ciriolo, M.R. MAPK14/P38α-Dependent Modulation of Glucose Metabolism Affects ROS Levels and Autophagy during Starvation. *Autophagy* **2014**, *10*, 1652–1665. [CrossRef]
114. Choi, C.-H.; Lee, B.-H.; Ahn, S.-G.; Oh, S.-H. Proteasome Inhibition-Induced P38 MAPK/ERK Signaling Regulates Autophagy and Apoptosis through the Dual Phosphorylation of Glycogen Synthase Kinase 3β. *Biochem. Biophys. Res. Commun.* **2012**, *418*, 759–764. [CrossRef]
115. Martina, J.A.; Jeong, E.; Puertollano, R. P38 MAPK-Dependent Phosphorylation of TFEB Promotes Monocyte-to-Macrophage Differentiation. *EMBO Rep.* **2023**, *24*, e55472. [CrossRef]
116. Li, W.; Zhu, J.; Dou, J.; She, H.; Tao, K.; Xu, H.; Yang, Q.; Mao, Z. Phosphorylation of LAMP2A by P38 MAPK Couples ER Stress to Chaperone-Mediated Autophagy. *Nat. Commun.* **2017**, *8*, 1763. [CrossRef]
117. Yao, R.; Shen, J. Chaperone-Mediated Autophagy: Molecular Mechanisms, Biological Functions, and Diseases. *MedComm* **2023**, *4*, e347. [CrossRef]
118. Bryant, K.L.; Stalnecker, C.A.; Zeitouni, D.; Klomp, J.E.; Peng, S.; Tikunov, A.P.; Gunda, V.; Pierobon, M.; Waters, A.M.; George, S.D.; et al. Combination of ERK and Autophagy Inhibition as a Treatment Approach for Pancreatic Cancer. *Nat. Med.* **2019**, *25*, 628–640. [CrossRef]
119. Yang, J.-Y.; Zong, C.S.; Xia, W.; Yamaguchi, H.; Ding, Q.; Xie, X.; Lang, J.-Y.; Lai, C.-C.; Chang, C.-J.; Huang, W.-C.; et al. ERK Promotes Tumorigenesis by Inhibiting FOXO3a via MDM2-Mediated Degradation. *Nat. Cell Biol.* **2008**, *10*, 138–148. [CrossRef]
120. Zhang, W.; Li, X.; Wang, S.; Chen, Y.; Liu, H. Regulation of TFEB Activity and Its Potential as a Therapeutic Target against Kidney Diseases. *Cell Death Discov.* **2020**, *6*, 32. [CrossRef]
121. Martinez-Lopez, N.; Athonvarangkul, D.; Mishall, P.; Sahu, S.; Singh, R. Autophagy Proteins Regulate ERK Phosphorylation. *Nat. Commun.* **2013**, *4*, 2799. [CrossRef]
122. Craig, J.E.; Miller, J.N.; Rayavarapu, R.R.; Hong, Z.; Bulut, G.B.; Zhuang, W.; Sakurada, S.M.; Temirov, J.; Low, J.A.; Chen, T.; et al. MEKK3-MEK5-ERK5 Signaling Promotes Mitochondrial Degradation. *Cell Death Discov.* **2020**, *6*, 107. [CrossRef]

123. Jo, M.; Lee, S.; Kim, K.; Lee, S.; Kim, S.R.; Kim, H.-J. Inhibition of MEK5 Suppresses TDP-43 Toxicity via the mTOR-Independent Activation of the Autophagy-Lysosome Pathway. *Biochem. Biophys. Res. Commun.* **2019**, *513*, 925–932. [CrossRef]
124. Gámez-García, A.; Bolinaga-Ayala, I.; Yoldi, G.; Espinosa-Gil, S.; Diéguez-Martínez, N.; Megías-Roda, E.; Muñoz-Guardiola, P.; Lizcano, J.M. ERK5 Inhibition Induces Autophagy-Mediated Cancer Cell Death by Activating ER Stress. *Front. Cell Dev. Biol.* **2021**, *9*, 742049. [CrossRef]
125. Yuan, H.-X.; Wang, Z.; Yu, F.-X.; Li, F.; Russell, R.C.; Jewell, J.L.; Guan, K.-L. NLK Phosphorylates Raptor to Mediate Stress-Induced mTORC1 Inhibition. *Genes. Dev.* **2015**, *29*, 2362–2376. [CrossRef]
126. Tejwani, L.; Jung, Y.; Kokubu, H.; Sowmithra, S.; Ni, L.; Lee, C.; Sanders, B.; Lee, P.J.; Xiang, Y.; Luttik, K.; et al. Reduction of Nemo-like Kinase Increases Lysosome Biogenesis and Ameliorates TDP-43-Related Neurodegeneration. *J. Clin. Invest.* **2023**, *133*, e138207. [CrossRef]
127. Kwon, I.; Song, W.; Jang, Y.; Choi, M.D.; Vinci, D.M.; Lee, Y. Elevation of Hepatic Autophagy and Antioxidative Capacity by Endurance Exercise Is Associated with Suppression of Apoptosis in Mice. *Ann. Hepatol.* **2020**, *19*, 69–78. [CrossRef]

antioxidants

MDPI

Review

Pexophagy and Oxidative Stress: Focus on Peroxisomal Proteins and Reactive Oxygen Species (ROS) Signaling Pathways

Xiaofan Wei †, Laxman Manandhar †, Hyunsoo Kim, Arun Chhetri, Jaetaek Hwang, Gyuho Jang, Channy Park and Raekil Park *

Department of Biomedical Science and Engineering, Gwangju Institute of Science and Technology, Gwangju 61005, Republic of Korea; weixiaofan1@gm.gist.ac.kr (X.W.); laxmanandhar@gm.gist.ac.kr (L.M.); ruyhyunsookim@gm.gist.ac.kr (H.K.); chhetri5@gm.gist.ac.kr (A.C.); isoul9103@gm.gist.ac.kr (J.H.); gyuho9008@gm.gist.ac.kr (G.J.); channypark@gist.ac.kr (C.P.)

* Correspondence: rkpark@gist.ac.kr; Tel.: +82-62-715-5361; Fax: +82-62-715-5309

† These authors contributed equally to this work.

Abstract: Peroxisomes generate reactive oxygen species (ROS) and also play a role in protecting cells from the damaging effects of such radicals. Dysfunctional peroxisomes are recognized by receptors and degraded by a selective type of macroautophagy called pexophagy. Oxidative stress is one of the signals that activates pexophagy through multiple signaling pathways. Conversely, impaired pexophagy results in the accumulation of damaged peroxisomes, which in turn leads to elevated ROS levels and oxidative stress, resulting as cellular dysfunction and the progression of diseases such as neurodegeneration, cancer, and metabolic disorders. This review explores the molecular mechanisms driving pexophagy and its regulation by oxidative stress with a particular focus on ROS. This highlights the role of peroxisomal proteins and ROS-mediated signaling pathways in regulating pexophagy. In addition, emerging evidence suggests that the dysregulation of pexophagy is closely linked to neurological disorders, underscoring its potential as a therapeutic target. Understanding the intricate crosstalk between pexophagy and oxidative stress provides new insights into the maintenance of cellular homeostasis and offers promising directions for addressing neurological disorders that are tightly associated with pexophagy and oxidative stress.

Keywords: peroxisome; pexophagy; autophagy; ROS

1. Introduction

The quality of organelle and balanced oxidative stress is critical for maintaining cellular homeostasis. The clearance of damaged organelles removes potentially toxic byproducts from the cells and reuses organelle components for bioenergetics. Therefore, defects in organelle clearance can be detrimental to cell health and contribute to cancer, neurodegeneration, and inflammatory diseases [1].

Autophagy is a fundamental cellular process that occurs at the basal level and plays an important role in cellular equilibrium and removing debris from damaged organelles or cells. It can also be activated in response to cellular stresses such as starvation, hypoxia, or exposure to anticancer agents and triggers a cell survival process that supplies energy to cells during energy depletion [2]. The process of autophagy involves sequestering cytoplasmic components into double-membrane vesicles known as autophagosomes. These autophagosomes then fuse with lysosomes to degrade their contents. These degradative processes are important not only for maintaining cellular homeostasis and removing excess or damaged organelles, aggregated proteins, or pathogens from cells, but also for providing energy to support cell survival and function. Defects in autophagy have been linked to a variety of human diseases, including cancer, neurodegeneration, and inflammatory diseases [3,4]. Organelle-specific autophagy can clear mitochondria, peroxisomes, lysosomes, endoplasmic reticulum (ER), chloroplasts, and the nucleus. The selective autophagy of organelles is important for maintaining the integrity and number of organelles in the context of various environments and stresses. Organelle clearance, or selective autophagy of organelles, is different from the bulk degradation process that occurs, for example, in starvation-induced autophagy. It is a selective process that involves the specific sequestration of cellular components. Various types of organelle clearance have been identified, all of which involve initiation by a signal that triggers downstream events, leading to the recognition and marking of the target organelle for degradation. Additionally, there are also specialized molecules that mark components as cargo for degradation and autophagy-related components, promoting their sequestration and removal. Several organelles, including mitochondria, peroxisomes, lysosomes, the ER, and the nucleus, have all been identified as cargo that can be degraded by autophagy across a variety of taxa [1].

Oxidative stress results from an imbalance between the production of reactive oxygen species (ROS), including free radicals, and cellular antioxidant defense. This imbalance can lead to the damage of cellular components such as proteins, lipids, and DNA, ultimately disrupting normal cellular function. ROS, generated as byproducts of normal cellular metabolism, particularly from peroxisomes and mitochondria, can function as signaling molecules [5]. Importantly, this process is crucial for maintaining cellular health by preventing the accumulation of impaired peroxisomes, which further contributes to metabolic disturbances and the exacerbation of oxidative stress [6–8]. Furthermore, the only currently available study comparing the relative ROS production of different cellular sources showed that the endoplasmic reticulum (ER) and peroxisomes may have a greater capacity to generate ROS than mitochondria, at least in rat liver [9]. The peroxisomal antioxidant defense system of mammalian peroxisomes contain a variety of ROS-metabolizing enzymes, including catalase, superoxide dismutase 1, peroxyredoxin 5, glutathione S-transferase kappa, 'microsomal' glutathione S-transferase, and epoxide hydrolase 2. There is also evidence that these organelles utilize non-enzymatic, low-molecular-weight antioxidant compounds [10].

Peroxisomes are highly dynamic oxidative organelles with important metabolic functions in cellular lipid metabolism, including the β-oxidation of fatty acids, the synthesis of myelin sheath lipids, and the regulation of cellular redox balance. The functional loss of peroxisomes causes serious metabolic disorders in humans, such as Zellweger syndrome and X-linked adrenoleukodystrophy [11–13]. The idea that peroxisomes can act as endogenous stress generator stems from the discovery that the long-term administration of peroxisome proliferators to rodents induced oxidative stress in hepatocytes [14]. Peroxisomes can also protect cells from oxidative stress [15]. For example, the absence of functional peroxisomes increases apoptosis in the developing mouse cerebella [16]. In addition, mammalian cells catalyze the first two steps of plasmalogen biosynthesis exclusively by peroxisomal enzymes [17]. Cells defective in the peroxisomal steps of plasmalogen biosynthesis are shown to be significantly more sensitive than control cells to ROS generated by UV irradiation [18,19].

Peroxisomes are both sources and targets of ROS, underscoring the importance of their regulated turnover through pexophagy in maintaining cellular homeostasis. Peroxisomes are essential organelles involved in lipid metabolism and ROS detoxification. However, peroxisomal dysfunction can lead to excessive oxidative stress, thus disrupting normal cellular function [20,21]. Damaged, excessive, or dysfunctional peroxisomes are recognized to degrade by a selective autophagic degradation process known as pexophagy [22,23]. Studies have consistently shown that impaired pexophagy results in the accumulation of ROS. In contrast, ROS, as signaling molecules, play an important role in regulating pexophagy by mediating several pathways, such as inducing the ubiquitination of peroxisomal membrane proteins (PMPs). These processes underscore the intricate relationship between ROS and pexophagy, highlighting their collaborative roles in mitigating oxidative damage and maintaining cellular balance.

Peroxisomes are selectively recognized by receptors through their ubiquitin-binding domains (UBDs), and those peroxisomes interact with the LC3-interacting region (LIR) to be delivered to autophagosomes for pexophagy [24–26]. Two mammalian pexophagy receptors have been identified: NBR1 and p62 [27,28], which interact with ubiquitinated peroxisomal membrane proteins (PMPs) and sequester target peroxisomes into autophagosome. In addition, peroxisomes can be delivered for degradation through protein–protein interactions independently of their ubiquitin status [29,30]. Although the mechanisms and functions of pexophagy have been well studied and extensively reviewed, a critical gap still exists in our understanding of the complex regulatory networks of this process in mammalian cells.

Pexophagy specifically targets peroxisomes to degrade them, working together with peroxisome biogenesis to maintain peroxisomal homeostasis. It is tightly regulated by various signaling pathways and can be triggered beyond its basal level by several factors such as cellular stress, changes in nutrient levels and environmental stimuli. Importantly, the accumulation of dysfunctional peroxisomes can lead to metabolic disturbances and increased oxidative stress.

There is a growing number of studies suggesting that dysregulated pexophagy contributes to the development and progression of neurological diseases [31]. While ROS have been well studied in the context of neurological diseases, the role of impaired pexophagy in these conditions highlight the need for further investigation into their interplay as potential therapeutic targets [32]. In this review, we discuss the current findings of molecular mechanisms driving pexophagy, emphasizing the role of peroxisomal proteins in its regulation. In addition, we explore how ROS function as signaling molecules that trigger pexophagy, aiming to offer insights into the involute relationship between pexophagy and oxidative stress.

2. Pexophagy-Related Peroxisomal Proteins

Peroxisomal proteins located in both the membrane and the matrix are critical for maintaining peroxisome homeostasis, which is regulated by peroxisome biogenesis and degradation [33]. Around 70–80% of peroxisomes are removed through pexophagy, a selective autophagy pathway [34]. Several proteins, such as PEX3, PEX5, and PEX16, are involved in peroxisome biogenesis. In addition, other proteins that localize or partially localize to peroxisomes and regulate pexophagy have been identified, including USP30, MARCH5, HSPA9, and p97/VCP-UBXD8 complex [35–41]. These proteins function differently to modulate pexophagy by regulating the ubiquitination status of peroxisomal proteins, potentially mediating the turnover of peroxisomal components, and contributing to the stress responses that influence pexophagy. Further research is necessary to fully elucidate the specific mechanisms involved in peroxisome dynamics and cellular homeostasis [35–39]. Defects or deficiencies in peroxisomal proteins can lead to metabolic disorders such as Zellweger syndrome, neonatal adrenoleukodystrophy, and other peroxisomal biogenesis disorders [42]. Although many of these proteins are involved in pexophagy, ongoing research continues to uncover additional factors and regulatory mechanisms that govern this selective autophagic pathway. As our understanding advances, the catalogue of peroxisomal proteins directly implicated in regulating pexophagy is expected to expand, reflecting ongoing discoveries in this field. Therefore, in this section, we will introduce the peroxisomal proteins involved in pexophagy and its associated pathways (Figure 1).

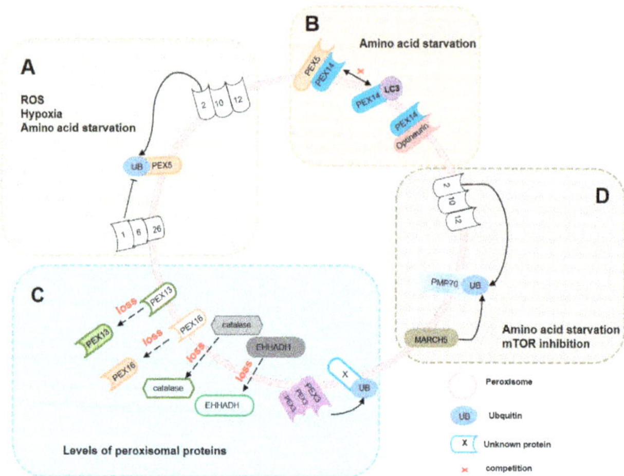

Figure 1. Pexophagy-related peroxisomal proteins. (**A**) PEX5 ubiquitination is a critical signal that promotes the initiation of pexophagy. This post-translational modification is triggered by various physiological conditions, including dysfunction of the AAA complex, amino acid starvation, and stimulation by ROS. (**B**) Under starvation conditions, PEX14 directly interacts with LC3, thereby promoting the initiation of pexophagy. Additionally, PEX14 serves as a molecular bridge linking Optineurin (OPTN) to the pexophagy pathway. (**C**) The expression levels of peroxisomal proteins significantly affect the pexophagy process. The loss of PEX13, PEX16, catalase, EHHADH, or the AAA complex leads to enhanced pexophagy. While this regulation is partially linked to ROS production and PEX5 ubiquitination, the precise mechanisms underlying these effects remain to be fully elucidated. Conversely, the overexpression of PEX3 has been shown to promote pexophagy through the ubiquitination of an unidentified protein. (**D**) PMP70, ubiquitinated by E3 ligases such as PEX2 and MARCH5, recruits pexophagy receptors, which facilitate pexophagy under diverse cellular conditions.

2.1. PEX5 Ubiquitination-Mediated Pexophagy

PEX5 plays a crucial role in peroxisomal biogenesis by facilitating the import of newly synthesized peroxisomal matrix proteins into peroxisomes. It recognizes peroxisomal targeting signal 1 (PTS1) present on the target proteins [43,44]. Once PEX5 binds to a protein carrying the PTS1 signal in the cytosol, it forms a complex with the cargo protein. This PEX5-cargo complex then docks to the peroxisomal membrane and interacts with membrane proteins such as PEX13 and PEX14 [44,45]. Upon cargo release into the peroxisome matrix, PEX5 undergoes ubiquitination and subsequent recognition by the peroxisomal membrane proteins PEX2, PEX10, and PEX12, thereby facilitating its extraction from the peroxisomal membrane and recycling for further rounds of import [46]. In addition, PEX5 plays a key role in the ubiquitination of peroxisomal membrane proteins, marking them for recognition by autophagic receptors, which then deliver damaged peroxisomes to the autophagic machinery. Several studies have demonstrated that PEX5 ubiquitination in response to several stimuli, including ROS accumulation, hypoxia, and amino acid starvation, recruits p62 and NBR1 to activate pexophagy [27,47,48]. The peroxisomal AAA ATPase complex (AAA complex) is essential for cycling PEX5 during peroxisomal matrix protein import. The disruption of the AAA complex leads to the accumulation of ubiquitinated PEX5 on the peroxisomal membrane, thereby triggering pexophagy [49]. PEX13, a component of the peroxisomal matrix import system, regulates pexophagy. The loss of

PEX13 results in the accumulation of ubiquitinated PEX5 in peroxisomes, promoting the initiation of pexophagy [50]. These coordinated processes highlight the interplay between the peroxisomal protein import machinery and pexophagy regulation, which is crucial for maintaining peroxisome function and cellular homeostasis (Figure 1A).

2.2. PEX14-Mediated Pexophagy

PEX14 is a peroxisomal membrane protein involved in peroxisomal biogenesis. It functions as a docking receptor, ensuring that proteins are correctly delivered to their destination [51,52]. Notably, PEX5 forms a complex with peroxisomal matrix proteins in the cytosol, facilitating their import into peroxisomes by docking to the peroxisomal membrane where they interact with PEX14. However, under conditions such as nutrient starvation, PEX14 has been reported to interact with LC3, a key component involved in autophagosome formation. This interaction aids in the recognition and degradation of damaged or unnecessary peroxisomes via pexophagy [29,53] (Figure 1B). Optineurin (OPTN) is a multifunctional adaptor involved in various autophagic pathways. Recent studies have suggested that the C-terminal domain of OPTN can bind to PEX14, thereby initiating a cell-type-specific process known as pexophagy. This interaction highlights the role of OPTN as a critical mediator in targeting peroxisomes for degradation under specific cellular conditions. PEX14 serves as an interface linking OPTN to cell-type-selective pexophagy [54]. Further exploration of the molecular mechanisms governing OPTN-mediated pexophagy helps to extend our knowledge of disorders linked to peroxisome dysfunction and OPTN-related abnormalities, which will provide valuable insights into potential therapeutic strategies for treating conditions associated with impaired peroxisomal function (Figure 1B).

2.3. Pexophagy Regulated by Different Expression Levels of Peroxisomal Proteins

PEX3 is a peroxisomal membrane protein and a key factor in peroxisome biogenesis that acts in collaboration with PEX16 and PEX19 to facilitate the import of peroxisomal membrane proteins and initiate peroxisome formation from the endoplasmic reticulum (ER) [43]. The overexpression of PEX3 induces pexophagy, which is characterized by the formation of ubiquitinated and clustered peroxisomes regardless of the ubiquitination status of PEX3. However, the specific ubiquitinated substrates during this process remain unidentified, and further investigation is needed to elucidate their precise molecular mechanisms [55] (Figure 1C). PEX16 plays a critical role in peroxisome biogenesis and is involved in the early stages of peroxisomal membrane assembly and growth. Research has indicated that PEX16 plays a role in regulating pexophagy, and that the depletion or dysfunction of PEX16 has been associated with the induction of pexophagy. This suggests that PEX16 participates in maintaining the balance between peroxisome proliferation and degradation via mechanisms that influence pexophagy regulation. Further studies are needed to fully understand the specific mechanisms by which PEX16 affects pexophagy and its implications in cellular homeostasis and diseases [56] (Figure 1C). Catalase, an enzyme located in the peroxisomal matrix, protects cells from oxidative damage by converting hydrogen peroxide to water and oxygen. Catalase deficiency, especially during serum starvation or fasting, can lead to elevated levels of ROS, which in turn activate pexophagy [6,57]. This process underscores the vital role of catalase in protecting cells from oxidative damage and maintaining peroxisome homeostasis (Figure 1C). Moreover, the peroxisomal L-bifunctional enzyme (EHHADH) has recently been identified as a regulator of pexophagy. EHHADH deficiency has been shown to induce pexophagy through increased ROS levels [58] (Figure 1C).

2.4. PMP70 Ubiquitination-Mediated Pexophagy

The 70-kDa peroxisomal membrane protein (PMP70), also known as ATP-binding cassette subfamily D member 3 (ABCD3), plays a pivotal role in peroxisome function by transporting crucial substrates across the peroxisomal membrane. The protein is essential for various metabolic processes such as fatty acid metabolism, bile acid synthesis, and the detoxification of xenobiotics. These functions are important for maintaining cellular balance and promoting the overall health of organisms [59–61]. Several studies have demonstrated that PMP70 is ubiquitinated in response to cellular stress or pharmacological treatment. Ubiquitinated PMP70 is recognized by autophagy receptors such as NBR1 and p62, which facilitate the targeting of peroxisomes for degradation through pexophagy [27,36]. Under amino acid starvation, PMP70 is a substrate of the ubiquitin ligase, PEX2, which leads to ubiquitination and triggers pexophagy [27]. In response to mTOR inhibition, the ubiquitin ligase MARCH5 binds to PEX19, targeting it to the peroxisome where it ubiquitinates PMP70 and inducing pexophagy [36] (Figure 1D).

3. Oxidative Stress and Pexophagy

An imbalance between ROS generation and antioxidant capacity leads to oxidative stress, resulting in excessive ROS levels. Chronic oxidative stress accelerates the aging process and leads to the development of several diseases, including diabetes, cancer, heart disease, and neurological disorders [62]. Peroxisomes play a vital role in generating and scavenging intracellular ROS. They produce ROS as byproducts of fatty acid oxidation (FAO) and contain detoxifying enzymes, such as catalase. ROS cause structural and functional abnormalities in peroxisomes by damaging many of the proteins and lipids in the peroxisomal membrane [63]. Oxidative damage is exacerbated when peroxisomes lose their function because they are unable to detoxify ROS. In recent years, several studies have suggested that ROS accumulation stimulates pexophagy [7,48]. Under oxidative stress, the N-terminal cysteine of ACAD10 is translocated to damaged peroxisomes, where it binds to p62 and subsequently recruits GABARAP or LC3 to autophagic membranes, inducing pexophagy [64]. This section summarizes the pexophagy pathways associated with oxidative stress, with a particular emphasis on the role of ROS (Figures 2 and 3).

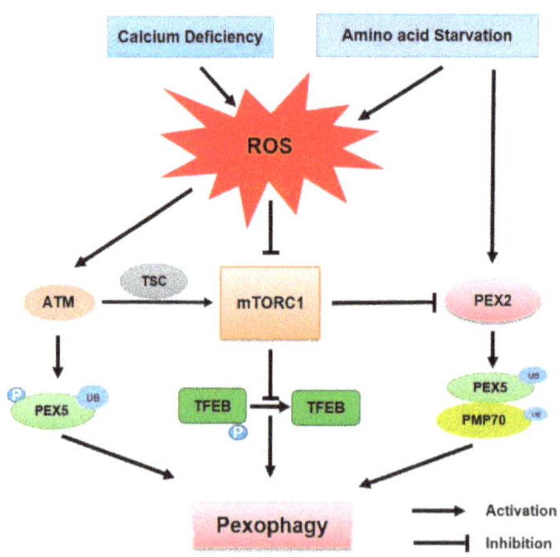

Figure 2. ROS function as signaling mediators in pexophagy. ROS induce pexophagy through the mTORC1 signaling pathway under oxidative stress conditions due to calcium deficiency and amino acid starvation. ROS activate ATM, which phosphorylates and ubiquitinates PEX5, leading to its degradation via pexophagy. ATM suppresses mTORC1 activity via the TSC complex. Simultaneously, ROS suppress mTORC1 activity, inducing the dephosphorylation of the transcription factor EB (TFEB), thereby promoting its nuclear translocation and transcriptional activation of autophagy-related genes, leading to pexophagy. Additionally, mTORC1 inhibition influences the ubiquitination of peroxisomal proteins, such as PMP70 and PEX5, which is mediated by PEX2, further promoting pexophagy.

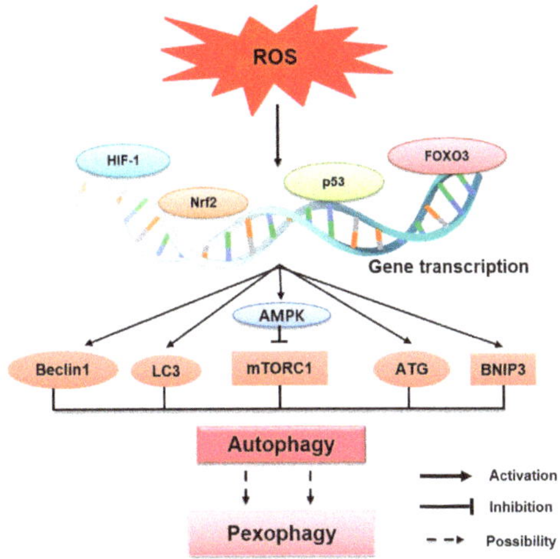

Figure 3. ROS regulate the transcription of genes involved in autophagy. ROS trigger various transcription factors, including HIF-1, Nrf2, p53, and FOXO3, to modulate gene transcription. These factors translocate to the nucleus and interact with different signaling pathways, including autophagy-related pathways such as the AMPK and mTORC1 signaling pathways. Autophagy-related proteins such as Beclin1, LC3, ATG proteins, and BNIP3 are regulated through these pathways in response to oxidative stress, which might regulate the selective autophagic degradation of peroxisomes, known as pexophagy.

3.1. ROS Originating from Various Cellular Compartments

Numerous biological components generate ROS from the ER, mitochondria, and peroxisomes known as the three major redox-sensitive organelles [65]. These organelles produce ROS that can be released via aquaporins or unknown protein channels [66]. Although ROS from peroxisomes and mitochondria have been well studied as contributors to pexophagy induction under stress conditions, the precise role of ER-derived ROS in pexophagy remains unclear. Mitochondrial ROS are generated in the electron transport chain during oxidative phosphorylation and act as signaling molecules. Studies have shown that the depletion of the mitochondrial protein HSPA9 in SH-SY5Y cells increases ROS levels [67], and the loss of HSPA9 in these cells induces pexophagy due to peroxisomal ROS accumulation [39]. This suggests that ROS diffuse from the mitochondria to the peroxisomes and promote pexophagy. In addition, elevated levels of ROS within the peroxisomal lumen can activate Stub1-mediated pexophagy [68]. Given the dynamic ROS transfer among mitochondria, peroxisomes, and the ER, ER-derived ROS may play a role in the regulation of pexophagy. Further studies are needed to clarify whether ER-derived ROS directly or indirectly influence pexophagy pathways.

3.2. ROS Enhance Pexophagy Through Various Signaling Pathways

ROS serve as critical triggers for the initiation of pexophagy by signaling through different pathways. Upon activation by ROS, ataxia–telangiectasia mutated (ATM) translocates to damaged peroxisomes, where it represses mTORC1 and facilitates the mono-ubiquitination of PEX5 [48]. Consequently, ubiquitinated PEX5 is recognized by pexophagy receptors, such as NBR1 and p62, to induce pexophagy [48] (Figure 2). During amino acid starvation, oxidative stress is induced as ROS levels markedly increase [27,69]. Under amino acid starvation conditions, PEX2 is upregulated and functions as an E3 ubiquitin ligase that ubiquitinates PEX5 and PMP70. Ubiquitinated proteins are subsequently recognized by NBR1 during pexophagy [27] (Figure 2). Calcium deficiency in the medium decreases the catalytic activity of peroxisomal catalase, resulting in the accumulation of ROS, which inhibits mTOR activity and activates the transcription factor EB (TFEB). The inactivation of mTORC1 inhibits TFEB phosphorylation and promotes its nuclear translocation into the nucleus. TFEB stimulates the transcription of genes involved in lysosomal biogenesis and autophagy, enhancing autophagic flux, which leads to pexophagy to remove the oxidative stress present within the cell [7] (Figure 2). Interestingly, in response to peroxisomal ROS, ATM activates the tuberous sclerosis complex (TSC), which localizes to peroxisomes, inhibits mTORC1, and promotes autophagy [70]. Given that the mTORC1 pathway has been implicated in the regulation of pexophagy by controlling PEX2 expression, these findings suggest that mTORC1 serves as a central regulator of pexophagy by coordinating cellular responses to oxidative stress and nutrient deprivation. Although these interactions highlight an important link between ROS, mTORC1 activity, and pexophagy, further studies are required to determine the precise mechanisms by which ROS regulate pexophagy.

3.3. *ROS Induce Autophagy by Regulating Gene Expression*

ROS trigger the activation of transcription factors such as hypoxia-inducible factor (HIF-1α), nuclear factor erythroid 2-related factor 2 (Nrf2), p53, and forkhead box O-3 (FOXO3) [71–74]. These transcription factors induce the expression of genes required for autophagy induction, including BECN1, LC3, and SQSTM1 [75–77] (Figure 3). HIF-1α is rapidly degraded by the oxygen-dependent prolyl hydrolases (PHDs), through ubiquitin–proteasome degradation in normal oxygen levels. However, this degradation is inhibited under hypoxic conditions, and HIF-1α is stabilized and accumulates [78]. The stabilized HIF-1α translocates to the nucleus, where it activates genes that support survival under hypoxia, such as those involved in angiogenesis and glucose metabolism. Notably, increased ROS levels can suppress PHDs, allowing HIF-1α to accumulate and activate target genes for pro-autophagic proteins such as BNIP3 and NIX [78,79], which are well-known mitophagy/pexophagy receptors that induce selective autophagy [80,81]. Under oxidative stress, Nrf2 is stabilized and translocated to the nucleus to activate the expression of antioxidant and cytoprotective genes to neutralize ROS and restore the cellular redox balance [82]. Additionally, Nrf2 directly regulates mTOR activity, establishing a connection between the oxidative stress response and autophagy [83,84]. p53 plays a dual role in promoting or inhibiting autophagy depending on its subcellular localization. When oxidative stress occurs, DNA damage leads to the activation of p53, which enhances AMPK activity and, in turn, inhibits mTOR signaling. This promotes autophagy as a protective response against oxidative damage [85]. In addition, nuclear p53 induces the transcriptional activation of autophagy-related genes, such as damage-regulated autophagy modulator (DRAM) and TP53-induced glycolysis and apoptosis regulator (TIGAR), further facilitating autophagy [86,87]. Similarly, oxidative stress triggers the nuclear translocation of FOXO3 and induces the transcription of autophagy-related genes such as LC3, BNIP3, and ATG. This activation helps to reduce oxidative stress by removing ROS and preventing further cellular damage [88] (Figure 3).

The upregulation of these autophagy-related genes promotes specific forms of autophagy such as pexophagy. The accumulation of ROS triggers cellular stress responses that activate autophagic pathways, including those that selectively degrade peroxisomes, helping to maintain cellular homeostasis and mitigate oxidative damage. However, the exact mechanism by which ROS regulate pexophagy has not yet been fully elucidated.

4. Role of Pexophagy and Oxidative Stress in Neurological Diseases

Both peroxisomes and oxidative status are critical for cellular stability, specifically in an organ with a high demand for energy such as the brain [89,90]. This notion indicates that the regulatory balance of pexophagy and oxidative stress is essential for supporting proper neuronal health, and disruptions in this balance contribute to the progression of neurodegenerative diseases.

Peroxisomes are crucial for the formation of cellular membranes and myelin sheaths in the CNS. In addition, the ether phospholipids produced by peroxisomes are essential for maintaining proper function of glia and neurons [91]. Pexophagy plays a critical role in protecting neurons from oxidative damage by selectively degrading dysfunctional peroxisomes that could otherwise contribute to excessive ROS production [20]. The dysregulation of pexophagy can exacerbate oxidative stress and cellular damage, contributing to disease progression. In addition to their role in lipid synthesis, peroxisomes are central to cellular oxidative metabolism, including the β-oxidation of very-long-chain fatty acids (VLCFAs) and the detoxification of ROS. Impaired pexophagy can lead to the accumulation of dysfunctional peroxisomes, resulting in elevated levels of ROS and VLCFAs, both of which are observed in neurodegenerative diseases such as Alzheimer's disease and Parkinson's disease [89,90]. Moreover, the failure to remove excessive or damaged peroxisomes may contribute to mitochondrial dysfunction, another critical factor in neurodegeneration. On the other hand, neurodegenerative diseases are characterized by the accumulation of misfolded proteins such as amyloid-β, tau, and α-synuclein [92]. Recent studies suggest that peroxisomal dysfunction and impaired pexophagy can indirectly affect proteostasis by influencing cellular redox states and lipid metabolism, indicating that the dysregulation of pexophagy may promote protein aggregation and neurotoxicity [90,93]. In addition, as a specialized form of autophagy, pexophagy is also influenced by general autophagy pathways, including those regulated by mTOR signaling. For example, in ALS, mutations in key autophagy regulators, such as TDP-43 and FUS, may also impair selective processes including pexophagy [94]. Similarly, reduced autophagic activity in aging may further contribute to the impaired autophagic degradation of peroxisomes, resulting in the progressive neuronal damage exacerbating neurodegeneration [95].

Several signs of neurodegeneration associated with pexophagy gene knockout include growth retardation, abnormal reflexes, premature death, and progressive motor deficits. These manifestations highlight the critical role of pexophagy genes in maintaining neural health and function [96–98]. Pharmacological promotion of pexophagy through the activation of key regulators may be beneficial for the treatment of neurological disorders [20]. In addition, targeting the mTOR signaling pathway may offer a therapeutic angle for neurodegenerative diseases since mTOR inhibition has been shown to induce pexophagy.

Certain proteins that regulate pexophagy have been implicated in neurological disorders, such as USP30, MARCH5, and HSPA9 [99–101]. However, there was no direct evidence linking their role in these disorders to their regulation of pexophagy. Despite growing interest in pexophagy and its effects in neurological diseases, its precise role in neurological diseases has not been well studied. The mechanisms underlying the pexophagy crosstalk in neurological pathology require further investigation, for example, identifying specific biomarkers for pexophagy dysregulation in neurodegenerative diseases. A deeper understanding of the molecular mechanisms and therapeutic potential of pexophagy may lead to novel treatments for neurodegenerative diseases and other diseases associated with peroxisomal dysfunction.

Oxidative stress refers to the imbalance between free radicals and antioxidants in the body. As the CNS consumes large amounts of oxygen and generates abundant free radicals, it is particularly sensitive to such imbalances, and they can contribute to the development and progression of neurological diseases. It is well known that oxidative stress induces protein misfolding and aggregation by promoting the oxidative modifications of proteins that hinder their proper folding and clearance. In addition, oxidative stress can impair the function of molecular chaperones and proteasomal activity, further disrupting proteostasis and accelerating neurodegeneration [102]. Mitochondria are both a major source and a target of ROS, and excessive ROS generated by damaged mitochondria can impair neuronal energy metabolism. For example, in Parkinson's disease, mutations in genes, such as PINK1 and Parkin, disrupt mitochondrial quality control, leading to oxidative damage and neuronal loss [103]. Moreover, lipid peroxidation products, such as malondialdehyde and 4-hydroxynonenal, are toxic messengers that propagate and amplify oxidative damage, which further contribute to neuronal dysfunction [104]. Inflammation and oxidative stress are closely interconnected and play pivotal roles in the pathogenesis of neurological diseases. Chronic neuroinflammation amplifies oxidative stress, and in turn, excessive oxidative stress exacerbates inflammation. This vicious cycle contributes to neuronal dysfunction and degeneration [105]. As oxidative stress is one of common features shared by several numerous neurodegenerative diseases such as Alzheimer's disease, Parkinson's disease, and amyotrophic lateral sclerosis [89], numerous preclinical and clinical investigations are exploring antioxidant therapeutic strategies. However, the effectiveness of antioxidant therapy for these conditions remains a topic of debate, largely due to inconclusive results from clinical trials.

Despite the growing recognition of the interplay between pexophagy and oxidative stress in neurological diseases, many aspects remain unexplored. Recently, TFEB activation was shown to be a promising therapeutic strategy for Alzheimer's disease. Pexophagy occurs through TFEB activation for functional adaptation to oxidative stress [7,106].

Like mitotherapy, which is a promising approach for preventing neurodegeneration [107], pexotherapy may constitute a new therapeutic axis to address aging but also to prevent and/or treat age-related diseases [108]. For example, 7-ketocholesterol (7KC) and 7β-hydroxycholesterol (7β-OHC) are toxic oxysterols produced by cholesterol autoxidation, which has been implicated in neurological disorders such as Alzheimer's disease [109,110]. These two oxysterols can induce oxidative stress and alter the quality, quantity, and function of peroxisomes [110–112]. However, treatment with certain molecules can prevent peroxisomal damages [108,110]. Although there is currently a lack of definitive evidence for peroxisome-targeted therapies, these findings provide a direction for future peroxisome-targeted therapies and may expand the exploration of pexophagy and oxidative stress, providing potential strategies for addressing neurological diseases.

5. Conclusions

In this review, we summarize the current state of the research on the regulatory mechanisms between pexophagy and the role of oxidative stress, particularly ROS. Although significant progress has been achieved in understanding the interplay between pexophagy and oxidative stress, it is far from being completely elucidated, and their relationship remains a critical but underexplored area in neurological disease research. Several questions still remain, including how oxidative stress signals are integrated into pexophagy pathways and the disease-specific dynamics of these interactions. Addressing these challenges requires innovative approaches, including the identification of specific biomarkers for peroxisomal health and advanced methods for distinguishing pexophagy from general autophagy. Further studies are needed to explore the precise mechanisms linking pexophagy and oxidative stress, which may aid in the development of novel therapeutic strategies aimed at restoring cellular homeostasis, reducing oxidative damage, and protecting neuronal function. Moreover, clinical interventions targeting these pathways would provide more effective and promising outcomes in the treatment of neurodegenerative diseases.

Author Contributions: Conceptualization, X.W., L.M. and C.P.; writing—original draft preparation, X.W., L.M., H.K., A.C., J.H., G.J. and C.P.; writing—review and editing, C.P. and R.P.; supervision,

R.P.; project administration, R.P.; funding acquisition, R.P. All authors have read and agreed to the published version of the manuscript.

Funding: This work was supported by the National Research Foundation of Korea (NRF) under grants funded by the Korean government (Grant No. 2022R1A2C3007463), and by a GIST Research Institute (GRI) Grant funded by GIST in 2023.

Conflicts of Interest: The authors declare no conflicts of interest.

References

1. Anding, A.L.; Baehrecke, E.H. Cleaning House: Selective Autophagy of Organelles. *Dev. Cell* **2017**, *41*, 10–22. [CrossRef] [PubMed]
2. Anding, A.L.; Baehrecke, E.H. Autophagy in Cell Life and Cell Death. *Curr. Top. Dev. Biol.* **2015**, *114*, 67–91. [CrossRef]
3. Mizushima, N.; Levine, B.; Cuervo, A.M.; Klionsky, D.J. Autophagy fights disease through cellular self-digestion. *Nature* **2008**, *451*, 1069–1075. [CrossRef] [PubMed]
4. Al Rawi, S.; Louvet-Vallée, S.; Djeddi, A.; Sachse, M.; Culetto, E.; Hajjar, C.; Boyd, L.; Legouis, R.; Galy, V. Postfertilization autophagy of sperm organelles prevents paternal mitochondrial DNA transmission. *Science* **2011**, *334*, 1144–1147. [CrossRef]
5. D'Autréaux, B.; Toledano, M.B. ROS as signalling molecules: Mechanisms that generate specificity in ROS homeostasis. *Nat. Rev. Mol. Cell Biol.* **2007**, *8*, 813–824. [CrossRef] [PubMed]
6. Lee, J.N.; Dutta, R.K.; Maharjan, Y.; Liu, Z.Q.; Lim, J.Y.; Kim, S.J.; Cho, D.H.; So, H.S.; Choe, S.K.; Park, R. Catalase inhibition induces pexophagy through ROS accumulation. *Biochem. Biophys. Res. Commun.* **2018**, *501*, 696–702. [CrossRef]
7. Manandhar, L.; Dutta, R.K.; Devkota, P.; Chhetri, A.; Wei, X.; Park, C.; Kwon, H.M.; Park, R. TFEB activation triggers pexophagy for functional adaptation during oxidative stress under calcium deficient-conditions. *Cell Commun. Signal.* **2024**, *22*, 142. [CrossRef] [PubMed]
8. Kim, Y.H.; Jo, D.S.; Park, N.Y.; Bae, J.E.; Kim, J.B.; Lee, H.J.; Kim, S.H.; Kim, S.H.; Lee, S.; Son, M.; et al. Inhibition of BRD4 Promotes Pexophagy by Increasing ROS and ATM Activation. *Cells* **2022**, *11*, 2839. [CrossRef] [PubMed]
9. Boveris, A.; Oshino, N.; Chance, B. The cellular production of hydrogen peroxide. *Biochem. J.* **1972**, *128*, 617–630. [CrossRef]
10. Kim, H.; Hwang, J.; Park, C.; Park, R. Redox system and ROS-related disorders in peroxisomes. *Free Radic. Res.* **2024**, *58*, 662–675. [CrossRef]
11. Kumar, R.; Islinger, M.; Worthy, H.; Carmichael, R.; Schrader, M. The peroxisome: An update on mysteries 3.0. *Histochem. Cell Biol.* **2024**, *161*, 99–132. [CrossRef] [PubMed]
12. Rafique, M.; Zia, S.; Rana, M.N.; Mostafa, O.A. Zellweger syndrome—A lethal peroxisome biogenesis disorder. *J. Pediatr. Endocrinol. Metab.* **2013**, *26*, 377–379. [CrossRef] [PubMed]
13. Cappa, M.; Todisco, T.; Bizzarri, C. X-linked adrenoleukodystrophy and primary adrenal insufficiency. *Front. Endocrinol.* **2023**, *14*, 1309053. [CrossRef] [PubMed]
14. Kasai, H.; Okada, Y.; Nishimura, S.; Rao, M.S.; Reddy, J.K. Formation of 8-hydroxydeoxyguanosine in liver DNA of rats following long-term exposure to a peroxisome proliferator. *Cancer Res.* **1989**, *49*, 2603–2605. [PubMed]
15. Fransen, M.; Nordgren, M.; Wang, B.; Apanasets, O. Role of peroxisomes in ROS/RNS-metabolism: Implications for human disease. *Biochim. Biophys. Acta* **2012**, *1822*, 1363–1373. [CrossRef]
16. Krysko, O.; Hulshagen, L.; Janssen, A.; Schütz, G.; Klein, R.; De Bruycker, M.; Espeel, M.; Gressens, P.; Baes, M. Neocortical and cerebellar developmental abnormalities in conditions of selective elimination of peroxisomes from brain or from liver. *J. Neurosci. Res.* **2007**, *85*, 58–72. [CrossRef] [PubMed]
17. Wallner, S.; Schmitz, G. Plasmalogens the neglected regulatory and scavenging lipid species. *Chem. Phys. Lipids* **2011**, *164*, 573–589. [CrossRef] [PubMed]
18. Zoeller, R.A.; Morand, O.H.; Raetz, C.R. A possible role for plasmalogens in protecting animal cells against photosensitized killing. *J. Biol. Chem.* **1988**, *263*, 11590–11596. [CrossRef] [PubMed]
19. Hoefler, G.; Paschke, E.; Hoefler, S.; Moser, A.B.; Moser, H.W. Photosensitized killing of cultured fibroblasts from patients with peroxisomal disorders due to pyrene fatty acid-mediated ultraviolet damage. *J. Clin. Investig.* **1991**, *88*, 1873–1879. [CrossRef]
20. Moruno-Manchon, J.F.; Uzor, N.E.; Kesler, S.R.; Wefel, J.S.; Townley, D.M.; Nagaraja, A.S.; Pradeep, S.; Mangala, L.S.; Sood, A.K.; Tsvetkov, A.S. Peroxisomes contribute to oxidative stress in neurons during doxorubicin-based chemotherapy. *Mol. Cell. Neurosci.* **2018**, *86*, 65–71. [CrossRef]
21. Uzor, N.-E.; McCullough, L.D.; Tsvetkov, A.S. Peroxisomal Dysfunction in Neurological Diseases and Brain Aging. *Front. Cell. Neurosci.* **2020**, *14*, 44. [CrossRef]
22. Shibata, M.; Oikawa, K.; Yoshimoto, K.; Kondo, M.; Mano, S.; Yamada, K.; Hayashi, M.; Sakamoto, W.; Ohsumi, Y.; Nishimura, M. Highly oxidized peroxisomes are selectively degraded via autophagy in Arabidopsis. *Plant Cell* **2013**, *25*, 4967–4983. [CrossRef] [PubMed]

23. Kim, J.; Lee, H.; Lee, H.N.; Kim, S.H.; Shin, K.D.; Chung, T. Autophagy-related proteins are required for degradation of peroxisomes in Arabidopsis hypocotyls during seedling growth. *Plant Cell* **2013**, *25*, 4956–4966. [CrossRef] [PubMed]
24. Yin, Z.; Popelka, H.; Lei, Y.; Yang, Y.; Klionsky, D.J. The Roles of Ubiquitin in Mediating Autophagy. *Cells* **2020**, *9*, 2025. [CrossRef]
25. Yokota, S.; Fahimi, H.D. Degradation of excess peroxisomes in mammalian liver cells by autophagy and other mechanisms. *Histochem. Cell Biol.* **2009**, *131*, 455–458. [CrossRef] [PubMed]
26. Yokota, S.; Himeno, M.; Roth, J.; Brada, D.; Kato, K. Formation of autophagosomes during degradation of excess peroxisomes induced by di-(2-ethylhexyl)phthalate treatment. II. Immunocytochemical analysis of early and late autophagosomes. *Eur. J. Cell Biol.* **1993**, *62*, 372–383. [PubMed]
27. Sargent, G.; van Zutphen, T.; Shatseva, T.; Zhang, L.; Di Giovanni, V.; Bandsma, R.; Kim, P.K. PEX2 is the E3 ubiquitin ligase required for pexophagy during starvation. *J. Cell Biol.* **2016**, *214*, 677–690. [CrossRef] [PubMed]
28. Deosaran, E.; Larsen, K.B.; Hua, R.; Sargent, G.; Wang, Y.; Kim, S.; Lamark, T.; Jauregui, M.; Law, K.; Lippincott-Schwartz, J.; et al. NBR1 acts as an autophagy receptor for peroxisomes. *J. Cell Sci.* **2013**, *126*, 939–952. [CrossRef] [PubMed]
29. Hara-Kuge, S.; Fujiki, Y. The peroxin Pex14p is involved in LC3-dependent degradation of mammalian peroxisomes. *Exp. Cell Res.* **2008**, *314*, 3531–3541. [CrossRef]
30. van Zutphen, T.; Veenhuis, M.; van der Klei, I.J. Pex14 is the sole component of the peroxisomal translocon that is required for pexophagy. *Autophagy* **2008**, *4*, 63–66. [CrossRef]
31. Zhu, W.; Zhang, W.; Young, J.; Barnes, A.P.; Alkayed, N.J. Abstract TP96: Pexophagy is Neuroprotective in Ischemic Brain. *Stroke* **2017**, *48*, ATP96. [CrossRef]
32. Fransen, M.; Revenco, I.; Li, H.; Costa, C.F.; Lismont, C.; Van Veldhoven, P.P. Peroxisomal Dysfunction and Oxidative Stress in Neurodegenerative Disease: A Bidirectional Crosstalk. *Adv. Exp. Med. Biol.* **2020**, *1299*, 19–30. [CrossRef] [PubMed]
33. Han, J.; Zheng, D.; Liu, P.S.; Wang, S.; Xie, X. Peroxisomal homeostasis in metabolic diseases and its implication in ferroptosis. *Cell Commun. Signal.* **2024**, *22*, 475. [CrossRef] [PubMed]
34. Komatsu, M.; Waguri, S.; Ueno, T.; Iwata, J.; Murata, S.; Tanida, I.; Ezaki, J.; Mizushima, N.; Ohsumi, Y.; Uchiyama, Y.; et al. Impairment of starvation-induced and constitutive autophagy in Atg7-deficient mice. *J. Cell Biol.* **2005**, *169*, 425–434. [CrossRef] [PubMed]
35. Verhoeven, N.; Oshima, Y.; Cartier, E.; Bippes, C.C.; Neutzner, A.; Boyman, L.; Karbowski, M. Outer mitochondrial membrane E3 Ub ligase MARCH5 controls de novo peroxisome biogenesis. *Dev. Cell* **2024**, *60*, 40–50. [CrossRef]
36. Zheng, J.; Chen, X.; Liu, Q.; Zhong, G.; Zhuang, M. Ubiquitin ligase MARCH5 localizes to peroxisomes to regulate pexophagy. *J. Cell Biol.* **2022**, *221*, e202103156. [CrossRef]
37. Riccio, V.; Demers, N.; Hua, R.; Vissa, M.; Cheng, D.T.; Strilchuk, A.W.; Wang, Y.; McQuibban, G.A.; Kim, P.K. Deubiquitinating enzyme USP30 maintains basal peroxisome abundance by regulating pexophagy. *J. Cell Biol.* **2019**, *218*, 798–807. [CrossRef]
38. Pan, W.; Wang, Y.; Bai, X.; Yin, Y.; Dai, L.; Zhou, H.; Wu, Q.; Wang, Y. Deubiquitinating enzyme USP30 negatively regulates mitophagy and accelerates myocardial cell senescence through antagonism of Parkin. *Cell Death Discov.* **2021**, *7*, 187. [CrossRef] [PubMed]
39. Jo, D.S.; Park, S.J.; Kim, A.K.; Park, N.Y.; Kim, J.B.; Bae, J.E.; Park, H.J.; Shin, J.H.; Chang, J.W.; Kim, P.K.; et al. Loss of HSPA9 induces peroxisomal degradation by increasing pexophagy. *Autophagy* **2020**, *16*, 1989–2003. [CrossRef]
40. Montes, I.D.; Amirthagunanathan, S.; Joshi, A.S.; Raman, M. The p97-UBXD8 complex maintains peroxisome abundance by suppressing pexophagy. *bioRxiv* **2024**, bioRxiv: 2024.2009.2024.614749. [CrossRef]
41. Koyano, F.; Yamano, K.; Hoshina, T.; Kosako, H.; Fujiki, Y.; Tanaka, K.; Matsuda, N. AAA+ ATPase chaperone p97/VCP(FAF2) governs basal pexophagy. *Nat. Commun.* **2024**, *15*, 9347. [CrossRef]
42. Delille, H.K.; Bonekamp, N.A.; Schrader, M. Peroxisomes and disease—An overview. *Int. J. Biomed. Sci.* **2006**, *2*, 308–314.
43. Ma, C.; Agrawal, G.; Subramani, S. Peroxisome assembly: Matrix and membrane protein biogenesis. *J. Cell Biol.* **2011**, *193*, 7–16. [CrossRef] [PubMed]
44. Williams, C.; Distel, B. Pex13p: Docking or cargo handling protein? *Biochim. Biophys. Acta* **2006**, *1763*, 1585–1591. [CrossRef] [PubMed]
45. Hasan, S.; Platta, H.W.; Erdmann, R. Import of proteins into the peroxisomal matrix. *Front. Physiol.* **2013**, *4*, 261. [CrossRef]
46. Di Cara, F. Peroxisomes: The current understanding. *Postdoc. J.* **2013**, *1*, 27–45. [CrossRef]
47. Nordgren, M.; Francisco, T.; Lismont, C.; Hennebel, L.; Brees, C.; Wang, B.; Van Veldhoven, P.P.; Azevedo, J.E.; Fransen, M. Export-deficient monoubiquitinated PEX5 triggers peroxisome removal in SV40 large T antigen-transformed mouse embryonic fibroblasts. *Autophagy* **2015**, *11*, 1326–1340. [CrossRef]
48. Zhang, J.; Tripathi, D.N.; Jing, J.; Alexander, A.; Kim, J.; Powell, R.T.; Dere, R.; Tait-Mulder, J.; Lee, J.H.; Paull, T.T.; et al. ATM functions at the peroxisome to induce pexophagy in response to ROS. *Nat. Cell Biol.* **2015**, *17*, 1259–1269. [CrossRef]
49. Law, K.B.; Bronte-Tinkew, D.; Di Pietro, E.; Snowden, A.; Jones, R.O.; Moser, A.; Brumell, J.H.; Braverman, N.; Kim, P.K. The peroxisomal AAA ATPase complex prevents pexophagy and development of peroxisome biogenesis disorders. *Autophagy* **2017**, *13*, 868–884. [CrossRef]

50. Demers, N.D.; Riccio, V.; Jo, D.S.; Bhandari, S.; Law, K.B.; Liao, W.; Kim, C.; McQuibban, G.A.; Choe, S.K.; Cho, D.H.; et al. PEX13 prevents pexophagy by regulating ubiquitinated PEX5 and peroxisomal ROS. *Autophagy* **2023**, *19*, 1781–1802. [CrossRef]
51. Meinecke, M.; Cizmowski, C.; Schliebs, W.; Krüger, V.; Beck, S.; Wagner, R.; Erdmann, R. The peroxisomal importomer constitutes a large and highly dynamic pore. *Nat. Cell Biol.* **2010**, *12*, 273–277. [CrossRef]
52. Reuter, M.; Kooshapur, H.; Suda, J.-G.; Gaussmann, S.; Neuhaus, A.; Brühl, L.; Bharti, P.; Jung, M.; Schliebs, W.; Sattler, M.; et al. Competitive Microtubule Binding of PEX14 Coordinates Peroxisomal Protein Import and Motility. *J. Mol. Biol.* **2021**, *433*, 166765. [CrossRef]
53. Jiang, L.; Hara-Kuge, S.; Yamashita, S.; Fujiki, Y. Peroxin Pex14p is the key component for coordinated autophagic degradation of mammalian peroxisomes by direct binding to LC3-II. *Genes Cells* **2015**, *20*, 36–49. [CrossRef]
54. Li, H.; Chen, S.; Claes, Z.; Lismont, C.; Vandewinkel, B.; Hussein, M.A.F.; Costa, C.F.; Imberechts, D.; Liu, Y.; Vandenberghe, W.; et al. PEX14 acts as the interface linking optineurin to cell type-selective pexophagy. *bioRxiv* **2024**, bioRxiv: 2024.2005.2031.596776. [CrossRef]
55. Yamashita, S.; Abe, K.; Tatemichi, Y.; Fujiki, Y. The membrane peroxin PEX3 induces peroxisome-ubiquitination-linked pexophagy. *Autophagy* **2014**, *10*, 1549–1564. [CrossRef] [PubMed]
56. Wei, X.; Maharjan, Y.; Dorotea, D.; Dutta, R.K.; Kim, D.; Kim, H.; Mu, Y.; Park, C.; Park, R. Knockdown of PEX16 Induces Autophagic Degradation of Peroxisomes. *Int. J. Mol. Sci.* **2021**, *22*, 7989. [CrossRef]
57. Dutta, R.K.; Maharjan, Y.; Lee, J.N.; Park, C.; Ho, Y.S.; Park, R. Catalase deficiency induces reactive oxygen species mediated pexophagy and cell death in the liver during prolonged fasting. *Biofactors* **2021**, *47*, 112–125. [CrossRef]
58. Kan, S.; Hou, Q.; Shi, J.; Zhang, M.; Xu, F.; Liu, Z.; Jiang, S. EHHADH deficiency regulates pexophagy and accelerates tubulointerstitial injury in diabetic kidney disease. *Cell Death Discov.* **2024**, *10*, 289. [CrossRef]
59. Chornyi, S.; Ijlst, L.; van Roermund, C.W.T.; Wanders, R.J.A.; Waterham, H.R. Peroxisomal Metabolite and Cofactor Transport in Humans. *Front. Cell Dev. Biol.* **2020**, *8*, 613892. [CrossRef] [PubMed]
60. Ranea-Robles, P.; Chen, H.; Stauffer, B.; Yu, C.; Bhattacharya, D.; Friedman, S.L.; Puchowicz, M.; Houten, S.M. The peroxisomal transporter ABCD3 plays a major role in hepatic dicarboxylic fatty acid metabolism and lipid homeostasis. *J. Inherit. Metab. Dis.* **2021**, *44*, 1419–1433. [CrossRef] [PubMed]
61. van Roermund, C.W.T.; Ijlst, L.; Wagemans, T.; Wanders, R.J.A.; Waterham, H.R. A role for the human peroxisomal half-transporter ABCD3 in the oxidation of dicarboxylic acids. *Biochim. Et Biophys. Acta (BBA)-Mol. Cell Biol. Lipids* **2014**, *1841*, 563–568. [CrossRef]
62. Hajam, Y.A.; Rani, R.; Ganie, S.Y.; Sheikh, T.A.; Javaid, D.; Qadri, S.S.; Pramodh, S.; Alsulimani, A.; Alkhanani, M.F.; Harakeh, S.; et al. Oxidative Stress in Human Pathology and Aging: Molecular Mechanisms and Perspectives. *Cells* **2022**, *11*, 552. [CrossRef]
63. Phaniendra, A.; Jestadi, D.B.; Periyasamy, L. Free radicals: Properties, sources, targets, and their implication in various diseases. *Indian J. Clin. Biochem.* **2015**, *30*, 11–26. [CrossRef] [PubMed]
64. Shim, S.M.; Choi, H.; Kwon, S.C.; Kim, H.Y.; Sung, K.W.; Jung, E.J.; Mun, S.R.; Bae, T.H.; Kim, D.H.; Son, Y.S.; et al. The Cys-N-degron pathway modulates pexophagy through the N-terminal oxidation and arginylation of ACAD10. *Autophagy* **2023**, *19*, 1642–1661. [CrossRef]
65. Forrester, S.J.; Kikuchi, D.S.; Hernandes, M.S.; Xu, Q.; Griendling, K.K. Reactive Oxygen Species in Metabolic and Inflammatory Signaling. *Circ. Res.* **2018**, *122*, 877–902. [CrossRef] [PubMed]
66. Yoboue, E.D.; Sitia, R.; Simmen, T. Redox crosstalk at endoplasmic reticulum (ER) membrane contact sites (MCS) uses toxic waste to deliver messages. *Cell Death Dis.* **2018**, *9*, 331. [CrossRef] [PubMed]
67. Bae, J.E.; Jang, S.; Kim, J.B.; Hyung, H.; Park, N.Y.; Kim, Y.H.; Kim, S.H.; Kim, S.H.; Ha, J.M.; Oh, G.S.; et al. Enhanced primary ciliogenesis via mitochondrial oxidative stress activates AKT to prevent neurotoxicity in HSPA9/mortalin-depleted SH-SY5Y cells. *Mol. Brain* **2023**, *16*, 41. [CrossRef] [PubMed]
68. Chen, B.H.; Yang, W.Y. Monitoring Stub1-Mediated Pexophagy. *Jove-J. Vis. Exp.* **2023**, *195*, e65010. [CrossRef]
69. Li, R.B.; Kato, H.; Fumimoto, C.; Nakamura, Y.; Yoshimura, K.; Minagawa, E.; Omatsu, K.; Ogata, C.; Taguchi, Y.; Umeda, M. Essential Amino Acid Starvation-Induced Oxidative Stress Causes DNA Damage and Apoptosis in Murine Osteoblast-like Cells. *Int. J. Mol. Sci.* **2023**, *24*, 15314. [CrossRef]
70. Zhang, J.W.; Kim, J.; Alexander, A.; Cai, S.L.; Tripathi, D.N.; Dere, R.; Tee, A.R.; Tait-Mulder, J.; Di Nardo, A.; Han, J.M.; et al. A tuberous sclerosis complex signalling node at the peroxisome regulates mTORC1 and autophagy in response to ROS. *Nat. Cell Biol.* **2013**, *15*, U1186–U1196. [CrossRef]
71. Movafagh, S.; Crook, S.; Vo, K. Regulation of Hypoxia-Inducible Factor-1a by Reactive Oxygen Species: New Developments in an Old Debate. *J. Cell. Biochem.* **2015**, *116*, 696–703. [CrossRef]
72. Ngo, V.; Duennwald, M.L. Nrf2 and Oxidative Stress: A General Overview of Mechanisms and Implications in Human Disease. *Antioxidants* **2022**, *11*, 2345. [CrossRef] [PubMed]
73. Shi, T.; van Soest, D.M.K.; Polderman, P.E.; Burgering, B.M.T.; Dansen, T.B. DNA damage and oxidant stress activate p53 through differential upstream signaling pathways. *Free Radic. Biol. Med.* **2021**, *172*, 298–311. [CrossRef]

74. Habrowska-Górczynska, D.E.; Koziel, M.J.; Urbanek, K.A.; Kowalska, K.; Piastowska-Ciesielska, A.W. FOXO3a/PI3K/Akt pathway participates in the ROS- induced apoptosis triggered by α-ZEL and β-ZEL. *Sci. Rep.* **2024**, *14*, 13281. [CrossRef] [PubMed]
75. Kimball, S.R.; Gordon, B.S.; Moyer, J.E.; Dennis, M.D.; Jefferson, L.S. Leucine induced dephosphorylation of Sestrin2 promotes mTORC1 activation. *Cell Signal.* **2016**, *28*, 896–906. [CrossRef] [PubMed]
76. Roberts, D.J.; Tan-Sah, V.P.; Ding, E.Y.; Smith, J.M.; Miyamoto, S. Hexokinase-II Positively Regulates Glucose Starvation-Induced Autophagy through TORC1 Inhibition. *Mol. Cell* **2014**, *53*, 521–533. [CrossRef] [PubMed]
77. Chang, K.C.; Liu, P.F.; Chang, C.H.; Lin, Y.C.; Chen, Y.J.; Shu, C.W. The interplay of autophagy and oxidative stress in the pathogenesis and therapy of retinal degenerative diseases. *Cell Biosci.* **2022**, *12*, 1. [CrossRef]
78. Li, Y.N.; Xi, M.M.; Guo, Y.; Hai, C.X.; Yang, W.L.; Qin, X.J. NADPH oxidase-mitochondria axis-derived ROS mediate arsenite-induced HIF-1alpha stabilization by inhibiting prolyl hydroxylases activity. *Toxicol. Lett.* **2014**, *224*, 165–174. [CrossRef]
79. Li, J.; Lin, Q.; Shao, X.; Li, S.; Zhu, X.; Wu, J.; Mou, S.; Gu, L.; Wang, Q.; Zhang, M.; et al. HIF1alpha-BNIP3-mediated mitophagy protects against renal fibrosis by decreasing ROS and inhibiting activation of the NLRP3 inflammasome. *Cell Death Dis.* **2023**, *14*, 200. [CrossRef]
80. Zhang, J.; Ney, P.A. Mechanisms and Biology of B-Cell Leukemia/Lymphoma 2/Adenovirus E1B Interacting Protein 3 and Nip-Like Protein X. *Antioxid. Redox Signal.* **2011**, *14*, 1959–1969. [CrossRef]
81. Wilhelm, L.P.; Zapata-Muñoz, J.; Villarejo-Zori, B.; Pellegrin, S.; Freire, C.M.; Toye, A.M.; Boya, P.; Ganley, I.G. BNIP3L/NIX regulates both mitophagy and pexophagy. *EMBO J.* **2022**, *41*, e111115. [CrossRef] [PubMed]
82. Tian, W.; de la Vega, M.R.; Schmidlin, C.J.; Ooi, A.; Zhang, D.D. Kelch-like ECH-associated protein 1 (KEAP1) differentially regulates nuclear factor erythroid-2-related factors 1 and 2 (NRF1 and NRF2). *J. Biol. Chem.* **2018**, *293*, 2029–2040. [CrossRef]
83. Bendavit, G.; Aboulkassim, T.; Hilmi, K.; Shah, S.; Batist, G. Nrf2 Transcription Factor Can Directly Regulate mTOR: LINKING CYTOPROTECTIVE GENE EXPRESSION TO A MAJOR METABOLIC REGULATOR THAT GENERATES REDOX ACTIVITY. *J. Biol. Chem.* **2016**, *291*, 25476–25488. [CrossRef]
84. Sun, W.; Yi, Y.; Xia, G.; Zhao, Y.; Yu, Y.; Li, L.; Hua, C.; He, B.; Yang, B.; Yu, C.; et al. Nrf2-miR-129-3p-mTOR Axis Controls an miRNA Regulatory Network Involved in HDACi-Induced Autophagy. *Mol. Ther.* **2019**, *27*, 1039–1050. [CrossRef]
85. Wang, H.L.; Guo, M.; Wei, H.D.; Chen, Y.H. Targeting p53 pathways: Mechanisms, structures, and advances in therapy. *Signal Transduct. Target. Ther.* **2023**, *8*, 92. [CrossRef]
86. Hu, W.L.; Chen, S.; Thorne, R.F.; Wu, M. TP53, TP53 Target Genes (DRAM, TIGAR), and Autophagy. *Adv. Exp. Med. Biol.* **2019**, *1206*, 127–149. [CrossRef] [PubMed]
87. Cao, W.Y.; Li, J.H.; Yang, K.P.; Cao, D.L. An overview of autophagy: Mechanism, regulation and research progress. *Bull. Du Cancer* **2021**, *108*, 304–322. [CrossRef]
88. Yao, J.Y.; Wang, J.B.; Xu, Y.; Guo, Q.L.; Sun, Y.I.; Liu, J.; Li, S.C.; Guo, Y.J.; Wei, L.B. CDK9 inhibition blocks the initiation of PINK1-PRKN-mediated mitophagy by regulating the SIRT1-FOXO3-BNIP3 axis and enhances the therapeutic effects involving mitochondrial dysfunction in hepatocellular carcinoma. *Autophagy* **2022**, *18*, 1879–1897. [CrossRef]
89. Houldsworth, A. Role of oxidative stress in neurodegenerative disorders: A review of reactive oxygen species and prevention by antioxidants. *Brain Commun.* **2024**, *6*, fcad356. [CrossRef]
90. Jo, D.S.; Park, N.Y.; Cho, D.H. Peroxisome quality control and dysregulated lipid metabolism in neurodegenerative diseases. *Exp. Mol. Med.* **2020**, *52*, 1486–1495. [CrossRef] [PubMed]
91. Cabeza, R. Cognitive neuroscience of aging: Contributions of functional neuroimaging. *Scand. J. Psychol.* **2001**, *42*, 277–286. [CrossRef]
92. Peng, C.; Trojanowski, J.Q.; Lee, V.M. Protein transmission in neurodegenerative disease. *Nat. Rev. Neurol.* **2020**, *16*, 199–212. [CrossRef] [PubMed]
93. Walker, C.L.; Pomatto, L.C.D.; Tripathi, D.N.; Davies, K.J.A. Redox Regulation of Homeostasis and Proteostasis in Peroxisomes. *Physiol. Rev.* **2018**, *98*, 89–115. [CrossRef] [PubMed]
94. Navone, F.; Genevini, P.; Borgese, N. Autophagy and Neurodegeneration: Insights from a Cultured Cell Model of ALS. *Cells* **2015**, *4*, 354–386. [CrossRef]
95. Metaxakis, A.; Ploumi, C.; Tavernarakis, N. Autophagy in Age-Associated Neurodegeneration. *Cells* **2018**, *7*, 37. [CrossRef]
96. Hara, T.; Nakamura, K.; Matsui, M.; Yamamoto, A.; Nakahara, Y.; Suzuki-Migishima, R.; Yokoyama, M.; Mishima, K.; Saito, I.; Okano, H.; et al. Suppression of basal autophagy in neural cells causes neurodegenerative disease in mice. *Nature* **2006**, *441*, 885–889. [CrossRef]
97. Komatsu, M.; Waguri, S.; Chiba, T.; Murata, S.; Iwata, J.; Tanida, I.; Ueno, T.; Koike, M.; Uchiyama, Y.; Kominami, E.; et al. Loss of autophagy in the central nervous system causes neurodegeneration in mice. *Nature* **2006**, *441*, 880–884. [CrossRef]
98. Komatsu, M.; Wang, Q.J.; Holstein, G.R.; Friedrich, V.L., Jr.; Iwata, J.; Kominami, E.; Chait, B.T.; Tanaka, K.; Yue, Z. Essential role for autophagy protein Atg7 in the maintenance of axonal homeostasis and the prevention of axonal degeneration. *Proc. Natl. Acad. Sci. USA* **2007**, *104*, 14489–14494. [CrossRef] [PubMed]

99. Fang, T.Z.; Sun, Y.; Pearce, A.C.; Eleuteri, S.; Kemp, M.; Luckhurst, C.A.; Williams, R.; Mills, R.; Almond, S.; Burzynski, L.; et al. Knockout or inhibition of USP30 protects dopaminergic neurons in a Parkinson's disease mouse model. *Nat. Commun.* **2023**, *14*, 7295. [CrossRef]
100. Nagashima, S.; Tokuyama, T.; Yonashiro, R.; Inatome, R.; Yanagi, S. Roles of mitochondrial ubiquitin ligase MITOL/MARCH5 in mitochondrial dynamics and diseases. *J. Biochem.* **2014**, *155*, 273–279. [CrossRef]
101. Chung, S.J.; Kim, M.J.; Ryu, H.S.; Kim, J.; Kim, Y.J.; Kim, K.; You, S.; Kim, S.Y.; Lee, J.H. Lack of association of mortalin (HSPA9) and other mitochondria-related genes with risk of Parkinson's and Alzheimer's diseases. *Neurobiol. Aging* **2017**, *49*, 215.e219–215.e210. [CrossRef] [PubMed]
102. Höhn, A.; Tramutola, A.; Cascella, R. Proteostasis Failure in Neurodegenerative Diseases: Focus on Oxidative Stress. *Oxidative Med. Cell. Longev.* **2020**, *2020*, 5497046. [CrossRef]
103. Ge, P.; Dawson, V.L.; Dawson, T.M. PINK1 and Parkin mitochondrial quality control: A source of regional vulnerability in Parkinson's disease. *Mol. Neurodegener.* **2020**, *15*, 20. [CrossRef]
104. Pizzimenti, S.; Ciamporcero, E.; Daga, M.; Pettazzoni, P.; Arcaro, A.; Cetrangolo, G.; Minelli, R.; Dianzani, C.; Lepore, A.; Gentile, F.; et al. Interaction of aldehydes derived from lipid peroxidation and membrane proteins. *Front. Physiol.* **2013**, *4*, 242. [CrossRef]
105. Dash, U.C.; Bhol, N.K.; Swain, S.K.; Samal, R.R.; Nayak, P.K.; Raina, V.; Panda, S.K.; Kerry, R.G.; Duttaroy, A.K.; Jena, A.B. Oxidative stress and inflammation in the pathogenesis of neurological disorders: Mechanisms and implications. *Acta Pharm. Sin. B* 2024, *in press*. [CrossRef]
106. Zheng, X.; Lin, W.; Jiang, Y.; Lu, K.; Wei, W.; Huo, Q.; Cui, S.; Yang, X.; Li, M.; Xu, N.; et al. Electroacupuncture ameliorates beta-amyloid pathology and cognitive impairment in Alzheimer disease via a novel mechanism involving activation of TFEB (transcription factor EB). *Autophagy* **2021**, *17*, 3833–3847. [CrossRef]
107. Nascimento-dos-Santos, G.; de-Souza-Ferreira, E.; Linden, R.; Galina, A.; Petrs-Silva, H. Mitotherapy: Unraveling a Promising Treatment for Disorders of the Central Nervous System and Other Systemic Conditions. *Cells* **2021**, *10*, 1827. [CrossRef] [PubMed]
108. Ghzaiel, I.; Zarrouk, A.; Essadek, S.; Martine, L.; Hammouda, S.; Yammine, A.; Ksila, M.; Nury, T.; Meddeb, W.; Tahri Joutey, M.; et al. Protective effects of milk thistle (*Sylibum marianum*) seed oil and α-tocopherol against 7β-hydroxycholesterol-induced peroxisomal alterations in murine C2C12 myoblasts: Nutritional insights associated with the concept of pexotherapy. *Steroids* **2022**, *183*, 109032. [CrossRef]
109. Anderson, A.; Campo, A.; Fulton, E.; Corwin, A.; Jerome, W.G., 3rd; O'Connor, M.S. 7-Ketocholesterol in disease and aging. *Redox Biol.* **2020**, *29*, 101380. [CrossRef] [PubMed]
110. Ghzaiel, I.; Maaloul, S.; Ksila, M.; Namsi, A.; Yammine, A.; Debbabi, M.; Badreddine, A.; Meddeb, W.; Pires, V.; Nury, T.; et al. In Vitro Evaluation of the Effects of 7-Ketocholesterol and 7β-Hydroxycholesterol on the Peroxisomal Status: Prevention of Peroxisomal Damages and Concept of Pexotherapy. *Adv. Exp. Med. Biol.* **2024**, *1440*, 437–452. [CrossRef]
111. Nury, T.; Sghaier, R.; Zarrouk, A.; Ménétrier, F.; Uzun, T.; Leoni, V.; Caccia, C.; Meddeb, W.; Namsi, A.; Sassi, K.; et al. Induction of peroxisomal changes in oligodendrocytes treated with 7-ketocholesterol: Attenuation by α-tocopherol. *Biochimie* **2018**, *153*, 181–202. [CrossRef] [PubMed]
112. Ghzaiel, I.; Zarrouk, A.; Pires, V.; de Barros, J.P.; Hammami, S.; Ksila, M.; Hammami, M.; Ghrairi, T.; Jouanny, P.; Vejux, A.; et al. 7β-Hydroxycholesterol and 7-ketocholesterol: New oxidative stress biomarkers of sarcopenia inducing cytotoxic effects on myoblasts and myotubes. *J. Steroid Biochem. Mol. Biol.* **2023**, *232*, 106345. [CrossRef] [PubMed]

antioxidants

MDPI

Review

Oxidative Stress in the Regulation of Autosis-Related Proteins

María Guerra-Andrés [1,2], Inés Martínez-Rojo [3], Alejandra Piedra-Macías [1,2], Elena Lavado-Fernández [3,4], Marina García-Macia [3,4,*] and Álvaro F. Fernández [1,2,5,*]

[1] Departamento de Bioquímica y Biología Molecular, Universidad de Oviedo, 33006 Oviedo, Spain; guerraamaria@uniovi.es (M.G.-A.); uo277802@uniovi.es (A.P.-M.)
[2] Instituto Universitario de Oncología del Principado de Asturias (IUOPA), 33006 Oviedo, Spain
[3] Instituto de Biología Funcional y Genómica (IBFG), Universidad de Salamanca/CSIC, 37007 Salamanca, Spain; inesmartinez21@usal.es (I.M.-R.); ellavadof@usal.es (E.L.-F.)
[4] Departamento de Bioquímica y Biología Molecular, Universidad de Salamanca, 37007 Salamanca, Spain
[5] Instituto de Investigación Sanitaria del Principado de Asturias (ISPA), 33011 Oviedo, Spain
* Correspondence: marinagarciamacia@usal.es (M.G.-M.); fernandezferalvaro@uniovi.es (Á.F.F.)

Abstract: Physiological levels of reactive oxygen species (ROS) play a crucial role as intracellular signaling molecules, helping to maintain cellular homeostasis. However, when ROS accumulate excessively, they become toxic to cells, leading to damage to lipids, proteins, and DNA. This oxidative stress can impair cellular function and lead to various forms of cell death, including apoptosis, necroptosis, ferroptosis, pyroptosis, paraptosis, parthanatos, and oxeiptosis. Despite their significance, the role of ROS in autosis (an autophagy-dependent form of cell death) remains largely unexplored. In this review, we gather current knowledge on autotic cell death and summarize how oxidative stress influences the activity of Beclin-1 and the Na^+,K^+-ATPase pump, both of which are critical effectors of this pathway. Finally, we discuss the theoretical potential for ROS to modulate this type of cell death, proposing a possible dual role for these species in autosis regulation through effectors such as HIF-1α, TFEB, or the FOXO family, and highlighting the need to experimentally address cellular redox status when working on autotic cell death.

Keywords: autosis; ROS; oxidative stress; Beclin-1; Na^+,K^+-ATPase; autophagy

1. Introduction

The oxidoreduction (redox) state of a cell is the center of its metabolism. Almost all metabolic pathways include redox reactions, which affect the redox state of the cell and, at the same time, are influenced by it [1]. The redox state of cells is primarily established by the ratios of the cofactors $NADH/NAD^+$, $NADPH/NADP^+$, and glutathione (GSH)/glutathione disulfide (GSSG), as well as the balance between reactive oxygen species (ROS) and antioxidants [2]. Maintaining these ratios is essential for cellular homeostasis, which is critical for its correct function and adaptation to environmental stressors. Interestingly, moderate levels of ROS are beneficial, as they preserve, modulate, and regulate cellular functions. However, excessive production of ROS causes oxidative stress, which provokes cellular damage and dysfunction, affecting different cellular mechanisms, including autophagy [3].

Autophagy is an evolutionarily well-conserved pathway essential for cell survival, characterized by the delivery of intracellular components to the lysosome for degradation and recycling. To date, three major forms of autophagy have been described: macroautophagy, microautophagy, and chaperone-mediated autophagy [4]. Amongst them, macroautophagy remains the most studied autophagy variant, and it is defined by the formation of double-membraned vesicles (termed "autophagosomes") that sequester cellular cargo. These autophagosomes eventually fuse with lysosomes, where pH-sensitive hydrolases mediate degradation of the enclosed material [5]. Autophagy is essential to maintain cellular homeostasis and viability, as it avoids the accumulation of damaged intracellular components and ensures the metabolic needs of the cell during stress and nutrient starvation conditions [6]. Furthermore, it also plays an important role in additional processes, such as intercellular communication, modulation of immune cell functions, and maintenance of tissue barrier integrity [4]. However, autophagy dysregulation or excessive autophagic flux can lead to autophagy-mediated cell death, as it occurs with autosis [7].

In this review, we summarize our current knowledge on autotic cell death and how oxidative stress influences the activity of Beclin-1 and the Na^+,K^+-ATPase pump, crucial mediators of autosis. Finally, we discuss the potential for ROS to modulate this type of cell death, hypothesizing a possible dual role for these species in autosis regulation and highlighting the need to address redox status when working on autotic cell death.

2. ROS and Oxidative Stress

Oxidative stress is a cellular phenomenon characterized by an imbalance between the production of ROS and the antioxidant defence mechanisms. Under normal physiological conditions, the presence of antioxidants neutralizes these reactive species, maintaining cellular homeostasis. However, some factors, such as radiation (e.g., UV), inflammation, and different metabolic processes, can disrupt this balance and lead to excessive ROS production [8]. These species are highly reactive and can cause damage to cellular components such as DNA, proteins, and lipids. These aggressions can lead to mutations in critical genes, alterations in signaling pathways, and impaired cellular functions [9,10]. For instance, the accumulation of DNA damage induced by ROS in cancer can contribute to genetic instability and the development of malignant tumors, promoting proliferation, angiogenesis, and resistance to cell death, providing favorable conditions for tumor growth and metastasis [11,12]. In addition to ROS, reactive nitrogen species (RNS) also play a significant role in oxidative stress, contributing to cellular and DNA damage and affecting mitochondrial functions [13].

Mitochondria are the primary intracellular source of reactive oxygen species (ROS). During oxidative phosphorylation, complexes I and III of the mitochondrial electron transport chain generate superoxide anions ($O_2^{\bullet -}$) as byproducts of electron leakage. These anions can be converted into hydrogen peroxide (H_2O_2), which, in the presence of transition metal ions such as Fe^{2+} or Cu^+, leads to the formation of highly reactive hydroxyl radicals ($^{\bullet}OH$) through the Fenton reaction [14]. In addition to this canonical pathway, mitochondria can also produce ROS via reverse electron transport (RET), a process in which electrons flow backwards from complex II to complex I. This phenomenon occurs under specific metabolic conditions, such as high substrate availability and elevated mitochondrial membrane potential, and results in a burst of superoxide production. RET has gained attention as a potent and regulated source of mitochondrial ROS, with implications in both physiological signaling and pathological oxidative damage [15]. Beyond mitochondria, several non-mitochondrial sources contribute to the intracellular generation of reactive oxygen species. One of the most prominent is NADPH oxidase (NOX), a key enzyme involved in inflammatory responses, particularly in immune cells such as neutrophils and macrophages, where it produces superoxide during the respiratory burst [16]. Furthermore, xanthine oxidase, involved in purine metabolism, also generates superoxide as a byproduct of its enzymatic activity [17]. Under pathological conditions, nitric oxide synthase (NOS) can shift from its normal function and contribute to oxidative stress by producing peroxynitrite (ONOO—) through the reaction of nitric oxide with superoxide [18]. Additionally, enzymes in the endoplasmic reticulum, such as members of the cytochrome P450 family, can generate ROS during the metabolism of xenobiotics, especially when ER stress or substrate overload occurs [19]. While all of these systems play essential roles in normal cellular physiology, their dysregulation can lead to excessive ROS accumulation and significant oxidative damage.

Oxidative stress has been related to many pathological conditions, such as cancer, cardiovascular diseases, diabetes, and neurodegenerative diseases [20–23]. In fact, it has been identified as a key mediator of cell death processes in several of these diseases. For example, oxidative stress can contribute to the emergence of ferroptosis cell death in some cardiovascular diseases, such as atherosclerosis or ischemia [24,25]. In addition, several cell death mechanisms that have been demonstrated to be related to oxidative stress, like apoptosis, necroptosis, or autophagy-dependent cell death, are also relevant in neurodegenerative diseases [26–28]. Cells activate different pathways when they detect ROS accumulation to prevent further damage, namely NF-κB, MAPK/p38, or JNK (c-Jun N-terminal kinase), which may induce apoptosis if necessary [29]. A less dramatic response can be mediated by autophagic activation, which would be induced by different pro-survival mediators, such as AMPK or nuclear factor erythroid 2-related factor 2 (NRF2), or directly activating autophagic proteins like ATG4 [30–32]. But autophagy can also result in cellular death when exacerbated [33], which could happen in response to uncontrolled oxidative stress. Thus, it is necessary to evaluate the possible interplay between ROS and autophagic cell death and clarify how these species regulate autophagic cell death modes such as autosis.

3. Autotic Cell Death

Autophagy is a conserved catabolic pathway that mediates the lysosomal degradation of intracellular threats and long-lived organelles, enabling cells to adapt to environmental stresses such as nutrient deprivation or hypoxia [34]. Even though autophagy has been mainly described as a pro-survival cellular mechanism, it was linked to cell death long ago. Historically, the classification of cell death has been based on morphological traits, distinguishing type I (apoptosis), type II (autophagic cell death), and type III (necrosis) [35]. Accordingly, the term "autophagic cell death" was first used upon ultrastructural features such as the accumulation of autophagosomes. However, autophagy can sometimes be induced during cell death as a protective mechanism, without being responsible for the final demise of the cell. For this reason, the Nomenclature Committee on Cell Death (NCCD) recommendation is to use the term "autophagic cell death" only when the causative role of autophagy has been proven, showing that it can be blocked by genetic or chemical inhibition of at least two components of the autophagic machinery [33] (Figure 1).

Autosis, a new form of cell demise that differs from "classical" autophagic cell death (Table 1), was originally described in 2013 following the aforementioned criteria. Moreover, pharmacological and genetic approaches demonstrated its high dependence on the Na^+,K^+-ATPase pump and the autophagy machinery. However, it is important to note that autosis was only inhibited when early stages of autophagy (but not autophagosome–lysosome fusion) were blocked. Interestingly, no autosis reduction was detected when either apoptosis or necroptosis was repressed, showing its independence from other types of cell death [7]. As previously mentioned, the biochemical signature of this process is its dependence on Na^+/K^+-ATPase. Accordingly, a large chemical screening identified cardiac glycosides, known natural antagonists of the pump, as potent inhibitors of autosis [7,36]. Further studies, such as a genome-wide siRNA screening, confirmed the implication of Na^+,K^+-ATPase in autosis and identified potential new drivers that need to be investigated in the future.

Additionally, these studies have also shown that the physical interaction between the pump and Beclin-1, a key autophagy protein, plays a crucial role in autosis [37,38].

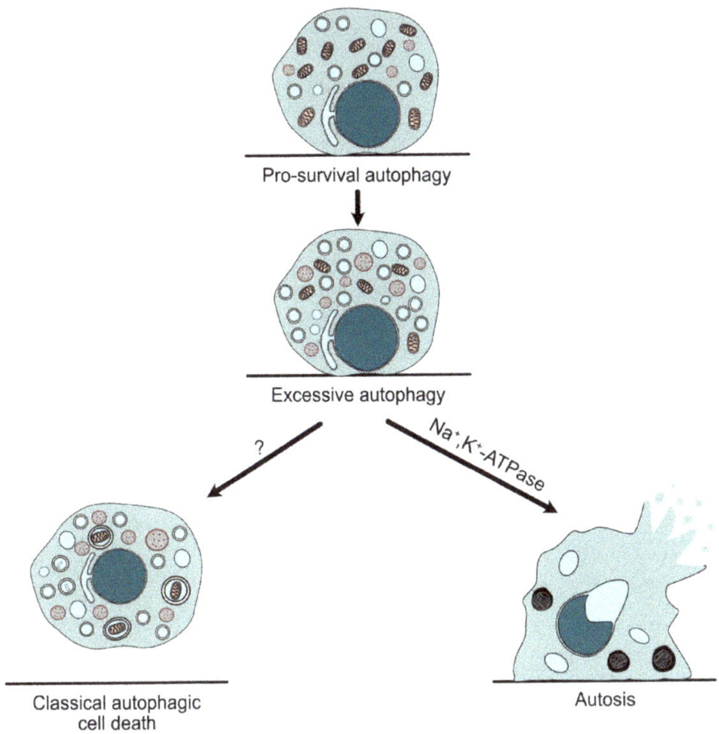

Figure 1. Autophagy in cell survival and cell death. Although autophagy often acts as a protective mechanism, its dysregulation can lead to an exacerbated response that results in autophagy-mediated cell death, such as autosis, which differs from other possible types of autophagic cell death due to its unique morphological features, as well as its dependence on Na^+,K^+-ATPase.

Table 1. Morphological differences between autophagy-dependent cell death and autosis.

Cellular Structure	"Classical" Autophagy-Dependent Cell Death	Autosis
Nucleus	Minor changes	Nuclear membrane convolution Detachment of inner and outer nuclear membranes Swollen perinuclear space and focal ballooning Focal concavity of the inner nuclear surface
Chromatin	Minor changes	Chromatin condensation
Plasma membrane	Plasma membrane rupture Occasional blebbing	Focal plasma membrane rupture
Autophagic structures	Numerous autophagic vesicles	Numerous autophagic vesicles in early stages
Organelles	Occasional ER, mitochondria and Golgi enlargement Occasional depletion of organelles	Electrodense and swollen mitochondria ER dilation, fragmentation (early stages) and disappearance (late stages)
Other features		Cell-substrate adhesion Na^+,K^+-ATPase dependence

From a morphological point of view, autosis can be divided into three phases, characterized by distinctive ultrastructural changes (Figure 2). In what has been called phase 1a, a gradual increase in vacuolar dynamics is observed, with autophagosome accumulation, endoplasmic reticulum dilation and fragmentation, and changes in mitochondria morphology. Later on, during phase 1b, the external and internal membranes separate, with this newly formed perinuclear space occasionally containing inclusions with density and granularity resembling the cytosol. Finally, phase 2 can be described as a rapid and abrupt collapse of the cell, characterized by the shrinkage of the nucleus, which acquires a concave morphology due to the ballooning of the perinuclear space where the nuclear membranes show their maximal separation [7]. Besides these unique features, the dying cell resembles a necrotic one, with swollen mitochondria, absence of the endoplasmic reticulum, and final rupture of the plasma membrane [7,36]. Interestingly, cells become more adherent during autosis and remain on the plate (not floating away) when growing in vitro. Even though light microscopy allows the observation of some of these features, electron microscopy remains the gold standard for the identification of autotic cells (for example, to correctly identify the separation between nuclear membranes) [39].

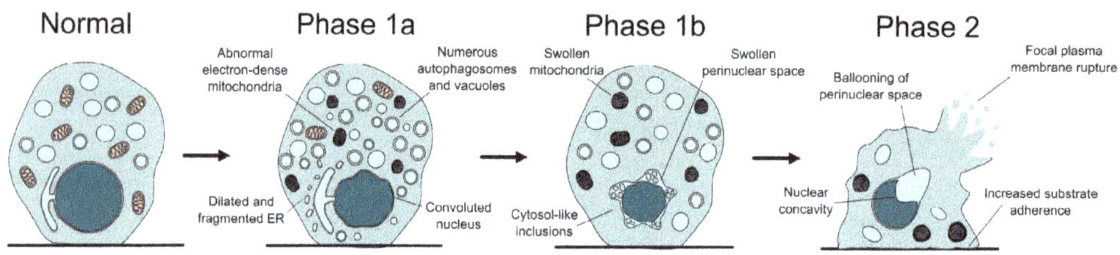

Figure 2. The different phases of autotic cell death. During autosis, the cell undergoes several morphological changes, some of which are distinctive of this process, like the separation of the nuclear membranes, the increased attachment to the substrate, or the formation of a balloon and a concavity in the surface of the nucleus.

The first observation of this type of death occurred in HeLa cells exposed to increasing doses of autophagy-inducing peptides such as Tat-beclin-1 and Tat-vFLIP $\alpha 2$, showing a time-dose dependent induction of cell death [7]. Additionally, this process has also been observed in other contexts, such as in vitro nutrient starvation and hypoxia, or different models of ischemia [7,37,40,41]. Interestingly, autosis has also been identified in the livers of patients with severe anorexia nervosa [42], as well as different immune and cancer cells [43–47]. Even in other vertebrates, like zebrafish, features similar to autosis have also been observed; however, they were not defined as such at that moment [48].

4. Oxidative Stress and Autosis

Even though it was first reported that antioxidants that block ROS-mediated cell death cannot repress autosis [7], recent reports have shown that the activity of essential autotic proteins (mainly, Beclin-1 and the Na^+,K^+-ATPase pump) can be altered by oxidative stress, as it is explained in the next subsections.

4.1. Beclin-1 and Oxidative Stress

Beclin-1 is an essential protein required for the formation of autophagosomes during macroautophagy. This process is initiated when the ULK1 complex, formed by ULK1/ATG13/ATG101/RB1CC1 (FIP200) proteins, is activated in membranes containing ATG9 [49–51]. ULK1, acting with the protein SRC, phosphorylates ATG9, promoting the translocation of ATG9-containing vesicles to the autophagy initiation sites [52]. This allows the incorporation of phospholipids from sources such as the endoplasmic reticulum (ER), recycling endosomes, and mitochondria, initiating the elongation of pre-autophagosomal membranes [53]. A complex with Class III phosphatidylinositol 3-kinase (PI3K) activity, containing Beclin-1/PK3C3 (VPS34)/PI3R4 (VPS15) proteins [54,55], is then recruited to these membranes by ATG14 and NRBF2 [56,57], resulting in the production of phosphatidylinositol 3-phosphate (PI3P) by PK3C3 (VPS34). The action of members of the WIPI family and the union of PI3P-binding proteins to these autophagosomal membranes sustain their expansion until their closure [58].

Recent studies have described that Beclin-1 modulation may influence cellular response towards oxidative stress. For instance, Guo et al. demonstrated that with prolonged glucose starvation and hypoxia, ROS levels increase and activate the ATM/CHK2/Beclin-1 axis, promoting autophagy to control excessive ROS accumulation, clear damaged mitochondria, and inhibit apoptosis. During this process, CHK2 phosphorylates Beclin-1 at Ser90/93 residues, which are located in the Bcl-2 binding domain. Thus, this phosphorylation disrupts the interaction between Beclin-1 and Bcl-2, promoting autophagy under oxidative stress [59]. In hepatocytes, the inhibition of PSMD14 (RPN11) deubiquitinase protects against hepatic steatosis and insulin resistance induced by a high-fat diet. This is caused, in part, by the stabilization of Beclin-1, supporting autophagy and decreasing oxidative stress in hepatic cells [60]. Another study shows that a sustained period of oxidative stress in the mammary glands of dairy cows suffering from ketosis is a major cause of injury during early lactation. The presence of oxidative stress is attributed to the supraphysiological circulating concentrations of non-esterified fatty acids (NEFA), which also enhance autophagy as a counteracting response [61]. Moreover, silencing of Beclin-1 attenuated autophagy activity and increased the levels of ROS, which once again suggests that Beclin-1 plays an important role against oxidative stress [62]. However, it has also been proven that ROS can inhibit autophagy initiation, specifically repressing Beclin-1 activity. For example, they can trigger TRPM2-dependent Ca^{2+} influx, which activates CAMK2 at both phosphorylation and oxidation levels, and subsequently phosphorylates Beclin-1 on Ser295. This phosphorylation, in turn, decreased the association of Beclin-1 with PK3C3 (VPS34) while increasing its interaction with BCL2, and thus inhibiting autophagy [63].

The relationship between Beclin-1 and oxidative stress is already being explored to develop therapeutic strategies against some diseases, such as cancer. An example is the antineoplastic agent cannabidiol, which promotes the dissociation of Beclin-1 and BCL2 (enhancing its interaction with PK3C3 (VPS34)) through ROS-induced autophagy [64,65].

4.2. Na^+,K^+-ATPase and Oxidative Stress

Na^+,K^+-ATPase is a fundamental enzyme for the maintenance of ionic homeostasis in cells and the regulation of the membrane potential [66]. This pump is a multimeric complex consisting of three subunits: α, β, and γ [67]. The α-subunit is the catalytic component, responsible for ATP hydrolysis and ion transport, while the β-subunit has no catalytic activity but regulates the enzymatic function of the pump and confers stability to the α-subunit [68]. There are four isoforms of the α-subunit in humans: $\alpha1$ is the dominant isoform and is widely expressed in almost all cell types [66], $\alpha2$-isoform is predominantly produced in both cardiac and skeletal muscle as well as in the brain (in astrocytes and glia cells) [66,69], $\alpha3$ is mainly located in neurons and cardiac cells (with gender-specific differences in the latter) [70,71], and $\alpha4$-isoform is only expressed in the testes, where it has been associated with sperm motility [72]. There are also three isoforms of the β-subunit [73]: $\beta1$ is found in most tissues [66], while $\beta2$ is expressed in the colon, neurons, and cardiac cells [69,74,75], and $\beta3$ is detected in the testes [76]. Finally, mammals express up to seven isoforms of the γ-subunit (also known as the FXYD family), and they are responsible for the regulation of the affinity of the enzyme to different ligands [77]. Besides modulating the ionic gradient of Na^+ and K^+, the pump also forms complexes with proteins from the plasma membrane, like caveolin, SRC, EGFR, or GPR35, which enable it to participate in different signaling pathways [78,79]. Furthermore, the pump can also modulate adhesion and migration between cells [80].

Many stimuli induce specific modifications in Na^+,K^+-ATPase and can change its activity [81,82], ROS being one of them. For example, Na^+,K^+-ATPase α1-subunit has been observed to be degraded during hypoxia-induced pulmonary edema due to mitochondria-generated ROS and the participation of the ubiquitin-conjugating system [83]. During some neurodegenerative diseases, such as Alzheimer's, trans fatty acids like linoelaidic acid enhance oxidative stress and decrease Na^+,K^+-ATPase activity. Furthermore, it highly reacts with amyloid β (Aβ) depositions, causing even more severe oxidative damage [84]. Also, long-term exposure to Aβ can change the thiol redox status of human neuroblastoma cells, inhibiting the pump and leading to the induction of glutathionylation of the α-subunit [85]. S-glutathionylation is, in fact, one of the most documented oxidative modifications of Na^+,K^+-ATPase. In the case of cardiac sarcolemma, the activation of the renin–angiotensin system also leads to the glutathionylation of the β1 subunit of the pump, causing its inhibition [86]. Similarly, oxidative stress from placental ischemia/reperfusion and hypoxia in preeclampsia also causes S-glutathionylation of the β1 subunit, hampering its function [87]. S-glutathionylation of cysteine residues of the α1 and β1 subunits can also reduce the α1/β1 association, causing conformational changes and blocking the α1 subunit's intracellular ATP-binding site, leading to the inhibition of its activity [88,89]. Nevertheless, the oxidative modifications of Na^+,K^+-ATPase appear to be reversible [90,91], which means its activity can be regulated in a redox-sensitive manner. Furthermore, members of the FXYD family can also reverse oxidative stress-induced inhibition of the pump activity by deglutathionylation of the β1 subunit [91]. Still, the exposure of the pump to free radicals increases its susceptibility to degradation by proteolytic enzymes [92,93].

Apart from ROS, RNS can also modify Na^+,K^+-ATPase activity. Peroxynitrite, for example, is produced when nitric oxide and superoxide react [94], and it can act as a potent irreversible inhibitor of the pump activity by both nitrating tyrosine residues in all three subunits and modifying cysteine residues [95]. Furthermore, the free radical nitric oxide (•NO) can also regulate Na^+,K^+-ATPase through the activation of soluble guanylate cyclase and cGMP in the central nervous system, modulating cerebral blood flow and synaptic transmission [96,97]. The regulation of the pump activity by •NO is also known in other tissues, such as the choroid plexus [98].

Interestingly, oxidative stress can also modulate the interaction of the pump with other proteins, like the Na^+,K^+-ATPase/SRC axis. The α1-subunit serves as a scaffold for proto-oncogene tyrosine kinase c-SRC, interacting with it and inhibiting its function [99]. However, when cardiac glucosides bind to the extracellular domain of the pump, a conformational change is produced, allowing SRC to be activated. In turn, it transactivates EGFR, which then activates RAS [100]. This can lead to the production of ROS by the mitochondria, resulting in the activation of nuclear factor kappa B (NF-κB) and initiating the MAPK cascade [101,102]. Furthermore, SRC may also be regulated by ROS through a reversible oxidation of cysteine residues, generating a positive feedback loop [90]. Some of these oxidized residues are located where the interaction between Na^+,K^+-ATPase and SRC takes place [99], inducing changes in either the pump, SRC, or both, which in turn might affect the interaction between them and, consequently, the downstream kinase cascade [103].

5. A New Layer in Autosis Regulation

A decade has passed since autosis was first described, yet our understanding of this specific type of cell death remains limited. While the Na^+,K^+-ATPase pump and certain components of the autophagy machinery are crucial for initiating this cellular response, the complete molecular pathway and its regulatory mechanisms are still largely unexplored. Most research has concentrated on potential ionic imbalances caused by dysregulated activity of the pump, as well as oxygen and nutrient deprivation, since both hypoxia and starvation can trigger autosis. However, in this review, we have displayed recent studies that indicate that ROS can also affect the function of autotic components. Therefore, we propose that the redox status of the cell should be considered when investigating the molecular and regulatory mechanisms of autosis.

In this regard, it is noteworthy that oxidative stress can inhibit both Beclin-1 and Na^+,K^+-ATPase [63,88,104–108], for example, by modifications such as S-glutathionylation, tyrosine nitration, and others [89,95,109]. This suggests that these species may actually prevent autotic induction at first, rather than promote it, as the repression of Beclin-1 and pump activities can effectively block autosis [7]. Depending on the context, ROS can act as important signaling molecules instead of toxins, helping to maintain cellular homeostasis by allowing cells to rapidly respond to various conditions for survival. In this sense, ROS may first negatively affect Beclin-1 and the pump, reducing their activity, preventing their binding, and hindering the autotic response. However, an overwhelming increase in ROS production could concurrently promote an exacerbated autophagic response that is triggered as an attempt to counteract oxidative stress [110], but that can ultimately lead to the initiation of autosis. This could be particularly relevant, for example, under hypoxic conditions, which are associated with both elevated ROS generation [111,112] and autotic cell death [7,37,38], potentially through HIF-1α. This is an essential transcription factor that can be activated and stabilized in response to hypoxia-induced ROS [113], resulting in the promotion of autophagy [114,115]. Another transcription factor that could be important in this process is TFEB, which is also activated under oxidative stress [116,117] and promotes the expression of autophagic and lysosomal genes [118]. Other interesting effectors that can activate autophagy in response to ROS (even under hypoxic conditions) are components of the FOXO family, such as FOXO1 and FOXO3 [119–123]. But how much oxidative stress would be needed to activate autosis? What is the threshold for this switch in the ROS-autosis interplay? These are complex questions that would need to be experimentally addressed. Nevertheless, it seems it could greatly depend on the context. For example, several studies have described that AMPK, one of the main autophagy regulators, can be both repressed and stimulated by oxidative stress, depending on whether ROS mediates the phosphorylation (positive regulation) or the oxidation (negative regulation) of its residues [124].

In conclusion, based on our current understanding of ROS and autotic-related proteins, we suggest that these species could have a dual role in autosis (Figure 3). First, ROS may function as molecular brakes for this type of cell death by inhibiting the activity of Beclin-1 and the Na^+,K^+-ATPase pump. However, when present in high concentrations, ROS can activate different autophagy-inducing signaling pathways (through mediators such as HIF-1α, TFEB, FOXO, or AMPK), exacerbating the autophagy response and leading to autosis initiation. Nevertheless, this conceptual model must be experimentally confirmed in the future to fully unveil the role of ROS and oxidative stress in this type of autophagy-dependent cell death. Therefore, we believe it is crucial to consider the redox status of the cell when examining the molecular and regulatory mechanisms of autosis, as it can influence the function of key effectors in the pathway.

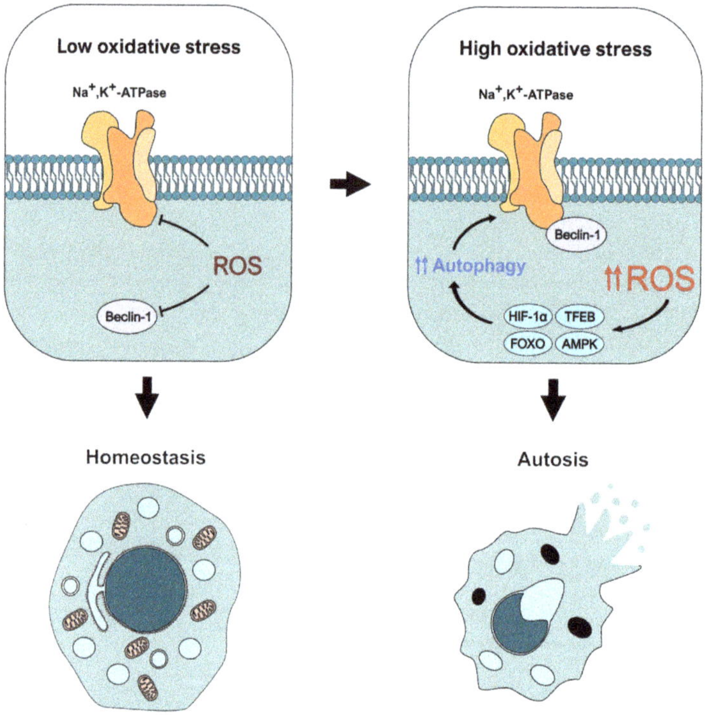

Figure 3. Theoretical model of the dual regulation of autosis-related effectors by oxidative stress. ROS would block autosis initiation early by inhibiting the activity of Beclin-1 and Na^+,K^+-ATPase. However, increased oxidative stress would trigger an intense autophagic response mediated by different effectors (such as HIF-1 α, TFEB, or AMPK) that could lead to autosis initiation.

Author Contributions: Conceptualization, M.G.-M. and Á.F.F.; writing—original draft preparation, M.G.-A., I.M.-R., A.P.-M. and E.L.-F.; writing—review and editing, M.G.-M. and Á.F.F.; supervision, M.G.-M. and Á.F.F. All authors have read and agreed to the published version of the manuscript.

Funding: M.G.A.'s contract is funded by a predoctoral grant from the University of Oviedo (PAPI-22-PF-21). E.L.F. has an FPI contract (PRE2023-138478) funded by the grant PID2022-138478OA-100. M.G.M. is a Ramón y Cajal researcher (grant RYC2021-033684-I, funded by MICIU/AEI/10.13039/501100011033 and by European Union NextGenerationEU/PRTR), and her research is funded by an Internationalization Project "CL-EI-2021-08-IBFG Unit of Excellence" from the Spanish National Research Council (CSIC), which is funded by the Junta de Castilla y León and co-financed by the European Regional Development Fund (ERDF "Europe drives our growth") and the grant PID2022-138478OA-100, funded by MICIU/AEI/10.13039/501100011033 and by FEDER, UE. Á.F.F.'s work is supported by grants CNS2024-154954 and PID2021-127534OB-I00, funded by MICIU/AEI/10.13039/501100011033 and by ERDF/EU.

Institutional Review Board Statement: Not applicable.

Informed Consent Statement: Not applicable.

Data Availability Statement: No new data were created or analyzed in this study. Data sharing is not applicable to this article.

Acknowledgments: We are members of and thank Women in Autophagy (WIA), Sociedad Española de Bioquímica y Biología Molecular (SEBBM), and Sociedad Española de Autofagia (SEFAGIA).

Conflicts of Interest: The authors declare no conflicts of interest.

Abbreviations

The following abbreviations are used in this manuscript:

Aβ	Amyloid β
AMPK	AMP-activated protein kinase
ATG9	Autophagy-related protein 9
ATG13	Autophagy-related protein 13
ATG14	Autophagy-related protein 14
ATG101	Autophagy-related protein 101
ATM	Serine protein kinase ATM
BCL2	Apoptosis regulator Bcl-2
CAMK2	Calcium/calmodulin-dependent protein kinase type II
cGMP	Cyclic guanosine monophosphate
CHK2	Serine/threonine-protein kinase Chk2
EGFR	Epidermal growth factor receptor
FIP200FOXO	FAK family kinase-interacting protein of 200 kDaForkhead box proteins
FXYD	FXYD domain-containing ion transport regulator
GPR35	G-protein coupled receptor 35
GSH	Glutathione
GSSG	Glutathione disulfide
H_2O_2	Hydrogen peroxide
HIF-1αJNK	Hypoxia-inducible factor 1-alphac-Jun N-terminal kinase
MAPK	Mitogen-activated protein kinase
NAD	Reactive oxygen species
NADP	Reactive nitrogen species
NCCD	Nomenclature Committee on Cell Death
NEFA	Non-esterified fatty acids
NF-κB	Nuclear factor kappa-light-chain-enhancer of activated B cells
NOS	Nitric oxide synthase
NOX	NADPH oxidase
NRBF2	Nuclear receptor-binding factor 2
$O_2^{\bullet-}$	Superoxide anion
ONOO—	Peroxynitrite
PI3K	Class III phosphatidylinositol 3-kinase
PI3P	Phosphatidylinositol 3-phosphate
PI3R4	Phosphoinositide 3-kinase regulatory subunit 4
PK3C3	Phosphatidylinositol 3-kinase catalytic subunit type 3
PSMD14	26S proteasome non-ATPase regulatory subunit 14
RAS	Rat sarcoma virus small GTPase
RB1CC1	RB1-inducible coiled-coil protein 1
RET	Reverse electron transport
RNS	Reactive nitrogen species
ROS	Reactive oxygen species
RPN11	26S proteasome regulatory subunit RPN11
SiRNA	Small interfering RNA
SRCTFEB	Proto-oncogene tyrosine-protein kinase SrcTranscription factor EB
TRPM2	Transient receptor potential cation channel subfamily M member 2
ULK1	Serine/threonine-protein kinase ULK1
UV	Ultraviolet
VPS15	Vacuolar protein sorting 15
VPS34	Vacuolar protein sorting 34
WIPI	WD repeat domain phosphoinositide-interacting
$^{\bullet}OH$	Hydroxyl radical
$^{\bullet}NO$	Nitric oxide

References

1. Lennicke, C.; Cochemé, H.M. Redox Metabolism: ROS as Specific Molecular Regulators of Cell Signaling and Function. *Mol. Cell* **2021**, *81*, 3691–3707. [CrossRef]
2. Zoccarato, A.; Nabeebaccus, A.A.; Oexner, R.R.; Santos, C.X.C.; Shah, A.M. The Nexus between Redox State and Intermediary Metabolism. *FEBS J.* **2022**, *289*, 5440–5462. [CrossRef] [PubMed]
3. Jomova, K.; Raptova, R.; Alomar, S.Y.; Alwasel, S.H.; Nepovimova, E.; Kuca, K.; Valko, M. Reactive Oxygen Species, Toxicity, Oxidative Stress, and Antioxidants: Chronic Diseases and Aging. *Arch. Toxicol.* **2023**, *97*, 2499–2574. [CrossRef] [PubMed]
4. Klionsky, D.J.; Petroni, G.; Amaravadi, R.K.; Baehrecke, E.H.; Ballabio, A.; Boya, P.; Pedro, J.M.B.; Cadwell, K.; Cecconi, F.; Choi, A.M.K.; et al. Autophagy in Major Human Diseases. *EMBO J.* **2021**, *40*, e108863. [CrossRef] [PubMed]
5. Miller, D.R.; Thorburn, A. Autophagy and Organelle Homeostasis in Cancer. *Dev. Cell* **2021**, *56*, 906–918. [CrossRef] [PubMed]
6. Rakesh, R.; PriyaDharshini, L.C.; Sakthivel, K.M.; Rasmi, R.R. Role and Regulation of Autophagy in Cancer. *Biochim. Biophys. Acta Mol. Basis Dis.* **2022**, *1868*, 166400. [CrossRef] [PubMed]
7. Liu, Y.; Shoji-Kawata, S.; Sumpter, R.M.; Wei, Y.; Ginet, V.; Zhang, L.; Posner, B.; Tran, K.A.; Green, D.R.; Xavier, R.J.; et al. Autosis Is a Na+,K+-ATPase-Regulated Form of Cell Death Triggered by Autophagy-Inducing Peptides, Starvation, and Hypoxia-Ischemia. *Proc. Natl. Acad. Sci. USA* **2013**, *110*, 20364–20371. [CrossRef]
8. Iqbal, M.J.; Kabeer, A.; Abbas, Z.; Siddiqui, H.A.; Calina, D.; Sharifi-Rad, J.; Cho, W.C. Interplay of Oxidative Stress, Cellular Communication and Signaling Pathways in Cancer. *Cell Commun. Signal.* **2024**, *22*, 7. [CrossRef]
9. Stefanou, D.T.; Kouvela, M.; Stellas, D.; Voutetakis, K.; Papadodima, O.; Syrigos, K.; Souliotis, V.L. Oxidative Stress and Deregulated DNA Damage Response Network in Lung Cancer Patients. *Biomedicines* **2022**, *10*, 1248. [CrossRef]
10. Foret, M.K.; Orciani, C.; Welikovitch, L.A.; Huang, C.; Cuello, A.C.; Do Carmo, S. Early Oxidative Stress and DNA Damage in Aβ-Burdened Hippocampal Neurons in an Alzheimer's-like Transgenic Rat Model. *Commun. Biol.* **2024**, *7*, 861. [CrossRef]
11. Bardelčíková, A.; Šoltys, J.; Mojžiš, J. Oxidative Stress, Inflammation and Colorectal Cancer: An Overview. *Antioxidants* **2023**, *12*, 901. [CrossRef] [PubMed]
12. Huang, Z.; Zhou, L.; Duan, J.; Qin, S.; Jiang, J.; Chen, H.; Wang, K.; Liu, R.; Yuan, M.; Tang, X.; et al. Oxidative Stress Promotes Liver Cancer Metastasis via RNF25-Mediated E-Cadherin Protein Degradation. *Adv. Sci.* **2024**, *11*, e2306929. [CrossRef] [PubMed]
13. Zaric, B.L.; Macvanin, M.T.; Isenovic, E.R. Free Radicals: Relationship to Human Diseases and Potential Therapeutic Applications. *Int. J. Biochem. Cell Biol.* **2023**, *154*, 106346. [CrossRef] [PubMed]
14. Scialo, F.; Sanz, A. Coenzyme Q Redox Signalling and Longevity. *Free Radic. Biol. Med.* **2021**, *164*, 187–205. [CrossRef]
15. Scialò, F.; Fernández-Ayala, D.J.; Sanz, A. Role of Mitochondrial Reverse Electron Transport in ROS Signaling: Potential Roles in Health and Disease. *Front. Physiol.* **2017**, *8*, 273331. [CrossRef]
16. Taylor, J.P.; Tse, H.M. The Role of NADPH Oxidases in Infectious and Inflammatory Diseases. *Redox Biol.* **2021**, *48*, 102159. [CrossRef] [PubMed]
17. Matsumoto, S.; Koshiishi, I.; Inoguchi, T.; Nawata, H.; Utsumi, H. Confirmation of Superoxide Generation via Xanthine Oxidase in Streptozotocin-Induced Diabetic Mice. *Free Radic. Res.* **2003**, *37*, 767–772. [CrossRef] [PubMed]
18. Radi, R. Peroxynitrite, a Stealthy Biological Oxidant. *J. Biol. Chem.* **2013**, *288*, 26464–26472. [CrossRef] [PubMed]
19. De Almeida, A.J.P.O.; De Oliveira, J.C.P.L.; Da Silva Pontes, L.V.; De Souza Júnior, J.F.; Gonçalves, T.A.F.; Dantas, S.H.; De Almeida Feitosa, M.S.; Silva, A.O.; De Medeiros, I.A. ROS: Basic Concepts, Sources, Cellular Signaling, and Its Implications in Aging Pathways. *Oxid. Med. Cell Longev.* **2022**, *2022*, 1225578. [CrossRef]
20. Moon, D.O.; Kim, M.O.; Choi, Y.H.; Hyun, J.W.; Chang, W.Y.; Kim, G.Y. Butein Induces G2/M Phase Arrest and Apoptosis in Human Hepatoma Cancer Cells through ROS Generation. *Cancer Lett.* **2010**, *288*, 204–213. [CrossRef]
21. Dai, D.F.; Hsieh, E.J.; Liu, Y.; Chen, T.; Beyer, R.P.; Chin, M.T.; MacCoss, M.J.; Rabinovitch, P.S. Mitochondrial Proteome Remodelling in Pressure Overload-Induced Heart Failure: The Role of Mitochondrial Oxidative Stress. *Cardiovasc. Res.* **2012**, *93*, 79–88. [CrossRef]
22. Chatterjee, K.; Pal, A.; Padhy, D.S.; Saha, R.; Chatterjee, A.; Bharadwaj, M.; Sarkar, B.; Mazumder, P.M.; Banerjee, S. Vitamin K2 Ameliorates Diabetes-Associated Cognitive Decline by Reducing Oxidative Stress and Neuroinflammation. *J. Neuroimmune Pharmacol.* **2024**, *19*, 56. [CrossRef]
23. Guan, L.; Mao, Z.; Yang, S.; Wu, G.; Chen, Y.; Yin, L.; Qi, Y.; Han, L.; Xu, L. Dioscin Alleviates Alzheimer's Disease through Regulating RAGE/NOX4 Mediated Oxidative Stress and Inflammation. *Biomed. Pharmacother.* **2022**, *152*, 113248. [CrossRef] [PubMed]
24. Hofmans, S.; Berghe, T.V.; Devisscher, L.; Hassannia, B.; Lyssens, S.; Joossens, J.; Van Der Veken, P.; Vandenabeele, P.; Augustyns, K. Novel Ferroptosis Inhibitors with Improved Potency and ADME Properties. *J. Med. Chem.* **2016**, *59*, 2041–2053. [CrossRef] [PubMed]
25. Baba, Y.; Higa, J.K.; Shimada, B.K.; Horiuchi, K.M.; Suhara, T.; Kobayashi, M.; Woo, J.D.; Aoyagi, H.; Marh, K.S.; Kitaoka, H.; et al. Protective Effects of the Mechanistic Target of Rapamycin against Excess Iron and Ferroptosis in Cardiomyocytes. *Am. J. Physiol. Heart Circ. Physiol.* **2018**, *314*, H659–H668. [CrossRef] [PubMed]

26. Zhang, Y.; Chen, D.; Tian, R.; Yan, X.; Zhou, Y. Resveratrol Alleviates Amyloid β-Induced Neuronal Apoptosis, Inflammation, and Oxidative and Endoplasmic Reticulum Stress by Circ_0050263/MiR-361-3p/PDE4A Axis during Alzheimer's Disease. *Chem. Biol. Drug Des.* **2023**, *102*, 1121–1132. [CrossRef] [PubMed]
27. Thadathil, N.; Nicklas, E.H.; Mohammed, S.; Lewis, T.L.; Richardson, A.; Deepa, S.S. Necroptosis Increases with Age in the Brain and Contributes to Age-Related Neuroinflammation. *Geroscience* **2021**, *43*, 2345. [CrossRef]
28. Zheng, L.; Terman, A.; Hallbeck, M.; Dehvari, N.; Cowburn, R.F.; Benedikz, E.; Kågedal, K.; Cedazo-Minguez, A.; Marcusson, J. Macroautophagy-Generated Increase of Lysosomal Amyloid β-Protein Mediates Oxidant-Induced Apoptosis of Cultured Neuroblastoma Cells. *Autophagy* **2011**, *7*, 1528–1545. [CrossRef]
29. Shi, S.; Chen, Y.; Luo, Z.; Nie, G.; Dai, Y. Role of Oxidative Stress and Inflammation-Related Signaling Pathways in Doxorubicin-Induced Cardiomyopathy. *Cell Commun. Signal.* **2023**, *21*, 61. [CrossRef]
30. Li, L.; Chen, Y.; Gibson, S.B. Starvation-Induced Autophagy Is Regulated by Mitochondrial Reactive Oxygen Species Leading to AMPK Activation. *Cell. Signal.* **2013**, *25*, 50–65. [CrossRef]
31. Komatsu, M.; Kurokawa, H.; Waguri, S.; Taguchi, K.; Kobayashi, A.; Ichimura, Y.; Sou, Y.S.; Ueno, I.; Sakamoto, A.; Tong, K.I.; et al. The Selective Autophagy Substrate P62 Activates the Stress Responsive Transcription Factor Nrf2 through Inactivation of Keap1. *Nat. Cell Biol.* **2010**, *12*, 213–223. [CrossRef]
32. Scherz-Shouval, R.; Shvets, E.; Fass, E.; Shorer, H.; Gil, L.; Elazar, Z. Reactive Oxygen Species Are Essential for Autophagy and Specifically Regulate the Activity of Atg4. *EMBO J.* **2007**, *26*, 1749–1760. [CrossRef] [PubMed]
33. Galluzzi, L.; Vitale, I.; Aaronson, S.A.; Abrams, J.M.; Adam, D.; Agostinis, P.; Alnemri, E.S.; Altucci, L.; Amelio, I.; Andrews, D.W.; et al. Molecular Mechanisms of Cell Death: Recommendations of the Nomenclature Committee on Cell Death 2018. *Cell Death Differ.* **2018**, *25*, 486–541. [CrossRef] [PubMed]
34. Levine, B.; Kroemer, G. Biological Functions of Autophagy Genes: A Disease Perspective. *Cell* **2019**, *176*, 11–42. [CrossRef] [PubMed]
35. Schweichel, J.-U.; Merker, H.-J. The Morphology of Various Types of Cell Death in Prenatal Tissues. *Teratology* **1973**, *7*, 253–266. [CrossRef] [PubMed]
36. Liu, Y.; Levine, B. Autosis and Autophagic Cell Death: The Dark Side of Autophagy. *Cell Death Differ.* **2015**, *22*, 367–376. [CrossRef] [PubMed]
37. Fernández, Á.F.; Liu, Y.; Ginet, V.; Shi, M.; Nah, J.; Zou, Z.; Zhou, A.; Posner, B.A.; Xiao, G.; Tanguy, M.; et al. Interaction between the Autophagy Protein Beclin 1 and Na+,K+-ATPase during Starvation, Exercise, and Ischemia. *JCI Insight* **2020**, *5*, e133282. [CrossRef] [PubMed]
38. Depierre, P.; Ginet, V.; Truttmann, A.C.; Puyal, J. Neuronal Autosis Is Na+/K+-ATPase Alpha 3-Dependent and Involved in Hypoxic-Ischemic Neuronal Death. *Cell Death Dis.* **2024**, *15*, 363. [CrossRef] [PubMed]
39. Kaludercic, N.; Maiuri, M.C.; Kaushik, S.; Fernández, Á.F.; De Bruijn, J.; Castoldi, F.; Chen, Y.; Ito, J.; Mukai, R.; Murakawa, T.; et al. Comprehensive Autophagy Evaluation in Cardiac Disease Models. *Cardiovasc. Res.* **2020**, *116*, 483–504. [CrossRef] [PubMed]
40. Chen, Y.; Henson, E.S.; Xiao, W.; Huang, D.; McMillan-Ward, E.M.; Israels, S.J.; Gibson, S.B. Tyrosine Kinase Receptor EGFR Regulates the Switch in Cancer Cells between Cell Survival and Cell Death Induced by Autophagy in Hypoxia. *Autophagy* **2016**, *12*, 1029–1046. [CrossRef]
41. Nah, J.; Zhai, P.; Huang, C.Y.; Fernández, Á.F.; Mareedu, S.; Levine, B.; Sadoshima, J. Upregulation of Rubicon Promotes Autosis during Myocardial Ischemia/Reperfusion Injury. *J. Clin. Investig.* **2020**, *130*, 2978–2991. [CrossRef] [PubMed]
42. Kheloufi, M.; Boulanger, C.M.; Codogno, P.; Rautou, P.E. Autosis Occurs in the Liver of Patients with Severe Anorexia Nervosa. *Hepatology* **2015**, *62*, 657–658. [CrossRef] [PubMed]
43. Zhang, G.; Luk, B.T.; Wei, X.; Campbell, G.R.; Fang, R.H.; Zhang, L.; Spector, S.A. Selective Cell Death of Latently HIV-Infected CD4+ T Cells Mediated by Autosis Inducing Nanopeptides. *Cell Death Dis.* **2019**, *10*, 419. [CrossRef] [PubMed]
44. Zheng, N.; Fang, J.; Xue, G.; Wang, Z.; Li, X.; Zhou, M.; Jin, G.; Rahman, M.M.; McFadden, G.; Lu, Y. Induction of Tumor Cell Autosis by Myxoma Virus-Infected CAR-T and TCR-T Cells to Overcome Primary and Acquired Resistance. *Cancer Cell* **2022**, *40*, 973–985.e7. [CrossRef] [PubMed]
45. Han, S.; Li, X.; Wang, K.; Zhu, D.; Meng, B.; Liu, J.; Liang, X.; Jin, Y.; Liu, X.; Wen, Q.; et al. PURPL Represses Autophagic Cell Death to Promote Cutaneous Melanoma by Modulating ULK1 Phosphorylation. *Cell Death Dis.* **2021**, *12*, 1070. [CrossRef] [PubMed]
46. Camuzard, O.; Trojani, M.-C.; Santucci-Darmanin, S.; Pagnotta, S.; Breuil, V.; Carle, G.; Pierrefite-Carle, V. Autophagy in Osteosarcoma Cancer Stem Cells Is Critical Process Which Can Be Targeted by the Antipsychotic Drug Thioridazine. *Cancers* **2020**, *12*, 3675. [CrossRef]
47. Zhang, X.; Shan, G.; Li, N.; Chen, J.; Ji, C.; Li, X.; Jiang, L.; Kin, T.; Lee, W.; Keng, V.W.; et al. An Autophagy-Inducing Stapled Peptide Induces Mitochondria Dysfunction and Triggers Autotic Cell Death in Triple-Negative Breast Cancer. *Cell Death Discov.* **2023**, *9*, 303. [CrossRef]

48. Santos-Ledo, A.; Garcia-Macia, M.; Campbell, P.D.; Gronska, M.; Marlow, F.L. Kinesin-1 Promotes Chondrocyte Maintenance during Skeletal Morphogenesis. *PLoS Genet.* **2017**, *13*, e1006918. [CrossRef]
49. Hosokawa, N.; Sasaki, T.; Iemura, S.I.; Natsume, T.; Hara, T.; Mizushima, N. Atg101, a Novel Mammalian Autophagy Protein Interacting with Atg13. *Autophagy* **2009**, *5*, 973–979. [CrossRef]
50. Ganley, I.G.; Lam, D.H.; Wang, J.; Ding, X.; Chen, S.; Jiang, X. ULK1.ATG13.FIP200 Complex Mediates MTOR Signaling and Is Essential for Autophagy. *J. Biol. Chem.* **2009**, *284*, 12297–12305. [CrossRef] [PubMed]
51. Karanasios, E.; Walker, S.A.; Okkenhaug, H.; Manifava, M.; Hummel, E.; Zimmermann, H.; Ahmed, Q.; Domart, M.C.; Collinson, L.; Ktistakis, N.T. Autophagy Initiation by ULK Complex Assembly on ER Tubulovesicular Regions Marked by ATG9 Vesicles. *Nat. Commun.* **2016**, *7*, 12420. [CrossRef]
52. Zhou, C.; Ma, K.; Gao, R.; Mu, C.; Chen, L.; Liu, Q.; Luo, Q.; Feng, D.; Zhu, Y.; Chen, Q. Regulation of MATG9 Trafficking by Src- and ULK1-Mediated Phosphorylation in Basal and Starvation-Induced Autophagy. *Cell Res.* **2016**, *27*, 184–201. [CrossRef]
53. Galluzzi, L.; Baehrecke, E.H.; Ballabio, A.; Boya, P.; Bravo-San Pedro, J.M.; Cecconi, F.; Choi, A.M.; Chu, C.T.; Codogno, P.; Colombo, M.I.; et al. Molecular Definitions of Autophagy and Related Processes. *EMBO J.* **2017**, *36*, 1811–1836. [CrossRef] [PubMed]
54. Kihara, A.; Noda, T.; Ishihara, N.; Ohsumi, Y. Two Distinct Vps34 Phosphatidylinositol 3-Kinase Complexes Function in Autophagy and Carboxypeptidase Y Sorting in Saccharomyces Cerevisiae. *J. Cell Biol.* **2001**, *152*, 519–530. [CrossRef] [PubMed]
55. Kihara, A.; Kabeya, Y.; Ohsumi, Y.; Yoshimori, T. Beclin-Phosphatidylinositol 3-Kinase Complex Functions at the Trans-Golgi Network. *EMBO Rep.* **2001**, *2*, 330–335. [CrossRef] [PubMed]
56. Itakura, E.; Kishi, C.; Inoue, K.; Mizushima, N. Beclin 1 Forms Two Distinct Phosphatidylinositol 3-Kinase Complexes with Mammalian Atg14 and UVRAG. *Mol. Biol. Cell* **2008**, *19*, 5360–5372. [CrossRef] [PubMed]
57. Lu, J.; He, L.; Behrends, C.; Araki, M.; Araki, K.; Jun Wang, Q.; Catanzaro, J.M.; Friedman, S.L.; Zong, W.X.; Fiel, M.I.; et al. NRBF2 Regulates Autophagy and Prevents Liver Injury by Modulating Atg14L-Linked Phosphatidylinositol-3 Kinase III Activity. *Nat. Commun.* **2014**, *5*, 3920. [CrossRef]
58. Dooley, H.C.; Razi, M.; Polson, H.E.J.; Girardin, S.E.; Wilson, M.I.; Tooze, S.A. WIPI2 Links LC3 Conjugation with PI3P, Autophagosome Formation, and Pathogen Clearance by Recruiting Atg12–5-16L1. *Mol. Cell* **2014**, *55*, 238. [CrossRef]
59. Guo, Q.; Wang, S.; Zhang, S.; Xu, H.; Li, X.; Guan, Y.; Yi, F.; Zhou, T.; Jiang, B.; Bai, N.; et al. ATM-CHK2-Beclin 1 Axis Promotes Autophagy to Maintain ROS Homeostasis under Oxidative Stress. *EMBO J.* **2020**, *39*, e103111. [CrossRef]
60. Zhou, B.; Luo, Y.; Bi, H.; Zhang, N.; Ma, M.; Dong, Z.; Ji, N.; Zhang, S.; Wang, X.; Liu, Y.; et al. Amelioration of Nonalcoholic Fatty Liver Disease by Inhibiting the Deubiquitylating Enzyme RPN11. *Cell Metab.* **2024**, *36*, 2228–2244.e7. [CrossRef]
61. Chang, R.; Sun, X.; Jia, H.; Xu, Q.; Dong, Z.; Tang, Y.; Luo, S.; Jiang, Q.; Loor, J.J.; Xu, C. Inhibiting Nuclear Factor Erythroid 2 Related Factor 2-Mediated Autophagy in Bovine Mammary Epithelial Cells Induces Oxidative Stress in Response to Exogenous Fatty Acids. *J. Anim. Sci. Biotechnol.* **2022**, *13*, 48. [CrossRef] [PubMed]
62. Liu, K.; Dong, Y.; Cao, L.; Li, G.; Yang, Z.; Luo, J.; Lei, L.; Du, X.; Song, Y.; Usman, M.; et al. Caveolin 1 Ameliorates Nonesterified Fatty Acid-Induced Oxidative Stress via the Autophagy Regulator Beclin 1 in Bovine Mammary Gland Epithelial Cells. *J. Dairy Sci.* **2024**, *108*, 928–942. [CrossRef] [PubMed]
63. Wang, Q.; Guo, W.; Hao, B.; Shi, X.; Lu, Y.; Wong, C.W.M.; Ma, V.W.S.; Yip, T.T.C.; Au, J.S.K.; Hao, Q.; et al. Mechanistic Study of TRPM2-Ca2+-CAMK2-BECN1 Signaling in Oxidative Stress-Induced Autophagy Inhibition. *Autophagy* **2016**, *12*, 1340–1354. [CrossRef] [PubMed]
64. Shrivastava, A.; Kuzontkoski, P.M.; Groopman, J.E.; Prasad, A. Cannabidiol Induces Programmed Cell Death in Breast Cancer Cells by Coordinating the Cross-Talk between Apoptosis and Autophagy. *Mol. Cancer Ther.* **2011**, *10*, 1161–1172. [CrossRef] [PubMed]
65. Kim, N.Y.; Shivanne Gowda, S.G.; Lee, S.G.; Sethi, G.; Ahn, K.S. Cannabidiol Induces ERK Activation and ROS Production to Promote Autophagy and Ferroptosis in Glioblastoma Cells. *Chem. Biol. Interact.* **2024**, *394*, 110995. [CrossRef] [PubMed]
66. Clausen, M.V.; Hilbers, F.; Poulsen, H. The Structure and Function of the Na,K-ATPase Isoforms in Health and Disease. *Front. Physiol.* **2017**, *8*, 257141. [CrossRef]
67. Mobasheri, A.; Avila, J.; Cózar-Castellano, I.; Brownleader, M.D.; Trevan, M.; Francis, M.J.O.; Lamb, J.F.; Martín-Vasallo, P. Na^+, K^+-ATPase Isozyme Diversity; Comparative Biochemistry and Physiological Implications of Novel Functional Interactions. *Biosci. Rep.* **2000**, *20*, 51–91. [CrossRef]
68. Da Silva, C.I.; Gonçalves-de-Albuquerque, C.F.; De Moraes, B.P.; Garcia, D.G.; Burth, P. Na/K-ATPase: Their Role in Cell Adhesion and Migration in Cancer. *Biochimie* **2021**, *185*, 1–8. [CrossRef]
69. Zlokovic, B.V.; Mackic, J.B.; Wang, L.; McComb, J.G.; McDonough, A. Differential Expression of Na,K-ATPase Alpha and Beta Subunit Isoforms at the Blood-Brain Barrier and the Choroid Plexus. *J. Biol. Chem.* **1993**, *268*, 8019–8025. [CrossRef]
70. Gaborit, N.; Varro, A.; Le Bouter, S.; Szuts, V.; Escande, D.; Nattel, S.; Demolombe, S. Gender-Related Differences in Ion-Channel and Transporter Subunit Expression in Non-Diseased Human Hearts. *J. Mol. Cell Cardiol.* **2010**, *49*, 639–646. [CrossRef]

71. Bøttger, P.; Tracz, Z.; Heuck, A.; Nissen, P.; Romero-Ramos, M.; Lykke-Hartmann, K. Distribution of Na/K-ATPase Alpha 3 Isoform, a Sodium-Potassium P-Type Pump Associated with Rapid-Onset of Dystonia Parkinsonism (RDP) in the Adult Mouse Brain. *J. Comp. Neurol.* **2011**, *519*, 376–404. [CrossRef]
72. Jimenez, T.; Sanchez, G.; McDermott, J.P.; Nguyen, A.N.; Kumar, T.R.; Blanco, G. Increased Expression of the Na,K-ATPase Alpha4 Isoform Enhances Sperm Motility in Transgenic Mice. *Biol. Reprod.* **2011**, *84*, 153–161. [CrossRef]
73. Geering, K. Functional Roles of Na,K-ATPase Subunits. *Curr. Opin. Nephrol. Hypertens.* **2008**, *17*, 526–532. [CrossRef] [PubMed]
74. Baker Bechmann, M.; Rotoli, D.; Morales, M.; Maeso, M.d.C.; García, M.d.P.; Ávila, J.; Mobasheri, A.; Martín-Vasallo, P. Na,K-ATPase Isozymes in Colorectal Cancer and Liver Metastases. *Front. Physiol.* **2016**, *7*, 9. [CrossRef] [PubMed]
75. Habeck, M.; Tokhtaeva, E.; Nadav, Y.; Zeev, E.B.; Ferris, S.P.; Kaufman, R.J.; Bab-Dinitz, E.; Kaplan, J.H.; Dada, L.A.; Farfel, Z.; et al. Selective Assembly of Na,K-ATPase A2β2 Heterodimers in the Heart: Distinct Functional Properties And Isoform-Selective Inhibitors. *J. Biol. Chem.* **2016**, *291*, 23159–23174. [CrossRef] [PubMed]
76. Arystarkhova, E.; Sweadner, K.J. Tissue-Specific Expression of the Na,K-ATPase Beta3 Subunit. The Presence of Beta3 in Lung and Liver Addresses the Problem of the Missing Subunit. *J. Biol. Chem.* **1997**, *272*, 22405–22408. [CrossRef]
77. Mishra, N.K.; Peleg, Y.; Cirri, E.; Belogus, T.; Lifshitz, Y.; Voelker, D.R.; Apell, H.J.; Garty, H.; Karlish, S.J.D. FXYD Proteins Stabilize Na,K-ATPase: Amplification of Specific Phosphatidylserine-Protein Interactions. *J. Biol. Chem.* **2011**, *286*, 9699–9712. [CrossRef]
78. Cui, X.; Xie, Z. Protein Interaction and Na/K-ATPase-Mediated Signal Transduction. *Molecules* **2017**, *22*, 990. [CrossRef]
79. Schneditz, G.; Elias, J.E.; Pagano, E.; Zaeem Cader, M.; Saveljeva, S.; Long, K.; Mukhopadhyay, S.; Arasteh, M.; Lawley, T.D.; Dougan, G.; et al. GPR35 Promotes Glycolysis, Proliferation, and Oncogenic Signaling by Engaging with the Sodium Potassium Pump. *Sci. Signal.* **2019**, *12*, eaau9048. [CrossRef]
80. Li, L.; Feng, R.; Xu, Q.; Zhang, F.; Liu, T.; Cao, J.; Fei, S. Expression of the B3 Subunit of Na+/K+-ATPase Is Increased in Gastric Cancer and Regulates Gastric Cancer Cell Progression and Prognosis via the PI3/AKT Pathway. *Oncotarget* **2017**, *8*, 84285. [CrossRef]
81. Chkadua, G.; Nozadze, E.; Tsakadze, L.; Shioshvili, L.; Leladze, M.; Arutinova, N.; Dzneladze, S.; Javakhishvili, M.; Kupradze, S. Some Kinetic Features of Na,K-ATPase and Sensitivity to Noradrenaline. *Cell Biochem. Biophys.* **2022**, *80*, 23–29. [CrossRef]
82. Mohan, S.; Tiwari, M.N.; Biala, Y.; Yaari, Y. Regulation of Neuronal Na+/K+-ATPase by Specific Protein Kinases and Protein Phosphatases. *J. Neurosci.* **2019**, *39*, 5440. [CrossRef]
83. Comellas, A.P.; Dada, L.A.; Lecuona, E.; Pesce, L.M.; Chandel, N.S.; Quesada, N.; Budinger, G.R.S.; Strous, G.J.; Ciechanover, A.; Sznajder, J.I. Hypoxia-Mediated Degradation of Na,K-ATPase via Mitochondrial Reactive Oxygen Species and the Ubiquitin-Conjugating System. *Circ. Res.* **2006**, *98*, 1314–1322. [CrossRef]
84. Tsai, S.J.; Liu, W.H.; Yin, M.C. Trans Fatty Acids Enhanced Beta-Amyloid Induced Oxidative Stress in Nerve Growth Factor Differentiated PC12 Cells. *Neurochem. Res.* **2012**, *37*, 786–794. [CrossRef]
85. Lakunina, V.A.; Petrushanko, I.Y.; Burnysheva, K.M.; Mitkevich, V.A.; Makarov, A.A. Alzheimer's Disease Aβ42 Peptide Induces an Increase in Na,K-ATPase Glutathionylation. *Dokl. Biochem. Biophys.* **2017**, *473*, 114–117. [CrossRef]
86. Rasmussen, H.H.; Hamilton, E.J.; Liu, C.C.; Figtree, G.A. Reversible Oxidative Modification: Implications for Cardiovascular Physiology and Pathophysiology. *Trends Cardiovasc. Med.* **2010**, *20*, 85–90. [CrossRef] [PubMed]
87. Liu, C.C.; Zhang, Y.; Kim, Y.J.; Hamilton, E.J.; Xu, B.; Limas, J.; McCracken, S.A.; Morris, J.M.; Makris, A.; Hennessy, A.; et al. B3-Adrenergic Agonist Counters Oxidative Stress and Na1 -K1 Pump Inhibitory S-Glutathionylation of Placental Cells: Implications for Preeclampsia. *Am. J. Physiol. Cell Physiol.* **2025**, *328*, C27–C39. [CrossRef] [PubMed]
88. Petrushanko, I.Y.; Yakushev, S.; Mitkevich, V.A.; Kamanina, Y.V.; Ziganshin, R.H.; Meng, X.; Anashkina, A.A.; Makhro, A.; Lopina, O.D.; Gassmann, M.; et al. S-Glutathionylation of the Na,K-ATPase Catalytic α Subunit Is a Determinant of the Enzyme Redox Sensitivity. *J. Biol. Chem.* **2012**, *287*, 32195–32205. [CrossRef] [PubMed]
89. Liu, C.C.; Garcia, A.; Mahmmoud, Y.A.; Hamilton, E.J.; Galougahi, K.K.; Fry, N.A.S.; Figtree, G.A.; Cornelius, F.; Clarke, R.J.; Rasmussen, H.H. Susceptibility of B1 Na^+-K^+ Pump Subunit to Glutathionylation and Oxidative Inhibition Depends on Conformational State of Pump. *J. Biol. Chem.* **2012**, *287*, 12353–12364. [CrossRef]
90. Yan, Y.; Shapiro, A.P.; Haller, S.; Katragadda, V.; Liu, L.; Tian, J.; Basrur, V.; Malhotra, D.; Xie, Z.J.; Abraham, N.G.; et al. Involvement of Reactive Oxygen Species in a Feed-Forward Mechanism of Na/K-ATPase-Mediated Signaling Transduction. *J. Biol. Chem.* **2013**, *288*, 34249–34258. [CrossRef]
91. Figtree, G.A.; Liu, C.C.; Bibert, S.; Hamilton, E.J.; Garcia, A.; White, C.N.; Chia, K.K.M.; Cornelius, F.; Geering, K.; Rasmussen, H.H. Reversible Oxidative Modification: A Key Mechanism of Na^+-K^+ Pump Regulation. *Circ. Res.* **2009**, *105*, 185–193. [CrossRef] [PubMed]
92. Thévenod, F.; Friedmann, J.M. Cadmium-Mediated Oxidative Stress in Kidney Proximal Tubule Cells Induces Degradation of Na+/K(+)-ATPase through Proteasomal and Endo-/Lysosomal Proteolytic Pathways. *FASEB J.* **1999**, *13*, 1751–1761. [CrossRef] [PubMed]

93. Zolotarjova, N.; Ho, C.; Mellgren, R.L.; Askari, A.; Huang, W. hsiung Different Sensitivities of Native and Oxidized Forms of Na+/K(+)-ATPase to Intracellular Proteinases. *Biochim. Biophys. Acta* **1994**, *1192*, 125–131. [CrossRef] [PubMed]
94. Prolo, C.; Piacenza, L.; Radi, R. Peroxynitrite: A Multifaceted Oxidizing and Nitrating Metabolite. *Curr. Opin. Chem. Biol.* **2024**, *80*, 102459. [CrossRef] [PubMed]
95. Reifenberger, M.S.; Arnett, K.L.; Gatto, C.; Milanick, M.A. The Reactive Nitrogen Species Peroxynitrite Is a Potent Inhibitor of Renal Na-K-ATPase Activity. *Am. J. Physiol. Renal Physiol.* **2008**, *295*, F1191–F1198. [CrossRef] [PubMed]
96. Mckee, M.; Scavone, C.; Nathanson, J.A. Nitric Oxide, CGMP, and Hormone Regulation of Active Sodium Transport. *Proc. Natl. Acad. Sci. USA* **1994**, *91*, 12056–12060. [CrossRef] [PubMed]
97. Ellis, D.Z.; Rabe, J.; Sweadner, K.J. Global Loss of Na,K-ATPase and Its Nitric Oxide-Mediated Regulation in a Transgenic Mouse Model of Amyotrophic Lateral Sclerosis. *J. Neurosci.* **2003**, *23*, 43–51. [CrossRef]
98. Ellis, D.Z.; Nathanson, J.A.; Sweadner, K.J. Carbachol Inhibits $Na(^{+})$-$K(^{+})$-ATPase Activity in Choroid Plexus via Stimulation of the NO/CGMP Pathway. *Am. J. Physiol. Cell Physiol.* **2000**, *279*. [CrossRef]
99. Nie, Y.; Bai, F.; Chaudhry, M.A.; Pratt, R.; Shapiro, J.I.; Liu, J. The Na/K-ATPase A1 and c-Src Form Signaling Complex under Native Condition: A Crosslinking Approach. *Sci. Rep.* **2020**, *10*, 6006. [CrossRef]
100. Haas, M.; Wang, H.; Tian, J.; Xie, Z. Src-Mediated Inter-Receptor Cross-Talk between the Na+/K+-ATPase and the Epidermal Growth Factor Receptor Relays the Signal from Ouabain to Mitogen-Activated Protein Kinases. *J. Biol. Chem.* **2002**, *277*, 18694–18702. [CrossRef]
101. Schoner, W.; Scheiner-Bobis, G. Endogenous Cardiac Glycosides: Hormones Using the Sodium Pump as Signal Transducer. *Semin. Nephrol.* **2005**, *25*, 343–351. [CrossRef]
102. Cai, L.; Pessoa, M.T.; Gao, Y.; Strause, S.; Banerjee, M.; Tian, J.; Xie, Z.; Pierre, S.V. The Na/K-ATPase A1/Src Signaling Axis Regulates Mitochondrial Metabolic Function and Redox Signaling in Human IPSC-Derived Cardiomyocytes. *Biomedicines* **2023**, *11*, 3207. [CrossRef] [PubMed]
103. Wang, Y.; Ye, Q.; Liu, C.; Xie, J.X.; Yan, Y.; Lai, F.; Duan, Q.; Li, X.; Tian, J.; Xie, Z. Involvement of Na/K-ATPase in Hydrogen Peroxide-Induced Activation of the Src/ERK Pathway in LLC-PK1 Cells. *Free Radic. Biol. Med.* **2014**, *71*, 415–426. [CrossRef] [PubMed]
104. Bogdanova, A.; Petrushanko, I.; Boldyrev, A.; Gassmann, M. Oxygen- and Redox-Induced Regulation of the Na/K ATPase. *Curr. Enzym. Inhib.* **2006**, *2*, 37–59. [CrossRef]
105. Dobrota, D.; Matejovicova, M.; Kurella, E.G.; Boldyrev, A.A. Na/K-ATPase under Oxidative Stress: Molecular Mechanisms of Injury. *Cell. Mol. Neurobiol.* **1999**, *19*, 141–149. [CrossRef]
106. Kurella, E.G.; Tyulina, O.V.; Boldyrev, A.A. Oxidative Resistance of Na/K-ATPase. *Cell Mol. Neurobiol.* **1999**, *19*, 133–140. [CrossRef]
107. Liu, J.; Nie, Y.; Chaudhry, M.; Bai, F.; Chuang, J.; Sodhi, K.; Shapiro, J.I. The Redox-Sensitive Na/K-ATPase Signaling in Uremic Cardiomyopathy. *Int. J. Mol. Sci.* **2020**, *21*, 1256. [CrossRef]
108. De Melo, A.D.; Freire, V.A.F.; Diogo, Í.L.; Santos, H.d.L.; Barbosa, L.A.; De Carvalho, L.E.D. Antioxidant Therapy Reduces Oxidative Stress, Restores Na,K-ATPase Function and Induces Neuroprotection in Rodent Models of Seizure and Epilepsy: A Systematic Review and Meta-Analysis. *Antioxidants* **2023**, *12*, 1397. [CrossRef]
109. Hill, S.M.; Wrobel, L.; Rubinsztein, D.C. Post-Translational Modifications of Beclin 1 Provide Multiple Strategies for Autophagy Regulation. *Cell Death Differ.* **2018**, *26*, 617–629. [CrossRef]
110. Filomeni, G.; De Zio, D.; Cecconi, F. Oxidative Stress and Autophagy: The Clash between Damage and Metabolic Needs. *Cell Death Differ.* **2014**, *22*, 377–388. [CrossRef]
111. Pialoux, V.; Mounier, R. Hypoxia-Induced Oxidative Stress in Health Disorders. *Oxid. Med. Cell Longev.* **2012**, *2012*, 940121. [CrossRef]
112. Tafani, M.; Sansone, L.; Limana, F.; Arcangeli, T.; De Santis, E.; Polese, M.; Fini, M.; Russo, M.A. The Interplay of Reactive Oxygen Species, Hypoxia, Inflammation, and Sirtuins in Cancer Initiation and Progression. *Oxid. Med. Cell Longev.* **2016**, *2016*, 3907147. [CrossRef] [PubMed]
113. Hielscher, A.; Gerecht, S. Hypoxia and Free Radicals: Role in Tumor Progression and the Use of Engineering-Based Platforms to Address These Relationships. *Free Radic. Biol. Med.* **2015**, *79*, 281–291. [CrossRef] [PubMed]
114. Asgari, R.; Yarani, R.; Mohammadi, P.; Emami Aleagha, M.S. HIF-1α in the Crosstalk Between Reactive Oxygen Species and Autophagy Process: A Review in Multiple Sclerosis. *Cell Mol. Neurobiol.* **2022**, *42*, 2121–2129. [CrossRef] [PubMed]
115. Wang, P.; Long, M.; Zhang, S.; Cheng, Z.; Zhao, X.; He, F.; Liu, H.; Ming, L. Hypoxia Inducible Factor-1α Regulates Autophagy via the P27-E2F1 Signaling Pathway. *Mol. Med. Rep.* **2017**, *16*, 2107–2112. [CrossRef] [PubMed]
116. Zhang, X.; Cheng, X.; Yu, L.; Yang, J.; Calvo, R.; Patnaik, S.; Hu, X.; Gao, Q.; Yang, M.; Lawas, M.; et al. MCOLN1 Is a ROS Sensor in Lysosomes That Regulates Autophagy. *Nat. Commun.* **2016**, *7*, 12109. [CrossRef] [PubMed]

117. Fang, S.; Wan, X.; Zou, X.; Sun, S.; Hao, X.; Liang, C.; Zhang, Z.; Zhang, F.; Sun, B.; Li, H.; et al. Arsenic Trioxide Induces Macrophage Autophagy and Atheroprotection by Regulating ROS-Dependent TFEB Nuclear Translocation and AKT/MTOR Pathway. *Cell Death Dis.* **2021**, *12*, 88. [CrossRef] [PubMed]
118. Settembre, C.; Di Malta, C.; Polito, V.A.; Arencibia, M.G.; Vetrini, F.; Erdin, S.; Erdin, S.U.; Huynh, T.; Medina, D.; Colella, P.; et al. TFEB Links Autophagy to Lysosomal Biogenesis. *Science* **2011**, *332*, 1429–1433. [CrossRef]
119. Klotz, L.O.; Sánchez-Ramos, C.; Prieto-Arroyo, I.; Urbánek, P.; Steinbrenner, H.; Monsalve, M. Redox Regulation of FoxO Transcription Factors. *Redox Biol.* **2015**, *6*, 51–72. [CrossRef]
120. Murtaza, G.; Khan, A.K.; Rashid, R.; Muneer, S.; Hasan, S.M.F.; Chen, J. FOXO Transcriptional Factors and Long-Term Living. *Oxid. Med. Cell Longev.* **2017**, *2017*, 3494289. [CrossRef]
121. Akasaki, Y.; Alvarez-Garcia, O.; Saito, M.; Caramés, B.; Iwamoto, Y.; Lotz, M.K. FoxO Transcription Factors Support Oxidative Stress Resistance in Human Chondrocytes. *Arthritis Rheumatol.* **2014**, *66*, 3349–3358. [CrossRef]
122. Cheng, Z. The FoxO–Autophagy Axis in Health and Disease. *Trends Endocrinol. Metab.* **2019**, *30*, 658–671. [CrossRef]
123. Chi, Y.; Shi, C.; Zhao, Y.; Guo, C. Forkhead Box O (FOXO) 3 Modulates Hypoxia-Induced Autophagy through AMPK Signalling Pathway in Cardiomyocytes. *Biosci. Rep.* **2016**, *36*, 345. [CrossRef]
124. Agostini, F.; Bisaglia, M.; Plotegher, N. Linking ROS Levels to Autophagy: The Key Role of AMPK. *Antioxidants* **2023**, *12*, 1406. [CrossRef]

antioxidants

MDPI

Article

Procyanidin A1 from Peanut Skin Exerts Anti-Aging Effects and Attenuates Senescence via Antioxidative Stress and Autophagy Induction

Yajing Li, Lan Xiang and Jianhua Qi *

College of Pharmaceutical Sciences, Zhejiang University, Yu Hang Tang Road 866, Hangzhou 310058, China; 12019045@zju.edu.cn (Y.L.); lxiang@zju.edu.cn (L.X.)
* Correspondence: qijianhua@zju.edu.cn

Abstract: The aging population is steadily increasing, with aging and age-related diseases serving as major risk factors for morbidity, mortality, and economic burden. Peanuts, known as the "longevity nut" in China, have been shown to offer various health benefits, with peanut skin extract (PSE) emerging as a key compound of interest. This study investigates the bioactive compound in PSE with anti-aging potential and explores its underlying mechanisms of action. Procyanidin A1 (PC A1) was isolated from PSE, guided by the K6001 yeast replicative lifespan model. PC A1 prolonged the replicative lifespan of yeast and the yeast-like chronological lifespan of PC12 cells. To further confirm its anti-aging effect, cellular senescence, a hallmark of aging, was assessed. In senescent cells induced by etoposide (Etop), PC A1 alleviated senescence by reducing ROS levels, decreasing the percentage of senescent cells, and restoring proliferative capacity. Transcriptomics analysis revealed that PC A1 induced apoptosis, reduced senescence-associated secretory phenotype (SASP) factors, and modulated the phosphatidylinositol 3-kinase (PI3K)/protein kinase B (Akt) signaling pathway. The antioxidative capacity of PC A1 was also evaluated, showing enhanced resistance to oxidative stress in PC12 cells by reducing reactive oxygen species (ROS) and malondialdehyde (MDA) levels and increasing superoxide dismutase (SOD) activity. Moreover, PC A1 induced autophagy, as evidenced by an increase in fluorescence-labeled autophagic compartments and confirmation via Western blot analysis of autophagy-related proteins. In addition, the treatment of an autophagy inhibitor abolished the antioxidative stress and senescence-alleviating effects of PC A1. These findings reveal that PC A1 extended lifespans and alleviated cellular senescence by enhancing oxidative stress resistance and inducing autophagy, positioning it as a promising candidate for further exploration as a geroprotective agent.

Keywords: aging; peanut skin; procyanidin A1; cell senescence; antioxidative stress; autophagy; PI3K/Akt signaling pathway

1. Introduction

Aging is a gradual and irreversible biological process characterized by a progressive loss of physiological integrity, which leads to declining function and increased susceptibility to age-related diseases such as cancer, cardiovascular disorders, and neurodegenerative diseases. With a global population that is living longer and becoming older, age-related diseases have emerged as significant contributors to morbidity, mortality, and social and economic burdens [1]. Despite the inevitability of death, the rate of aging can be modulated, thus making healthy aging attainable. Numerous compounds have demonstrated significant anti-aging activity, particularly natural products, which often exhibit superior safety and efficacy [2]. Therefore, the exploration of anti-aging molecules derived from natural products presents great potential for the prevention and treatment of aging and age-related diseases.

During the screening of active compounds with anti-aging potential, aging models play a crucial role in evaluating the efficacy of potential therapeutics and understanding their interactions with biological systems. The yeast *Saccharomyces cerevisiae* has been a prominent model organism for studying pathways relevant to aging. Two different paradigms of aging have been established using yeast: the replicative lifespan (RLS) and chronological lifespan (CLS). The RLS of a yeast cell, which is based on the replicative potential of the cells, is defined as the number of daughter cells produced from a single mother cell before death. This metric may correlate with the aging of mitotically active cells in multicellular organisms [3]. The K6001 strain, a genetically modified strain of yeast derived from W303, is particularly useful for conducting RLS assays, as only the mother cells can reproduce offspring in glucose medium, whereas daughter cells cannot [4]. The second paradigm, CLS, measures the duration of survival for non-dividing yeast cells and may parallel the aging of non-dividing cells in higher organisms [5]. However, the yeast chronological senescence does not perfectly align with cellular senescence in mammals. To address this, a yeast-like CLS assay for mammalian cells has been developed to evaluate chronological senescence [6]. Significantly, the same signal transduction pathways that drive yeast-like chronological senescence also influence aging in other organisms. Inhibitors that attenuate the senescent phenotype are found to decelerate yeast-like chronological senescence, establishing this model as a valuable tool for drug discovery focused on anti-aging effects [6].

Cell senescence is a hallmark of aging [7]. Senescence cells accumulate in aged organisms and contribute to the progression of aging and age-related diseases. Cell senescence is a state characterized by irreversible cell cycle arrest. In addition to cell cycle blockade and proliferation defects, senescent cells also have the following features: increased cell size and flattening, impaired mitochondrial function and membrane integrity, elevated levels of reactive oxygen species (ROS), heightened activity of senescence-associated β-galactosidase (SA-β-gal) at a pH of 6, the development of a senescence-associated secretory phenotype (SASP), and nuclear alterations such as DNA damage. Numerous stressors can induce cellular senescence, including replicative stress, genotoxic agents, oncogene activation, oxidative stress, and metabolic stress [8]. Cell senescence has attracted increasing attention, and it is considered a potential target for preventing or treating age-related diseases and extending healthspan. Senotherapeutic strategies that target senescent cells can be classified into two categories: senolytic treatments, which involve the clearance of senescent cells, and senomorphic treatments, which aim to reduce the effects of SASP [9].

ROS are generally small, short-lived, and highly reactive molecules formed by the incomplete one-electron reduction in oxygen. ROS include superoxide, peroxide, and hydroxyl radicals and singlet oxygen. When tightly controlled, ROS serve as signaling molecules. However, when the redox balance is disrupted, excess ROS can lead to oxidative stress, resulting in damage to lipids, proteins, DNA, and carbohydrates. Antioxidants are substances that play a crucial role in delaying, preventing, or removing oxidative damage to target molecules. A variety of antioxidants are present in biological systems, including enzymes (such as superoxide dismutase (SOD)) and various small molecules. The supplementation of antioxidants has been advocated as a strategy to reduce cellular oxidative stress and potentially extend lifespans in different organisms [10,11].

Autophagy is a cellular process that delivers cytoplasmic substrates, including proteins, DNA, and organelles, to lysosomes for degradation. This process can be broadly divided into several stages: initiation, nucleation, elongation, fusion, degradation, and recycling. Autophagy promotes cellular growth and development, protects cells from metabolic stress and oxidative damage, and plays a crucial role in maintaining cellular homeostasis, as well as the synthesis, degradation, and recycling of cellular products [12,13]. Research has shown that autophagy capacity declines with aging, and the regulation of autophagy is vital for lifespan maintenance [14]. Several pharmacological autophagy inducers, such as rapamycin (Rapa), spermidine, flavonoid 4,4′-dimethoxychalcone, and urolithin A, have been shown to prolong lifespans [15–18].

Arachis hypogaea Linn., commonly known as peanut or groundnut, is a significant oilseed and food crop in many tropical and subtropical regions. It is extensively processed into oil, snacks, and peanut paste. China stands as the largest producer of peanuts, accounting for approximately 38% of global production [19]. In Chinese culture, peanuts are referred to as the "longevity nut". The skin of the peanut, a by-product of the roasting process, has been utilized in Traditional Chinese Medicine (TCM) for centuries to treat various disorders, including hemophilia, hemorrhage, primary and secondary thrombocytopenic purpura, ulcers, inflammation, kidney issues, and hypertension. Recent studies have demonstrated that peanut skin extracts (PSEs) exhibit anti-obesity, anti-atherosclerotic, anti-inflammation, and antioxidant effects in mice. Additionally, PSE contributes to the maintenance of gut microbiota [20–23]. In this study, a compound that is capable of prolonging the yeast RLS was isolated from the skin of *Arachis hypogaea* Linn. This compound was identified as procyanidin A1 (PC A1) through spectral analysis, with comparisons made to published data. The anti-aging effects and underlying mechanisms of PC A1 were further explored, with findings indicating that it alleviates cell senescence, enhances oxidative stress resistance, and induces autophagy.

2. Materials and Methods

2.1. General

Analytical pure reagents (methanol, ethanol, dichloromethane) were acquired from Sinopharm Chemical Reagent Co., Ltd. (Shanghai, China). Chromatographic-grade methanol was obtained from the TEDIA Company, LLC. (Fairfield, OH, USA). Silica gel (200–300 mesh) was purchased from the Yantai Research Institute of Chemical Industry (Yantai, China). Reversed-phase C18 (Octadecylsilyl, ODS) silica gel (Cosmosil 75C18-OPN) was from Nacalai Tesque, Inc. (Kyoto, Japan). Develosil ODS-UG-5 (Nomura Chemical Co., Ltd., Aichi, Japan) and Supersil Phenyl (Dalian Elite Analytical Instruments Co., Ltd., Dalian, China) packed columns were used for the isolation and purification of the natural products. Thin-layer chromatography (TLC) analysis was performed using the TLC silica gel plates (Yantai Jiangyou Silicone Development Co., Ltd., Yantai, China) and TLC silica gel 60 RP-18 F254s 25 glass plates (0.25 mm) (Merck KGaA, Darmstadt, Germany). CD_3OD (Cambridge Isotope Laboratories Inc., Andover, WA, USA) was used as the solvent for ^1H NMR. ^1H NMR spectra and HR ESI-TOF-MS data were obtained using a Bruker AV III-500 spectrometer (Bruker Corporation, Karlsruhe, Germany) and Agilent 6224A LC/MS (Agilent Technologies Inc., Beijing, China), respectively.

The following reagents and compounds were purchased from the indicated manufacturer and used in biological experiments: dimethyl sulfoxide (DMSO) from Merck KGaA (Darmstadt, Germany). Resveratrol (Res), rapamycin (Rapa), etoposide (Etop), and chloroquine (CQ) were obtained from Shanghai Yuanye Bio-Technology Co., Ltd. (Shanghai, China). SBI-0206965 was from MedChemExpress LLC. (Shanghai, China).

2.2. Isolation and Structure Identification of PC A1

The PSE was prepared according to the previous literature [20]. Under the guidance of K6001 yeast replicative lifespan assay, 1 g of PSE was subjected to ODS open-column chromatography with a methanol/water solvent system (10/90, 30/70, 50/50, 70/30, 100/0). Fractions were combined into 11 fractions according to TLC analysis, and the active fraction (348.1 mg) was obtained from a 30% aqueous methanol elution. Then, 100 mg of this fraction was taken out and subjected to silica open-column chromatography with a dichloromethane/methanol elution system (100/0, 90/10, 70/30, 50/50, 30/70, 10/90, 0/100). Then, 7 samples were obtained. Sample 1 (15.4 mg), obtained from dichloromethane/methanol (90/10), was purified first through HPLC (Develosil ODS-UG-5 ($\phi \cdot 10 \times 250$ mm), methanol: water = 18:100, 100 min, 3 mL/min, 280 nm) to obtain sample 2 (5 mg, $t_R = 75$ min). Sample 2 was then purified again by another HPLC (Supersil Phenyl ($\phi \cdot 10 \times 200$ mm), methanol: water = 20:100, 20 min, 3 mL/min, 280 nm) to obtain PC A1 (3 mg, $t_R = 16$ min) as colorless needles. The isolation scheme of PC A1 from PSE is shown in Supplementary Figure S1. The chemical structure of PC A1 was identified by comparing the ^{1}H NMR spectra and MS with the literature [24]: ^{1}H NMR (500 MHz, CD_3OD): δ_H = 7.13 (1H, d, J = 2.1 Hz), 7.01 (1H, dd, J = 8.3, 2.1 Hz), 6.91 (1H, s), 6.81 (3H, m), 6.08 (1H, s), 6.06 (1H, d, J = 2.3 Hz), 5.95 (1H, d, J = 2.3 Hz), 4.73 (1H, d, J = 7.8 Hz), 4.23 (1H, d, J = 3.5 Hz), 4.15 (1H, m), 4.07 (1H, d, J = 3.5 Hz), 2.94 (1H, dd, J = 16.5, 5.6 Hz), and 2.57 (1H, dd, J = 16.4, 8.3 Hz). The ^{1} H NMR spectrum of PC A1 is shown in Supplementary Figure S2. High-resolution ESI-TOF-MS *m/z* 577.1344 was calculated for $C_{30}H_{25}O_{12}$ $[M+H]^+$ 577.1341. The high-resolution ESI-MS chromatograms of PC A1 is shown in Supplementary Figure S3.

2.3. Cell Lines

The PC12 cell line was purchased from the Cell Bank of the Chinese Academy of Sciences (Shanghai, China) and cultured in Dulbecco's Modified Eagle Medium (DMEM, Cellmax Cell Technology (Beijing) Co., Ltd. (Beijing, China)) supplemented with 10% horse serum (Gibco (Herndon, VA, USA)), 7.5% fetal bovine serum (Cellmax Cell Technology (Beijing) Co., Ltd. (Beijing, China)), and 1% antibiotic–antimycotic solution (Beijing Solarbio Science & Technology Co., Ltd. (Beijing, China)). The NIH/3T3 cell line was generously given from MeilunBio (Dalian, China) and cultured in DMEM containing 10% fetal bovine serum and 1% antibiotic–antimycotic solution. All cells were cultured at 37 °C in a humidified incubator of 5% CO_2. Etoposide-induced senescence (ETIS) was triggered in NIH/3T3 and PC12 cells after culturing for 2 d in the presence of different concentrations of Etop (0.3 and 7.5 μM, respectively). Oxidative stress was triggered in PC12 cells after culturing for 2 h in the presence of 0.7 mM H_2O_2. All cell lines tested negative for microbial contamination and were routinely authenticated with STR assays.

2.4. Yeast Replicative Lifespan Assay

K6001 yeast was cultured in galactose liquid medium, which comprised 3% galactose, 2% hipolypeptone, and 1% yeast extract. Following incubation for 24 h with continuous shaking (180 rpm, 28 °C), a total of 4000 cells were washed and then evenly distributed on yeast peptone dextrose (YPD) agar plates, which were formulated with 2% glucose, 2% hipolypeptone, 1% yeast extract, and 2% agar and supplemented with Res or varying concentrations of PC A1. After incubation for 48 h at 28 °C, forty microcolonies from the agar plate were randomly selected for observation under an optical microscope (Olympus, Tokyo, Japan), and the number of daughter cells produced by one mother cell was counted.

2.5. Yeast-like Chronological Lifespan Assay

The yeast-like chronological lifespan (CLS) assay was performed according to the reference [6]. The principle of this assay is based on the observation that, over time, a densely overgrown cell culture loses its ability to survive and re-enter the growth phase when transferred to a fresh nutrient-rich medium. This loss of viability occurs in a density-dependent and time-dependent (chronological) manner, reflecting the aging process of the cells. In detail, PC12 cells were seeded at a high density of 8×10^4 cells per well in 96-well plates, with each well containing 0.2 mL of culture medium. After 24 h, the culture medium was replaced with serum-free medium supplemented with either 0.5% DMSO (vehicle control), 200 nM of rapamycin (Rapa, positive control), or procyanidin A1 (PC A1) at concentrations of 1, 3, and 10 μM. After 4 days, the medium, including any floating cells, was carefully aspirated. The adherent cells were then trypsinized using 0.2 mL of trypsin solution. Subsequently, an equivalent volume of the cell culture (4 μL of aliquot), representing approximately 2% of the total adherent (viable) cells, was transferred into 6-well plates containing 4 mL of fresh medium per well. The cells were cultured for an additional 15 days for colony formation. To assess cellular viability, the resulting colonies were fixed with 4% paraformaldehyde for 15 min and subsequently stained with a 0.1% (*w*/*v*) crystal violet solution for 20 min. Following staining, the cells were thoroughly rinsed with water and allowed to air dry. The number of viable colonies, which serves as a quantitative indicator of chronological lifespan, was enumerated and subsequently analyzed for statistical significance.

2.6. Cell Viability Assay

An MTT assay was performed to measure the cell viability. In general, 5000 cells were seeded into each well of a 96-well plate and cultured under the indicated treatment. Then, 100 μL of serum-free DMEM containing 500 μg/mL of MTT (Richu BioScience Co., Ltd. (Shanghai, China)) was added and incubated for 4 h followed by the removal of the medium carefully and an addition of 100 μL of DMSO. The plates were read with the absorbance at 570 nm using a plate reader (BioTek Synergy H1, Agilent, Winooski, VT, USA).

2.7. Senescence-Associated β-Galactosidase (SA-β-gal) Assay

SA-β-gal staining was performed using the senescence β-galactosidase staining kit (Beyotime Biotechnology Inc., Shanghai, China), adhering strictly to the manufacturer's protocols. For the assessment of SA-β-gal activity, approximately 50,000 PC12 cells or 20,000 NIH/3T3 cells were seeded into each well of a 24-well plate. Then, cells were exposed to various test samples; 0.5% dimethyl sulfoxide (DMSO) was employed as the negative control, while Rapa served as the positive control. After 24 h, cells were treated with Etop for 2 days. After the treatment, cells were gently washed, fixed, and stained with the provided dyeing solution as directed. Cells were examined under a bright-field microscope (BX63, Olympus, Japan, 20× objective). SA-β-gal$^+$ percentages were quantified by counting the number of SA-β-gal-positive cells per visual field.

2.8. Cell Proliferation Assay

The 5-Ethynyl-2′-deoxyuridine (EdU) incorporation assay was conducted to evaluate cellular proliferation. For this purpose, the BeyoClick™ EdU Cell Proliferation Kit with Alexa Fluor 488, supplied by Beyotime Biotechnology Inc. in Shanghai, China, was utilized, and the assay was carried out in accordance with the manufacturer's guidelines. Following treatment, the cells were incubated with EdU at a concentration of 10 μM for 2 h and subsequently fixed and permeabilized, then cells were treated with the click reaction additive solution for 30 min. Following this step, the cells were counterstained with Hoechst 33342 for 10 min. After a thorough washing process, the EdU-positive cells were visualized using a fluorescence microscope (BX63, Olympus, Japan) equipped with a 20× objective lens. The proliferating cells were then quantified based on the fluorescence signals observed.

2.9. RNA Extract, RNA-Seq, and Data Analysis

NIH/3T3 cells (4×10^5 cells) at passage 5 were seeded into each 10 cm dish. The next day, the cells were treated with or without 10 μM of PC A1 for 2 days before exposure to 0.3 μM of Etop for 2 days. The control group was treated with the same medium containing an equal amount of DMSO. Total RNA was extracted using the TRIzon reagent (Jiangsu Cowin Biotech Co., Ltd. (Taizhou, China)).

The processes of quality control, cDNA library construction, and sequencing were expertly handled by ShenZhen BGI Genomics Co., Ltd. (Shenzhen, China). Three biological replicates were used for each group. Quality control of the RNA samples was conducted using a Fragment Analyzer, while sequencing was performed on the DNBSEQ platform. The raw data obtained from sequencing were filtered using SOAPnuke to obtain clean data. The clean reads were then aligned to the reference genome using HISAT and to the gene set using Bowtie2. The reference species used for this study was *Mus musculus*, and the specific reference genome version is GCF_000001635.27_GRCm39, sourced from the NCBI database. Differential gene expression analysis was conducted using the DESeq2 method, identifying genes with a Q value (adjusted p value) ≤ 0.05 and a $\log_2$(Fold Change (FC)) ≥ 0.5 or ≤ -0.5 as differentially expressed genes (DEGs). For comprehensive data analysis and visualization, including the Kyoto Encyclopedia of Genes and Genomes (KEGG) pathway enrichment analysis and the Gene Ontology (GO) biological process enrichment analysis, the online bioinformatic platform tool Dr. Tom provided by BGI (https://biosys.bgi.com (accessed on 18 November 2024)) was utilized. Additionally, volcano plots and heatmaps were carried out using another online platform, CNSKnowall (https://cnsknowall.com (accessed on 20 February 2025)).

2.10. ROS Assay

A ROS assay was performed using a ROS Assay Kit (Beyotime Biotechnology Inc., Shanghai, China), following the manufacturer's instructions. Generally, 50,000 cells were seeded into each well of a 24-well plate. Then, cells were treated with PC A1 (1, 3, 10, and 30 μM) for 18 h, and then with H_2O_2 for 2 h or Etop for 2 days. Then, DCFH-DA, at a final concentration of 10 μM, was added and incubated with cells for 30 min. After washing with phosphate-buffered saline (PBS), fluorescence was observed using a fluorescence microscope (IX53, Olympus, Japan, 20× objective).

2.11. MDA Quantifications and SOD Assay

Approximately 10^6 of the PC12 cells were seeded in a 60 mm culture dish. Then, cells were treated with Res (10 μM) or PC A1 (1, 3, 10, and 30 μM) for 18 h, and then with 0.7 mM H_2O_2 for another 2 h. The MDA quantification and SOD assay were determined using the MDA assay kit and SOD assay kit (Nanjing Jiancheng Bioengineering Institute, Nanjing, China) in accordance with the manufacturer's instructions, respectively.

2.12. Autophagy Detection

At first, approximately 80,000 PC12 cells were seeded in each well of a 24-well plate. After 24 h, cells were treated with CQ (10 μM, as a negative control), Rapa (500 nM) plus CQ (as a positive control), and PC A1 (at doses of 0, 3, 10, and 30 μM) plus CQ. After 18 h, the cells were stained with the CYTO-ID® Autophagy Detection Kit (Enzo Life Sciences,

Inc., New York, NY, USA), according to the manufacturer's instructions. Briefly, the culture medium was removed, and the cells were rinsed twice with an assay buffer supplemented with 5% fetal bovine serum. Subsequently, 250 μL of assay buffer, containing 0.2% green detection reagent and 0.1% Hoechst 33342 nuclear stain, was added to each well. Following a 30 min incubation, the cells were fixed, washed with the assay buffer, and then examined under a confocal microscope (BX61, Olympus, Japan) with a 20× objective lens.

2.13. Western Blot Analysis

Whole-cell lysates were prepared using the RIPA lysis buffer containing a 1% complete protease inhibitor cocktail (Jiangsu Cowin Biotech Co., Ltd. (Taizhou, China)), 1% phosphatase inhibitor cocktail II, and 1% phosphatase inhibitor cocktail III (Abcam Limited. (Cambridge, UK)) and homogenized and centrifuged at 12,000× g for 20 min at 4 °C. The protein concentration of cell lysates was determined by the BCA protein assay kit. Cell lysates were added with thr SDS-PAGE sample loading buffer and heated for 10 min at 100 °C. Then, 20 μg of protein of each sample was separated by electrophoresis on sodium dodecyl sulfate (SDS) polyacrylamide gels and transferred to an Immun-Blot PVDF membrane (Bio-Rad Laboratories Inc., Hercules, CA, USA). Membranes were incubated with primary and then secondary antibodies. Primary antibodies against phosphoinositide 3-kinase (PI3K) (#4249, 1:1000), phospho-PI3K (#4228, 1:1000), mammalian target of rapamycin (mTOR, #2983, 1:1000), phospho-mTOR (#5536, 1:1000), unc-51 like autophagy activating kinase 1 (ULK1, #8054, 1:1000), phospho-ULK1 (Ser757, #14202, 1:1000), p62 (#5114, 1:1000), microtubule-associated protein 1 light chain 3 (LC3B, #2775, 1:1000), protein kinase B (Akt, #9272, 1:1000), and phospho-Akt (#9271, 1:1000) were procured from Cell Signaling Technology, Inc. (Boston, MA, USA). Beclin-1 (#HA721216, 1:1000) was purchased from Hangzhou HuaAn Biotechnology Co., Ltd. (Hangzhou, China). p21 (#AP021, 1:200) was from Beyotime Biotechnology Co., Ltd. (Shanghai, China). β-Actin (#CW0096, 1:1000) was from Jiangsu Cowin Biotech Co., Ltd. (Taizhou, China). HRP-conjugated goat anti-rabbit IgG (#CW0103S, 1:5000) and anti-mouse IgG (#CW0102S, 1:5000) were from Jiangsu Cowin Biotech Co., Ltd. (Taizhou, China). Finally, antigens were visualized using the SuperPico ECL Chemiluminescence Kit (Nanjing Vazyme Biotech Co., Ltd., Nanjing, China). The Bio-Rad ChemiDoc™ MP Imaging System (Bio-Rad Laboratories, Inc., Hercules, CA, USA) was used for the detection of proteins of interest, and the blot density was quantified utilizing Image Lab software (Version 6.1, Bio-Rad Laboratories, Inc., Hercules, CA, USA).

2.14. Statistical Analysis

Statistical analyses were performed using the GraphPad Prism software (Version 9.0, GraphPad Software, LLC, San Diego, CA, USA). To assess differences among multiple groups, ordinary one-way ANOVA was conducted, followed by Dunnett's multiple comparisons test for post hoc analysis. For pairwise comparisons between the treatment group and the control group in the replicative lifespan assay, two-tailed, unpaired Student's t-tests were employed. Statistical significance was defined as $p < 0.05$. Each experiment was repeated three times, and data for each experiment are shown as mean ± SEM.

3. Results

3.1. PC A1 Extended the Replicative Lifespan of K6001 Yeast and Yeast-like Chronological Lifespan of PC12 Cells

Due to its convenience and speed, the K6001 yeast RLS assay was utilized as a guide to isolate compounds with potential anti-aging activity. In this study, PC A1 was isolated and purified from PSE under the guidance of the yeast RLS system. The isolation scheme and the chemistry structure of PC A1 are presented in Supplementary Figure S1 and Figure 1a, respectively. In the yeast RLS assay, Res was employed as a positive control for its stimulating effects on SIRTI and its ability to prolong the lifespan in yeast [25]. The results in Figure 1b demonstrate that PC A1 (0.1, 0.3, 1, 3, and 10 μM) and Res significantly slowed the replicative aging of yeast. However, PC A1 at 30 μM exhibited toxicity to the yeast. Furthermore, yeast-like CLS assays were conducted on PC12 cells to evaluate the lifespan-extending effect of PC A1 at the mammalian cell level. The results in Figure 1c,d indicate that PC A1 (1 and 3 μM) and Rapa (as a positive control) increased the number of colonies, demonstrating that PC A1 could prevent the senescence-mediated decline of clonogenic survival in highly confluent PC12 cells [6]. Collectively, these findings suggest that PC A1 prolongs both yeast RLS and yeast-like CLS in mammalian cells.

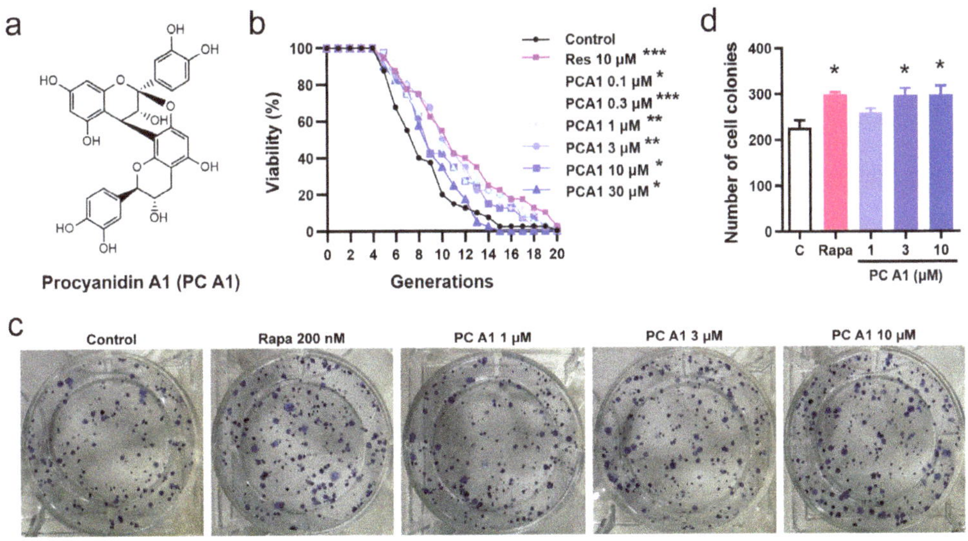

Figure 1. Procyanidin A1 (PC A1) isolated and purified from peanut skin extended the replicative lifespan of K6001 yeast and the yeast-like chronological lifespan of PC12 cells. (**a**) The chemical structure of PC A1. (**b**) The effect of PC A1 on the replicative lifespan of K6001 yeast. Resveratrol (Res) at 10 μM was used as the positive control. The experiment was conducted three independent times, with each replicate involving 40 individual mother cells per treatment group. The replicative lifespan was determined by counting the number of daughter cells produced by each mother cell. To assess the significance of the results, a two-sided Student's t-test was used to compare the number of daughter cells in each treatment group to the control group. (**c**,**d**) The colony formation of PC12 cells treated with PC A1 (1, 3, and 10 μM) and rapamycin (Rapa, 200 nM) for testing the yeast-like chronological lifespan of PC12 cells. The representative images of colony-forming units (CFUs) (**c**) and quantification (**d**) are shown. Rapamycin (Rapa) was used as the positive control. Experiments were repeated three times. Data represent mean ± SEM. Significant difference was obtained with ordinary one-way ANOVA followed by Dunnett's multiple comparisons test. *, **, and *** indicate significant differences at $p < 0.05$, $p < 0.01$, and $p < 0.001$ compared with the control (C) group, respectively.

3.2. PC A1 Alleviated Cellular Senescence Induced by Etoposide

3.2.1. PC A1 Alleviated Cellular Senescence Induced by Etoposide in PC12 Cells

The evaluation of cellular senescence as a hallmark of aging was conducted. Cellular senescence is characterized by elevated levels of ROS, an increased expression of SA-β-gal, and arrested cell proliferation. Etoposide (Etop), a chemotherapy agent, inhibits topoisomerase II, destroys the rejoining of DNA after superhelical unwinding, induces DNA damage, and subsequently leads to cell cycle arrest and senescence. Therefore, Etop was employed to model the pathological conditions associated with cellular senescence. The PC12 cell line, derived from a pheochromocytoma of the rat adrenal medulla, is widely utilized in neuroscience research, including studies on neuroprotection, neurosecretion, neuroinflammation, and synaptogenesis [26]. Recent studies also demonstrated that PC12 cells are valuable in simulating the cellular changes associated with nervous system aging [27]. Initially, the viability of PC12 cells following treatment with PC A1 was assessed. The results indicated that PC A1 (at concentrations of 1, 3, 10, and 30 μM) did not exhibit any significant cytotoxic effects on normal PC12 cells, whereas the treatment of PC A1 at 100 μM resulted in a 50% reduction in cellular viability (Figure 2a). Subsequently, PC12 cells were pre-treated with PC A1 (at 1, 3, 10, and 30 μM) for one day and then exposed to Etop (7.5 μM) for 2 days to evaluate the protective effect of PC A1 against cell senescence. Rapa at 500 nM was used as a positive control due to its known geroprotective effects [15]. Cell viability was assessed using the MTT assay, and the results demonstrated that PC A1 (at 1, 3, and 10 μM) and Rapa (500 nM) significantly mitigated the loss of cellular viability caused by Etop (Figure 2b). Furthermore, the level of ROS was found to be elevated by Etop; however, treatment with PC A1 (1, 3, 10, and 30 μM) and Rapa (500 nM) significantly reduced ROS levels (Figure 2c,d). Subsequently, SA-β-gal staining was performed, as shown in Figure 2e,f, and quantitative analysis revealed that over 70% of Etop-treated cells exhibited a senescent phenotype characterized by SA-β-gal-positive cells. In contrast, the pre-treatment of PC A1 (at 1, 3, 10, and 30 μM) significantly decreased the number of SA-β-gal-positive PC12 cells. Cell cycle arrest, another hallmark of cell senescence, was assessed using the EdU cell proliferation kit. EdU, a thymidine analog, was incorporated into DNA during synthesis, followed by a click reaction with a green fluorescence-labeled azide probe, thereby labeling newly synthesized DNA for the detection of proliferating cells. To visualize all cells, nuclei were stained with Hoechst 33342. As shown in Figure 2g,h, nearly 25% of the PC12 cells in the control group were EdU positive, exhibiting green fluorescence, whereas this percentage dropped to 4% in Etop-induced senescent cells. The pre-treatment of PC A1 (1, 3, and 10 μM) and Rapa (500 nM) protected against the proliferative impairment caused by Etop. These experimental findings suggest that PC A1 effectively prevented cellular viability loss, reduced ROS levels, decreased the number of SA-β-gal-positive senescent cells, and restored proliferative capacity, thereby alleviating Etop-induced senescence in PC12 cells.

3.2.2. PC A1 Alleviated Cell Senescence Induced by Etoposide in NIH/3T3 Cells

To further confirm the cell senescence alleviation effect of PC A1, we then induced cell senescence using Etop in the NIH/3T3 cell line. The NIH/3T3 mouse embryonic fibroblast cell line serves as a vital model for in vitro research, particularly in the fields of cellular senescence and cell cycle studies. Considering that NIH/3T3 cells exhibit greater sensitivity to Rapa and Etop, the concentration of Rapa was adjusted to 50 nM to serve as a positive control, whereas the dose of Etop was reduced to 0.3 μM. The effect of PC A1 on cellular viability was also assessed. As shown in Figure 3a, PC A1 (at 1, 3, 10, and 30 μM) demonstrated no toxicity to NIH/3T3 cells. Following this, NIH/3T3 cells were pre-treated with PC A1, subsequently inducing cell senescence with Etop for 2 days, and then we evaluated cellular viability, the expression of p21, ROS levels, and SA-β-gal activity. The results in Figure 3b show that the pre-treatment of PC A1 (1, 3, 10, and 30 μM) and Rapa (50 nM) significantly protected NIH/3T3 cells from the loss of viability. The expression levels of p21, a biomarker of cellular senescence, were then assessed. As shown in Figure 3c, PC A1 at 30 μM and Rapa reduced p21 levels elevated by Etop. The results of ROS assays (Figure 3d,e) and SA-β-gal staining (Figure 3f,g) were consistent with those obtained from the PC12 cells, demonstrating that both PC A1 and Rapa significantly decreased ROS levels and the number of senescent cells, as indicated by SA-β-gal-positive cells. In conclusion, PC A1 alleviated cellular senescence induced by Etop in both PC12 and NIH/3T3 cells.

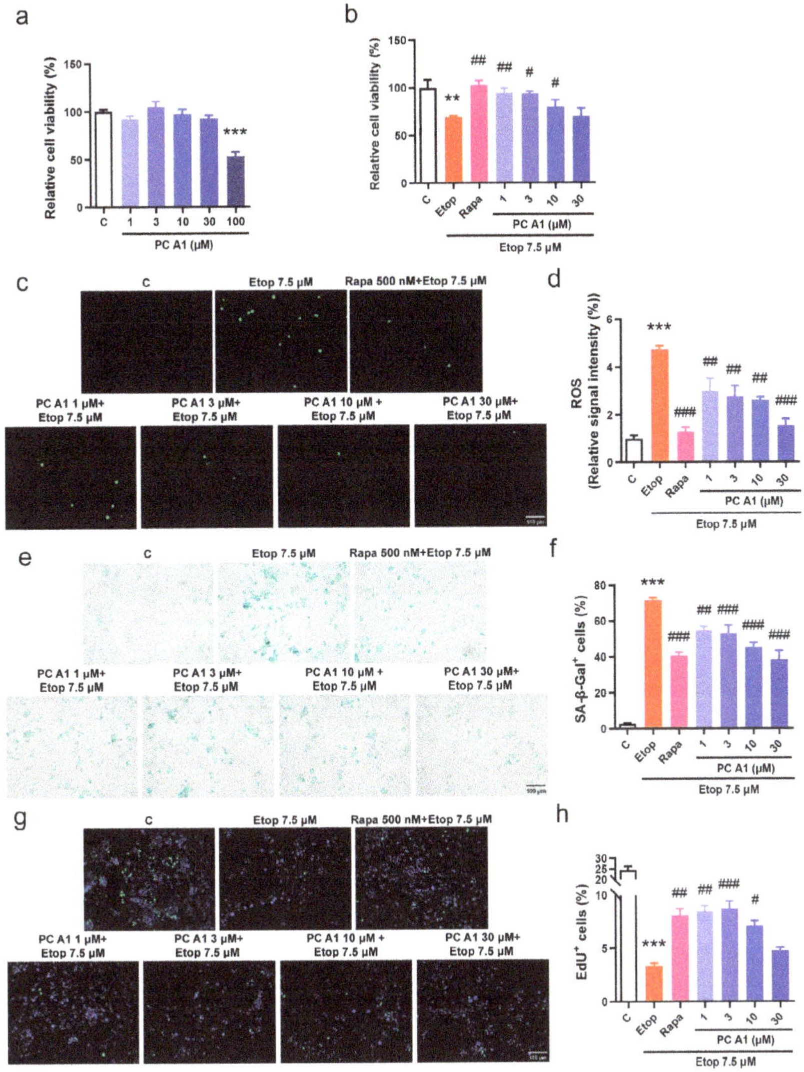

Figure 2. Procyanidin A1 (PC A1) alleviated Etop-induced senescence in PC12 cells. (**a**) The cell viability of PC12 cells after treatment with PC A1 (1, 3, 10, 30, and 100 μM) for 24 h. (**b**–**h**) PC12 cells were pre-treated with PC A1 (1, 3, 10, and 30 μM) for 24 h followed by 7.5 μM of etoposide (Etop) for 48 h. The cellular viability was determined (**b**), and ROS level (**c**,**d**), senescence-associated β-galactosidase (SA-β-gal) staining (**e**,**f**), and cell proliferation (**g**,**h**) are pictured and quantified. Proliferating cells were labeled with green fluorescence, and nuclei were stained with Hoechst 33342. Scale bar: 100 μm. Data represent mean ± SEM, $n = 3$ for each group. ** and *** indicate significant differences at $p < 0.01$ and $p < 0.001$ compared with the control (C) group, respectively; #, ##, and ### indicate significant differences at $p < 0.05$, $p < 0.01$, and $p < 0.001$ compared with the etoposide (Etop) group, respectively.

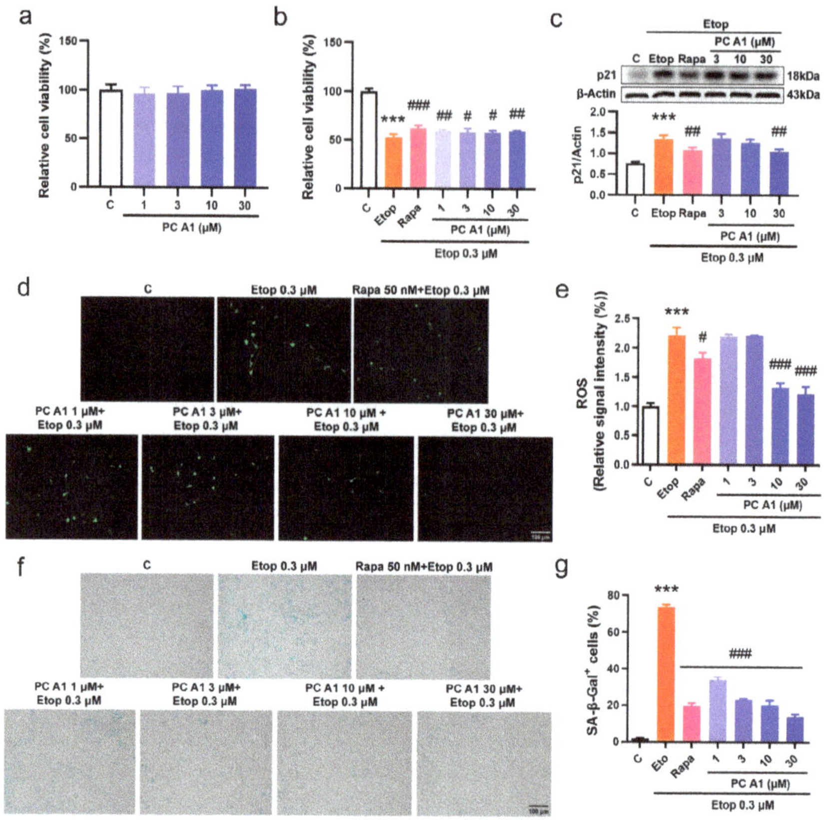

Figure 3. Procyanidin A1 (PC A1) alleviated Etop-induced senescence in NIH/3T3 cells. (**a**) The cell viability of NIH/3T3 cells after treatment with PC A1 (1, 3, 10, and 30 μM) for 24 h. (**b**–**g**) NIH/3T3 cells were pre-treated with PC A1 (1, 3, 10, and 30 μM) for 24 h followed by 0.3 μM of etoposide (Etop) for 48 h. The cellular viability was determined (**b**), the expression levels of p21 were evaluated (**c**), and ROS levels (**d**,**e**) and senescence-associated β-galactosidase (SA-β-gal) staining (**f**,**g**) were pictured and quantified. Scale bar: 100 μm. The experimental samples and controls used for the comparative analysis in (**c**) were run on the same blot/gel. Data represent mean ±SEM, n = 3. *** indicates significant differences at $p < 0.001$ compared with the control (C) group; #, ##, and ### indicate significant differences at $p < 0.05$, $p < 0.01$, and $p < 0.001$, compared with the etoposide (Etop) group, respectively.

3.2.3. The PI3K/Akt Signaling Pathway Played a Role in the Alleviation Effect of PC A1 on Cell Senescence

To further understand how PC A1 mitigates cell senescence, gene expression profiling of NIH/3T3 cells was performed through RNA sequencing. As shown in Figure 4a–c, a total of 5724 differentially expressed genes (DEGs) ($\log_2$FoldChange (FC) ≥ 0.5 or ≤ -0.5, Q value ≤ 0.05) were identified between the Etop-treated group and control group, with 3175 genes upregulated and 2549 genes downregulated in Etop-treated cells compared to the control group. Additionally, 181 DEGs were found between the Etop + PC A1 group and the Etop-only group, with 113 genes upregulated and 68 downregulated in the PC A1 pre-treatment group compared to the Etop group.

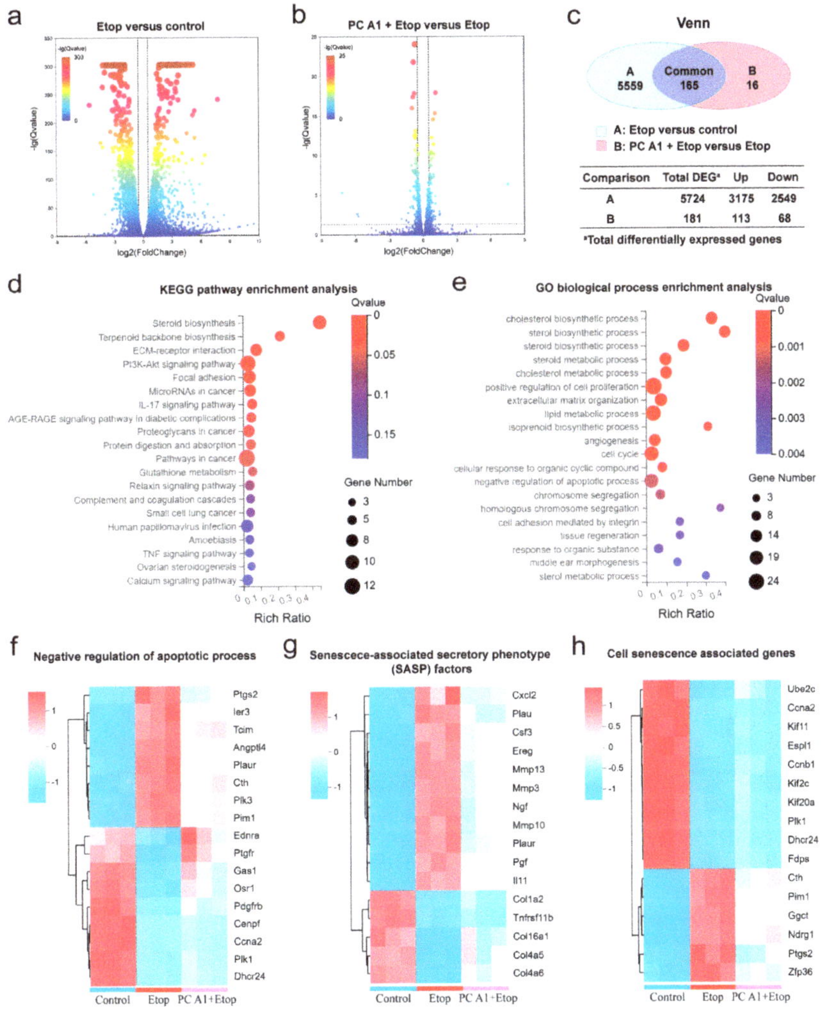

Figure 4. RNA sequencing analysis on senescent NIH/3T3 cells treated with procyanidin A1 (PC A1). NIH/3T3 cells were pre-treated with PC A1 (10 µM) for 24 h followed by 0.3 µM of etoposide (Etop) for 48 h. RNA was extracted from cells lysis for RNA sequencing analysis. (**a**) Volcano plot of gene expression in the Etop group compared to the control group. (**b**) Volcano plot of gene expression in the PC A1 + Etop group compared to the Etop group. In the volcano plot, the two vertical dashed lines indicate log2(FoldChange) values of −0.5 and 0.5, while the horizontal dashed line represents a Q-value threshold of 0.05. Genes with log2(FoldChange) ≥ 0.5 or ≤−0.5 and a Q value ≤ 0.05 were identified as differentially expressed. (**c**) Venn diagram showing the number of differentially expressed genes (DEGs, with $\log_2$FoldChange (FC) ≥ 0.5 or ≤−0.5, Q value ≤ 0.05, calculated by raw count value) and overlapped genes between A and B (A. Etop group versus control group; B. PC A1 + Etop group versus Etop group). (**d**) KEGG pathway enrichment analysis of the overlapped 165 common differentially expressed genes. (**e**) GO biological processes associated with the 165 common differentially expressed genes. (**f**) Heatmaps of genes associated with negative regulation of the apoptosis process. (**g**) Heatmaps of genes associated with senescence associated secretory phenotype (SASP) factors in different groups. (**h**) Heatmaps of cell senescence-related genes according to the CellAge database. *n* = 3 for each group. *n* stands for the number of samples in a group.

The 165 genes that were differentially expressed in both comparisons were analyzed using the KEGG pathways and GO enrichment analysis. As shown in Figure 4d, the KEGG pathway analysis identified several significantly enriched pathways associated with the effects of PC A1 treatment on Etop-induced senescence. Among these pathways, the PI3K/Akt signaling pathway, focal adhesion, ECM–receptor interaction, and pathways in cancer were prominently represented. Notably, the PI3K/Akt signaling pathway exhibited the highest number of enriched genes and a low Q value. Therefore, we propose that the PI3K/Akt signaling pathway plays a crucial role in the anti-aging effect of PC A1.

The DEGs were annotated using the GO terms from the GO database to enhance our understanding of their molecular characteristics. As shown in Figure 4e, the DEGs were annotated using the GO terms from the GO database to further discover their molecular characterization. The DEGs were categorized into three main areas: biological processes, molecular functions, and cellular components. Within the biological process category, the DEGs were implicated in the positive regulation of cell proliferation, the cell cycle, and the negative regulation of the apoptotic process. We further analyzed the transcriptomic expression profile. As shown in Figure 4f, 17 genes were associated with the negative regulation of the apoptotic process. We observed that the expression of eight genes associated with apoptosis resistance increased with Etop treatment but was reduced upon treatment with PC A1. These genes included *Ptgs2, Ier3, Tcim, Angpt14, Plaur, Cth, Plk3,* and *Pim*. Additionally, we noted a significant upregulation of several SASP factors (including *Cxcl2, Plau, Csf3, Ereg, Mmp3, Mmp10, Mmp13, Ngf, Plaur, Pgf,* and *Il11*) during cellular senescence, which were substantially downregulated by PC A1. Four genes (*Col16a1, Col1a2, Col4a5,* and *Col4a6*), encoding members of the collagen family, along with *Tnfrsf11b,* were found to be downregulated in senescent cells but substantially upregulated by treatment with PC A1 (Figure 4g). Furthermore, a search of gene expression databases, specifically CellAge [28], revealed 16 genes associated with cell senescence that were regulated by Etop but alleviated by PC A1 treatment (Figure 4h). Overall, these findings confirm that PC A1 ameliorates cell senescence induced by Etop by promoting apoptosis in senescent cells, regulating the gene transcription levels of SASP factors and restoring proliferative capacity. Moreover, the PI3K/Akt signaling pathway appears to play a role in the protective effect of PC A1 against cellular senescence.

3.3. *PC A1 Remedied Oxidative Stress in H_2O_2-Exposed PC12 Cells*

In organisms, the aging process is associated with progressive mitochondrial dysfunction, leading to an increased production of ROS. The pathological level of ROS contributes to further mitochondrial deterioration and widespread cellular damage, including harm to DNA, proteins, and lipids, which are significant factors in aging and age-related diseases [29,30]. Therefore, we investigated the ability of PC A1 to reduce ROS and protect PC12 cells from oxidative stress. H_2O_2, the most commonly used endogenous source of cellular oxidative stress, was employed to induce this condition. Initially, the appropriate concentration of H_2O_2 was pre-tested. After incubating cells with varying doses of H_2O_2 for 2 h, cell viability was assessed using the MTT assay. As shown in Figure 5a, H_2O_2 at 0.7 mM resulted in a 50% reduction in cell viability compared to the control and was chosen as an appropriate concentration for further experiments. Cells were subsequently treated with different doses of PC A1 for 24 h, followed by exposure to 0.7 mM H_2O_2 for 2 h. The findings in Figure 5b indicate that the reduction in cell viability caused by H_2O_2 was alleviated by the pre-treatment with PC A1 (1, 3, and 10 μM). Res was utilized as a positive control due to its well-established antioxidant properties [31]. The level of MDA, a common indicator in oxidative stress studies, was also assessed. As shown in Figure 5c, pre-treatment with Res (10 μM) and PC A1 (1, 3, 10, and 30 μM) significantly lowered the elevated MDA levels induced by H_2O_2. Furthermore, ROS levels were evaluated using DCFH-DA, a probe that undergoes hydrolysis and oxidation to produce fluorescent DCF. As shown in Figure 5d,e, H_2O_2 produced a marked increase in ROS levels, which were significantly reduced by pre-treatment with Res and PC A1 (at 1, 3, 10, and 30 μM). SOD is a crucial endogenous antioxidant enzyme that scavenges superoxide anion free radicals and protects cells from oxidative damage. The activities of total SOD, SOD1, and SOD2 were measured. The results in Figure 5f–h demonstrate the PC A1 enhanced SOD2 activity but did not affect SOD1 activity. In conclusion, PC A1 protects PC12 cells from oxidative damage induced by H_2O_2 by increasing SOD2 activity and reducing both ROS and MDA levels.

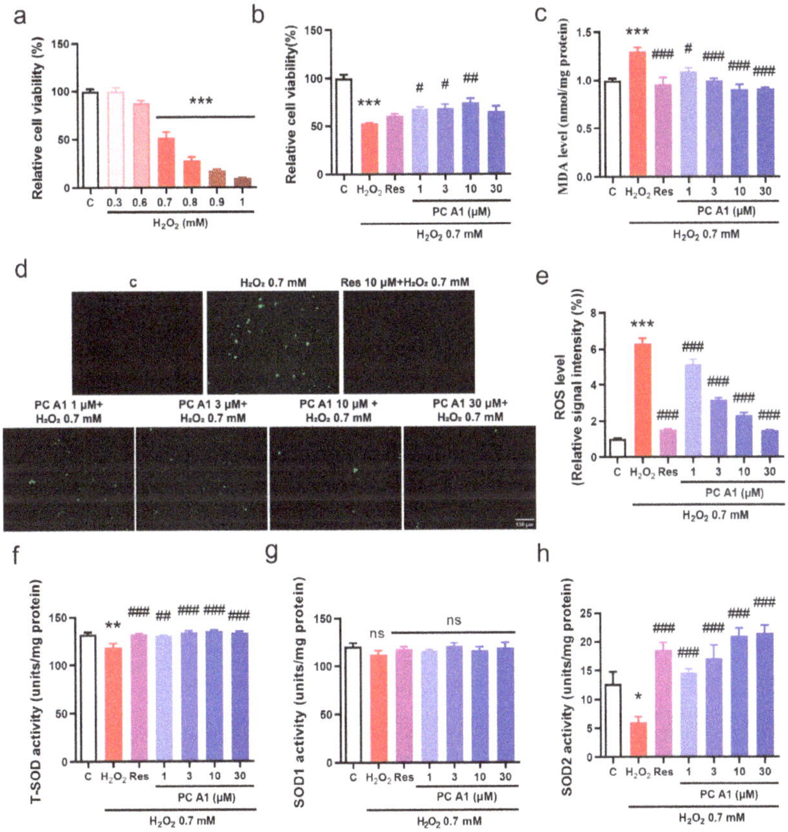

Figure 5. Antioxidative stress effect of procyanidin A1 (PC A1). (**a**) PC12 cell viability change caused by different doses of H_2O_2. (**b**–**h**) PC A1 reduced H_2O_2-induced toxicity and attenuated oxidative stress. PC12 cells were pre-treated with PC A1 (1, 3, 10, and 30 μM) for 24 h followed by 0.7 mM H_2O_2 for 2 h. Then, the cellular viability (**b**), MDA level (**c**), ROS level (**d**), and its digital result (**e**) and total SOD (**f**), SOD1 (**g**), and SOD2 activities (**h**) of PC12 cells were assessed. Scale bar: 100 μm. Data represent mean ± SEM, $n = 3$ for each group. ns, *, **, and *** indicate significant differences at $p > 0.05$, $p < 0.05$, $p < 0.01$, and $p < 0.001$ compared with the control (C) group, respectively; ns, #, ##, and ### indicate significant differences at $p > 0.05$, $p < 0.05$, $p < 0.01$, and $p < 0.001$ compared with the H_2O_2 group, respectively.

3.4. *PC A1 Induced Autophagy in PC12 Cells*

Impaired microautophagy has been proposed as a hallmark of aging [7]. Autophagy is the cellular process by which portions of the cell, including macromolecules and entire organelles, are degraded within lysosome. CYTO-ID® green dye, a fluorescent probe, serves as an effective marker for vesicles produced during autophagy. To assess the capacity of PC A1 to induce autophagy, CQ was employed to block the conversion from autophagosomes to autolysosomes by elevating the lysosomal/vacuolar pH. Rapa was used as a positive control for its known capacity to induce autophagy by inhibiting TOR (in particular, TOR complex 1) activity [15]. As shown in Figure 6a,b, Rapa (500 nM) and PC A1 (3 and 10 μM) significantly increased the fluorescent intensity of autophagic vacuoles. Given that the conversion from autophagosomes to autolysosomes was blocked by CQ, we conclude that PC A1 effectively induces autophagy in PC12 cells.

Then, the expressions of autophagy-associated proteins mTOR, ULK1, Beclin-1, p62, and LC3 were evaluated through Western blot analysis to confirm the intracellular autophagy. PC12 cells were incubated with varying doses of PC A1 (0.3, 1, 3, 10, and 30 μM) for 18 h to assess dose dependence. As illustrated in Figure 6c, the levels of phospho-mTOR (Ser2448) were reduced by both PC A1 and Rapa. Meanwhile, the levels of Beclin-1 and the ratio of LC3II/LC3I were upregulated, whereas the p62 levels were decreased in response to PC A1. The digital results of Figure 6c are shown in Figure 6e–i. Additionally, PC12 cells were incubated with 3 μM of PC A1 for varying time periods to assess time dependence, and the Western blot results for mTOR, ULK1, Beclin-1, p62, and LC3 are shown in Supplementary Figure S4a. These results further confirm that PC A1 induces autophagy in a dose- and time-dependent manner.

Then, the PI3K/Akt signaling pathway, serving as an upstream signaling pathway in the induction of autophagy, was also explored. As shown in Figure 6d, PC A1 decreased the level of the phosphorylated form of PI3K p85 (Tyr458) and p55 (Tyr199), as well as Akt (Ser473), in a dose-dependent manner. The digital results are presented in Figure 6j–l. Time dependence was similarly assessed, and the Western blot results are shown in Supplementary Figure S4b. These findings suggest that PC A1 enhances autophagy, in which the PI3K/Akt signaling pathway was involved.

3.5. *Autophagy Inhibitor Abolished Antioxidative Stress and Cell Senescence Alleviation Effects of PC A1*

Studies have indicated that many features of aging are interconnected. The impairment of autophagy or genetic defects in autophagy in young cells can lead to a loss of proteostasis, heightened mitochondrial dysfunction, and increased oxidative stress, ultimately resulting in cellular senescence [12]. To test whether the antioxidative stress and cell senescence alleviation effects of PC A1 could be negated by impaired autophagy, SA-β-gal staining and ROS assays were conducted. The selective ULK1 kinase inhibitor SBI-0206965, used to inhibit autophagy in vitro, was administered [32]. The results in Figure 7a indicated that PC A1 at 10 μM distinctly reduced the SA-β-gal$^+$ cell percentage promoted by Etop. However, SBI-0206965 negated this effect of PC A1. The evaluation of ROS yielded results consistent with the SA-β-gal assay. As shown in Figure 7b, Etop at 0.3 μM induced elevated levels of ROS in NIH/3T3 cells; pre-treatment with Rapa (50 nM) and PC A1 (10 μM) reduced ROS levels. Conversely, SBI-0206965 abrogated the ROS scavenging effect of PC A1. The results confirm that there is a crosstalk between autophagy and oxidative stress, as well as cellular senescence. The inhibition of autophagy can obstruct the ROS scavenging and cell senescence elimination effects of PC A1.

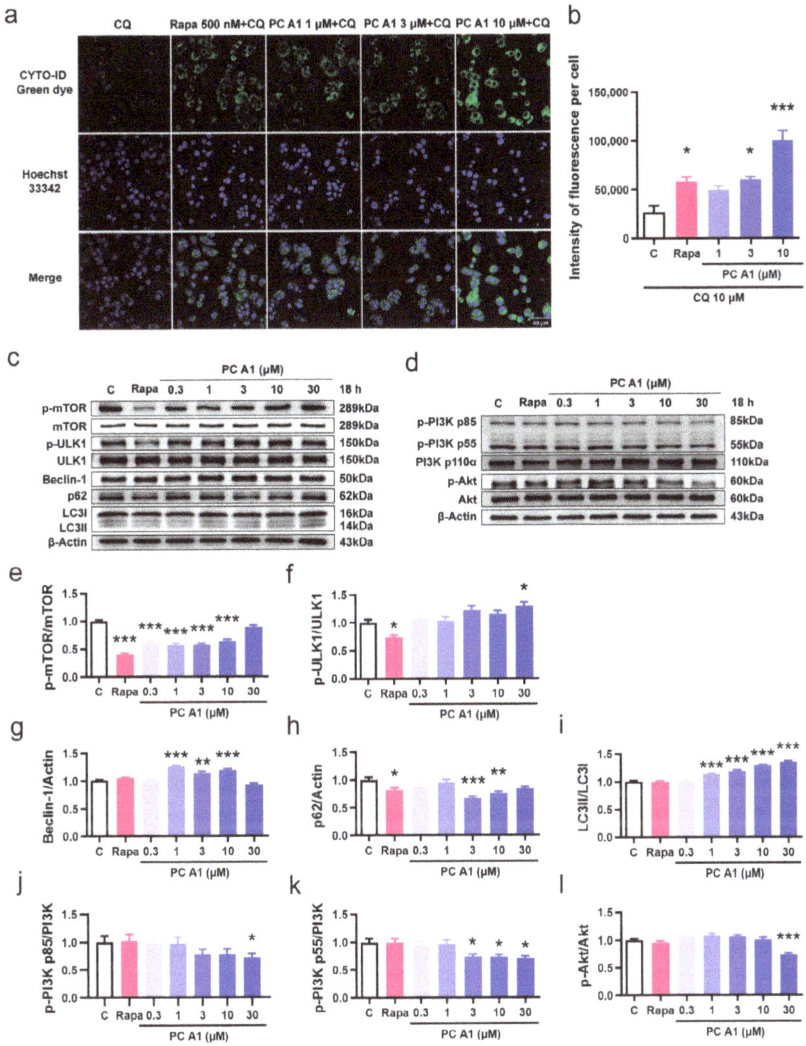

Figure 6. Procyanidin A1 (PC A1) induced autophagy in PC12 cells. (**a**) Staining of the autophagic vesicles with a fluorescent dye in PC12 cells after treatment with rapamycin (Rapa) and PC A1. Scale bar: 40 μm. (**b**) The fluorescence intensity quantification results of (**a**). (**c**) The Western blot results of p-mTOR (Ser2448), mTOR, p-ULK1 (Ser757), ULK1, Beclin-1, p62, and LC3 compared with β-Actin in PC12 cells after treatment with 500 nM of Rapa and different doses of PC A1 for 18 h. (**d**) The Western blot results of p-PI3K (p85 (Tyr458)/p55 (Tyr199)), PI3K, p-Akt (Ser473), and Akt in PC12 cells after treatment with 500 nM of Rapa and different doses of PC A1 for 18 h. (**e–i**) The digital Western blot results of p-mTOR (Ser2448)/mTOR (**e**), p-ULK1 (Ser757)/ULK1 (**f**), Beclin-1 (**g**), p62 (**h**), and LC3II/I (**i**). (**j–l**) The digital Western blot results of p-PI3K p85 (Tyr458)/PI3K (**j**), p-PI3K p55 (Tyr199)/PI3K (**k**), and p-Akt (Ser473)/Akt (**l**). The samples used for the Western blot analysis in (**c**,**d**) on different proteins are derived from the same experiment or parallel experiments and the blots are processed in parallel. *, **, and *** represent significant differences compared with the negative control ($p < 0.05$, $p < 0.01$, and $p < 0.001$, respectively). The experiments were repeated three times, and data from each experiment are displayed as mean ± SEM.

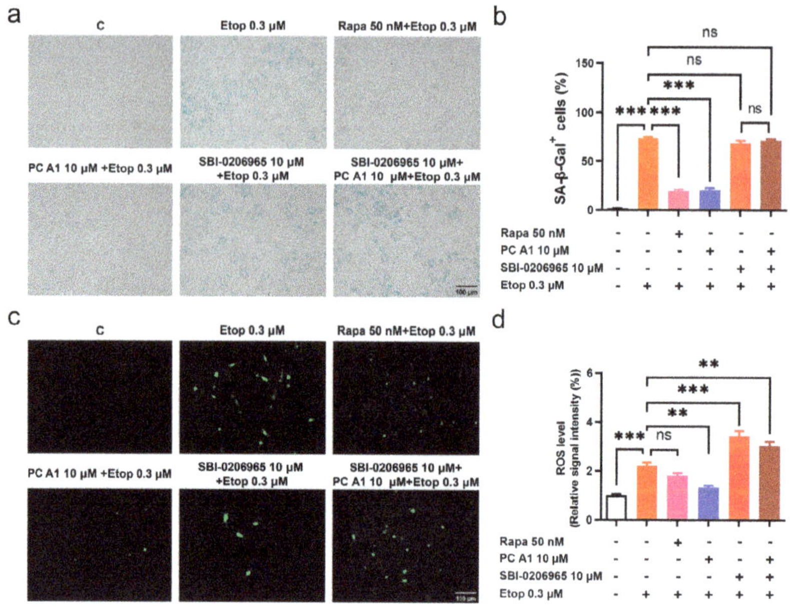

Figure 7. The autophagy inhibitor SBI-0206965 abolished antioxidative stress and the cell senescence alleviation effect of procyanidin A1 (PC A1). (**a–d**) NIH-3T3 cells were pre-treated with PC A1 at 10 μM with or without SBI-0206965 for 24 h followed by 0.3 μM of etoposide (Etop) for 48 h. Rapa (50 nM) was used as a positive control. The senescence-associated β-galactosidase (SA-β-gal) staining (**a**,**b**) and ROS level (**c**,**d**) are pictured and quantified. Scale bar: 100 μm. Data represent mean ± SEM, $n = 3$ for each group. ns, **, and *** indicate significant differences at $p > 0.05$, $p < 0.01$, and $p < 0.001$ compared with the designated group, respectively.

4. Discussion

The aging population is steadily increasing, highlighting the importance of identifying phytochemical senotherapeutics compounds with significant potential. In China, peanuts are known as the "longevity nut" and PSE is recognized as a form of TCM. Modern pharmacological studies have demonstrated that PSE offers multiple benefits against various age-related vulnerabilities. However, the potential anti-aging effects of the bioactive molecules from PSE remain not fully understood. In this study, we utilized K6001 yeast RLS as a guiding model to isolate PC A1 from PSE. Our research findings indicate that PC A1 can extend the RLS, as well as the CLS of mammalian cells. Additionally, we observed that PC A1 provides a protective effect against cellular senescence and oxidative stress and induces autophagy.

PC A1 is classified as an A-type procyanidin dimer, which is a part of the proanthocyanidin class of flavonoids. The constituent units of procyanidins are catechin and/or epicatechin. A-type procyanidins (linked via C_4-C_6 or C_4-C_8 and C_2-O-C_7) and B-type procyanidins (linked via C_4-C_6 or C_4-C_8) are categorized based on the specific interflavan linkages among their constituent units. Previous studies have identified peanut skin as a rich source of procyanidins, including monomers, dimers, trimers, and tetramers, with a particular abundance of A-type procyanidins [33]. Studies have shown that A-type procyanidins demonstrate prebiotic-like, antioxidative, anti-inflammation, anti-diabetic, antiviral, neuroprotective, and autophagy- and apoptosis-inducing effects [34]. Notably, some studies have also indicated that procyanidins may have the potential to extend lifespans and alleviate age-related pathologies [35,36]. However, different procyanidins may exhibit inverse phenotypes. For example, procyanidin C1 was shown to increase ROS in senescent cells, but not for procyanidin B2 [36]. Thereby, the anti-aging mechanism of PC A1 was further investigated.

A fundamental aging mechanism that has attracted increasing attention is cellular senescence. Senescent cells accumulate with age, and if persistent, can adversely affect tissue function due to the SASP that they develop. Despite the cytotoxic microenvironment they create, senescent cells evade death by regulating pro-survival and anti-apoptotic pathways, such as the PI3K/Akt signaling pathway. Senolytic agents, which selectively eliminate senescent cells, and senomorphic agents, which reduce the SASP, have shown promise as interventions for aging and treating age-related diseases [9]. In this study, Etop, a DNA topoisomerase inhibitor, was utilized to induce cellular senescence. This treatment elevated the expression of p21, increased ROS production, resulted in a rise in the number of SA-β-gal-positive cells, and caused cell cycle arrest, while the treatment of PC A1 alleviated these changes (Figures 2 and 3). To further investigate the mechanisms of PC A1, we conducted RNA-sequencing analysis. The results revealed that PC A1 regulates the PI3K/Akt signaling pathway. Furthermore, PC A1 downregulated the expression of anti-apoptosis genes that had been increased by Etop (Figure 4f) and reduced many SASP factors produced by senescent cells (Figure 4g). Thus, it is believed that PC A1 exhibited both senolytic and senomorphic functions, with the PI3K/Akt signaling pathway playing a significant role in the senotherapeutic effects of PC A1.

Oxidative stress is a prevalent theme among the key features associated with the aging process. It can lead to various hallmarks of aging, including the accumulation of damaged proteins, telomere attrition, epigenetic alterations, cellular senescence, and mitochondrial dysfunction, contributing to aging and age-related diseases. While antioxidants may act as scavengers of ROS to maintain the biological redox homeostasis, they may play a protective role in aging and age-related diseases [29]. In this study, H_2O_2 was used to induce oxidative stress in PC12 cells, and the treatment of PC A1 significantly improved cell viability under oxidative stress and reduced ROS levels. MDA, a harmful end product of lipid peroxidation, was also assessed as an indicator of oxidative damage. The results indicated that PC A1 decreased MDA production. As a primary defense against ROS-mediated damage, SODs were also evaluated. We observed an increase in total SOD and SOD2 activity following the treatment with PC A1; however, SOD1 activity remained unchanged (Figure 5). Notably, elevated ROS levels were also observed in senescent cells, and pre-treatment with PC A1 significantly reduced ROS levels in both senescent PC12 cells and NIH/3T3 cells (Figures 2c and 3d).

Disabled macroautophagy is one of the hallmarks of aging [7]. The term 'autophagic flux' refers to the entire process of autophagic degradation, including the formation of autophagosome and the subsequent degradation of the cargo within lysosomes. To assess the ability to induce autophagy, we blocked the fusion of lysosome and autophagosome using CQ and evaluated the autophagy flux by labeling autophagic compartments with a CYTO-ID fluorescence dye [37]. The results indicated that PC A1 increased autophagy (Figure 6a,b). Consistently, the expression levels of autophagy-related proteins, including p62, Beclin-1, and LC3II/I, also confirmed the activation of autophagy (Figure 6c). Furthermore, the upstream signaling pathway that regulates autophagy was tested through Western blot analysis, which revealed that PC A1 downregulated the levels of phosphorylated PI3K and Akt (Figure 6d).

Studies have demonstrated that impaired autophagy leads to oxidative stress and cellular senescence [12]. In this study, we observed that Rapa, as an autophagy inducer, also reduced ROS levels in senescent cells (Figures 2c and 3d). Conversely, SBI-0206965, a highly selective ULK1 kinase inhibitor and autophagy inhibitor, exacerbated the senescence phenotype. Cells treated with both SBI-0206965 and Etop were even bigger and flatter than those treated with Etop alone (Figure 7a). Additionally, SBI-0206965 elevated ROS levels in senescent cells. Notably, the ability of PC A1 to scavenge ROS and decrease the number of SA-β-gal-positive cells was diminished by SBI-0206965 (Figure 7). These findings support the notion that autophagy deficiency plays a critical role in oxidative stress and cellular senescence. Meanwhile, ULK1, a conserved kinase involved in autophagy initiation, emerges as a necessary component in the anti-aging mechanism of PC A1.

The PI3K/Akt signaling pathway regulates signal transduction and biological processes such as cell growth, proliferation, survival, apoptosis, autophagy, and metabolism [38,39]. Previous research has shown that PI3K inhibition can alleviate aging in Drosophila and reduce cardiac aging and immune senescence in older adults [40–42]. In this work, the levels of phosphorylated PI3K and Akt were reduced by PC A1 (Figure 3d). Furthermore, RNA-seq analysis indicated that the PI3K/Akt signaling pathway is implicated in the senescence-alleviating effects of PC A1 (Figure 6d). Therefore, we propose that the PI3K/Akt signaling pathway plays a role in the anti-aging effects of PC A1. However, further data are needed to substantiate this in our future work. Additionally, this investigation into the anti-aging effects of PC A1 is currently limited to the cellular level and requires validation at the animal level. Given the low concentration of PC A1 in peanut skin, alternative sources must be explored for its isolation.

5. Conclusions

Overall, our findings highlight the potential of PC A1 as an anti-aging agent. Isolated from PSE, PC A1 demonstrates significant efficacy, including an extension of the RLS of yeast and the CLS of mammalian cells, as well as alleviating cell senescence, mitigating oxidative stress, and inducing autophagy. Furthermore, the PI3K/Akt signaling pathway plays a role in the anti-aging effects of PC A1. Given these promising results, further investigation into PC A1 as a potential geroprotective agent is warranted.

Supplementary Materials: The following supporting information can be downloaded at: https://www.mdpi.com/article/10.3390/antiox14030322/s1, Figure S1: Isolation scheme of procyanidin A1 (PC A1) from peanut skin extract (PSE). Figure S2: The ^{1}H NMR spectrum of procyanidin A1 (PC A1) (500 MHz, CD_3OD). Figure S3: The HR ESI-TOF-MS chromatogram of procyanidin A1 (PC A1). Figure S4: Procyanidin A1 (PC A1) induced autophagy in PC12 cells, time dependently. (**a**) The Western blot results of p-mTOR (Ser2448), mTOR, p-ULK1 (Ser757), ULK1, Beclin-1, p62, and LC3 compared with β-Actin in PC12 cells after treatment with 500 nM of rapamycin (Rapa) and 3 μM of PC A1 for different times (0, 0.5, 1, 2, 4, 8, 18, 24, and 48 h). (**b**) The Western blot results of p-PI3K (p85 (Tyr458)/p55 (Tyr199)), PI3K, p-Akt (Ser473), and Akt in PC12 cells after treatment with 500 nM of rapamycin (Rapa) and 3 μM of PC A1 for different times (0, 0.5, 1, 2, 4, 8, 18, 24, and 48 h). (**c**–**g**) The digital Western blot results of p-mTOR (Ser2448)/mTOR (**c**), p-ULK1 (Ser757)/ULK1 (**d**), Beclin-1 (**e**), p62 (**f**), and LC3II/I (**g**). (**h**–**j**) The digital Western blot results of p-PI3K p85 (Tyr458)/PI3K (**h**), p-PI3K p55 (Tyr199)/PI3K (**i**), and p-Akt (Ser473)/Akt (**j**). The samples used for the Western blot analysis in (**a**,**b**) on different proteins are derived from the same experiment or parallel experiments and the blots were processed in parallel. *, **, and *** represent significant difference compared with the negative control ($p < 0.05$, $p < 0.01$, and $p < 0.001$). The experiments were repeated three times, and data from each experiment are displayed as mean ± SEM.

Author Contributions: Conceptualization, J.Q. and L.X.; methodology, Y.L. and L.X.; investigation and writing—original draft preparation, Y.L.; project administration, J.Q. and L.X.; funding acquisition, J.Q. All authors have read and agreed to the published version of the manuscript.

Funding: This research was funded by National Key R&D Program of China, grant number 2022YFE0104000.

Institutional Review Board Statement: Not applicable.

Informed Consent Statement: Not applicable.

Data Availability Statement: All figures and data used to support this study are included within this article; further inquiries can be directed to the corresponding authors.

Acknowledgments: We thank Shuangshuang Liu, Qiong Huang, Jingyao Chen, Xin Shen, Hongying Shen, and Liyan Wang from the Core Facilities, Zhejiang University School of Medicine for their technical support. We also thank Dan Wu, Jianyang Pan from the Research and Service Center, College of Pharmaceutical Sciences, Zhejiang university for their technical support.

Conflicts of Interest: The authors declare no conflicts of interest. The funders had no role in the design of the study; in the collection, analyses, or interpretation of data; in the writing of the manuscript; or in the decision to publish the results.

Abbreviations

The following abbreviations are used in this manuscript:

CLS	chronological lifespan
CQ	chloroquine
DEGs	differentially expressed genes
EdU	5-ethynyl-2′ -deoxyuridine
Etop	etoposide
ETIS	etoposide-induced senescence
FC	fold change
MDA	malondialdehyde
PC A1	procyanidin A1
PSE	peanut skin extracts
Rapa	rapamycin
Res	resveratrol
RLS	replicative lifespan
ROS	reactive oxygen species
SA-β-gal	senescence-associated β-galactosidase
SASP	senescence-associated secretory phenotype
SOD	superoxide dismutase
TCM	Traditional Chinese Medicine
YPD	yeast peptone dextrose

References

1. Guo, J.; Huang, X.; Dou, L.; Yan, M.; Shen, T.; Tang, W.; Li, J. Aging and aging-related diseases: From molecular mechanisms to interventions and treatments. *Signal Transduct. Target. Ther.* **2022**, *7*, 391. [CrossRef] [PubMed]
2. Shen, C.-Y.; Jiang, J.-G.; Yang, L.; Wang, D.-W.; Zhu, W. Anti-ageing active ingredients from herbs and nutraceuticals used in traditional Chinese medicine: Pharmacological mechanisms and implications for drug discovery. *Br. J. Pharmacol.* **2017**, *174*, 1395–1425. [CrossRef] [PubMed]
3. Longo, V.D.; Shadel, G.S.; Kaeberlein, M.; Kennedy, B. Replicative and Chronological Aging in Saccharomyces cerevisiae. *Cell Metab.* **2012**, *16*, 18–31. [CrossRef] [PubMed]
4. Jarolim, S.; Millen, J.; Heeren, G.; Laun, P.; Goldfarb, D.S.; Breitenbach, M. A novel assay for replicative lifespan in Saccharomyces cerevisiae. *FEMS Yeast Res.* **2004**, *5*, 169–177. [CrossRef]
5. Mirisola, M.G.; Braun, R.J.; Petranovic, D. Approaches to study yeast cell aging and death. *FEMS Yeast Res.* **2014**, *14*, 109–118. [CrossRef]
6. Leontieva, O.V.; Blagosklonny, M.V. Yeast-like chronological senescence in mammalian cells: Phenomenon, mechanism and pharmacological suppression. *Aging* **2011**, *3*, 1078–1091. [CrossRef]
7. López-Otín, C.; Blasco, M.A.; Partridge, L.; Serrano, M.; Kroemer, G. Hallmarks of aging: An expanding universe. *Cell* **2023**, *186*, 243–278. [CrossRef]
8. Huang, W.; Hickson, L.J.; Eirin, A.; Kirkland, J.L.; Lerman, L.O. Cellular senescence: The good, the bad and the unknown. *Nat. Rev. Nephrol.* **2022**, *18*, 611–627. [CrossRef]

9. Chaib, S.; Tchkonia, T.; Kirkland, J.L. Cellular senescence and senolytics: The path to the clinic. *Nat. Med.* **2022**, *28*, 1556–1568. [CrossRef]
10. Anisimov, V.N.; Egorov, M.V.; Krasilshchikova, M.S.; Lyamzaev, K.G.; Manskikh, V.N.; Moshkin, M.P.; Novikov, E.A.; Popovich, I.G.; Rogovin, K.A.; Shabalina, I.G.; et al. Effects of the mitochondria-targeted antioxidant SkQ1 on lifespan of rodents. *Aging* **2011**, *3*, 1110–1119. [CrossRef]
11. Bou-Teen, D.; Kaludercic, N.; Weissman, D.; Turan, B.; Maack, C.; Di Lisa, F.; Ruiz-Meana, M. Mitochondrial ROS and mitochondria-targeted antioxidants in the aged heart. *Free Radic. Biol. Med.* **2021**, *167*, 109–124. [CrossRef] [PubMed]
12. Galluzzi, L.; Bravo-San Pedro, J.M.; Levine, B.; Green, D.R.; Kroemer, G. Pharmacological modulation of autophagy: Therapeutic potential and persisting obstacles. *Nat. Rev. Drug Discov.* **2017**, *16*, 487–511. [CrossRef] [PubMed]
13. Ornatowski, W.; Lu, Q.; Yegambaram, M.; Garcia, A.E.; Zemskov, E.A.; Maltepe, E.; Fineman, J.R.; Wang, T.; Black, S.M. Complex interplay between autophagy and oxidative stress in the development of pulmonary disease. *Redox Biol.* **2020**, *36*, 101679. [CrossRef]
14. Madeo, F.; Tavernarakis, N.; Kroemer, G. Can autophagy promote longevity? *Nat. Cell Biol.* **2010**, *12*, 842–846. [CrossRef] [PubMed]
15. Juricic, P.; Lu, Y.-X.; Leech, T.; Drews, L.F.; Paulitz, J.; Lu, J.; Nespital, T.; Azami, S.; Regan, J.C.; Funk, E.; et al. Long-lasting geroprotection from brief rapamycin treatment in early adulthood by persistently increased intestinal autophagy. *Nat. Aging* **2022**, *2*, 824–836. [CrossRef]
16. Eisenberg, T.; Knauer, H.; Schauer, A.; Büttner, S.; Ruckenstuhl, C.; Carmona-Gutierrez, D.; Ring, J.; Schroeder, S.; Magnes, C.; Antonacci, L.; et al. Induction of autophagy by spermidine promotes longevity. *Nat. Cell Biol.* **2009**, *11*, 1305–1314. [CrossRef]
17. Carmona-Gutierrez, D.; Zimmermann, A.; Kainz, K.; Pietrocola, F.; Chen, G.; Maglioni, S.; Schiavi, A.; Nah, J.; Mertel, S.; Beuschel, C.B.; et al. The flavonoid 4,4′-dimethoxychalcone promotes autophagy-dependent longevity across species. *Nat. Commun.* **2019**, *10*, 651. [CrossRef]
18. Ryu, D.; Mouchiroud, L.; Andreux, P.A.; Katsyuba, E.; Moullan, N.; Nicolet-dit-Félix, A.A.; Williams, E.G.; Jha, P.; Lo Sasso, G.; Huzard, D.; et al. Urolithin A induces mitophagy and prolongs lifespan in C. elegans and increases muscle function in rodents. *Nat. Med.* **2016**, *22*, 879–888. [CrossRef]
19. Peanut 2025 World Production. Available online: https://ipad.fas.usda.gov/cropexplorer/cropview/commodityView.aspx?cropid=2221000&sel_year=2025&rankby=Production (accessed on 9 February 2025).
20. Xiang, L.; Wu, Q.; Cheng, L.; Sun, K.; Li, J.; Yoshida, M.; Qi, J. Leptin and Adiponectin Signaling Pathways Are Involved in the Antiobesity Effects of Peanut Skin Extract. *Oxid. Med. Cell. Longev.* **2019**, *2019*, 2935315. [CrossRef]
21. Xu, M.; Lv, C.; Wang, H.; Lu, Q.; Ye, M.; Zhu, X.; Liu, R. Peanut skin extract ameliorates high-fat diet-induced atherosclerosis by regulating lipid metabolism, inflammation reaction and gut microbiota in ApoE−/− mice. *Food Res. Int.* **2022**, *154*, 111014. [CrossRef]
22. Xiang, L.; Wu, Q.; Osada, H.; Yoshida, M.; Pan, W.; Qi, J. Peanut skin extract ameliorates the symptoms of type 2 diabetes mellitus in mice by alleviating inflammation and maintaining gut microbiota homeostasis. *Aging* **2020**, *12*, 13991–14018. [CrossRef] [PubMed]
23. Kim, M.Y.; Kim, H.-J.; Lee, Y.-Y.; Kim, M.H.; Lee, J.Y.; Kang, M.S.; Koo, B.C.; Lee, B.W. Antioxidant and anti-inflammatory effects of Peanut (*Arachishypogaea* L.) skin extracts of various cultivars in oxidative-damaged HepG2 cells and LPS-induced raw 264.7 macrophages. *Food Sci. Nutr.* **2021**, *9*, 973–984. [CrossRef]
24. Lou, H.; Yamazaki, Y.; Sasaki, T.; Uchida, M.; Tanaka, H.; Oka, S. A-type proanthocyanidins from peanut skins. *Phytochemistry* **1999**, *51*, 297–308. [CrossRef]
25. Howitz, K.T.; Bitterman, K.J.; Cohen, H.Y.; Lamming, D.W.; Lavu, S.; Wood, J.G.; Zipkin, R.E.; Chung, P.; Kisielewski, A.; Zhang, L.-L.; et al. Small molecule activators of sirtuins extend Saccharomyces cerevisiae lifespan. *Nature* **2003**, *425*, 191–196. [CrossRef] [PubMed]
26. Wiatrak, B.; Kubis-Kubiak, A.; Piwowar, A.; Barg, E. PC12 Cell Line: Cell Types, Coating of Culture Vessels, Differentiation and Other Culture Conditions. *Cells* **2020**, *9*, 958. [CrossRef]
27. Shen, Q.-q.; Jv, X.-h.; Ma, X.-z.; Li, C.; Liu, L.; Jia, W.-t.; Qu, L.; Chen, L.-l.; Xie, J.-x. Cell senescence induced by toxic interaction between α-synuclein and iron precedes nigral dopaminergic neuron loss in a mouse model of Parkinson's disease. *Acta Pharmacol. Sin.* **2024**, *45*, 268–281. [CrossRef]
28. Avelar, R.A.; Ortega, J.G.; Tacutu, R.; Tyler, E.J.; Bennett, D.; Binetti, P.; Budovsky, A.; Chatsirisupachai, K.; Johnson, E.; Murray, A.; et al. A multidimensional systems biology analysis of cellular senescence in aging and disease. *Genome Biol.* **2020**, *21*, 91. [CrossRef]
29. López-Otín, C.; Blasco, M.A.; Partridge, L.; Serrano, M.; Kroemer, G. The Hallmarks of Aging. *Cell* **2013**, *153*, 1194–1217. [CrossRef]
30. Lee, Y.H.; Kuk, M.U.; So, M.K.; Song, E.S.; Lee, H.; Ahn, S.K.; Kwon, H.W.; Park, J.T.; Park, S.C. Targeting Mitochondrial Oxidative Stress as a Strategy to Treat Aging and Age-Related Diseases. *Antioxidants* **2023**, *12*, 934. [CrossRef]

31. Fukui, M.; Choi, H.J.; Zhu, B.T. Mechanism for the protective effect of resveratrol against oxidative stress-induced neuronal death. *Free Radic. Biol. Med.* **2010**, *49*, 800–813. [CrossRef]
32. Egan, D.F.; Chun, M.G.H.; Vamos, M.; Zou, H.; Rong, J.; Miller, C.J.; Lou, H.J.; Raveendra-Panickar, D.; Yang, C.-C.; Sheffler, D.J.; et al. Small Molecule Inhibition of the Autophagy Kinase ULK1 and Identification of ULK1 Substrates. *Mol. Cell* **2015**, *59*, 285–297. [CrossRef]
33. Bodoira, R.; Cecilia Cittadini, M.; Velez, A.; Rossi, Y.; Montenegro, M.; Martínez, M.; Maestri, D. An overview on extraction, composition, bioactivity and food applications of peanut phenolics. *Food Chem.* **2022**, *381*, 132250. [CrossRef] [PubMed]
34. Zeng, Y.; Zhao, L.; Wang, K.; Renard, C.M.G.C.; Le Bourvellec, C.; Hu, Z.; Liu, X. A-type proanthocyanidins: Sources, structure, bioactivity, processing, nutrition, and potential applications. *Compr. Rev. Food Sci. Food Saf.* **2024**, *23*, e13352. [CrossRef] [PubMed]
35. Xiao, Y.; Dong, J.; Yin, Z.; Wu, Q.; Zhou, Y.; Zhou, X. Procyanidin B2 protects against d-galactose-induced mimetic aging in mice: Metabolites and microbiome analysis. *Food Chem. Toxicol.* **2018**, *119*, 141–149. [CrossRef]
36. Xu, Q.; Fu, Q.; Li, Z.; Liu, H.; Wang, Y.; Lin, X.; He, R.; Zhang, X.; Ju, Z.; Campisi, J.; et al. The flavonoid procyanidin C1 has senotherapeutic activity and increases lifespan in mice. *Nat. Metab.* **2021**, *3*, 1706–1726. [CrossRef]
37. Guo, S.; Liang, Y.; Murphy, S.F.; Huang, A.; Shen, H.; Kelly, D.F.; Sobrado, P.; Sheng, Z. A rapid and high content assay that measures cyto-ID-stained autophagic compartments and estimates autophagy flux with potential clinical applications. *Autophagy* **2015**, *11*, 560–572. [CrossRef]
38. Fruman, D.A.; Chiu, H.; Hopkins, B.D.; Bagrodia, S.; Cantley, L.C.; Abraham, R.T. The PI3K Pathway in Human Disease. *Cell* **2017**, *170*, 605–635. [CrossRef] [PubMed]
39. Liu, Y.; Liu, Q.; Zhang, Z.; Yang, Y.; Zhou, Y.; Yan, H.; Wang, X.; Li, X.; Zhao, J.; Hu, J.; et al. The regulatory role of PI3K in ageing-related diseases. *Ageing Res. Rev.* **2023**, *88*, 101963. [CrossRef]
40. Abdellatif, M.; Eisenberg, T.; Heberle, A.M.; Thedieck, K.; Kroemer, G.; Sedej, S. Cardiac PI3K p110α attenuation delays aging and extends lifespan. *Cell Stress* **2022**, *6*, 72–75. [CrossRef]
41. Sapey, E.; Greenwood, H.; Walton, G.; Mann, E.; Love, A.; Aaronson, N.; Insall, R.H.; Stockley, R.A.; Lord, J.M. Phosphoinositide 3-kinase inhibition restores neutrophil accuracy in the elderly: Toward targeted treatments for immunosenescence. *Blood* **2014**, *123*, 239–248. [CrossRef]
42. Danilov, A.; Shaposhnikov, M.; Plyusnina, E.; Kogan, V.; Fedichev, P.; Moskalev, A. Selective anticancer agents suppress aging in Drosophila. *Oncotarget* **2013**, *4*, 1507–1526. [CrossRef]

antioxidants

MDPI

Article

The Survival of Human Intervertebral Disc Nucleus Pulposus Cells under Oxidative Stress Relies on the Autophagy Triggered by Delphinidin

Md Entaz Bahar [1], Jin Seok Hwang [1], Trang Huyen Lai [1], June-Ho Byun [2], Dong-Hee Kim [3,*] and Deok Ryong Kim [1,*]

[1] Department of Biochemistry and Convergence Medical Sciences, Institute of Medical Science, College of Medicine, Gyeongsang National University, Jinju 52727, Republic of Korea; mdentaz87@gnu.ac.kr (M.E.B.); cloud8104@naver.com (J.S.H.); tranghuyen20493@gmail.com (T.H.L.)

[2] Department of Oral and Maxillofacial Surgery, Institute of Medical Science, College of Medicine, Gyeongsang National University Hospital, Gyeongsang National University, Jinju 52727, Republic of Korea; surbyun@gnu.ac.kr

[3] Department of Orthopaedic Surgery, Institute of Medical Science, College of Medicine, Gyeongsang National University Hospital, Gyeongsang National University, Jinju 52727, Republic of Korea

* Correspondence: dhkim8311@gnu.ac.kr (D.-H.K.); drkim@gnu.ac.kr (D.R.K.)

Abstract: Delphinidin (Delp), a natural antioxidant, has shown promise in treating age-related ailments such as osteoarthritis (OA). This study investigates the impact of delphinidin on intervertebral disc degeneration (IVDD) using human nucleus pulposus cells (hNPCs) subjected to hydrogen peroxide. Various molecular and cellular assays were employed to assess senescence, extracellular matrix (ECM) degradation markers, and the activation of AMPK and autophagy pathways. Initially, oxidative stress (OS)-induced hNPCs exhibited notably elevated levels of senescence markers like p53 and p21, which were mitigated by Delp treatment. Additionally, Delp attenuated IVDD characteristics including apoptosis and ECM degradation markers in OS-induced senescence (OSIS) hNPCs by downregulating MMP-13 and ADAMTS-5 while upregulating COL2A1 and aggrecans. Furthermore, Delp reversed the increased ROS production and reduced autophagy activation observed in OSIS hNPCs. Interestingly, the ability of Delp to regulate cellular senescence and ECM balance in OSIS hNPCs was hindered by autophagy inhibition using CQ. Remarkably, Delp upregulated SIRT1 and phosphorylated AMPK expression while downregulating mTOR phosphorylation in the presence of AICAR (AMPK activator), and this effect was reversed by Compound C, AMPK inhibitor. In summary, our findings suggest that Delp can safeguard hNPCs from oxidative stress by promoting autophagy through the SIRT1/AMPK/mTOR pathway.

Keywords: delphinidin; IVDD; oxidative stress; senescence; apoptosis; ECM degradation; autophagy

1. Introduction

Age-related conditions such as osteoarthritis (OA) and intervertebral disc degeneration (IVDD) are closely associated with oxidative stress (OS). In particular, OS exacerbates during IVDD, significantly contributing to its progression [1]. Various pathophysiological pathways, including matrix metabolism, inflammation, apoptosis, autophagy, and disc cell senescence, play crucial roles in this progression [2]. The involvement of hydrogen peroxide (H_2O_2)-induced OS in the intervertebral disc (IVD) has been extensively studied due to its association with reactive oxygen species (ROSs). Hydrogen peroxide accelerates ROS generation and DNA damage in senescent nucleus pulposus (NP) cells within the IVD [3]. Senescent NP cells experience impaired proliferation due to accumulated cellular damage and permanent cell cycle arrest [4]. Stimulation of the ATM-Chk2-p53-p21-Rb and p16-Rb signaling pathways in NP cells induces premature cellular senescence [5,6].

Hydrogen peroxide can also induce a catabolic phenotype in senescent cells, characterized by increased expression of extracellular matrix-degrading enzymes (MMP-1, MMP-2, MMP-9, and ADAMTS-5), and by the decreased levels of their suppressors (TIMPs) and proteoglycans like aggrecan [5]. Moreover, H_2O_2 activates various signaling pathways, including p38 MAPKs, ERKs, and JNKs, and leads to the translocation of NF-κB and Nrf2 to the nucleus [5]. Additionally, hydrogen peroxide accelerates premature aging of cartilage endplate cells via the p53-p21-Rb pathway [7]. The marker p53 is associated with cellular aging [8]. Although various stressors contribute to cellular senescence in IVDD, significant knowledge gaps remain in this area, presenting opportunities for the development of therapeutic interventions for age-related IVDD.

OA and IVDD are also characterized by heightened inflammation, which is pivotal in the onset and progression of various diseases, influencing their pathophysiology [9]. Understanding the role of inflammation in OA and IVDD highlights the importance of focusing on inflammatory pathways for therapeutic intervention. Researchers are exploring anti-inflammatory drugs, including cytokine inhibitors and antioxidants, to slow the progression of these degenerative conditions and alleviate symptoms [10,11].

Autophagy, a cellular catabolic process, serves as the cellular quality control system by engulfing and breaking down damaged or dysfunctional cellular components. It acts as a fundamental process in maintaining cellular homeostasis and adapting to various environmental stresses. When cells encounter stressors like nutritional deficiency, viral infection, hypoxia, or oxidative and genotoxic stress, autophagy is upregulated to help mitigate the damage and restore cellular balance. Through this process, cells can recycle cytoplasmic components, including proteins and organelles, to generate energy and essential building blocks for survival [12]. Recent studies have shed light on the potential therapeutic implications of autophagy modulation in age-related degenerative diseases such as intervertebral disc degeneration and osteoarthritis [13,14]. While excessive autophagy may contribute to cellular dysfunction and disease progression, maintaining an optimal level of autophagic activity could potentially alleviate the pathological processes associated with these conditions. Thus, understanding the intricate regulation of autophagy and its role in disease pathogenesis holds promise for the development of novel therapeutic strategies targeting age-related degenerative disorders.

Anthocyanins exhibit heightened sensitivity to H_2O_2-induced oxidative stress and demonstrate superior capability in scavenging H_2O_2 compared to other phenolics, as reported in various studies [15,16]. Notably, the remarkable antioxidative activity of anthocyanins has led to their utilization as a distinct dietary supplement for free radical scavenging, thereby gaining prominence in addressing age-related ailments, including intervertebral disc degeneration [17]. Among these anthocyanins, delphinidin, renowned for its potent antioxidant properties, stands out as one of the most beneficial polyphenols. Previous research, including our own, has demonstrated the efficacy of delphinidin in protecting chondrocytes against oxidative stress associated with age-related conditions such as osteoarthritis (OA) [18,19]. Our previous findings indicated that delphinidin shields C28/I2 chondrocyte cells from ROS-induced apoptosis through the activation of Nrf2 and NF-κB pathways, while promoting protective autophagy mechanisms [18]. Despite delphinidin being a prominent bioactive compound within anthocyanins, the precise mechanisms underlying its protective effects against oxidative stress-induced senescence in age-related diseases remain inadequately characterized. We postulate that senescent cells may accumulate within the intervertebral disc with age and progressive disc degeneration. To elucidate the mechanisms underlying NP senescence, we employed H_2O_2 as an inducer of oxidative stress in human NP cells.

2. Materials and Methods

2.1. Human Nucleus Pulposus Cells Culture

Human nucleus pulposus cells (hNPCs) were purchased from ScienCell Research Laboratories (4800, ScienCell, Carlsbad, TX, USA) and cultured in Nucleus Pulposus Cell

Medium (NPCM, ScienCell, Carlsbad, TX, USA) supplemented with 2% fetal bovine serum (FBS; ScienCell, Carlsbad, CA, USA), 1% penicillin/streptomycin (P/S; ScienCell, Carlsbad, CA, USA), and nucleus pulposus cell growth supplement (NPCGS; ScienCell, Carlsbad, CA, USA).

2.2. Hydrogen Peroxide (H_2O_2) Treatment

The hNPCs were cultured in 96-well plates at 1×10^4 cells/well with 150 μL of NPCM in the presence of various doses of H_2O_2 (0 to 1000 μM) for 24 h to determine the cytotoxicity and inhibitory concentration (IC_{50}) of H_2O_2. Cell viability was measured via a Cell Counting Kit test (CCK-8) (CK04-13; Dojindo, Kumamoto, Japan). The hNPCs (700 cells) were cultured in 6-well plates with 1.5 mL of NPCM in the presence of various doses of H_2O_2 (0, 110, 185, and 250 μM) for 24 h, followed by 7 days of recovery. Clonogenicity was measured by crystal violet staining assay.

2.3. Delphinidin Treatment

The hNPCs were cultured in 96-well plates at 1×10^4 cells/well with 150 μL of NPCM in the presence of various doses of Delp (0 to 200 μM) at 24 h to determine the IC_{50} value of Delp. Cell viability was measured by the CCK-8 assay and crystal violet assay. The hNPCs were cultured in 96-well plates with 150 μL of NPCM in the presence of various doses of Delp (0, 2.5, 5, 10, 20, and 40 μM) or 5 mM of N-acetyl cysteine (NAC) at 12 and 24 h before 185 μM of H_2O_2 was added to determine the dose- and time-dependent effects of Delp. The hNPCs (700 cells) were cultured in 6-well plates with 1.5 mL of NPCM supplemented with 40 μM of Delp or 5 mM of NAC for 24 h before 185 μM of H_2O_2 was added for 24 h, followed by 7 days of recovery. Clonogenicity was determined by crystal violet staining assay.

2.4. Establishment of Oxidative Stress-Induced Senescence (OSIS)

H_2O_2 was employed to induce oxidative stress-induced senescence (OSIS), following previously established protocols with slight modifications (Figure S1) [20–22]. Primary human nucleus pulposus cells at a population doubling (PD) of 3.5 and a population doubling time (PDT) of 2.8 in passage 1 (P1) were utilized to establish the OSIS model. Treatment commenced 24 h post-seeding by incubating 3×10^5 cells in a 6-well plate with 2 mL of culture medium. Cells were cultured under normal conditions (nOSIS-control) or treated with delphinidin (nOSIS-Delp) or subjected to H_2O_2 treatment (OSIS-control), and H_2O_2 treatment with delphinidin (OSIS-Delp). Briefly, cells were incubated for 24 h in 6-well plates with 2 mL of NPCM containing 2% FBS supplemented with or without 40 μM of delphinidin before exposure to 250 μM of H_2O_2 for 4 h in passage 2 (P2). In passage 3 (P3), cells were pretreated with or without 20 μM of delphinidin for 24 h after being split into a 1:3 ratio and exposed to 185 μM of H_2O_2 for 4 h, followed by 24 h of recovery. Similarly, in passage 4 (P4), cells pretreated with 10 μM of delphinidin for 24 h or not were exposed to 110 μM of H_2O_2 for 4 h, followed by 24 h of recovery. The senescence model was confirmed through SA-β-gal assay, Western blotting, and other assays. For mechanistic evaluation, OSIS cells were cultured with normal media, delphinidin (20 μM), chloroquine (10 μM CQ; autophagy inhibitor), 5-Aminoimidazole-4-carboxamide ribonucleotide (1 mM, AICAR; AMPK inducer), or compound C (10 μM, CC; AMPK inhibitor) for 72 h.

2.5. Cell Population Doubling Time (CPDT)

The hNPCs were seeded at a constant density (2500 cells/mL) on the surface of a 10 cm culture plate containing NPCM in a humidified incubator (37 °C, 5% CO_2) for 10 days to assess the phenotypic and morphological alterations of the in vitro OSIS model. After seeding cells, the entire cultural medium was swapped out for a fresh one every three days. Trypan blue exclusion was used to assess the in vitro proliferative potential of hNPCs [23]. The numbers of cell population doubling (NCPD) [24] and cell population doubling time (CPDT) were then calculated based on the following equations (Equations (1) and (2)) [25]:

$$NCPD = 3.322 * (\log Nt - \log Ni) \quad (1)$$

$$CPDT = (t - ti)/NCPD \quad (2)$$

where Nt and Ni are the cell numbers at a specific time point t (10 days) and at the initial time point ti (0 days), respectively.

2.6. Cell Viability Assay

Cell viability analysis was conducted using the CCK-8 assay. hNPCs were seeded in 96-well plates and incubated with varying concentrations of delphinidin, H_2O_2 alone, or a combination of both as indicated. Subsequently, 150 μL of media comprising 135 μL of NPCM and 15 μL of CCK-8 solution (CK04-13; Dojindo, Kumamoto, Japan) was added to each well and incubated for 120 min at 37 °C. Following incubation, absorbance was measured at 450 nm using a microplate reader.

2.7. Crystal Violet Staining Assay

The cells were allowed to proliferate for the crystal violet proliferation assay for the specified duration. Following this, the media were aspirated, and the cells were washed twice with 1X Phosphate Buffered Saline (PBS). Subsequently, a solution of 10% formalin in 1X PBS was added and incubated for 20 min at room temperature. After incubation, the formalin solution was removed, and 0.1% (w/v) crystal violet (# C0775-25G, Sigma, St. Louis, MO, USA) was added to each well and incubated for an additional 20 min at room temperature. The crystal violet solution was then discarded, and the plates were thoroughly washed with tap water, followed by air-drying at room temperature. For quantification purposes, 1% SDS was added to each well and incubated at room temperature for 30 min. The extracted solution was transferred to a 96-well plate and quantified by measuring the optical density (OD) at 590 nm.

2.8. Clonogenic Survival Assay

To evaluate the cells' clonogenic survival capability, the exposure medium was aspirated, and cells were detached using trypsin and counted using a hemocytometer. Subsequently, cells were seeded at a density of approximately 700 cells in 2.0 mL of medium per well in 6-well plates. The plates were then incubated for 7 to 10 days at 37 °C with 5% CO_2. Following the incubation period, clonogenic activity was assessed using the crystal violet proliferation assay described earlier.

2.9. Measurement of Reactive Oxygen Species (ROSs)

To measure reactive oxygen species levels, a dichlorodihydrofluorescein diacetate cellular ROS assay kit (ab113851) from Abcam was employed following the manufacturer's instructions. hNPCs were cultured on Poly-L-lysine-coated 96-well plates, and dichlorodihydrofluorescein diacetate was added to the cultures 30 min before the end of the recovery period. Following washing steps, fluorescence intensity was measured at 485/535 nm using a microplate reader.

2.10. Senescence-Associated β-Galactosidase Staining (SA-β-Gal Staining)

To assess the aging process of hNPCs, a cellular senescence activity assay (catalog#: ENZ-KIT129, Enzo Life Sciences, Lausen, Switzerland) was conducted following the manufacturer's protocol. Initially, cells were seeded at a density of 1×10^4 cells per well in a 96-well plate and incubated for 72 h. Subsequently, the medium was aspirated, and after washing with PBS, hNPCs were lysed on ice using a lysis buffer and incubated at 4 °C for 5 min. The entire lysate was then transferred to a microcentrifuge tube and centrifuged at 14,000× g for 10 min at 4 °C to collect the supernatant as cell lysate. A quantity of 50 μL of the cell lysate was transferred to a 96-well plate, followed by the addition of 50 µL of freshly prepared assay buffer. The plate was then incubated at 37 °C, shielded from light, for 2 h. After incubation, 50 µL of the reaction mixture was transferred to a separate 96-well plate suitable for fluorescence measurement. The reaction was stopped by adding 200 µL of stop solution. Fluorescence intensity was measured using a fluorescence plate reader with excitation at 360 nm and emission at 465 nm.

2.11. *Autophagy Flux Detection*

The autophagic flux in response to Delp therapy was assessed using the CYTO-ID Autophagy detection kit (#ENZ-51031, Enzo Life Sciences, Lausen, Switzerland), according to the manufacturer's protocol. Briefly, human nucleus pulposus cells (hNPCs) were cultured in a 37 °C incubator with 5% CO_2 during the experimental period. The cells were then rinsed twice with PBS at room temperature and subjected to centrifugation at 400× *g* for 5 min at room temperature. After removing the supernatant, the cell pellets were resuspended in 200 µL of PBS at room temperature for 20 min. Next, 0.4 µL of Cyto-ID Green stain solution was added, and the cells were stained for 5 min at room temperature. This was followed by the addition of 0.2 µL of Hoechst 33342 stain solution for a 20 min incubation. The autophagic flux was quantified by collecting the cells and staining them with Cyto-ID Green fluorescent dye, which was detected at an excitation wavelength of approximately 480 nm and an emission wavelength of approximately 530 nm.

2.12. *Interleukin 1 Beta (IL-1β) Measurement*

The cellular IL-1β level was assessed using the ELISA assay (#ADI-900-130A, Enzo Life Sciences, Farmingdale, NY, USA) according to the manufacturer's guidelines. In brief, homogenized cell lysates (50 µL) were incubated with 100 µL of human IL-1β biotin conjugate solution in wells coated with human IL-1β antibody on a 96-well strip-well plate at room temperature for 2 h. A standard curve was generated using different concentrations of a human IL-1β standard (ranging from 0 to 250 pg/mL). Following washing steps, 100 µL of streptavidin–peroxidase substrate solution was added to each well (excluding the chromogen blanks) and incubated for 30 min at room temperature. The reaction was halted by adding 100 µL of stop solution to each well. Optical densities were measured at 450 nm using a microplate reader within 2 h after the addition of the stop solution. IL-1β concentrations were determined by comparing the optical densities to the standard curve generated using GraphPad Prism 8 software (GraphPad Software Inc., San Diego, CA, USA).

2.13. *Western Blotting*

Cells were harvested and lysed using RIPA lysis and extraction buffer (#89900, Thermo Fisher Scientific, Waltham, MA, USA) supplemented with 1× Halt Protease and Phosphatase Inhibitor Cocktail (#78441, Thermo Fisher Scientific). The protein concentration in the total cell lysates was determined using Pierce BCA Protein Assay Kits (#89900, Thermo Fisher Scientific) following the manufacturer's protocol. Subsequently, the protein samples were separated on an SDS-PAGE gel and transferred onto a PVDF membrane (GE Healthcare-Amersham Biosciences, Chicago, IL, USA) using a semi-dry transfer system (Bio-Rad, Hercules, CA, USA). The membrane was then blocked with 5% skim milk in TBST for 45 min at room temperature. After overnight incubation with primary antibodies (refer to Table S1) at 4 °C in skim milk, the membrane was washed three times in TBST for 10 min each and incubated with secondary antibodies (refer to Table S1) in TBST for one hour. Following three additional washes with TBST for 10 min each, the signal was detected using an Enhanced Chemiluminescence (ECL) detection system (#34080, Thermo Fisher Scientific). Protein quantification was performed using ImageJ® software (Version 1.53e, NIH, Bethesda, MD, USA). The graphical representations depict the mean values (±SD) derived from at least three independent experiments.

2.14. Statistical Analysis

All experimental data were analyzed using the GraphPad Prism 8 software program (San Diego, CA, USA) based on the number of replicates and group design. Ordinary one-way ANOVA or two-way ANOVA with Tukey's multiple comparisons test was employed for the analysis, as specified in each figure legend.

3. Results

3.1. Effects of H_2O_2 on Human Nucleus Pulposus Cells (hNPCs) Growth, Stress-Responsive ROS, Autophagy, and Cell Death

A significant decrease in cell viability was observed with H_2O_2 concentrations of 100 µM or higher after 24 h of incubation. H_2O_2 treatment (100–1000 µM) resulted in a significant reduction in hNPC cell viability (30–85%) compared to controls (Figure 1a). The IC_{30}, IC_{50}, and IC_{60} values of H_2O_2 for hNPCs were determined to be 110.7 µM, 185.0 µM, and 236.6 µM, respectively (Figure 1b). Exposure to 185 µM H_2O_2 led to increased ROS production between 12 and 24 h, suggesting the presence of oxidative stress (Figure 1c). These results indicate that H_2O_2 treatment significantly impaired hNPC proliferation, as corroborated by the in vitro clonogenic assay (Figure 1d,e). Furthermore, treatment with H_2O_2 significantly elevated the expression of apoptotic proteins, cleaved caspase-3, and reduced the expression of the anti-apoptotic protein, Bcl-2, compared to controls (Figure 1f) during the 12 to 24-h period. Additionally, our findings revealed significant alterations in the AMPK pathway following H_2O_2 treatment, as evidenced by the upregulation of p-AMPK and SIRT1, and downregulation of p-mTOR protein expression between 12 and 24 h (Figure 1g). Moreover, H_2O_2 treatment significantly suppressed autophagy flux, as indicated by reduced expression of LC3-II and Beclin-1, and increased p62 protein expression between 12 and 24 h (Figure 1h).

Overall, these results highlight the induction of oxidative stress and apoptosis, as well as alterations in cellular pathways including autophagy and AMPK signaling in hNPCs upon exposure to H_2O_2. This finding underscores the significance of oxidative stress in the biology of hNPCs and suggests potential therapeutic strategies for intervertebral disc degeneration associated with oxidative stress.

3.2. Effects of Delp on H_2O_2-Induced Oxidative Stress in hNPCs

Delphinidin was administered to hNPCs at various concentrations for 24 h, and its cytotoxic effect on hNPCs was assessed using the crystal violet assay. As depicted in Figure 2a, Delp significantly reduced hNPC viability at concentrations exceeding 100 µM, while showing no effect at concentrations below 50 µM. The IC_{20}, IC_{30}, and IC_{50} values of Delp in hNPCs at 24 h were determined to be 49.00 µM, 57.55 µM, and 74.10 µM, respectively (Figure 2b). These values offer crucial insights into the potency of Delp in modulating hNPC viability, thereby guiding further investigations into its mechanism of action and potential therapeutic applications. Given that H_2O_2 concentrations above 100 µM decreased hNPC activity, with inhibition increasing with higher concentrations (Figure 1a), we selected 185 µM H_2O_2 for pretreatment in combination with 5 mM NAC and 2.5, 5, 10, 20, and 40 µM Delp. Figure 2c demonstrates that doses of 20 and 40 µM Delp were effective at 12 and 24 h, with 10 µM also showing efficacy at 24 h. Remarkably, ROS production increased significantly at 185 µM H_2O_2 ($\geq$2.5-fold), while Delp pretreatment led to a substantial reduction (30 to 40%) in H_2O_2-induced ROS levels (Figure 2d,e). Furthermore, while H_2O_2 treatment decreased the cell survival rate of hNPCs, Delp treatment effectively rescued their clonogenic survival ability (Figure 2f,g). These findings underscore the potential of Delp in mitigating the adverse effects of H_2O_2 on hNPCs, highlighting its prospective therapeutic utility in oxidative stress-related conditions.

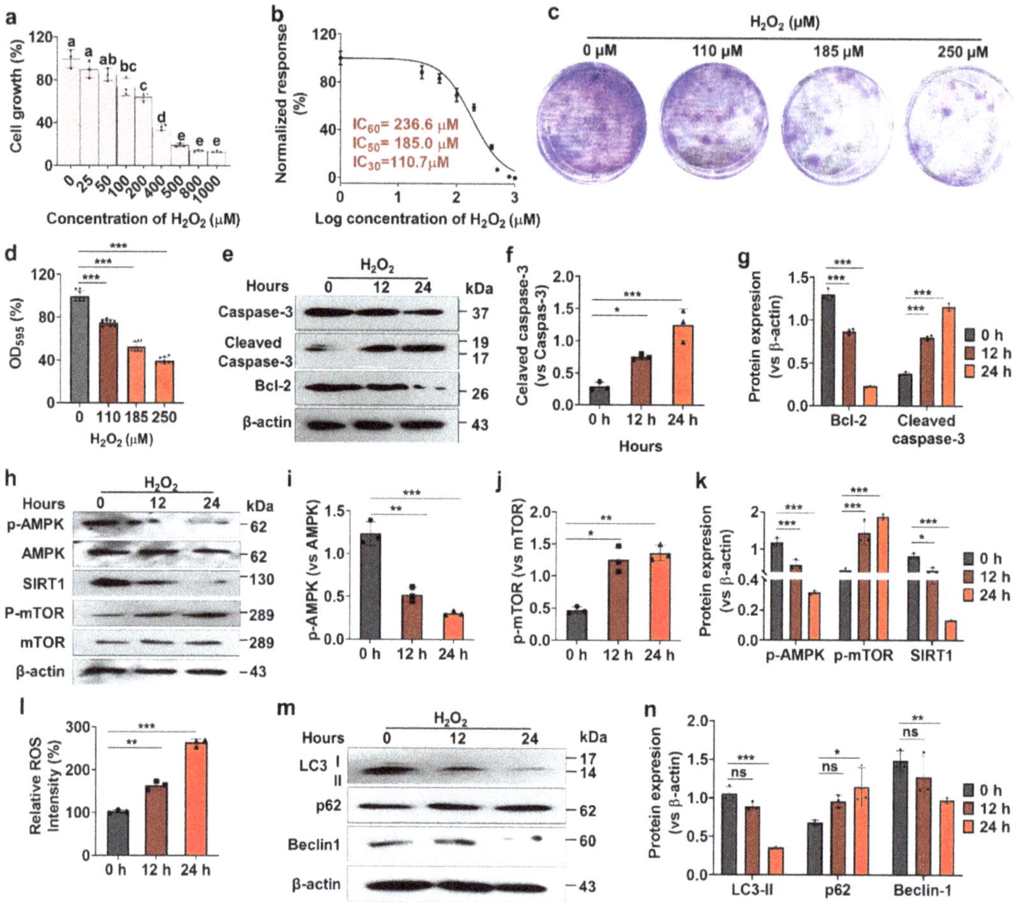

Figure 1. H_2O_2-induced oxidative stress decreases cell viability, increases ROS generation and cell death, and manipulates AMPK signaling and autophagy flux. (**a**) Cell growth rate following H_2O_2 treatment on hNPCs was assessed using the CCK-8 assay. Distinct letters indicate statistically significant variances. (**b**) The inhibitory concentration (IC) of H_2O_2 was determined to assess its cytotoxic effect on cells. (**c**) Clonogenic assay was employed to evaluate proliferative potential. (**d**) Proliferation ability was quantified using crystal violet by measuring absorbance at 590 nm. (**e**) Western blot analysis was conducted to detect protein levels of caspase-3, cleaved caspase-3, and Bcl-2 proteins. (**f**) Cleaved caspase-3/caspase-3 ratio. (**g**) Expression level of cleaved caspase-3 and Bcl-2 relative to β-actin. (**h**) Western blot analysis was performed to detect protein levels of p-AMPK, AMPK, SIRT1, p-mTOR, and mTOR. (**i**) p-AMPK/AMPK ratio. (**j**) p-mTOR/mTOR ratio. (**k**) Expression level of p-AMPK, SIRT1 and p-mTOR relative to β-actin. (**l**) Fluorescence intensity was analyzed using a fluorescence microplate spectrophotometer. (**m**) Western blot analysis was conducted to detect protein levels of LC-3I/II, p62, and Beclin-1. (**n**) Expression level of LC-3II, p62, and Beclin-1 relative to β-actin. h: hours. Values are presented as mean ± SD (n = 3 or >3), and statistical significance was determined using ordinary one-way ANOVA with Tukey's multiple comparisons in (**d**,**f**,**i**,**j**,**l**) and two-way ANOVA with Tukey's multiple comparisons in (**g**,**k**) and (**n**). * $p < 0.01$ ** $p < 0.001$, and *** $p < 0.0001$ were considered statistically significant. ns: not significant.

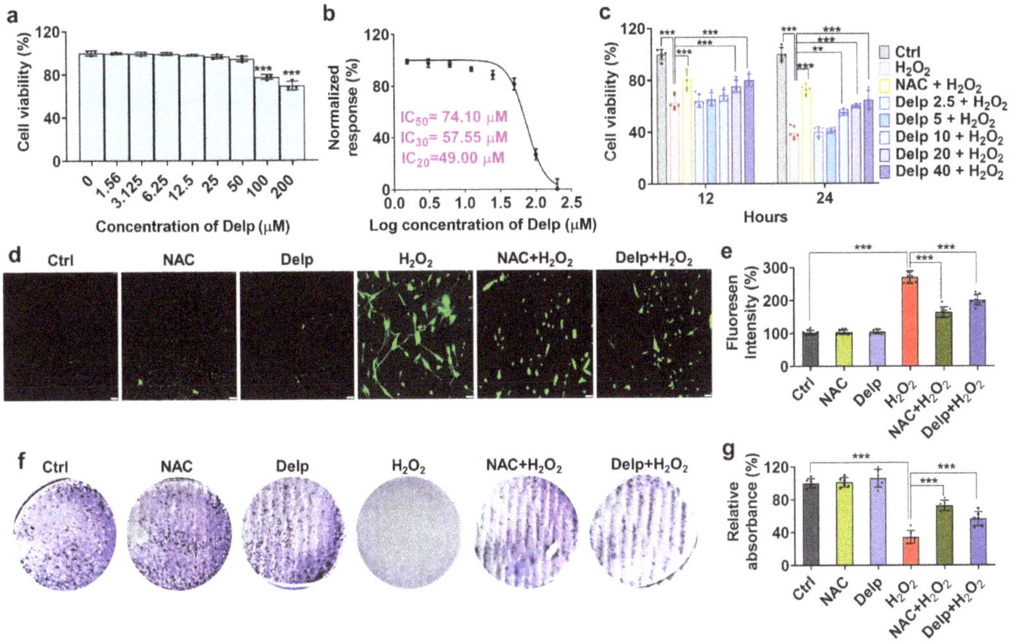

Figure 2. Delp increases cell viability and reduces oxidative stress in H_2O_2-treated hNPCs. (**a**) The cell growth rate following Delp treatment on hNPCs was assessed using the CCK-8 assay. (**b**) The inhibitory concentration (IC) of Delp was determined to identify an effective and safe dose for hNPCs. (**c**) Cell viability was evaluated using the CCK-8 assay with different doses of Delp (2.5, 5, 10, 20, and 40 μM) and 5 mM of NAC in 185 μM of H_2O_2 treated hNPCs at 12 and 24 h. (**d**) 2′,7′-dichlorodihydrofluorescein diacetate (DCFH2-DA) green fluorescence staining was performed to evaluate oxidative stress-induced ROS activity, with a scale bar of 50 μm. (**e**) Fluorescence intensity was analyzed using a fluorescence microplate spectrophotometer. (**f**) The clonogenic assay was utilized to assess proliferative potential. (**g**) Proliferation ability was quantified using crystal violet solution by measuring absorbance at 590 nm. Values are presented as mean ± SD (n = 3 or >3), and statistical significance was determined using ordinary one-way ANOVA with Tukey's multiple comparisons in (**a**,**e**,**g**), and two-way ANOVA with Tukey's multiple comparisons in (**c**). ** $p < 0.001$, and *** $p < 0.0001$ were considered statistically significant.

3.3. Confirmation of H_2O_2-Treated Oxidative Stress-Induced Senescence (OSIS) Model in hNPCs

We established an H_2O_2-induced oxidative stress-induced senescence (OSIS) model, which could serve as a valuable tool for comprehending the impact of Delp on cell growth and potentially studying intervertebral disc degeneration characterized by similar alterations in cell proliferation rates. In the OSIS model, we observed an increase in Cell Population Doubling Time (CPDT) (Figure 3a). Compared to the nOSIS control group, the OSIS control group exhibited a significant approximately 3- to 4-fold increase in CPDT (2.84 ± 0.10 vs. 10.40 ± 0.39 days, Figure 3a). Intriguingly, Delp substantially inhibited H_2O_2-induced CPDT by approximately 2-fold compared to the control (4.80 ± 1.69 vs. 10.40 ± 0.39 days, Figure 3a) in the OSIS model. However, when administering Delp in the nOSIS model, we did not observe any differences in CPDT compared to the control group (2.82 ± 0.08 vs. 2.84 ± 0.10 days, Figure 3a).

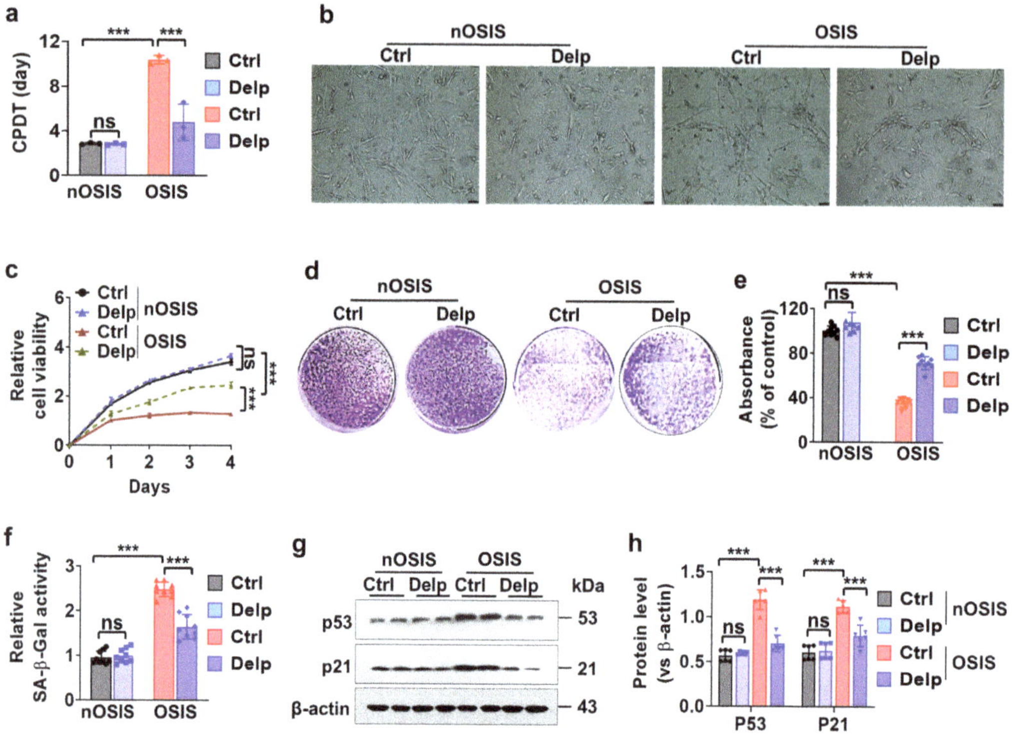

Figure 3. Delp induces cell proliferation and inhibits cellular senescence in OSIS hNPCs. (**a**) Cell population doubling time (CPDT) was determined to assess cellular aging. (**b**) Morphological evaluation was conducted under light microscopy, with a scale bar of 50 μm. (**c**) Relative cell viability was measured using the CCK-8 assay over a 4-day period. (**d**) The clonogenic assay was performed to evaluate proliferative potential. (**e**) The absorbance percentage of the blue-violet color at 590 nm was measured in the crystal violet assay. (**f**) Senescence activity was assessed using the senescence-associated-β-galactosidase (SA-β-gal) kit. (**g**) Western blot analysis was employed to evaluate the protein levels of p53 and p21. (**h**) Quantification of p53 and p21 protein levels relative to β-actin was conducted. Values are presented as mean ± SD (n = 3 or >3), and statistical significance was determined using ordinary one-way ANOVA with Tukey's multiple comparisons in (**a**,**c**,**e**,**f**), and two-way ANOVA with Tukey's multiple comparisons in (**h**). *** $p < 0.0001$ were considered statistically significant. ns: not significant.

Next, we examined the morphological changes of hNPCs in both nOSIS and OSIS models. In the nOSIS model, hNPCs displayed a spindle-shaped morphology, characteristic of actively proliferating cells (Figure 3b). Conversely, in the OSIS model, hNPCs underwent morphological alterations, transitioning from a spindle-like shape to enlarged, flattened, and irregular shapes, indicative of reduced cell growth rates (suggesting cellular senescence). Notably, Delp treatment significantly impeded this transition and maintained a spindle-like shape (Figure 3b).

Furthermore, the relative cell viability was notably reduced in the OSIS model, whereas Delp treatment significantly restored cell proliferation activity (Figure 3c). OSIS hNPCs exhibited substantially lower proliferation rates, as evidenced by diminished clonogenic cell growth (Figure 3d), indicating cellular senescence. Delp treatment significantly ameliorated the clonogenic survival capacity of OSIS hNPCs (Figure 3d,e).

Moreover, senescence-associated β-galactosidase (SA-β-Gal) activity was higher in the OSIS model, while Delp treatment resulted in lower SA-β-Gal activity (Figure 2f). SA-β-Gal is a widely used marker of cellular senescence, reflecting the presence of senescent cells. Additionally, we evaluated the expression levels of two key senescence-related proteins, p53 and p21, in OSIS hNPCs. Both p53 and p21 are established regulators of cellular senescence pathways. Western blot analysis revealed elevated expression of senescence markers, including p53 and p21, in H_2O_2-induced hNPCs (Figure 3g, h). Conversely, Delp pretreatment markedly reduced the expression of these markers (Figure 3g,h).

3.4. Delp Protects hNPCs from OSIS via Controlling ROS Production, ECM Synthesis, and Autophagy

We delved deeper into the effects of Delp therapy on OSIS in hNPCs, particularly focusing on its influence on cellular responses related to oxidative stress and autophagy, as well as its impact on IVDD phenotypes. Initially, we examined how Delp affected two crucial aspects of oxidative stress: superoxide dismutase (SOD) activity and reactive oxygen species (ROS) production. SOD serves as a vital antioxidant enzyme, neutralizing superoxide radicals to safeguard cells from oxidative damage. Our findings revealed a decrease in SOD activity in OSIS hNPCs compared to nOSIS conditions (Figure 4a), indicating diminished antioxidant capacity in OSIS cells, rendering them more vulnerable to oxidative damage. Remarkably, treatment with Delp significantly enhanced SOD activity in OSIS hNPCs (Figure 4a), suggesting an augmentation in the cells' ability to neutralize superoxide radicals, potentially mitigating oxidative stress-induced damage. Moreover, we observed ROS overproduction in OSIS hNPCs compared to nOSIS conditions (Figure 4b,c), a hallmark of oxidative stress. Notably, Delp treatment markedly attenuated ROS overproduction in OSIS hNPCs, indicating its potential to alleviate oxidative stress by reducing excessive ROS generation within the cells.

Subsequently, we investigated the role of autophagy in our senescence model, given its established role in mitigating oxidative stress. Our results revealed a significant reduction in autophagy activation in the OSIS model compared to nOSIS conditions (Figure 4d), suggesting an impaired autophagic process, possibly due to elevated oxidative stress or other cellular dysfunctions. However, treatment with Delp rescued autophagy flux in the OSIS model (Figure 4d), indicating its ability to restore or enhance the autophagic process under senescent conditions. Furthermore, we examined the expression levels of key autophagy-related proteins, LC3-I/II, Beclin-1, and p62, in OSIS hNPCs. Increasing expression levels of LC3 and Beclin-1, along with decreased expression of p62, signified significant restoration of autophagy activation in OSIS hNPCs upon Delp treatment (Figure 4e,f), suggesting that Delp-mediated rescue of autophagy flux may involve modulation of these key autophagy-related proteins.

Additionally, we explored the effect of Delp treatment on IVDD phenotypes using the OSIS model in hNPCs. We aimed to evaluate how Delp influences various molecular markers associated with IVDD. Our results demonstrated elevated levels of interleukin-1 beta (IL-1β), a pro-inflammatory cytokine implicated in IVDD pathology, in the OSIS model compared to nOSIS conditions (Figure 4g), indicative of increased inflammation associated with IVDD. However, treatment with Delp resulted in a reduction of IL-1β levels induced by oxidative stress (Figure 4g), suggesting its anti-inflammatory properties that may alleviate IVDD-related inflammation. Moreover, Western blot analysis revealed alterations in the expression levels of key ECM proteins associated with IVDD, including COL2A1, aggrecan, MMP-13, and ADAMTS-5, in the OSIS model. Delp treatment promoted COL2A1 and aggrecan expression while inhibiting MMP-13 and ADAMTS-5 expression in OSIS hNPCs (Figure 4h,i), indicating its potential to protect against IVDD by enhancing the synthesis of structural proteins and inhibiting enzymes responsible for disc degradation, thereby preserving disc integrity and function.

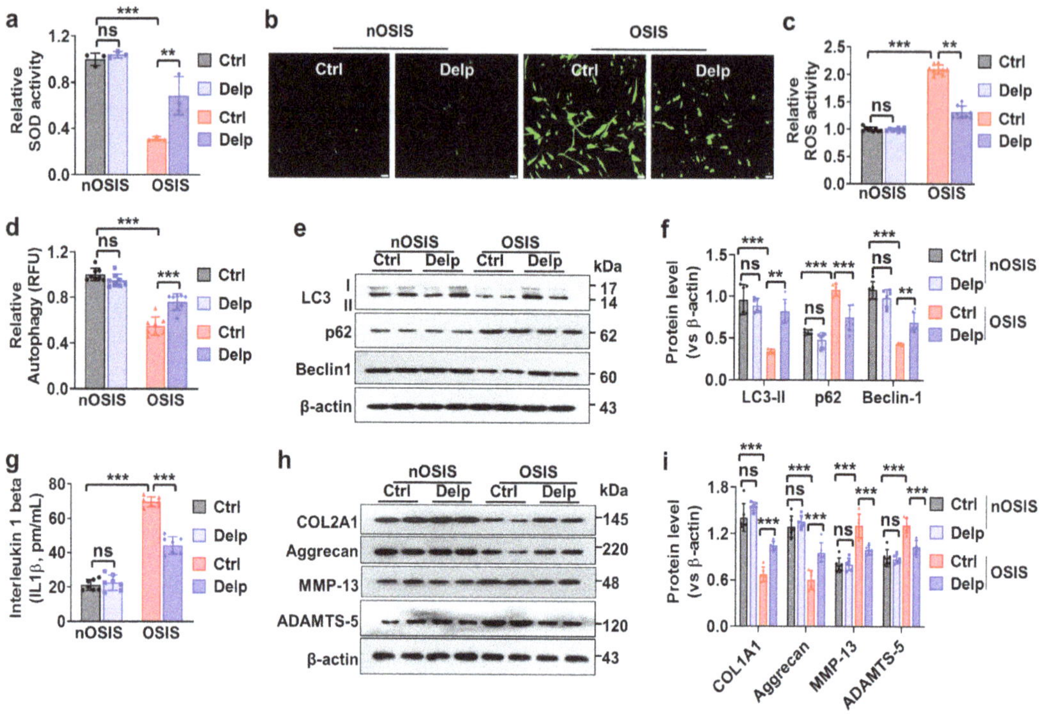

Figure 4. Delphinidin reduces oxidative stress and ECM degradation with increasing autophagy flux in OSIS hNPCs. (**a**) SOD activity was assessed to evaluate the antioxidant properties of Delp. (**b**) The green fluorescence staining of 2′,7′-dichlorodihydrofluorescein diacetate (DCFH2-DA) was performed to evaluate oxidative stress-induced ROS levels, with a scale bar of 50 μm. (**c**) Fluorescence intensity was analyzed using a fluorescence microplate spectrophotometer. (**d**) Relative autophagy flux was evaluated using an autophagy kit. (**e**) Western blot analysis was conducted to assess the expression of LC3-I/II, p62, and Beclin-1 proteins. (**f**) The expression levels of LC3-I/II, p62, and Beclin-1 proteins relative to β-actin were quantified. (**g**) The amount of interleukin 1 beta (IL-1β) was measured to evaluate IVDD phenotype in OSIS hNPCs. (**h**) Western blot analysis was performed to measure the expression of COL2A1, Aggrecan, MMP-13, and ADAMTS-5 proteins. (**i**) The expression levels of COL2A1, Aggrecan, MMP-13, and ADAMTS-5 proteins relative to β-actin were quantified. Values are presented as mean ± SD (n = 3 or >3), and statistical significance was determined using ordinary one-way ANOVA with Tukey's multiple comparisons in (**a**,**c**,**d**,**g**), and two-way ANOVA with Tukey's multiple comparisons in (**f**,**i**). ** $p < 0.001$, and *** $p < 0.0001$ were considered statistically significant. ns: not significant.

3.5. Autophagy Enhanced the Inhibitory Effect of Delp on the Senescence and ECM Degradation in OSIS hNPCs

To confirm the involvement of autophagy in cellular senescence and extracellular matrix (ECM) degradation in OSIS hNPCs, we employed chloroquine (CQ), a known autophagy inhibitor, to block the autophagic process and observe its effects on Delp-mediated autophagy activation and associated protein expression. Initially, Delp treatment activated autophagy in OSIS hNPCs, as evidenced by increased expression of key autophagy-related proteins such as Beclin-1, alongside decrease of p62 protein (Figure 5a–c). This indicates that Delp effectively induced autophagy in OSIS hNPCs, potentially contributing to cellular protection against oxidative stress and senescence. Subsequently, co-treatment of OSIS hNPCs with CQ abolished Delp-mediated autophagy activation, as evidenced by a significant reduction in the expression of Beclin-1 and the increased level of p62 protein (Figure 5a–c), suggesting that CQ effectively inhibited the autophagic process initiated by Delp, leading to the accumulation of autophagy-related proteins and disruption of autophagic flux.

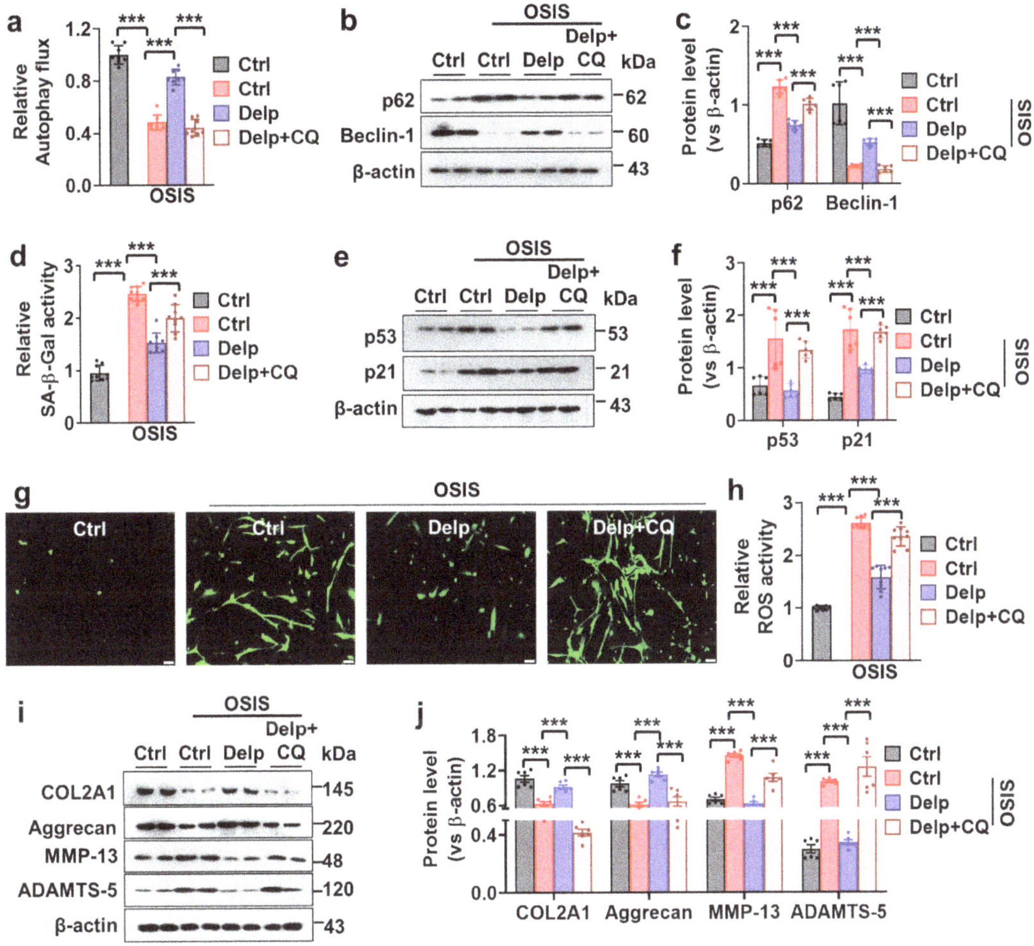

Figure 5. Inhibition of autophagy abolished the protective effect of Delp in OSIS hNPCs. (**a**) The reduction of Delp-induced autophagy by CQ treatment was assessed by evaluating the relative autophagy flux using an autophagy kit. (**b**) Western blot analysis was conducted to evaluate the expression levels of p62 and Beclin-1. (**c**) The expression levels of p62 and Beclin-1 proteins relative to β-actin were quantified. (**d**) Senescence activity was measured using a senescence-associated-β-galactosidase (SA-β-gal) kit. (**e**) Western blot analysis was performed to evaluate the protein levels of p53 and p21. (**f**) The expression levels of p53 and p21 proteins relative to β-actin were quantified. (**g**) The green fluorescence staining of 2′,7′-dichlorodihydrofluorescein diacetate (DCFH2-DA) was performed to evaluate oxidative stress-induced ROS levels, with a scale bar of 50 μm. (**h**) Fluorescence intensity was analyzed using a fluorescence microplate spectrophotometer. (**i**) Western blot analysis was conducted to measure the expression levels of COL2A1, Aggrecan, MMP-13, and ADAMTS-5 proteins. (**j**) The expression levels of COL2A1, Aggrecan, MMP-13, and ADAMTS-5 proteins relative to β-actin were quantified. Values are presented as mean ± SD ($n = 3$ or >3), and statistical significance was determined using ordinary one-way ANOVA with Tukey's multiple comparisons in (**a**,**d**,**h**), and two-way ANOVA with Tukey's multiple comparisons in (**c**,**f**,**j**). *** $p < 0.0001$ was considered statistically significant.

We continued our investigation into the role of autophagy in attenuating the cellular senescence of hNPCs subjected to OSIS. Inhibition of autophagy by CQ had significant consequences on several senescence-related parameters in OSIS hNPCs treated with Delp. Firstly, the attenuation of SA-β-Gal activity by Delp was reversed upon treatment with CQ (Figure 5d), indicating that the inhibition of autophagy by CQ interfered with the ability of Delp to attenuate cellular senescence. Additionally, Delp treatment effectively reduced the expression of p53 and p21 in the OSIS model, indicative of its ability to mitigate senescence-associated signaling pathways (Figure 5e,f). However, the inhibitory effect of Delp on p53 and p21 expression was significantly attenuated by CQ treatment, suggesting that the inhibition of autophagy compromises Delphinidin regulation of senescence-related protein expression in OSIS hNPCs (Figure 5e,f).

Furthermore, we explored how autophagy inhibition influenced the effects of Delp on ROS production in hNPCs subjected to OSIS. Delp treatment significantly reduced ROS overproduction in OSIS hNPCs, indicating its antioxidant properties and ability to mitigate oxidative stress-induced damage (Figure 5g,h). However, co-administration of CQ with Delp reversed the effect of Delp on ROS production (Figure 5g,h), suggesting that autophagy inhibition interferes with Delp's antioxidant mechanisms, leading to the restoration of ROS overproduction in OSIS hNPCs.

Finally, we investigated the impact of autophagy inhibition on the effects of Delp on IVDD phenotypes in OSIS hNPCs. Delp treatment promoted the expression of ECM synthesis proteins, such as COL2A1 and aggrecan, while inhibiting the expression of ECM degradation proteins, including MMP-13 and ADAMTS-5, in the OSIS model (Figure 5i,j), indicating its potential to promote ECM homeostasis and protect against IVDD. However, co-administration of Delp and CQ reversed the Delp-mediated effects on ECM homeostasis (Figure 5i,j), suggesting that autophagy inhibition interfered with Delp-dependent regulation of ECM synthesis and degradation proteins in OSIS hNPCs.

3.6. Activation of the AMPK Pathway Is Important for Delp-Induced Autophagy in the OSIS hNPCs

Based on our findings, it appears that treatment with chloroquine (CQ) reduces the autophagy induced by Delp in OSIS hNPCs, suggesting the crucial role of Delp-induced autophagy in its protective effect. We further explored the potential mechanisms underlying the autophagy-inducing effect of Delp in OSIS hNPCs. AMPK is recognized for its role in governing protective autophagy, enabling cells to counteract diverse stressors. By phosphorylating autophagy-related protein complexes, AMPK actively promotes autophagy across various regulatory stages. We hypothesized that Delp triggers autophagy in OSIS cells through activation of the AMPK signaling pathway. To investigate this hypothesis, we utilized compound C (CC), a potential inhibitor of AMPK, and AICAR, an analog of AMPK. As expected, like AICAR, Delp remarkably activated phosphorylated AMPK (p-AMPK) and SIRT1 proteins, while reducing phosphorylated mTOR (p-mTOR) protein expression in the OSIS hNPCs model (Figure 6a–d). Furthermore, Delp-mediated SIRT1/AMPK-mTOR activation was negated by CC treatment. Notably, the induction of autophagy by Delp was significantly diminished with CC treatment, evidenced by decreased levels of LC3-I/II and Beclin-1, along with elevated p62 protein expression in OSIS hNPCs (Figure 6e–g). These results strongly suggest that Delp-induced AMPK activation leads to autophagy activation in OSIS hNPCs. Moreover, our data revealed that AMPK activation by either AICAR or Delp notably reduced the overproduction of reactive oxygen species (ROS), whereas CC treatment increased ROS production suppressed by Delp (Figure 6h,i). Moreover, inhibition of the AMPK signaling pathway by CC markedly induced the attenuation of SA-β-gal activity in OSIS hNPCs (Figure 6j). Correspondingly, Western blot data indicated that CC treatment reversed the effects of Delp on the expression of senescence proteins p53 and p21 in the OSIS model (Figure 6j,k). Additionally, the Western blot analysis of IVDD candidate proteins showed significant reductions in COL2A1 and Aggrecan in the Delp plus CC-treated group, alongside increases in MMP-13 and ADAMTS-5 (Figure 6l,m). These findings underscore the critical role of AMPK signaling in mediating the effects of Delp on autophagy, ROS production, and senescence in OSIS hNPCs, highlighting its potential as a therapeutic target for IVDD. Taken together, our findings indicate that Delp activates autophagy through AMPK and reduces oxidative stress-induced senescence and IVDD phenotypes.

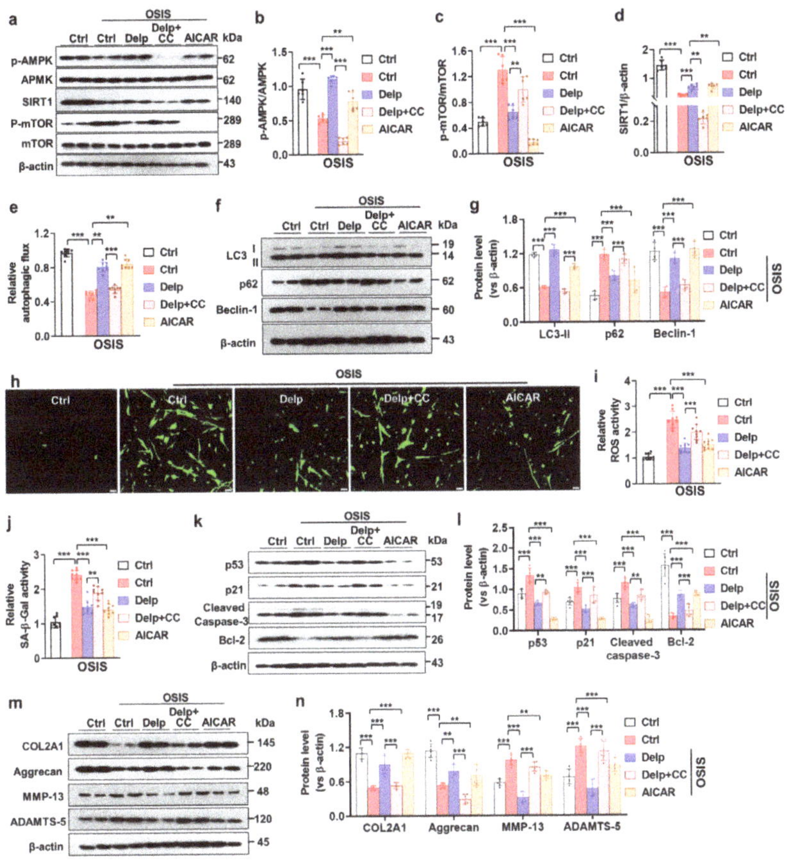

Figure 6. The AMPK pathway mediates Delp-induced autophagy in OSIS hNPCs. (**a**) Protein levels of p-AMPK, AMPK, SIRT1, p-mTOR, and mTOR were assessed using Western blot analysis. (**b**) The ratios of phospho-AMPK to AMPK were calculated. (**c**) The ratios of phospho-mTOR to mTOR were determined. (**d**) The expression level of SIRT1 relative to β-actin was quantified. (**e**) The relative autophagy flux was measured to assess the effect of CC on Delp-induced autophagy. (**f**) Western blot analysis was performed to evaluate the expression levels of LC3-I/II, p62, and Beclin-1. (**g**) The expression levels of LC3-II, p62, and Beclin-1 relative to β-actin were quantified. (**h**) 2′,7′-dichlorodihydrofluorescein diacetate (DCFH2-DA) staining was used to evaluate oxidative stress-induced ROS, with a scale bar of 50 µm. (**i**) Fluorescence intensity was analyzed using a fluorescence microplate spectrophotometer. (**j**) Senescence activity was measured using a senescence-associated-β-galactosidase (SA-β-gal) kit. (**k**) Western blot analysis was conducted to evaluate the protein levels of p53, p21, cleaved caspase-3, and Bcl-2. (**l**) The expression levels of p53, p21, cleaved caspase-3, and Bcl-2 relative to β-actin were quantified. (**m**) Protein levels of COL2A1, Aggrecan, MMP-13, and ADAMTS-5 were assessed using Western blot analysis. (**n**) The expression levels of COL2A1, Aggrecan, MMP-13, and ADAMTS-5 relative to β-actin were quantified. Values are presented as mean ± SD (n = 3 or >3), and statistical significance was determined using ordinary one-way ANOVA with Tukey's multiple comparisons in (**b–e**,**i**,**j**), and two-way ANOVA with Tukey's multiple comparisons in (**g**,**l**,**n**). ** $p < 0.001$, and *** $p < 0.0001$ were considered statistically significant.

4. Discussion

Our study demonstrated that Delp exerts antioxidant effects by mitigating ROS-induced oxidative stress and cellular senescence in human IVD NPC cells. Moreover, Delp simultaneously induces autophagy, fostering cell growth and ECM synthesis while suppressing ROS overproduction and cellular senescence. Inhibition of autophagy using CQ in hNPCs diminished the protective effect of Delphinidin on ROS overproduction, cellular senescence, and ECM degradation. This protective autophagy induction by Delp is mediated via the activation of the SIRT1/AMPK-mTOR signaling pathway in hNPCs.

Hydrogen peroxide (H_2O_2) was selected as a ROS inducer to simulate an in vitro oxidative stress condition in our study. We established an "H_2O_2-induced OSIS" model to investigate the effects of Delp on cell growth under oxidative stress conditions relevant to IVDD. This model is tailored to mimic oxidative stress-induced conditions in IVDD, providing insights into how Delp influences cell growth under such circumstances.

Oxidative stress, driven by ROS generation, triggers redox imbalance and lipid peroxidation, contributing to cellular cytotoxicity when exceeding the cell's repair capacity [26]. In degenerative disorders lacking sufficient antioxidant defense mechanisms, ROS production substantially disrupts cell homeostasis, leading to the accumulation of damaged DNA with molecular alterations [27]. Delphinidin, a polyphenol from the anthocyanin group, has been shown in previous studies to protect against age-related oxidative stress, playing a critical role in preventing osteoarthritis development and progression [28–31]. Consistent with prior reports, our study demonstrated the cytoprotective effect of Delp against oxidative stress, highlighting its potential as a clinical cytoprotective agent.

Prolonged ROS release induces oxidative stress, triggering premature senescence, apoptosis, and eventual cell death [32]. In our study, Delp modulated SA-β-gal enzymatic activity and regulated the expression of senescence-related proteins p53 and p21, mediating cell growth through a cytoprotective pathway. Autophagy initiation has been suggested to protect against apoptosis in IVDD, underscoring its cytoprotective role [33,34]. While current research predominantly supports autophagy's preventive role in IVDD, some studies suggest its potential to accelerate the condition [35]. Autophagy reduces NP cell apoptosis, ECM degradation, senescence, and CEP inflammation and calcification, maintaining IVD ECM balance to prevent IVDD [36–40].

Numerous signaling pathways regulate autophagy induction, with AMP-activated protein kinase (AMPK) being a key player impacted by ROS. AMPK serves as a significant indicator of cellular energy status and a central regulator of autophagy and lysosomal activity [41]. Several natural compounds regulate autophagy through the AMPK pathway in NP cells against oxidative stress-induced senescence, ECM degradation, and apoptosis [42–44]. Our study explored the molecular mechanism of Delp-induced autophagy and its relationship with the AMPK pathway. Delp upregulated SIRT1 function upstream of AMPK phosphorylation, affecting mTOR phosphorylation downstream of AMPK, thereby rescuing autophagy. Compound C, an AMPK inhibitor, notably reduced Delp-mediated autophagy activation [45]. This highlights its protective effect on hNPCs through the AMPK pathway, linking cell proliferation and autophagy induction. Further in vivo experiments are warranted to validate these findings.

5. Conclusions

This study presents the initial evidence suggesting that Delp has the potential to safeguard hNP cells against senescence, apoptosis, and ECM degradation induced by oxidative stress-driven ROS overload by activating autophagy. This protective effect is likely mediated through the ROS–AMPK–mTOR axis, as illustrated in Figure 7. The emerging therapeutic role of Delp in combating oxidative stress in hNPCs could pave the way for novel treatment strategies of IVDD. Nevertheless, the exact mechanism underlying Delphinidin action requires further investigation, and these findings need validation in in vivo settings.

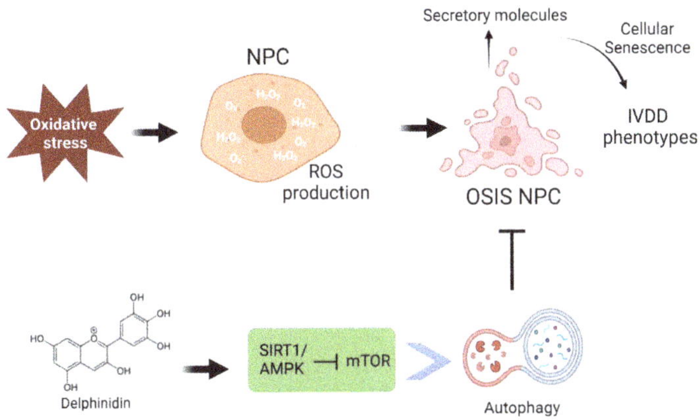

Figure 7. The proposed molecular mechanism involved in Delphinidin treatment in OSIS hNPCs. Hydrogen peroxide (H_2O_2) serves as a source of reactive oxygen species (ROS), inducing oxidative stress conditions and mimicking intervertebral disc degeneration (IVDD) phenotypes in human nucleus pulposus cells (hNPCs), leading to a state of oxidative stress-induced senescence (OSIS). Delphinidin (Delp) mitigated OSIS in H_2O_2-exposed hNPCs by enhancing cellular autophagy through activation of the SIRT1/AMPK/mTOR axis.

Supplementary Materials: The following supporting information can be downloaded at: https://www.mdpi.com/article/10.3390/antiox13070759/s1.

Author Contributions: M.E.B. conceptualized, performed experiments, wrote the manuscript, provided financial support, and created all original figures. J.S.H. edited the manuscript and analyzed data. T.H.L. edited the manuscript. J.-H.B. edited the manuscript. D.-H.K. edited the manuscript and provided financial support. D.R.K. conceptualized, provided financial support, edited all figures, and contributed to writing the manuscript. All authors have read and agreed to the published version of the manuscript.

Funding: This study was supported by grants from the Basic Science Research Program through the National Research Foundation of Korea (RS-2023-00219399, RS-2023-00238051) and by the National Research Foundation of Korea (NRF) grant funded by the Ministry of Education, Science, and Technology (2021R1F1A1059969).

Institutional Review Board Statement: Not applicable.

Informed Consent Statement: Not applicable.

Data Availability Statement: Data is contained within the article and Supplementary Materials.

Acknowledgments: We thank all the lab members for their thoughtful feedback on this study.

Conflicts of Interest: The authors declare no conflict of interest.

References

1. Feng, C.; Yang, M.; Lan, M.; Liu, C.; Zhang, Y.; Huang, B.; Liu, H.; Zhou, Y. ROS: Crucial Intermediators in the Pathogenesis of Intervertebral Disc Degeneration. *Oxid. Med. Cell Longev.* **2017**, *2017*, 5601593. [CrossRef]
2. Cao, G.; Yang, S.; Cao, J.; Tan, Z.; Wu, L.; Dong, F.; Ding, W.; Zhang, F. The Role of Oxidative Stress in Intervertebral Disc Degeneration. *Oxid. Med. Cell Longev.* **2022**, *2022*, 2166817. [CrossRef]
3. Kim, K.W.; Chung, H.N.; Ha, K.Y.; Lee, J.S.; Kim, Y.Y. Senescence mechanisms of nucleus pulposus chondrocytes in human intervertebral discs. *Spine J.* **2009**, *9*, 658–666. [CrossRef]
4. Silwal, P.; Nguyen-Thai, A.M.; Mohammad, H.A.; Wang, Y.; Robbins, P.D.; Lee, J.Y.; Vo, N.V. Cellular Senescence in Intervertebral Disc Aging and Degeneration: Molecular Mechanisms and Potential Therapeutic Opportunities. *Biomolecules* **2023**, *13*, 686. [CrossRef]
5. Dimozi, A.; Mavrogonatou, E.; Sklirou, A.; Kletsas, D. Oxidative stress inhibits the proliferation, induces premature senescence and promotes a catabolic phenotype in human nucleus pulposus intervertebral disc cells. *Eur. Cell Mater.* **2015**, *30*, 89–102; discussion 103. [CrossRef]

6. Krupkova, O.; Handa, J.; Hlavna, M.; Klasen, J.; Ospelt, C.; Ferguson, S.J.; Wuertz-Kozak, K. The Natural Polyphenol Epigallocatechin Gallate Protects Intervertebral Disc Cells from Oxidative Stress. *Oxid. Med. Cell Longev.* **2016**, *2016*, 7031397. [CrossRef] [PubMed]
7. Zhou, N.; Lin, X.; Dong, W.; Huang, W.; Jiang, W.; Lin, L.; Qiu, Q.; Zhang, X.; Shen, J.; Song, Z.; et al. SIRT1 alleviates senescence of degenerative human intervertebral disc cartilage endo-plate cells via the p53/p21 pathway. *Sci. Rep.* **2016**, *6*, 22628. [CrossRef]
8. Xu, J.; Li, H.; Yang, K.; Guo, S.; Wang, J.; Feng, C.; Chen, H. Hyper-osmolarity environment-induced oxidative stress injury promotes nucleus pulposus cell senescence in vitro. *Biosci. Rep.* **2019**, *39*, BSR20191711. [CrossRef]
9. Tossetta, G.; Fantone, S.; Licini, C.; Marzioni, D.; Mattioli-Belmonte, M. The multifaced role of HtrA1 in the development of joint and skeletal disorders. *Bone* **2022**, *157*, 116350. [CrossRef] [PubMed]
10. Shnayder, N.A.; Ashhotov, A.V.; Trefilova, V.V.; Novitsky, M.A.; Medvedev, G.V.; Petrova, M.M.; Narodova, E.A.; Kaskaeva, D.S.; Chumakova, G.A.; Garganeeva, N.P.; et al. High-Tech Methods of Cytokine Imbalance Correction in Intervertebral Disc Degeneration. *Int. J. Mol. Sci.* **2023**, *24*, 3333. [CrossRef] [PubMed]
11. Costachescu, B.; Niculescu, A.G.; Teleanu, R.I.; Iliescu, B.F.; Radulescu, M.; Grumezescu, A.M.; Dabija, M.G. Recent Advances in Managing Spinal Intervertebral Discs Degeneration. *Int. J. Mol. Sci.* **2022**, *23*, 6460. [CrossRef] [PubMed]
12. Filomeni, G.; De Zio, D.; Cecconi, F. Oxidative stress and autophagy: The clash between damage and metabolic needs. *Cell Death Differ.* **2015**, *22*, 377–388. [CrossRef] [PubMed]
13. Li, Z.; Shao, Z.; Chen, S.; Huang, D.; Peng, Y.; Chen, S.; Ma, K. TIGAR impedes compression-induced intervertebral disc degeneration by suppressing nucleus pulposus cell apoptosis and autophagy. *J. Cell Physiol.* **2020**, *235*, 1780–1794. [CrossRef] [PubMed]
14. Lee, D.Y.; Bahar, M.E.; Kim, C.W.; Seo, M.S.; Song, M.G.; Song, S.Y.; Kim, S.Y.; Kim, D.R.; Kim, D.H. Autophagy in Osteoarthritis: A Double-Edged Sword in Cartilage Aging and Mechanical Stress Response: A Systematic Review. *J. Clin. Med.* **2024**, *13*, 5. [CrossRef] [PubMed]
15. Bi, X.; Zhang, J.; Chen, C.; Zhang, D.; Li, P.; Ma, F. Anthocyanin contributes more to hydrogen peroxide scavenging than other phenolics in apple peel. *Food Chem.* **2014**, *152*, 205–209. [CrossRef] [PubMed]
16. Blando, F.; Calabriso, N.; Berland, H.; Maiorano, G.; Gerardi, C.; Carluccio, M.A.; Andersen, O.M. Radical Scavenging and Anti-Inflammatory Activities of Representative Anthocyanin Groupings from Pigment-Rich Fruits and Vegetables. *Int. J. Mol. Sci.* **2018**, *19*, 169. [CrossRef] [PubMed]
17. Bai, X.; Jiang, M.; Wang, J.; Yang, S.; Liu, Z.; Zhang, H.; Zhu, X. Cyanidin attenuates the apoptosis of rat nucleus pulposus cells and the degeneration of intervertebral disc via the JAK2/STAT3 signal pathway in vitro and in vivo. *Pharm. Biol.* **2022**, *60*, 427–436. [CrossRef] [PubMed]
18. Lee, D.Y.; Park, Y.J.; Song, M.G.; Kim, D.R.; Zada, S.; Kim, D.H. Cytoprotective Effects of Delphinidin for Human Chondrocytes against Oxidative Stress through Activation of Autophagy. *Antioxidants* **2020**, *9*, 83. [CrossRef] [PubMed]
19. Haseeb, A.; Chen, D.; Haqqi, T.M. Delphinidin inhibits IL-1beta-induced activation of NF-kappaB by modulating the phosphorylation of IRAK-1(Ser376) in human articular chondrocytes. *Rheumatology* **2013**, *52*, 998–1008. [CrossRef]
20. Maharajan, N.; Ganesan, C.D.; Moon, C.; Jang, C.H.; Oh, W.K.; Cho, G.W. Licochalcone D Ameliorates Oxidative Stress-Induced Senescence via AMPK Activation. *Int. J. Mol. Sci.* **2021**, *22*, 7324. [CrossRef]
21. Wang, Z.; Wei, D.; Xiao, H. Methods of cellular senescence induction using oxidative stress. *Methods Mol. Biol.* **2013**, *1048*, 135–144. [CrossRef] [PubMed]
22. Chen, J.H.; Stoeber, K.; Kingsbury, S.; Ozanne, S.E.; Williams, G.H.; Hales, C.N. Loss of proliferative capacity and induction of senescence in oxidatively stressed human fibroblasts. *J. Biol. Chem.* **2004**, *279*, 49439–49446. [CrossRef]
23. Strober, W. Trypan Blue Exclusion Test of Cell Viability. *Curr. Protoc. Immunol.* **2015**, *111*, A3.B.1–A3.B.3. [CrossRef] [PubMed]
24. Stolzing, A.; Jones, E.; McGonagle, D.; Scutt, A. Age-related changes in human bone marrow-derived mesenchymal stem cells: Consequences for cell therapies. *Mech. Ageing Dev.* **2008**, *129*, 163–173. [CrossRef] [PubMed]
25. Yang, Y.K.; Ogando, C.R.; Wang See, C.; Chang, T.Y.; Barabino, G.A. Changes in phenotype and differentiation potential of human mesenchymal stem cells aging in vitro. *Stem Cell Res. Ther.* **2018**, *9*, 131. [CrossRef] [PubMed]
26. Bhattacharyya, A.; Chattopadhyay, R.; Mitra, S.; Crowe, S.E. Oxidative stress: An essential factor in the pathogenesis of gastrointestinal mucosal diseases. *Physiol. Rev.* **2014**, *94*, 329–354. [CrossRef]
27. Afzal, S.; Abdul Manap, A.S.; Attiq, A.; Albokhadaim, I.; Kandeel, M.; Alhojaily, S.M. From imbalance to impairment: The central role of reactive oxygen species in oxidative stress-induced disorders and therapeutic exploration. *Front. Pharmacol.* **2023**, *14*, 1269581. [CrossRef]
28. Ritschel, W.A.; Agrawala, P.; Kappes, J.K.; Kraeling, M.; Hussain, S.A. Effect of age on the pharmacokinetics of coumarin. *Arzneimittelforschung* **1988**, *38*, 1466–1468.
29. Noda, Y.; Kaneyuki, T.; Mori, A.; Packer, L. Antioxidant activities of pomegranate fruit extract and its anthocyanidins: Delphinidin, cyanidin, and pelargonidin. *J. Agric. Food Chem.* **2002**, *50*, 166–171. [CrossRef]
30. Chen, C.Y.; Yi, L.; Jin, X.; Mi, M.T.; Zhang, T.; Ling, W.H.; Yu, B. Delphinidin attenuates stress injury induced by oxidized low-density lipoprotein in human umbilical vein endothelial cells. *Chem. Biol. Interact.* **2010**, *183*, 105–112. [CrossRef]
31. Jin, X.; Chen, M.; Yi, L.; Chang, H.; Zhang, T.; Wang, L.; Ma, W.; Peng, X.; Zhou, Y.; Mi, M. Delphinidin-3-glucoside protects human umbilical vein endothelial cells against oxidized low-density lipoprotein-induced injury by autophagy upregulation via the AMPK/SIRT1 signaling pathway. *Mol. Nutr. Food Res.* **2014**, *58*, 1941–1951. [CrossRef] [PubMed]

32. Schieber, M.; Chandel, N.S. ROS function in redox signaling and oxidative stress. *Curr. Biol.* **2014**, *24*, R453–R462. [CrossRef]
33. Kritschil, R.; Scott, M.; Sowa, G.; Vo, N. Role of autophagy in intervertebral disc degeneration. *J. Cell Physiol.* **2022**, *237*, 1266–1284. [CrossRef] [PubMed]
34. Luo, J.; Yang, Y.; Wang, X.; Chang, X.; Fu, S. Role of Pyroptosis in Intervertebral Disc Degeneration and Its Therapeutic Implications. *Biomolecules* **2022**, *12*, 1804. [CrossRef] [PubMed]
35. Bahar, M.E.; Hwang, J.S.; Ahmed, M.; Lai, T.H.; Pham, T.M.; Elashkar, O.; Akter, K.M.; Kim, D.H.; Yang, J.; Kim, D.R. Targeting Autophagy for Developing New Therapeutic Strategy in Intervertebral Disc Degeneration. *Antioxidants* **2022**, *11*, 1571. [CrossRef] [PubMed]
36. Zheng, G.; Pan, Z.; Zhan, Y.; Tang, Q.; Zheng, F.; Zhou, Y.; Wu, Y.; Zhou, Y.; Chen, D.; Chen, J.; et al. TFEB protects nucleus pulposus cells against apoptosis and senescence via restoring autophagic flux. *Osteoarthr. Cartil.* **2019**, *27*, 347–357. [CrossRef]
37. Jiang, W.; Zhang, X.; Hao, J.; Shen, J.; Fang, J.; Dong, W.; Wang, D.; Zhang, X.; Shui, W.; Luo, Y.; et al. SIRT1 protects against apoptosis by promoting autophagy in degenerative human disc nucleus pulposus cells. *Sci. Rep.* **2014**, *4*, 7456. [CrossRef] [PubMed]
38. Gong, C.Y.; Zhang, H.H. Autophagy as a potential therapeutic target in intervertebral disc degeneration. *Life Sci.* **2021**, *273*, 119266. [CrossRef] [PubMed]
39. Chen, J.; Xie, J.J.; Jin, M.Y.; Gu, Y.T.; Wu, C.C.; Guo, W.J.; Yan, Y.Z.; Zhang, Z.J.; Wang, J.L.; Zhang, X.L.; et al. Sirt6 overexpression suppresses senescence and apoptosis of nucleus pulposus cells by inducing autophagy in a model of intervertebral disc degeneration. *Cell Death Dis.* **2018**, *9*, 56. [CrossRef]
40. Chen, J.W.; Ni, B.B.; Li, B.; Yang, Y.H.; Jiang, S.D.; Jiang, L.S. The responses of autophagy and apoptosis to oxidative stress in nucleus pulposus cells: Implications for disc degeneration. *Cell Physiol. Biochem.* **2014**, *34*, 1175–1189. [CrossRef]
41. Agostini, F.; Bisaglia, M.; Plotegher, N. Linking ROS Levels to Autophagy: The Key Role of AMPK. *Antioxidants* **2023**, *12*, 1406. [CrossRef] [PubMed]
42. Xie, C.; Shi, Y.; Chen, Z.; Zhou, X.; Luo, P.; Hong, C.; Tian, N.; Wu, Y.; Zhou, Y.; Lin, Y.; et al. Apigenin Alleviates Intervertebral Disc Degeneration via Restoring Autophagy Flux in Nucleus Pulposus Cells. *Front. Cell Dev. Biol.* **2021**, *9*, 787278. [CrossRef] [PubMed]
43. Wang, X.H.; Zhu, L.; Hong, X.; Wang, Y.T.; Wang, F.; Bao, J.P.; Xie, X.H.; Liu, L.; Wu, X.T. Resveratrol attenuated TNF-alpha-induced MMP-3 expression in human nucleus pulposus cells by activating autophagy via AMPK/SIRT1 signaling pathway. *Exp. Biol. Med.* **2016**, *241*, 848–853. [CrossRef]
44. Chen, Y.; Zheng, Z.; Wang, J.; Tang, C.; Khor, S.; Chen, J.; Chen, X.; Zhang, Z.; Tang, Q.; Wang, C.; et al. Berberine suppresses apoptosis and extracellular matrix (ECM) degradation in nucleus pulposus cells and ameliorates disc degeneration in a rodent model. *Int. J. Biol. Sci.* **2018**, *14*, 682–692. [CrossRef]
45. Gao, S.; Li, N.; Chen, R.; Su, Y.; Song, Y.; Liang, S. Bushen Huoxue Formula Modulates Autophagic Flux and Inhibits Apoptosis to Protect Nucleus Pulposus Cells by Restoring the AMPK/SIRT1 Pathway. *Biomed. Res. Int.* **2022**, *2022*, 8929448. [CrossRef]

antioxidants

MDPI

Article

The Probiotic Yeast, Milmed, Promotes Autophagy and Antioxidant Pathways in BV-2 Microglia Cells and *C. elegans*

Federica Armeli [1,2], Beatrice Mengoni [1], Emily Schifano [3], Thomas Lenz [4], Trevor Archer [4], Daniela Uccelletti [3,5] and Rita Businaro [1,*]

1 Department of Medico-Surgical Sciences and Biotechnologies, Sapienza University of Rome, 04100 Latina, Italy; federica.armeli@uniroma1.it (F.A.); beatrice.mengoni@uniroma1.it (B.M.)
2 Department of Human Sciences, European University of Rome, 00163 Rome, Italy
3 Department of Biology and Biotechnologies "C. Darwin", Sapienza University of Rome, 00185 Rome, Italy; emily.schifano@uniroma1.it (E.S.); daniela.uccelletti@uniroma1.it (D.U.)
4 Milmed Unico AB, 11139 Stockholm, Sweden; thomas.lenz@milmed.se (T.L.); trevorcsarcher49@gmail.com (T.A.)
5 NMR-Based Metabolomics Laboratory (NMLab), Sapienza University of Rome, 00185 Rome, Italy
* Correspondence: rita.businaro@uniroma1.it

Abstract: Background: Autophagy, a catabolic process essential for maintaining cellular homeostasis, declines with age and unhealthy lifestyles, contributing to neurodegenerative diseases. Probiotics, including Milmed yeast, have demonstrated anti-inflammatory and antioxidant properties. This study evaluated the activity of Milmed on BV-2 microglial cells in vitro and in the in vivo model of *Caenorhabditis elegans* (*C. elegans*) in restoring autophagic processes. **Methods:** BV-2 microglial cells were incubated with *S. cerevisiae* (Milmed treated yeast or untreated yeast) and then stimulated with lipopolysaccharide (LPS). mRNAs of the autophagic factors and antioxidant enzymes were assessed by qPCR; mTOR and NRF2 were evaluated by ELISA. pNRF2 compared with cytosolic NRF2 was evaluated by immunofluorescence. The longevity, body size, and reactive oxygen species (ROS) levels of *C. elegans* were measured by fluorescence microscopy. **Results:** Treatment with Milmed YPD cultured yeast or the dried powder obtained from it promoted autophagic flux, as shown by the increased expression of the *Beclin-1*, *ATG7*, *LC3*, and *p62* mRNAs and the inhibition of mTOR, as evaluated by ELISA. It also enhanced the antioxidant response by increasing the expression of *NRF2*, *SOD1*, and *GPX*; moreover, pNRF2 expression compared with cytosolic NRF2 expression was enhanced, as shown by immunofluorescence. Milmed dietary supplementation prolonged the survival of *C. elegans* and reduced the age-related ROS accumulation without changing the expression of *gst-4*. The pro-longevity effect was found to be dependent on SKN-1/Nrf2 activation, as shown by the absence of benefit in *skn-1* mutants. **Conclusions:** Milmed yeast demonstrates significant pro-autophagy and antioxidant activity with significant pro-longevity effects in *C. elegans*, thereby extending the lifespan and improving stress resistance, which, together with the previously demonstrated anti-inflammatory activity, highlights its role as a highly effective probiotic for its beneficial health effects. Activation of the SKN-1/NRF2 pathway and the modulation of autophagy support the therapeutic potential of Milmed in neuroprotection and healthy aging.

Keywords: yeast; microglia; neuroinflammation; autophagy; oxidative stress; NRF2; *Caenorhabditis elegans*; probiotic; longevity; ROS

1. Introduction

Autophagy, as an evolution-restricted, lysosome-dependent catabolic process present in all eukaryotic cells, plays an essential maintenance role in the homeostatic response to stress and other extrinsic and intrinsic strains placed upon an organism, promoting cell survival and degrading damaged and dysfunctional intracellular organelles [1–3]. Nevertheless, autophagic efficacy deteriorates with advancing age, sedentary lifestyle and unrestricted, nonselective nutrition leading to chronic disease states such as obesity, sarcopenia, type 2 diabetes, inflammaging, and oxidative stress [4–6]. Neuronal survival, homeostatic processes, and the regulation of nutrient uptake and energy balance necessitate an ongoing autophagy [7,8]. The links between autophagy and aging processes have been established in longevity models of *Caenorhabditis elegans* whereby neurodegenerative propensities and a decline in health parameters and longevity are associated with compromised autophagy with concomitant expressions of inflammaging and oxidative stress [9].

Probiotic agents, living microorganisms with minimal or the absence of adverse reactions, have been applied for the treatment of a wide range of disease/disorder states as well as offering generalized health benefits and protective advantages [10–12]. It has been shown that probiotics induce health-enhancing effects by engaging a variety of mechanisms including lowering the intestinal pH, decreasing colonization and invasion by pathogenic organisms, and modifying the host immune response. In this context, it has been implied that probiotics may redress existing bacterial-fungal gut microbiome actions, thereby reducing the inflammatory and/or toxic propensities [13–15]. These agents have been shown to induce preventative/protective actions in several animal models of tissue disorder including intestinal damage, intestinal injury gastroenteritis, cardiovascular tissue damage, and improved renal function following injury [16–19]. The probiotic, *Lactiplantibacillus plantarum* NJAU-01, was found to produce ameliorative effects upon D-galactose-induced hepatic oxidative stress through the induction of the hepatic total antioxidant capacity and antioxidant enzyme activities involved in superoxide dismutase, glutathione peroxidase, and catalase [20]. In a systematic review presenting the beneficial effects of probiotics through the promotion of autophagy and a comparison of the intestinal cell lines and/or tissue with other types of cell lines and tissue, Nemati et al. (2021) postulated that autophagy effectively describes a viable mechanism to describe the health benefits of probiotic actions over a range of tissue substrates [21]. An effective yeast probiotic, a *Saccharomyces cerevisiae* strain isolated from a traditional Korean fermentation initiator, was found to reduce the levels of interleukin-1β and interferon-γ. Furthermore, the probiotic yeast, *Saccharomyces boulardii*, was administered to transgenic APP/PS1 mice expressing neuroinflammation arising from activated microglia and the toll-like receptor pathway; this treatment alleviated dysbiosis and improved cognitive impairment [15]. Yeasts have contributed to the understanding of fundamental aspects of lifespan regulation including the roles of nutrient response, global protein translation rates and quality, DNA damage, oxidative stress, mitochondrial function and dysfunction as well as autophagy [22].

It was previously found that the treated yeast, Milmed, exerted both neuroprotective and neurorestorative effects both functionally and neurochemically in a lower, repeated dose, progressive administration of -methyl-4-phenyl-1,2,3,6-tetrahydropyridine (MPTP), a selective dopamine neurotoxin, as a laboratory animal model of Parkinson's disease [23,24]. Yeast cells that have undergone treatment with millimeter-wavelength electromagnetic waves (range: 1 GHz to 300 GHz), so-called Milmed, were found to exert a high level of anti-allergy efficacy among suffering patients [25]. Furthermore, patients presenting with irritable bowel syndrome and symptoms of inflammatory bowel disease (IBS-IBD) reported fewer symptoms following treatment compared with patients who had a placebo (untreated yeast preparation) and expressed fewer symptoms compared with their pre-treatment report [26–28]. Armeli et al. (2022) demonstrated that Milmed yeast, derived from *S. cerevisiae* exposed to millimeter wavelengths (as developed by Golant 1994 and Golant et al. 1994 [28,29]), induced a shift in LPS-M1-polarized microglia toward an anti-inflammatory phenotype. This transition was evidenced morphologically by the restoration of the resting microglial phenotype, as shown by the reduced inducible nitric oxide synthase (iNOS) and the reduced mRNA levels of IL-1β, IL-6, and TNF-α [27].

Furthermore, Milmed stimulates the secretion of interleukin-10 and the expression of arginase-1, which provides cell markers of M2 anti-inflammatory polarized cells. Among racehorses in training presenting with physiological health problems, mainly 'common-cold' and inflammation symptoms remain a constant setback. In two studies, I and II, the time to reduce the pulse to 130 and pulse rate after 15-minutes were estimated both before and after the Milmed treatment, and the levels of improvement on a scale of 1–10 as well as judgements of vigor, general health, and performance following several weeks of Milmed administration were assessed [26,30].

In both studies, it was indicated that the Milmed-treated racehorses presenting poor health showed an improved physiological health responses, underlying the utility of several weeks of Milmed yeast treatment for the alleviation of mainly respiratory conditions among racehorses under the relatively stressful training and racing season. Remarkably, no evidence of toxicity, neither in vitro nor in vivo, has ever been obtained with the Milmed yeast [31].

Taking into account the several health-rendering observations attributed to the Milmed yeast, it was contended that the probiotic may promote the advancement of autophagic processes among cell cultures. Thus, in all the observations, liposaccharide (LPS) was applied to induce cellular damage/toxicity in order to assess the Milmed propensities for anti-inflammatory, autophagic, and antioxidant properties: the direct anti-inflammatory effect through the augmentation of arginine-1 following the exposure of BV-2 microglia to pro-inflammatory LPS was assessed. The promotion of autophagy was measured through Beclin-1, a protein that is encoded by the BECN1 gene in humans, which promotes the induction of autophagy, and ATG7, which recruits proteins related to autophagy. The formation of the phagophore begins, which enlarges to become an autophagosome factor as well as P62, a multifunctional ubiquitinated binding protein that is involved in the signaling pathways of many cell life activities including autophagy and has an impact upon cell survival [32–35]. NRF2, a basic leucine zipper (bZip) transcription factor with a Cap'n'collar (CNC) structure, accumulates in the cytoplasm and then shifts into the nucleus to activate the transcription of downstream genes that code for antioxidant enzymes, which protect cells from oxidative damage. It facilitates the transcription of the downstream antioxidant genes in disc cells by binding to antioxidant response elements (AREs) in promoter regions [36–38]. Evaluation and mRNA analysis of the factors involved in autophagic flux (RT-PCR) and enzyme linked immunosorbent assay (ELISA) were performed in BV-2 cells [32].

Given the well-established role of oxidative stress in aging and neurodegenerative processes, model organisms such as *Caenorhabditis elegans* provide an invaluable system for studying the molecular mechanisms underlying stress resistance and longevity [39]. *C. elegans* is widely recognized for its genetic tractability, short lifespan, and highly conserved stress response pathways, making it a powerful tool for investigating the effects of dietary and pharmacological interventions on oxidative homeostasis and lifespan regulation [40]. In this study, we utilized nematodes to evaluate the potential antioxidant and pro-longevity effects of Milmed in vivo. The transgenic *gst-4*::GFP worm strain, a well-established reporter strain for assessing the activation of the SKN-1/NRF2 pathway, which is a central regulator of cellular redox balance, was employed. Additionally, we analyzed the lifespan of *skn-1* mutant strains to determine the contribution of these stress-responsive pathways to the observed effects. Reactive oxygen species (ROS) levels were measured at different time points to assess whether yeast supplementation influenced the oxidative damage accumulation over time. By integrating different approaches in the BV-2 microglia cells and *C. elegans* in vivo model, this study aimed to elucidate the potential mechanisms through which Milmed yeast may promote cellular stress resistance and longevity, providing new insights into the interplay between dietary factors, oxidative stress, and autophagy.

2. Materials and Methods

2.1. Cell Culture and Treatment

The BV-2 murine microglial cell line, kindly provided by Dr. Mangino, Sapienza University of Rome (Italy), was cultured in Dulbecco's modified Eagle's medium (DMEM, Euroclone, Pero, MI, Italy) supplemented with 10% fetal bovine serum (FBS; Sigma-Aldrich, St. Louis, MO, USA) and 1% penicillin-streptomycin (Sigma-Aldrich, St. Louis, MO, USA) at 37 °C in a humidified incubator under 5% CO_2 until they reached 90% confluence. Cells were seeded in 6-well plates (cell density of 10^6 cells/well) and incubated at 37° C with 10^3 Milmed yeast, a commercial probiotic (Alnozine™) obtained from *Saccharomyces cerevisiae* after exposure to millimeter electromagnetic wavelengths (range: 1 GHz to 300 GHz) [28,29]. The dried yeast preparation was produced by the established yeast manufacturer, Jästbolaget AB, Sollentuna, Sweden. The yeast was treated in a suspension by applying an apparatus that generated electromagnetic millimeter waves, followed by the intensification of the suspension yeast manufactured, and then drying it to a powder through an air-drying technique. Milmed was administered to the microglia cultures either in liquid form (Milmed) or in the liquid form of dried powder regrown in YPD medium (Milmed YPD), or as a powder directly added to the cultures (dried Milmed). Prior to each treatment, a viability assay was performed to count the live yeast cells/each treatment. Microglia cultures were also incubated with the common *S. cerevisiae* strain (untreated yeast) as a control. After 45 min, the BV-2 cells were added with lipopolysaccharide (LPS, strain 0111:B4, Sigma-Aldrich, St. Louis, MO, USA) at a concentration of 1 ng/mL and compared with the control.

2.2. Real-Time Quantitative PRC Analysis

The total RNA was extracted from both the BV2 control and treated cells using the miRNeasy Micro Kit (Qiagen, Hilden, Germany) and quantified by a NanoDrop One/OneC (Thermo Fisher Scientific, Waltham, MA, USA). The cDNA was synthesized using a high-throughput reverse transcription kit. Quantitative real-time PCR (qPCR) was performed for each sample in triplicate on an Applied Biosystems 7900HT fast real-time PCR system (Applied Biosystem, Cheshire, UK) using Power SYBR® Green PCR Master Mix (Applied Biosystem, Cheshire, UK). Primers for real-time PCR amplification were designed through the UCSC Genome Browser https://genome.cse.ucsc.edu/ (accessed on 1 November 2022); University of California, Santa Cruz, CA, USA) (Table 1). Analysis of the real-time PCR data was performed using the comparative threshold cycle (CT) method. The target quantity, normalized against the endogenous β-actin reference primer (ΔCT) and against the untreated control calibrator (ΔΔCT), was calculated by the $2^{-\Delta\Delta CT}$ equation.

2.3. ELISA Assay

To distinguish the LC3-II form from the LC3-I form, the LC3-II antigen was analyzed by the ELISA assay. Cell lysates were prepared and analyzed according to the Autophagy

ELISA Kit (LC3-II Quantitation, Cell Biolabs, INC, San Diego, CA, USA). To quantify mTOR kinase and NRF2, cell lysates were prepared and analyzed according to mTOR KLM1703 GENLISA™ Mouse Mammalian Target of Rapamicyn ELISA 96T (KRISHGEN BioSystems Mumbai, India), and according to the Autophagy ELISA Kit LC3-II Quantitation CBA-5116 (Cell Biolabs, San Diego, CA, USA). The absorbance (450 nm) was determined by a Varioskan™ LUX Multimode Microplate Reader Thermo Scientific (Waltham, MA, USA).

Table 1. List of primers.

GENE	Forward Primer (5′–3′)	Reverse Primer (5′–3′)	Accession Numbers	bp
mLC3	TTCTTCCTCCTGGTGAATGG	GTCTCCTGCGAGGCATAAAC	NM_026160	2455
mBeclin-1	CAGCCTCTGAAACTGGACACGA	CTCTCCTGAGTTAGCCTCTTCC	NM_019584	2072
mNrf2	TCTGAGCCAGGACTACGACG	GAGGTGGTGGTGGTGTCTCTGC	NM_010902	2347
mp62	CCTTGCCCTACAGCTGAGTC	CCACACTCTCCCCCACATTC	NM_001290769	1916
mATG7	CAATGAGATCTGGGAAGCCATAA	AGGTCAAGAGCAGAAACTTGTTGA	NM_001253717	3872
mβ-Actin	GGCTGTATTCCCCTCCATCG	CCAGTTGGTAACAATGCCATGT	NM_007393.5	1935

2.4. *Immunofluorescence*

A total of 30,000 BV2 cells/well of the chamber slides were plated in 200 μL of 10% DMEM FBS and stimulated with 10^3 Milmed, dried Milmed, and untreated yeast in the presence and absence of LPS 1 ng/mL for 24 h. After 3 washes in PBS, cells were fixed in 4% paraformaldehyde for 30′ RT. After 3 washes, TritonX-100 0.1% × 5′ was added. Two washes in PBS were performed, and glycine 0.1 M was added for 20′ RT. After 2 further washes in PBS, the cells were incubated with Primary Antibody 1:100 in PBS 01% BSA O.N. 4 °C for anti-NRF2 (NRF2 (A-10), Santa Cruz Biotechnology, Dallas, TX, USA) and anti-pNRF2 (NRF2 phospho Ser40, GeneTex, Irvine, CA, USA). After 3 washes in PBS, the cells were incubated with the fluoresceinated secondary antibody (Rb CF488-a goat anti-Rb Ig(H+L) 20012, Biotium) for 30′ RT (1:100 in PBS) in the dark. After washing off the excess, the slides were sealed with Vectashield® Antifade Mounting Medium with DAPI (Newark, NJ, USA). Qualitative images were acquired using a confocal ZEISS Ism 980 with ZEISS Zen Microscopy Software 3.6 (Carl Zeiss Inc., Ober Kochen, Germany). Fluorescence intensity was quantified with ImageJ software, version 1.48.

2.5. *C. elegans Strains and Lifespan Analysis*

The *C. elegans* strains used in this study were wild-type N2, CL2166 (dvIs19 [(pAF15)gst-4p::GFP::NLS] III), and QV225 *skn-1* (zj15). Synchronized nematodes were prepared as described in Schifano et al. (2022) [41] on NGM plates spread with 60 μL of *S. cerevisiae* BY4741, untreated yeast, or Milmed at a final concentration of 10^8 cells/mL. Yeast strains were cultured in YPD broth and incubated at 28 °C overnight aerobically. Lifespan analysis was conducted at 16 °C, with worms transferred daily to fresh plates seeded with newly prepared yeast lawns. Worms were scored dead when they no longer responded to gentle touch with a platinum wire. A minimum of 80 nematodes per condition was used in each experiment. All lifespan assays were performed in triplicate.

2.6. *Body Size Analysis*

Synchronized N2 worms were incubated at 16 °C on NGM plates seeded with Milmed or *S. cerevisiae* BY4741, prepared as previously described, allowing the embryos to hatch and develop. For body length measurements, animals were photographed at 1- and 8-days post-hatching using a ZEISS Axiovert 25 microscope connected to an Axiocam 208 color camera. The worm body length was determined using ZEISS ZEN Microscopy Software

2011 and compared with the BY4741-fed worms. At least 30 nematodes were analyzed per dataset, with a minimum of three independent experiments conducted.

2.7. Fluorescence Analysis of *C. elegans* Transgenic Strains

At day 4 of adulthood, synchronized *gst-4*::GFP transgenic worms fed with Milmed or untreated yeast from embryo hatching were anesthetized with sodium azide (20 mmol L^{-1}) (Sigma-Aldrich, St. Louis, MO, USA) and observed using a ZEISS Axiovert 25 microscope, as described in Schifano et al. (2022) [41]. Each experiment was repeated three times, with 15 worms per group analyzed in each replicate. Images were acquired with an exposure time of 0.2 s, and the fluorescence intensity was quantified using ImageJ software. Scale bars were added using Zeiss ZEN Microscopy Software 2011.

2.8. Evaluation of Reactive Oxygen Species (ROS) Levels

The ROS levels in 1- and 10-day-old adult worms, fed with Milmed or untreated yeast from embryo hatching, were measured using the fluorescent probe 2′,7′-dichlorofluorescein diacetate (H_2DCFDA), according to Ficociello et al. (2023) [42]. Briefly, worms were collected in triplicate in a 96-well microplate and washed with M9 buffer. The H_2DCFDA probe (Sigma-Aldrich, Milan, Italy) was added to each sample to a final concentration of 50 μM. After 1 h of incubation in the dark at 20 °C, fluorescence was measured using a multiple reader (Promega, Glomax Multidetection System, Madison, WI, USA) at excitation/emission wavelengths of 485/520 nm. Fluorescence was detected in whole worms because the H_2DCFDA probe is cell-permeable and undergoes hydrolysis by intracellular esterases, followed by oxidation by reactive oxygen species (ROS), leading to fluorescence. It should be taken into account that in worm homogenates, the fluorescence signal can be significantly reduced or absent because the esterases might be inactivated or lost during homogenization, and the ROS levels may be lower or more rapidly degraded in the disrupted cellular environment. Several works have reported the measurements of *C. elegans* ROS in entire animals [43,44].

2.9. Statistical Analyses

Data were expressed as the mean values ± standard deviations (SD) or mean values ± SEM from at least three independent experiments. Statistical analyses were performed using the unpaired Student's *t* test (GraphPad Software Inc., San Diego, CA, USA). All results were considered statistically significant with $p < 0.05$. For the *C. elegans* experiments, the statistical significance was performed by the Student's t-test or one-way ANOVA analysis coupled with a Bonferroni post-test (GraphPad Prism 9.0 software, GraphPad Software Inc., La Jolla, CA, USA). Differences with p values < 0.05 were considered significant and were indicated as follows: * $p < 0.05$, ** $p < 0.01$, and *** $p < 0.001$. Experiments were performed at least in triplicate. Data were presented as the mean ± SD. For the fluorescence images, the mean fluorescence intensity was analyzed using ImageJ software, measuring the ratio of pixels per area of the worm.

3. Results

3.1. MILMED Restores Autophagic Processes in LPS-Treated BV2 Cells

As known, the autophagic process is composed of several steps that lead to the degradation of misfolded proteins and the elimination of damaged organelles. We evaluated the expression of the genes that promote autophagosome formation, namely ATG7, which is involved in the formation of the pre-autophagosomal structures; the Beclin-1 factor, which intervenes in the initial stages of nucleation and forms a complex that facilitates the recruitment of other ATG proteins; and LC3 and LC3II markers of autophagosome vescicles. Our results showed that cells incubated with Milmed increased the expression of *Beclin-1* mRNA by 50% also in the presence of LPS, which by itself induced a 20% decrement of *Beclin-1* mRNA expression. An analogous increase in *Beclin-1* mRNA was observed after the addition of Milmed dried powder. Cells supplemented with the untreated yeast showed no difference compared with the control cells. Milmed and Milmed dried powder increased the expression of *ATG7* by 50% compared with the control cells but Milmed dried powder regrown in YPD showed a 100% increase in *ATG7* mRNA (Figure 1).

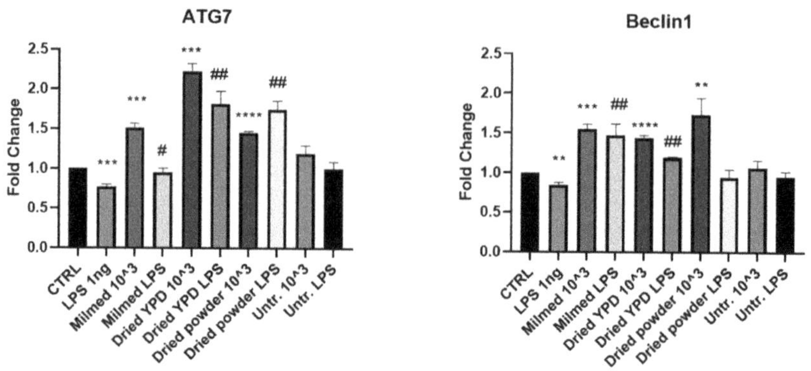

Figure 1. mRNA expression of *Beclin-1* and *ATG7* in BV-2 cells after yeast pre-treatment and LPS stimulation. mRNA expressions of *Beclin-1* and *ATG7* were evaluated in BV-2 cells after pre-treatment with Milmed or untreated yeast for 45 min and incubated with LPS 1 ng/mL for 4 h by qRT-PCR. Data are shown as the mean ± SD from three independent experiments performed in triplicate. Expression profiles were determined using the $2^{-\Delta\Delta CT}$ method. vs. CTRL ** $p < 0.01$, *** $p < 0.001$, **** $p < 0.0001$. vs. LPS # $p < 0.05$, ## $p < 0.01$.

The interaction between p62 and LC3 represents the specific and necessary signal to direct cytosolic elements to degradation. Analysis of *LC3* and *p62* mRNA expression, as shown in Figure 2, demonstrated that the presence of the LPS inflammatory stimulus significantly reduced the expression of these two key factors of autophagic flux compared with the CTRL group. After treatment with Milmed, both *LC3* and *p62* mRNA expression increased in the BV2 cells. Milmed treatment also increased the *p62* mRNA expression in the presence of LPS. The addition of dried yeast regrown in YPD significantly increased the expression of *LC3* and *p62* in the presence of the inflammatory stimulus. Addition of the Milmed dried powder directly to the BV2 cell culture increased the *p62* expression both in the absence and presence of LPS. The untreated yeast decreased *LC3* expression compared with the CTRL group and had no effect on *p62* expression.

mTOR is a major repressor of autophagic flux. The addition of Milmed as such or in the form of dried powder inhibited mTOR stimulated by the incubation of BV2 microglia with LPS, thereby removing one of the main pathways of inhibition of autophagic flux. Protein expression analysis of mTOR (Figure 3) significantly increased in the presence of LPS while drastically decreasing after 24 h after treatment with modified yeast (Milmed, dried YPD, and dried powder). There was also a slight decrease in the untreated yeast treatment in the presence of LPS. In the absence of LPS, there was no significant difference with the CTRL.

LC3 is a protein involved in autophagy that exists in two main forms: LC3-I, which is present in the cytoplasm, and LC3-II, which is associated with the membranes of autophagosomes. In response to stress signals, such as amino acid deficiency, autophagy is activated, increasing the conversion of LC3-I to LC3-II. This process indicates the formation of autophagosomes, making LC3-II a reliable marker for monitoring autophagy activity [45]. A commonly accepted signal for the induction or activation of autophagy refers to increased levels of LC3-II or decreased levels of p62, an autophagic substrate that is degraded through the autophagic process [46].

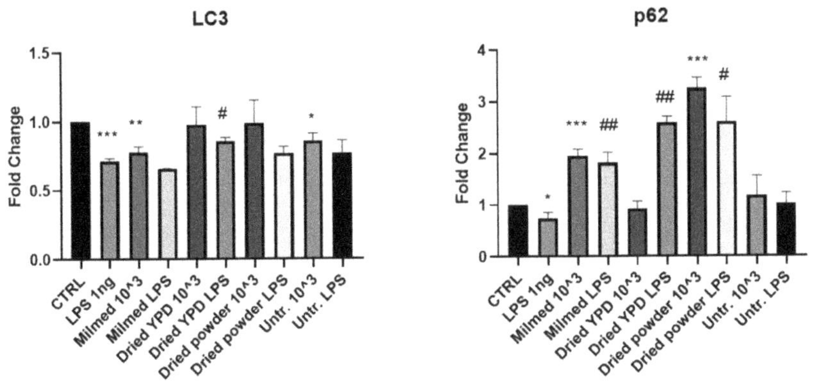

Figure 2. mRNA expression of *LC3* and *p62* in BV-2 cells after yeast pre-treatment and LPS stimulation. mRNA expressions of *LC3* and *p62* were evaluated in BV-2 cells after pre-treatment with Milmed or untreated yeast for 45 min and incubated with LPS 1 ng/mL for 4 h by qRT-PCR. Data are shown as the mean ± SD from three independent experiments performed in triplicate. Expression profiles were determined using the $2^{-\Delta\Delta CT}$ method. vs. CTRL * $p < 0.05$, ** $p < 0.01$, *** $p < 0.001$; vs. LPS # $p < 0.05$, ## $p < 0.01$.

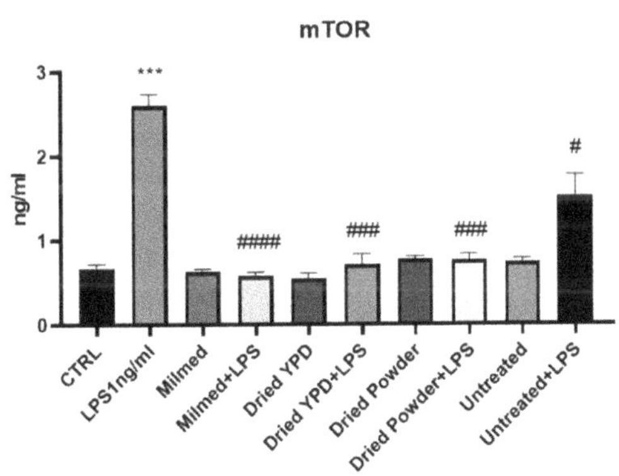

Figure 3. mTOR: a major repressor of autophagic flux. ELISA assay of mTOR was evaluated in BV-2 cells after pre-treatment with Milmed or untreated yeast for 45 min and incubated with LPS 1 ng/mL for 24 h. Data are shown as the mean ± SD from three independent experiments performed in duplicate using the unpaired Student's *t* test. *** $p < 0.001$, # $p < 0.05$, ### $p < 0.001$, #### $p < 0.0001$ * vs. CTRL; # vs. LPS.

In Figure 4, it can be seen that LPS treatment significantly decreased the LC3-II protein expression while modified yeast significantly increased the LC3-II protein expression compared with both the untreated BV2 cells (CTRL) and BV2 cells treated only with LPS. Untreated yeast added to cultures did not modulate LC3-II expression in the presence or in the absence of LPS.

3.2. Antioxidant Effect of Milmed in BV2 Cells

Nrf2 is a transcription factor present in all cells that is activated by oxidative stress. It binds to the antioxidant response element (ARE), an enhancer sequence found in the regulatory regions of antioxidant genes such as *SOD1* and *GPX* [47].

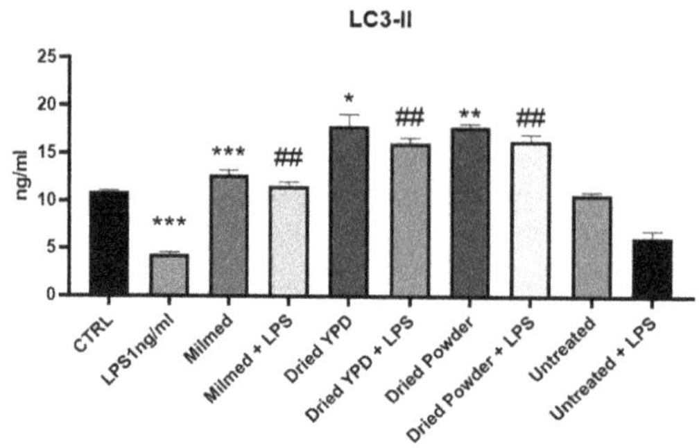

Figure 4. LC3-II is a reliable marker for monitoring autophagy activity. ELISA assay of LC3-II was evaluated in BV-2 cells after pre-treatment with Milmed or untreated (control) yeast for 45 min and incubated with LPS 1 ng/mL for 24 h. Data are shown as the mean ± SD from three independent experiments performed in duplicate using the unpaired Student's t test. * $p < 0.05$, ** $p < 0.01$, *** $p < 0.001$, ## $p < 0.01$ * vs. CTRL; # vs. LPS.

The analysis of *Nrf2* mRNA expression 4 h after pretreatment with Milmed yeast in the presence and absence of LPS demonstrated that both liquid Milmed and the dried form regrown in YPD significantly increased *Nrf2* expression in both the presence and absence of the inflammatory LPS stimuli. Powder directly added to the culture did not modulate *Nrf2* expression. Pre-treatment with untreated yeast decreased *Nrf2* mRNA expression in the presence of LPS compared with BV2 cells treated with LPS alone. Treatment with LPS significantly reduced the mRNA expression of *SOD1* and *GPX*. After 4 h after pretreatment, as shown in Figure 5, there was an increase in the mRNA expression of *SOD1* and *GPX* in the liquid Milmed conditions both in the presence and absence of LPS. *SOD1* mRNA expression increased significantly in BV2 cells treated with dried YPD and dried powder in the presence of LPS while *GPX* mRNA expression increased significantly in cells treated with dried YPD and dried powder compared with the CTRL group. In the presence of LPS, an increase in *GPX* mRNA expression was observed to be significant with the addition of dried powder. Treatment with untreated yeast significantly decreased *SOD1* mRNA expression both in the presence and absence of LPS. The same treatment did not appear to modulate *GPX* expression.

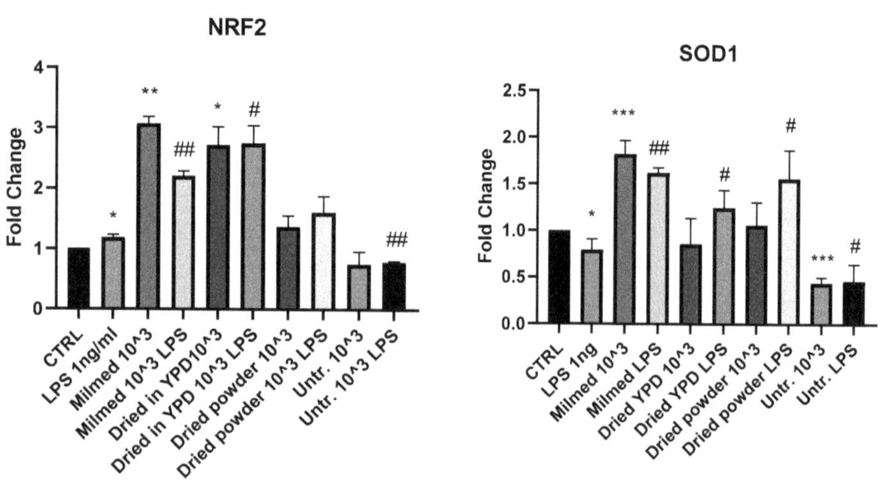

Figure 5. *Cont.*

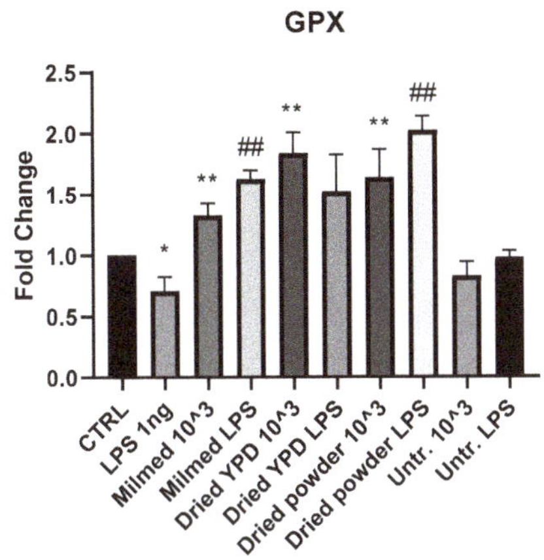

Figure 5. mRNA expression of *Nrf2, SOD1*, and *GPX* in BV-2 cells after yeast pre-treatment and LPS stimulation. mRNA expressions of *Nrf2, SOD1*, and *GPX* were evaluated in BV-2 cells after pre-treatment with Milmed or untreated yeast for 45 min and incubated with LPS 1 ng/mL for 4 h by qRT-PCR. Data are shown as the mean ± SD from three independent experiments performed in triplicate. Expression profiles were determined using the $2^{-\Delta\Delta CT}$ method. vs. CTRL * $p < 0.05$, ** $p < 0.01$, *** $p < 0.001$; vs. LPS # $p < 0.05$, ## $p < 0.01$.

Analysis of the active form of NRF2, phosphorylated NRF2 (pNRF2), was evaluated by immunuofluorescence, and in Figure 6, it is possible to observe that only a few conditions showed more pronounced changes on pNRF2 expression. In particular, two conditions showed a significant increase compared with the others, which were dried grown in YPD compared with CTRL. Both the dried YPD form and dried powder in the presence of LPS significantly increased the expression of pNRF2. The dried powder condition showed a reduction compared with CTRL, although this was not found to be significant.

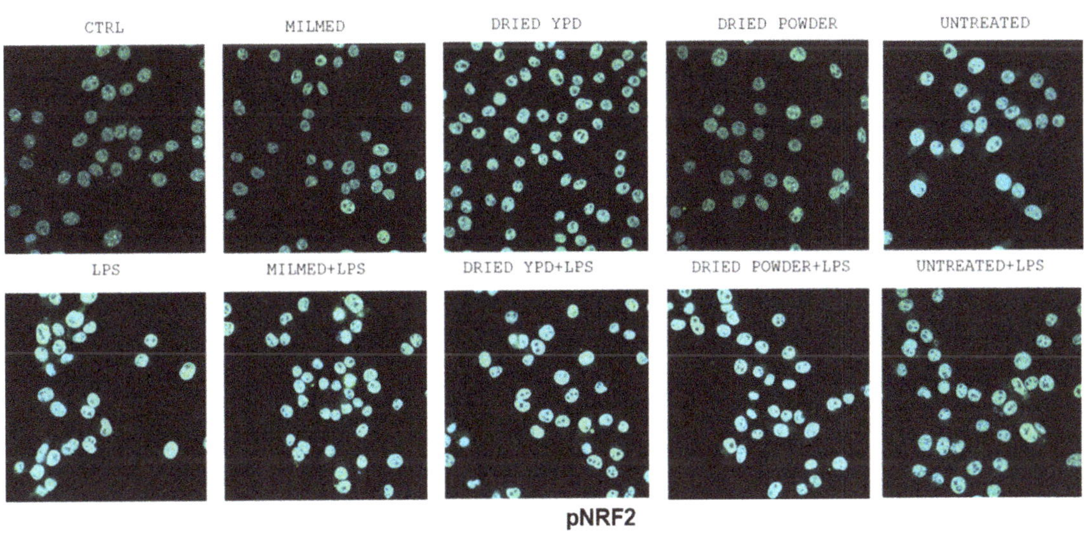

Figure 6. *Cont.*

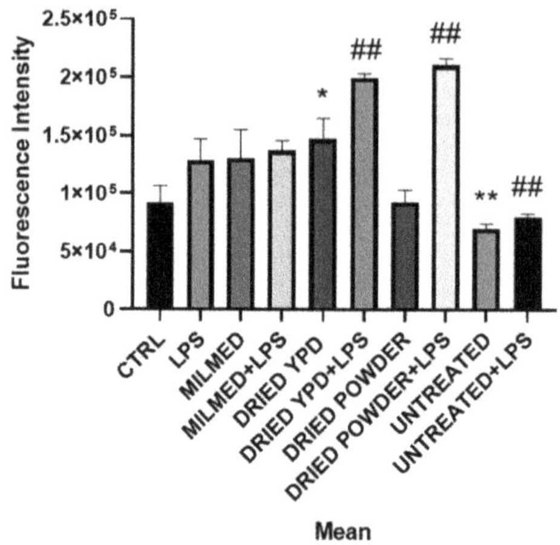

Figure 6. The bar graph shows the fluorescence intensity related to pNRF2 expression under different experimental conditions. Data are shown as the mean ± SD from three independent experiments (24 h). Magnification 63×. vs. LPS ## $p < 0.01$; vs. CTRL * $p < 0.05$, ** $p < 0.01$.

3.3. *Milmed Yeast Extends Lifespan and Modulates Growth in C. elegans*

To investigate the effects of yeast on *C. elegans* physiology, we first examined the survival rate (Figure 7A). The median lifespan of wild-type nematodes fed with Milmed yeast from embryo hatching was significantly extended compared with the *S. cerevisiae* BY4741-fed controls. Indeed, the 50% survival rate in the Milmed-fed worms was recorded at day 13, whereas it was observed at day 11 and day 9 in the untreated and BY4741-fed animals, respectively. Microscopic analysis of larval development revealed that the Milmed diet slightly affected the body size (Figure 7B). Body length analysis showed a slight reduction at day 1 of adulthood, but progressively increased with age in both conditions. However, at later stages, the body length of the Milmed-fed worms became comparable to that of the control group.

A

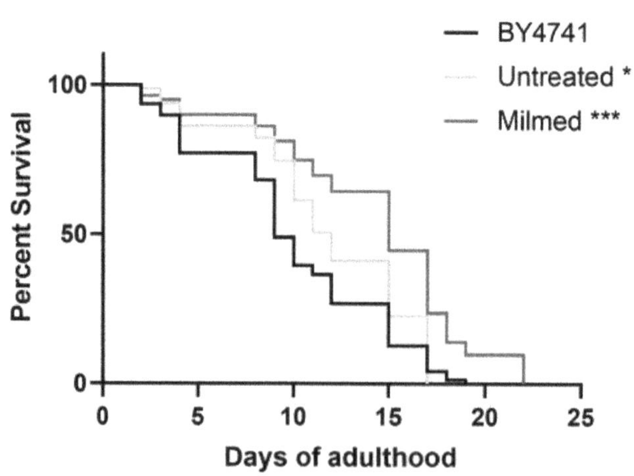

Figure 7. *Cont.*

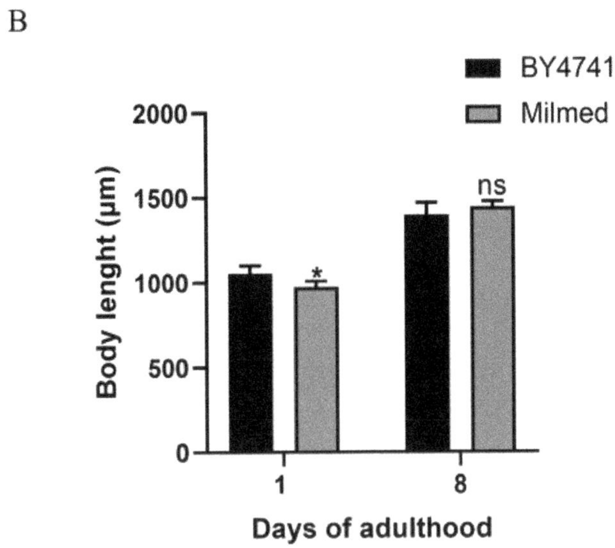

Figure 7. Effect of Milmed yeast on nematode lifespan and body length. (**A**) Kaplan–Meier survival plot of N2 worms fed with Milmed or untreated yeast compared with the *S. cerevisiae* BY4741-fed worms used as controls. $n = 80$ per data point in individual experiments. (**B**) Effect of yeast feeding on the body size of *C. elegans*. Worms were grown in the presence of Milmed yeast, untreated yeast, or *S. cerevisiae* BY4741 (control), and their body lengths were measured from head to tail at the indicated time points. Bars represent the mean of three independent experiments. Asterisks indicate statistically significant differences (* $p < 0.05$, *** $p < 0.001$); ns: not significant.

3.4. Milmed Yeast Supplementation Reduces Age-Related Oxidative Stress in C. elegans

Since excessive oxidative damage can impair cellular function and has been shown to increase with age [48], and given that reactive oxygen species (ROS) are one of the primary causes of aging, the ROS levels were analyzed in *C. elegans* following yeast-based dietary supplementation (Figure 8). These ROS are known to induce oxidative damage to essential cellular components including DNA, proteins, and lipids [41]. At day 2 of adulthood, the ROS levels in Milmed-fed worms were approximately twice as high as in the control group (Figure 8). However, by day 10 of adulthood, while the ROS levels in control worms had doubled compared with the young adults—as typically observed during aging—the Milmed-fed nematodes exhibited an over 80% reduction in ROS levels. This suggests that the Milmed diet may enhance cellular antioxidant defenses, thereby mitigating age-related oxidative stress and contributing to the observed lifespan extension.

In *C. elegans*, the oxidative stress response is primarily controlled by the SKN-1/Nrf2 transcription factor, which plays a key role in maintaining redox balance by regulating the expression of various antioxidant genes. The *gst-4* (glutathione S-transferase) gene encodes a phase II detoxification enzyme that is strongly induced in a SKN-1-dependent manner [42].

In this study, we utilized transgenic *C. elegans* expressing the *gst-4::GFP* reporter to assess potential differences in the expression of this detoxifying enzyme (Figure 9). However, during aging, no significant variations were observed, as further confirmed by the mean fluorescence intensity (MFI) analysis.

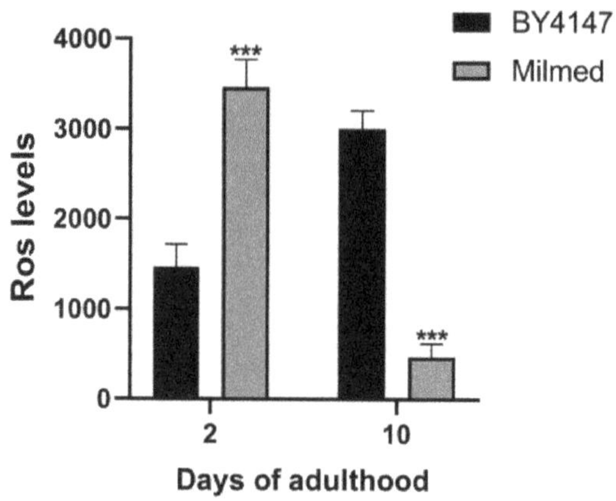

Figure 8. Measurement of ROS levels in Milmed-fed worms at 2 and 10 days of adulthood. Worms fed *S. cerevisiae* BY4741 were taken as the control. Statistical analysis was evaluated by one-way ANOVA with the Bonferroni post-test; asterisks indicate significant differences (*** $p < 0.001$). Bars represent the mean of three independent experiments.

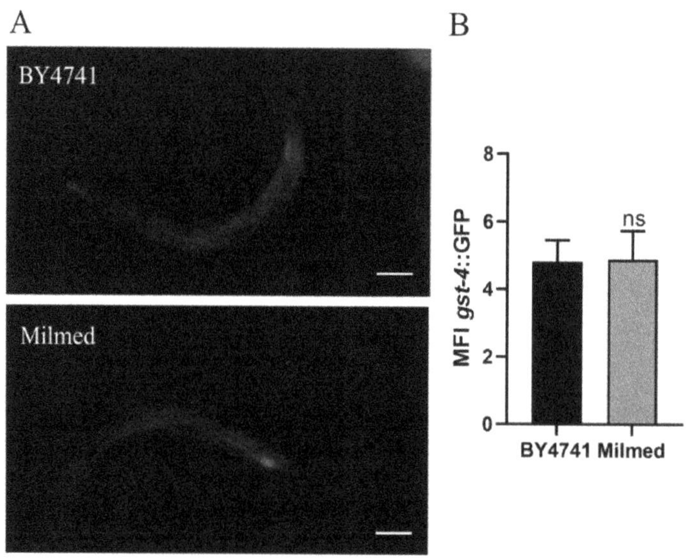

Figure 9. Fluorescence microscopy of *gst-4*::GFP transgenic strain. (**A**) Fluorescence microscopy of *gst-4*::GFP worm strain fed with Milmed from embryo hatching and (**B**) related MFI. Scale bar = 100 µm. Untreated yeast-fed worms were taken as the control. Statistical analysis was evaluated by one-way ANOVA with the Bonferroni post-test; ns: not significant. Bars represent the mean of three independent experiments.

3.5. Milmed Yeast Extends Lifespan in C. elegans Through Activation of SKN-1/Nrf2

On the other hand, the viability was further examined by administering Milmed yeast to worms carrying mutations in the *skn-1* gene, which encodes the transcription factor involved in the p38 MAPK pathway (Figure 10). The median lifespan of *skn-1* mutant nematodes treated with Milmed from embryo hatching was not only deprived of the pro-longevity effect, but was also significantly reduced (Figure 10). In particular, the 50% survival rate in Milmed-fed *skn-1* mutants was recorded at day 8 compared with day 9 in the control worms. Thus, Milmed did not induce a pro-longevity effect in these mutants as observed in the wild-type animals, demonstrating that the beneficial effects of Milmed are mediated through the activation of the transcription factor SKN-1/Nrf2.

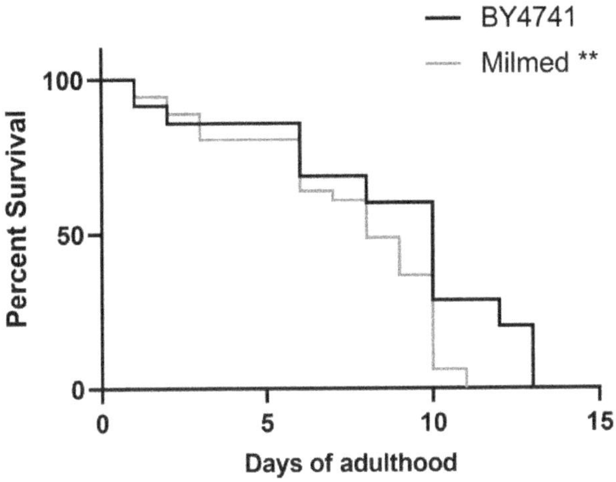

Figure 10. Effect of Milmed on *skn-1* mutant animals. Kaplan–Meier survival plot of *skn-1* mutant worms fed Milmed yeast from embryo hatching. Lifespans of untreated-fed worms (control) were taken as the reference; $n = 80$ for each data point of the single experiments (** $p < 0.01$). The experiment was performed in triplicate.

4. Discussion

As outlined above, modulation of microglia activity has recently been proposed as a therapeutic strategy to slow down the progression of neurodegenerative diseases. Gut microbiota has been shown to play an important role in the modulation of neuroinflammation and neurodegeneration; moreover, dysbiosis has been related to neurodegenerative acceleration. Our previous results showed that Milmed yeast, obtained from *S. cerevisiae*, after exposure to electromagnetic millimeter wavelenghts, induced a reversal of LPS-M1 polarized microglia toward an anti-inflammatory phenotype as demonstrated by the decrease in the mRNAs of IL-1β, IL-6, and TNF-α and in the expression of iNOS as well as by the increase in IL-10 mRNA and the expression of arginase-1 [27]. Recently, the importance of disabled macro-autophagy in aging and in the development of neurodegenerative diseases, including AD and PD, has been highlighted [49]. Several findings showed a direct correlation between dysbiosis, neuroinflammation, and the development of several neurodegenerative diseases including AD, PD, dementia, and depression [50]. Furthermore, a direct correlation has been hypothesized between aging and mitochondrial dysfunction, cellular senescence, disabled macro-autophagy, chronic inflammation, and dysbiosis [51]. Non-communicable diseases (NCDs) represent 77% of all deaths in Europe and remain the most widespread and without effective therapy; many of them share pathogenetic mechanisms and show a high degree of molecular connectivity. The study of these interconnections occurs through the identification of one or more mechanisms underlying the disease and its comorbidities. This approach, thanks to the regulation of a common molecular target can provide, at least partially, a therapeutic benefit to regulate different altered cellular responses. These alterations constitute a mosaic of significantly unbalanced processes that end up influencing each other, disrupting mechanisms that should guarantee the homeostasis of the cells. Therefore, an interdependence between these different alterations is created, whereby the accentuation or attenuation of one specific hallmark usually also affects other hallmarks.

The onset and development of several neurodegenerative diseases, including Alzheimer's disease, Parkinson's disease, schizophrenia and depression, have been related to neuroinflammation [52]. Neuroinflammation is characterized by the polarization of microglial cells toward a pro-inflammatory phenotype, M1 or classically activated phenotype, which releases inflammatory cytokines and chemokines, showing a decreased phagocytic capability and an increased chemotactic activity. The process is induced and amplified by oxidative stress, targeting the transcription factors that bind to the promoter regions of inflammatory genes. For all these reasons, the modulation of microglia activity has recently been proposed as a therapeutic strategy to slow down the progression of neurodegenerative diseases [53].

Our present study focused on Milmed actions that promote autophagy in microglia cells exposed to an inflammatory microenvironment and to promote longevity, as shown in the *C. elegans* experimental model. Disabled macro-autophagy accelerates the aging process, whereas, in contrast, autophagy is a major anti-aging mechanism involved in pro-longevity pathways [54]. In a recent review published in 2023, the importance of disabled macro-autophagy, chronic inflammation, and dysbiosis in accelerating the aging process was highlighted. The interdependence of aging hallmarks implies that the experimental accentuation or attenuation of one specific hallmark usually affects other hallmarks concurrently. Our findings demonstrate that Milmed exerted significant pro-longevity effects in *C. elegans*, extending the lifespan and improving stress resistance. The rise in ROS levels observed on the first day of adulthood seems to indicate a positive effect rather than a harmful one and appears to trigger oxidative defense systems, which help lower the ROS levels during aging and may contribute to a longer lifespan This was further confirmed by previous studies highlighting the role of probiotics, including yeast-based supplements, in modulating oxidative stress and inflammation [55,56]. The present results align with these findings and suggest that Milmed yeast may function as a bioactive dietary component capable of enhancing cellular stress responses. Notably, the ability of Milmed to lower ROS accumulation in aging worms suggests a potential protective mechanism against age-related oxidative damage, which is a hallmark of cellular aging and neurodegenerative diseases [57]. The observed reduction in ROS levels (Figure 8) among the aged worms and the loss of the pro-longevity effect in *skn-1* mutants (Figure 10) indicated that the p38 MAPK signaling cascade plays a crucial role in mediating these anti-aging effects. This contention is further supported by previous studies highlighting the role of probiotics, including yeast-based supplements, in modulating oxidative stress and inflammation [55,56]. The present results conform with these findings and suggest that Milmed yeast may function as a bioactive dietary component capable of enhancing cellular anti-stress responses. Notably, the ability of Milmed to lower ROS accumulation in aging worms suggests a potential protective mechanism against age-related oxidative damage, which is a hallmark of cellular aging and neurodegenerative diseases [57].

Autophagy also plays a key role in extending longevity. A proteostasis (protein homeostasis) imbalance may result from the dysregulation of autophagy, a well-known clearance mechanism of aggregated proteins, due to changes in mTOR/AMPK activity [58,59]. Indeed, mTOR inhibition with rapamycin reduces toxicity in animal models of NDs [60,61]. Additionally, given that autophagy has a central role in the removal of defective mitochondria, its regulation by mTOR/AMPK may also be associated with mitochondrial homeostasis and respiration [62,63]. In a previous study, *S. cerevisiae*-derived vacuoles added to LPS-treated human neuroblastoma cells reduced phosphorylated tau and β-amyloid expression and confirmed our previous data showing that Milmed decreased the expression of pro-inflammatory cytokines as well as iNOS. Furthermore, it was shown that *S. cerevisiae*-derived vacuoles regulated NF-kBp65 translocation to the nucleus [64]. The administration of *Saccharomyces boulardi* to Drosophila that were exposed to paraquat, a mitochondrial toxin, resulted in improved longevity and motor function. The main activity resulted in increased lysosomal degradation of dysfunctional mitochondria, which is mitophagy, outlining the potential therapeutic benefit of probiotic administration to patients with Parkinson's disease [65]. In recent years, it has been shown that the autophagy machinery is used for cellular activities independent from lysosomal degradation, opening a new chapter in understanding the broad spectrum of functions of autophagy, outlining the pro-survival role of autophagy [66,67].

It has been evidenced repeatedly that oxidative stress presents one of the main factors promoting chronic degenerative diseases, and several environmental conditions favoring the increase in ROS inside cells have been included among the main risk factors for the development of cardiovascular and neurodegenerative diseases; therefore it is of fundamental importance for pro-longevity interventions to contain the cellular concentrations of ROS within the physiological limits [68]. Our study demonstrated that Milmed is able to enhance the antioxidant defenses of the cell, as demonstrated by the modulation of the expression of NRF2, SOD3, and GPX, even in the presence of LPS and the translocation of phosphorilated-NRF2 to the nucleus of the cell. The in vivo *C. elegans* model confirmed the antioxidant effects of Milmed in the reduction of ROS. Concomitantly, the antioxidant potential of some strains of *S. cerevisiae* has also been demonstrated in other studies [69]. For example, Siesto et al. showed the antioxidant potential of *Saccharomyces cerevisiae* used in wine fermentation and correlated this activity to the content of beta-glucans [70]. Yeast β-glucan has various biological properties including immunomodulatory, anti-inflammatory, and antioxidant [71]. As a matter of fact, our study confirms the activity of Milmed as a powerful antioxidant.

5. Conclusions

Milmed yeast demonstrated a notable and marked pro-autophagic and antioxidant activity which, combined with the previously demonstrated anti-inflammatory activity, highlights its role as a highly effective probiotic for its beneficial effects on health and longevity.

Author Contributions: Conceptualization, R.B., D.U. and T.A.; Methodology, F.A. and E.S.; Software, F.A.; Validation, R.B., D.U. and T.A.; Formal analysis, F.A., B.M. and E.S.; Resources, R.B. and T.L.; Data curation, F.A., B.M. and E.S.; Writing—original draft preparation R.B., D.U., T.A. and F.A.; Writing—review and editing, R.B. and D.U.; Supervision, R.B.; Project administration, R.B. and D.U.; Funding acquisition, R.B. and T.L. All authors have read and agreed to the published version of the manuscript.

Funding: This research was funded by Sapienza Ateneo, grant number RM12218167C03EB5, to R.B.

Institutional Review Board Statement: Not applicable.

Informed Consent Statement: Not applicable.

Data Availability Statement: The original contributions presented in this study are included in the article. Further inquiries can be directed to the corresponding author.

Acknowledgments: The *C. elegans* strains were provided by the CGC, which is funded by the NIH Office of Research Infrastructure Programs (P40 OD010440).

Conflicts of Interest: Thomas Lenz and Trevor Archer are inventors of the following patent for Milmed: Yeast for promoting longevity and/or antiaging, Reference P154400001/MW; application number 2450665-1, submission number 1000238271. The remaining authors declare that the research was conducted in the absence of any commercial or financial relationships that could be construed as potential conflicts of interest.

References

1. Aman, Y.; Schmauck-Medina, T.; Hansen, M.; Morimoto, R.I.; Simon, A.K.; Bjedov, I.; Palikaras, K.; Simonsen, A.; Johansen, T.; Tavernarakis, N.; et al. Autophagy in Healthy Aging and Disease. *Nat. Aging* **2021**, *1*, 634–650. [CrossRef] [PubMed]
2. Kitada, M.; Koya, D. Autophagy in Metabolic Disease and Ageing. *Nat. Rev. Endocrinol.* **2021**, *17*, 647–661. [CrossRef]
3. Pinto, C.; Ninfole, E.; Benedetti, A.; Marzioni, M.; Maroni, L. Involvement of Autophagy in Ageing and Chronic Cholestatic Diseases. *Cells* **2021**, *10*, 2772. [CrossRef]
4. Kaushik, S.; Tasset, I.; Arias, E.; Pampliega, O.; Wong, E.; Martinez-Vicente, M.; Cuervo, A.M. Autophagy and the Hallmarks of Aging. *Ageing Res. Rev.* **2021**, *72*, 101468. [CrossRef]
5. Mizushima, N.; Levine, B. Autophagy in Human Diseases. *N. Engl. J. Med.* **2020**, *383*, 1564–1576. [CrossRef] [PubMed]
6. Wong, S.Q.; Kumar, A.V.; Mills, J.; Lapierre, L.R. Autophagy in Aging and Longevity. *Hum. Genet.* **2020**, *139*, 277–290. [CrossRef] [PubMed]
7. Aveleira, C.A.; Botelho, M.; Carmo-Silva, S.; Pascoal, J.F.; Ferreira-Marques, M.; Nóbrega, C.; Cortes, L.; Valero, J.; Sousa-Ferreira, L.; Álvaro, A.R.; et al. Neuropeptide Y Stimulates Autophagy in Hypothalamic Neurons. *Proc. Natl. Acad. Sci. USA* **2015**, *112*, E1642–E1651. [CrossRef]
8. Xiao, X.; Yeoh, B.S.; Vijay-Kumar, M. Lipocalin 2: An Emerging Player in Iron Homeostasis and Inflammation. *Annu. Rev. Nutr.* **2017**, *37*, 103–130. [CrossRef]
9. Konstantinidis, G.; Tavernarakis, N. Autophagy of the Nucleus in Health and Disease. *Front. Cell Dev. Biol.* **2022**, *9*, 814955. [CrossRef]
10. Abdel-Latif, M.A.; Abd El-Hack, M.E.; Swelum, A.A.; Saadeldin, I.M.; Elbestawy, A.R.; Shewita, R.S.; Ba-Awadh, H.A.; Alowaimer, A.N.; Abd El-Hamid, H.S. Single and Combined Effects of Clostridium Butyricum and Saccharomyces Cerevisiae on Growth Indices, Intestinal Health, and Immunity of Broilers. *Animals* **2018**, *8*, 184. [CrossRef]
11. Costanza, A.C.; Moscavitch, S.D.; Faria Neto, H.C.C.; Mesquita, E.T. Probiotic Therapy with Saccharomyces Boulardii for Heart Failure Patients: A Randomized, Double-Blind, Placebo-Controlled Pilot Trial. *Int. J. Cardiol.* **2015**, *179*, 348–350. [CrossRef]
12. Whelan, K.; Quigley, E.M.M. Probiotics in the Management of Irritable Bowel Syndrome and Inflammatory Bowel Disease. *Curr. Opin. Gastroenterol.* **2013**, *29*, 184–189. [CrossRef]
13. Shi, T.; Nishiyama, K.; Nakamata, K.; Aryantini, N.P.D.; Mikumo, D.; Oda, Y.; Yamamoto, Y.; Mukai, T.; Sujaya, I.N.; Urashima, T.; et al. Isolation of Potential Probiotic *Lactobacillus Rhamnosus* Strains from Traditional Fermented Mare Milk Produced in Sumbawa Island of Indonesia. *Biosci. Biotechnol. Biochem.* **2012**, *76*, 1897–1903. [CrossRef] [PubMed]
14. Webberley, T.S.; Masetti, G.; Bevan, R.J.; Kerry-Smith, J.; Jack, A.A.; Michael, D.R.; Thomas, S.; Glymenaki, M.; Li, J.; McDonald, J.A.K.; et al. The Impact of Probiotic Supplementation on Cognitive, Pathological and Metabolic Markers in a Transgenic Mouse Model of Alzheimer's Disease. *Front. Neurosci.* **2022**, *16*, 843105. [CrossRef] [PubMed]
15. Ye, T.; Yuan, S.; Kong, Y.; Yang, H.; Wei, H.; Zhang, Y.; Jin, H.; Yu, Q.; Liu, J.; Chen, S.; et al. Effect of Probiotic Fungi against Cognitive Impairment in Mice via Regulation of the Fungal Microbiota–Gut–Brain Axis. *J. Agric. Food Chem.* **2022**, *70*, 9026–9038. [CrossRef]
16. Zaylaa, M.; Alard, J.; Al Kassaa, I.; Peucelle, V.; Boutillier, D.; Desramaut, J.; Rosenstiel, P.; Nguyend, H.T.T.; Dabboussi, F.; Pot, B.; et al. Autophagy: A Novel Mechanism Involved in the Anti-Inflammatory Abilities of Probiotics. *Cell. Physiol. Biochem.* **2019**, *53*, 774–793. [CrossRef]
17. Candela, M.; Perna, F.; Carnevali, P.; Vitali, B.; Ciati, R.; Gionchetti, P.; Rizzello, F.; Campieri, M.; Brigidi, P. Interaction of Probiotic Lactobacillus and Bifidobacterium Strains with Human Intestinal Epithelial Cells: Adhesion Properties, Competition against Enteropathogens and Modulation of IL-8 Production. *Int. J. Food Microbiol.* **2008**, *125*, 286–292. [CrossRef] [PubMed]
18. Yang, L.; Zhang, J.; Wang, J.; Zhao, H.; Xie, X.; Wu, Q. Probiotic or Probiotics Add Supplement Interferes with Coronary Heart Disease: A Meta-analysis of Randomized Controlled Trials. *eFood* **2023**, *4*, e120. [CrossRef]
19. Vitetta, L.; Gobe, G. Uremia and Chronic Kidney Disease: The Role of the Gut Microflora and Therapies with pro- and Prebiotics. *Mol. Nutr. Food Res.* **2013**, *57*, 824–832. [CrossRef]
20. Jin, S.; Chen, P.; Yang, J.; Li, D.; Liu, X.; Zhang, Y.; Xia, Q.; Li, Y.; Chen, G.; Li, Y.; et al. *Phocaeicola Vulgatus* Alleviates Diet-Induced Metabolic Dysfunction-Associated Steatotic Liver Disease Progression by Downregulating Histone Acetylation Level via 3-HPAA. *Gut Microbes* **2024**, *16*, 2309683. [CrossRef]
21. Nemati, M.; Omrani, G.R.; Ebrahimi, B.; Montazeri-Najafabady, N. The Beneficial Effects of Probiotics via Autophagy: A Systematic Review. *BioMed Res. Int.* **2021**, *2021*, 2931580. [CrossRef] [PubMed]
22. Legon, L.; Rallis, C. Genome-Wide Screens in Yeast Models towards Understanding Chronological Lifespan Regulation. *Brief. Funct. Genom.* **2022**, *21*, 4–12. [CrossRef]

23. Archer, T.; Fredriksson, A. The Yeast Product Milmed Enhances the Effect of Physical Exercise on Motor Performance and Dopamine Neurochemistry Recovery in MPTP-Lesioned Mice. *Neurotox. Res.* **2013**, *24*, 393–406. [CrossRef] [PubMed]
24. Archer, T.; Garcia, D.; Fredriksson, A. Restoration of MPTP-Induced Deficits by Exercise and Milmed® Co-Treatment. *PeerJ* **2014**, *2*, e531. [CrossRef] [PubMed]
25. Archer, T. Milmed Treatment Alleviates Symptoms of Allergy and Improves General Health. *J. Immunol. Allergy* **2021**, *1*, 1–11. [CrossRef]
26. Archer, T. Anti-Inflammatory Action of the Treated-Yeast, Milmed, Under IBS-IBD Conditions. *J. Immunol. Allergy* **2022**, 3. [CrossRef]
27. Armeli, F.; Mengoni, B.; Maggi, E.; Mazzoni, C.; Preziosi, A.; Mancini, P.; Businaro, R.; Lenz, T.; Archer, T. Milmed Yeast Alters the LPS-Induced M_1 Microglia Cells to form M_2 Anti-Inflammatory Phenotype. *Biomedicines* **2022**, *10*, 3116. [CrossRef]
28. Golant, M.B.; Kuznetsov, A.P.; Bozhanova, T.P. The mechanism of synchronizing yeast cell cultures with EHF-radiation. *Biofizika* **1994**, *39*, 490–495.
29. Golant, M.B.; Mudrik, D.G.; Kruglyakova, O.P.; Izvol'skaya, V.E. Effect of EHF-Radiation Polarization on Yeast Cells. *Radiophys. Quantum Electron.* **1994**, *37*, 82–84. [CrossRef]
30. Archer, T. Physiologic And Subjective Health Benefits of Milmed Among Racehorses in Training. *J. Immunol. Allergy* **2022**, *3*, 1–9. [CrossRef]
31. Maggi, E.; Armeli, F.; Mengoni, B.; Leo, M.; Filetici, P.; Mancini, P.; Lenz, T.; Businaro, R.; Archer, T. Milmed Saccharomyces Cerevisiae Activity on Central Nervous System Cells. *J. Toxicol. Pharmacol.* **2022**, *5*, 1–8.
32. Zhang, Z.; Yang, X.; Song, Y.-Q.; Tu, J. Autophagy in Alzheimer's Disease Pathogenesis: Therapeutic Potential and Future Perspectives. *Ageing Res. Rev.* **2021**, *72*, 101464. [CrossRef] [PubMed]
33. Mizushima, N.; Yoshimori, T.; Ohsumi, Y. Role of the Apg_{12} Conjugation System in Mammalian Autophagy. *Int. J. Biochem. Cell Biol.* **2003**, *35*, 553–561. [CrossRef]
34. Liu, J.; Li, L. Targeting Autophagy for the Treatment of Alzheimer's Disease: Challenges and Opportunities. *Front. Mol. Neurosci.* **2019**, *12*, 203. [CrossRef]
35. Huang, X.; Zhang, J.; Yao, J.; Mi, N.; Yang, A. Phase Separation of P62: Roles and Regulations in Autophagy. *Trends Cell Biol.* **2025**, *25*, s0962-8924(25)00033-9. [CrossRef] [PubMed]
36. Xiang, Q.; Zhao, Y.; Lin, J.; Jiang, S.; Li, W. The Nrf_2 Antioxidant Defense System in Intervertebral Disc Degeneration: Molecular Insights. *Exp. Mol. Med.* **2022**, *54*, 1067–1075. [CrossRef]
37. Jalouli, M.; Rahman, M.A.; Biswas, P.; Rahman, H.; Harrath, A.H.; Lee, I.-S.; Kang, S.; Choi, J.; Park, M.N.; Kim, B. Targeting Natural Antioxidant Polyphenols to Protect Neuroinflammation and Neurodegenerative Diseases: A Comprehensive Review. *Front. Pharmacol.* **2025**, *16*, 1492517. [CrossRef] [PubMed]
38. La Torre, A.; Lo Vecchio, F.; Angelillis, V.S.; Gravina, C.; D'Onofrio, G.; Greco, A. Reinforcing Nrf_2 Signaling: Help in the Alzheimer's Disease Context. *Int. J. Mol. Sci.* **2025**, *26*, 1130. [CrossRef]
39. Lin, Y.; Lin, C.; Cao, Y.; Chen, Y. Caenorhabditis Elegans as an in Vivo Model for the Identification of Natural Antioxidants with Anti-Aging Actions. *Biomed. Pharmacother.* **2023**, *167*, 115594. [CrossRef]
40. Chen, X.; Bahramimehr, F.; Shahhamzehei, N.; Fu, H.; Lin, S.; Wang, H.; Li, C.; Efferth, T.; Hong, C. Anti-Aging Effects of Medicinal Plants and Their Rapid Screening Using the Nematode Caenorhabditis Elegans. *Phytomedicine* **2024**, *129*, 155665. [CrossRef]
41. Schifano, E.; Conta, G.; Preziosi, A.; Ferrante, C.; Batignani, G.; Mancini, P.; Tomassini, A.; Sciubba, F.; Scopigno, T.; Uccelletti, D.; et al. 2-Hydroxyisobutyric Acid (2-HIBA) Modulates Ageing and Fat Deposition in Caenorhabditis Elegans. *Front. Mol. Biosci.* **2022**, *9*, 986022. [CrossRef] [PubMed]
42. Ficociello, G.; Schifano, E.; Di Nottia, M.; Torraco, A.; Carrozzo, R.; Uccelletti, D.; Montanari, A. Silencing of the Mitochondrial Ribosomal Protein L-24 Gene Activates the Oxidative Stress Response in Caenorhabditis Elegans. *Biochim. Biophys. Acta BBA-Gen. Subj.* **2023**, *1867*, 130255. [CrossRef] [PubMed]
43. Yoon, D.; Lee, M.-H.; Cha, D. Measurement of Intracellular ROS in Caenorhabditis Elegans Using 2′,7′-Dichlorodihydrofluorescein Diacetate. *BIO-Protoc.* **2018**, *8*, e2774. [CrossRef]
44. Van Raamsdonk, J.M.; Hekimi, S. Reactive Oxygen Species and Aging in *Caenorhabditis Elegans*: Causal or Casual Relationship? *Antioxid. Redox Signal.* **2010**, *13*, 1911–1953. [CrossRef] [PubMed]
45. Liang, C.; E, X.; Jung, J.U. Downregulation of Autophagy by Herpesvirus Bcl-2 Homologs. *Autophagy* **2008**, *4*, 268–272. [CrossRef]
46. Klionsky, D.J.; Abdelmohsen, K.; Abe, A.; Abedin, M.J.; Abeliovich, H.; Acevedo Arozena, A.; Adachi, H.; Adams, C.M.; Adams, P.D.; Adeli, K.; et al. Guidelines for the Use and Interpretation of Assays for Monitoring Autophagy (3rd Edition). *Autophagy* **2016**, *12*, 1–222. [CrossRef]
47. Armeli, F.; Mengoni, B.; Laskin, D.L.; Businaro, R. Interplay among Oxidative Stress, Autophagy, and the Endocannabinoid System in Neurodegenerative Diseases: Role of the Nrf_2-P62/SQSTM1 Pathway and Nutraceutical Activation. *Curr. Issues Mol. Biol.* **2024**, *46*, 6868–6884. [CrossRef]

48. Pompa, L.; Montanari, A.; Tomassini, A.; Bianchi, M.M.; Aureli, W.; Miccheli, A.; Uccelletti, D.; Schifano, E. In Vitro Probiotic Properties and In Vivo Anti-Ageing Effects of Lactoplantibacillus Plantarum PFA2018AU Strain Isolated from Carrots on Caenorhabditis Elegans. *Microorganisms* **2023**, *11*, 1087. [CrossRef]
49. Liu, M.; Liu, S.; Lin, Z.; Chen, X.; Jiao, Q.; Du, X.; Jiang, H. Targeting the Interplay Between Autophagy and the Nrf_2 Pathway in Parkinson's Disease with Potential Therapeutic Implications. *Biomolecules* **2025**, *15*, 149. [CrossRef]
50. Fabi, J.P. The Connection between Gut Microbiota and Its Metabolites with Neurodegenerative Diseases in Humans. *Metab. Brain Dis.* **2024**, *39*, 967–984. [CrossRef]
51. López-Otín, C.; Blasco, M.A.; Partridge, L.; Serrano, M.; Kroemer, G. Hallmarks of Aging: An Expanding Universe. *Cell* **2023**, *186*, 243–278. [CrossRef] [PubMed]
52. Zhang, W.; Xiao, D.; Mao, Q.; Xia, H. Role of Neuroinflammation in Neurodegeneration Development. *Signal Transduct. Target. Ther.* **2023**, *8*, 267. [CrossRef] [PubMed]
53. Yang, X.; Wang, J.; Jia, X.; Yang, Y.; Fang, Y.; Ying, X.; Li, H.; Zhang, M.; Wei, J.; Pan, Y. Microglial Polarization in Alzheimer's Disease: Mechanisms, Implications, and Therapeutic Opportunities. *J. Alzheimer's Dis.* **2025**, *104*, 3–13. [CrossRef]
54. Humeau, J.; Leduc, M.; Cerrato, G.; Loos, F.; Kepp, O.; Kroemer, G. Phosphorylation of Eukaryotic Initiation Factor-2α (eIF2α) in Autophagy. *Cell Death Dis.* **2020**, *11*, 433. [CrossRef] [PubMed]
55. Romanin, D.E.; Llopis, S.; Genovés, S.; Martorell, P.; Ramón, V.D.; Garrote, G.L.; Rumbo, M. Probiotic Yeast Kluyveromyces Marxianus CIDCA 8154 Shows Anti-Inflammatory and Anti-Oxidative Stress Properties in in Vivo Models. *Benef. Microbes* **2016**, *7*, 83–94. [CrossRef]
56. Goyache, I.; Yavorov-Dayliev, D.; Milagro, F.I.; Aranaz, P. Caenorhabditis Elegans as a Screening Model for Probiotics with Properties against Metabolic Syndrome. *Int. J. Mol. Sci.* **2024**, *25*, 1321. [CrossRef]
57. Korovesis, D.; Rubio-Tomás, T.; Tavernarakis, N. Oxidative Stress in Age-Related Neurodegenerative Diseases: An Overview of Recent Tools and Findings. *Antioxidants* **2023**, *12*, 131. [CrossRef]
58. Bjedov, I.; Toivonen, J.M.; Kerr, F.; Slack, C.; Jacobson, J.; Foley, A.; Partridge, L. Mechanisms of Life Span Extension by Rapamycin in the Fruit Fly Drosophila Melanogaster. *Cell Metab.* **2010**, *11*, 35–46. [CrossRef]
59. Madeo, F.; Tavernarakis, N.; Kroemer, G. Can Autophagy Promote Longevity? *Nat. Cell Biol.* **2010**, *12*, 842–846. [CrossRef]
60. Bové, J.; Martínez-Vicente, M.; Vila, M. Fighting Neurodegeneration with Rapamycin: Mechanistic Insights. *Nat. Rev. Neurosci.* **2011**, *12*, 437–452. [CrossRef]
61. Menzies, F.M.; Huebener, J.; Renna, M.; Bonin, M.; Riess, O.; Rubinsztein, D.C. Autophagy Induction Reduces Mutant Ataxin-3 Levels and Toxicity in a Mouse Model of Spinocerebellar Ataxia Type 3. *Brain* **2010**, *133*, 93–104. [CrossRef] [PubMed]
62. Swinnen, E.; Ghillebert, R.; Wilms, T.; Winderickx, J. Molecular Mechanisms Linking the Evolutionary Conserved TORC1-Sch9 Nutrient Signalling Branch to Lifespan Regulation in *Saccharomyces cerevisiae*. *FEMS Yeast Res.* **2014**, *14*, 17–32. [CrossRef]
63. Mihaylova, M.M.; Shaw, R.J. The AMPK Signalling Pathway Coordinates Cell Growth, Autophagy and Metabolism. *Nat. Cell Biol.* **2011**, *13*, 1016–1023. [CrossRef] [PubMed]
64. Thi Nguyen, N.-H.; Kim, J.H.; Lee, S.-M.; Cho, B.-K.; Kim, Y.-H.; Min, J. Inhibition of Tau Phosphorylation and Aβ Accumulation by S. Cerevisiae-Derived Vacuoles in LPS-Induced SH-SY5Y Cells. *J. Biotechnol.* **2023**, *376*, 45–52. [CrossRef]
65. Hawrysh, P.J.; Gao, J.; Tan, S.; Oh, A.; Nodwell, J.; Tompkins, T.A.; McQuibban, G.A. PRKN/Parkin-Mediated Mitophagy Is Induced by the Probiotics *Saccharomyces boulardii* and *Lactococcus lactis*. *Autophagy* **2023**, *19*, 2094–2110. [CrossRef] [PubMed]
66. Yu, G.; Klionsky, D.J. Life and Death Decisions—The Many Faces of Autophagy in Cell Survival and Cell Death. *Biomolecules* **2022**, *12*, 866. [CrossRef]
67. Zhang, T.; Zhou, L.; Makarczyk, M.J.; Feng, P.; Zhang, J. The Anti-Aging Mechanism of Metformin: From Molecular Insights to Clinical Applications. *Molecules* **2025**, *30*, 816. [CrossRef]
68. Kaur, J.; Sharma, V.; Khan, H.; Singh, S.; Singh, T.G. Intersecting Molecular Pathways in Synucleinopathies and Amyloidogenesis: Exploring Shared Mechanisms and Therapeutic Potential. *Brain Res.* **2025**, *1855*, 149568. [CrossRef]
69. Menezes, A.G.T.; Ramos, C.L.; Cenzi, G.; Melo, D.S.; Dias, D.R.; Schwan, R.F. Probiotic Potential, Antioxidant Activity, and Phytase Production of Indigenous Yeasts Isolated from Indigenous Fermented Foods. *Probiotics Antimicrob. Proteins* **2020**, *12*, 280–288. [CrossRef]
70. Siesto, G.; Pietrafesa, R.; Infantino, V.; Thanh, C.; Pappalardo, I.; Romano, P.; Capece, A. In Vitro Study of Probiotic, Antioxidant and Anti-Inflammatory Activities among Indigenous Saccharomyces Cerevisiae Strains. *Foods* **2022**, *11*, 1342. [CrossRef]
71. Xu, C.; Zhang, Y.; Li, H.; Zhang, Z.; Sheng, W.; Zhang, S.; Li, P.; Zhang, X.; Li, X.; Lin, H.; et al. Carboxymethylated Yeast β-Glucan: Biological Activity Screening in Zebrafish, Sprayable Hydrogel Preparation, and Wound Healing Study in Diabetic Mice. *Int. J. Biol. Macromol.* **2025**, *285*, 138178. [CrossRef] [PubMed]

antioxidants

MDPI

Review

Crosstalk Between Autophagy and Oxidative Stress in Hematological Malignancies: Mechanisms, Implications, and Therapeutic Potential

Antonio José Cabrera-Serrano [1,2,†], José Manuel Sánchez-Maldonado [1,2,3,†], Carmen González-Olmedo [1,4], María Carretero-Fernández [1,2], Leticia Díaz-Beltrán [1,4], Juan Francisco Gutiérrez-Bautista [1,2,5,6], Francisco José García-Verdejo [1,4], Fernando Gálvez-Montosa [1,4], José Antonio López-López [1,4], Paloma García-Martín [2,7], Eva María Pérez [1,2,7], Pedro Sánchez-Rovira [1,4], Fernando Jesús Reyes-Zurita [1,3,*] and Juan Sainz [1,2,3,8,*]

1 Genomic Oncology Area, GENYO, Centre for Genomics and Oncological Research: Pfizer/University of Granada/Andalusian Regional Government, PTS, 18016 Granada, Spain; antonio.cabrera@genyo.es (A.J.C.-S.); josemanuel.sanchez@genyo.es (J.M.S.-M.); cgonzalezolmedo@fibao.es (C.G.-O.); maria.carretero@genyo.es (M.C.-F.); ldiaz@fibao.es (L.D.-B.); juanfrety@gmail.com (J.F.G.-B.); fjgverdejo@gmail.com (F.J.G.-V.); fernando.galvez.sspa@juntadeandalucia.es (F.G.-M.); josea.lopez.l.sspa@juntadeandalucia.es (J.A.L.-L.); evam.perez.sspa@juntadeandalucia.es (E.M.P.); pedro.sanchez.rovira.sspa@juntadeandalucia.es (P.S.-R.)
2 Instituto de Investigación Biosanitaria IBs.Granada, 18012 Granada, Spain; paloma.garcia.martin.sspa@juntadeandalucia.es
3 Department of Biochemistry and Molecular Biology I, Faculty of Sciences, University of Granada, 18012 Granada, Spain
4 Medical Oncology Unit, University Hospital of Jaén, 23007 Jaén, Spain
5 Servicio de Análisis Clínicos e Inmunología, University Hospital Virgen de las Nieves, 18014 Granada, Spain
6 Department of Biochemistry, Molecular Biology and Immunology III, University of Granada, 18016 Granada, Spain
7 Campus de la Salud Hospital, PTS, 18016 Granada, Spain
8 CIBER Epidemiología y Salud Pública (CIBERESP), 28029 Madrid, Spain
* Correspondence: ferjes@ugr.es (F.J.R.-Z.); jsainz@ugr.es (J.S.); Tel.: +34-958243252 (F.J.R.-Z.); +34-958241383 (J.S.)
† These authors contributed equally to this work.

Abstract: Autophagy is a fundamental cellular process that maintains homeostasis by degrading damaged components and regulating stress responses. It plays a crucial role in cancer biology, including tumor progression, metastasis, and therapeutic resistance. Oxidative stress, similarly, is key to maintaining cellular balance by regulating oxidants and antioxidants, with its disruption leading to molecular damage. The interplay between autophagy and oxidative stress is particularly significant, as reactive oxygen species (ROS) act as both inducers and by-products of autophagy. While autophagy can function as a tumor suppressor in early cancer stages, it often shifts to a pro-tumorigenic role in advanced disease, aiding cancer cell survival under adverse conditions such as hypoxia and nutrient deprivation. This dual role is mediated by several signaling pathways, including PI3K/AKT/mTOR, AMPK, and HIF-1α, which coordinate the balance between autophagic activity and ROS production. In this review, we explore the mechanisms by which autophagy and oxidative stress interact across different hematological malignancies. We discuss how oxidative stress triggers autophagy, creating a feedback loop that promotes tumor survival, and how autophagic dysregulation leads to increased ROS accumulation, exacerbating tumorigenesis. We also examine the therapeutic implications of targeting the autophagy–oxidative stress axis in cancer. Current strategies involve modulating autophagy through specific inhibitors, enhancing ROS levels with pro-oxidant compounds, and combining these approaches with conventional therapies to overcome drug resistance. Understanding the complex relationship between autophagy and oxidative stress provides critical insights into novel therapeutic strategies aimed at improving cancer treatment outcomes.

Keywords: autophagy; oxidative stress; reactive oxygen species; crosstalk; hematological malignancies; cancer treatment outcomes; therapeutic opportunities

1. Introduction

Cancer represents a significant challenge in modern society, posing substantial public health and economic burdens in the 21st century. Globally, it accounts for nearly one in six deaths (16.8%) and approximately one in four deaths (22.8%) attributed to non-communicable diseases. Furthermore, cancer is responsible for 30.3% of premature deaths from non-communicable diseases among individuals aged 30–69 years, making it one of the three leading causes of mortality in this age group in 177 out of 183 countries [1]. A recent study based on the 2022 GLOBOCAN estimates highlighted significant geographic variability in cancer incidence and mortality across 20 world regions, focusing on the 10 most common cancer types (https://gco.iarc.who.int/today, 20 November 2024). It further explored new opportunities for global cancer prevention and control and underscored the critical need for new targeted prevention strategies.

Given the complexity and heterogeneity of tumors, autophagy and oxidative stress have emerged in recent years as critical cellular processes in cancer development and progression. These mechanisms play pivotal roles in human health. Autophagy is an essential mechanism for maintaining cellular homeostasis [2,3], for preventing metabolic imbalance and the accumulation of cytotoxic elements within cells, and for prolonging cell survival [4–8]. On the other hand, oxidative stress arises from an imbalance between the production of reactive oxygen species (ROS) and the effectiveness of cellular antioxidant defenses. This imbalance often leads to DNA damage, genomic instability, cellular dysfunction, and disease [3,9]. While autophagy can limit oxidative stress by degrading damaged mitochondria (mitophagy), excessive levels of ROS can trigger autophagic activity to promote cell survival under adverse conditions [3,10]. Autophagy and oxidative stress are deeply interconnected in biology, with their roles oscillating between protective and pathological depending on the context [11]. This review explores the intricate relationship between autophagy and oxidative stress, examining their dual roles in tumorigenesis, their implications for therapeutic intervention, and potential future research directions to further elucidate these complex processes that may exhibit a synergistic and dual role, acting as both tumor suppressors and promoters depending on the specific cellular and microenvironmental context [12–15].

2. Mechanisms of Autophagy

Autophagy, a fundamental catabolic process in cellular homeostasis, acts in close coordination with other crucial mechanisms of cellular control, such as apoptosis and the proteasome system, to maintain cellular integrity and function [16]. This highly regulated pathway unfolds through a series of well-orchestrated steps, each mediated by a complex network of genes and proteins. Among the most extensively studied are the autophagy-related genes (ATG), which play a pivotal role in the autophagy process [17]. Additionally, key regulators such as the mechanistic target of rapamycin complex 1 (mTORC1), a serine/threonine kinase, and the phosphatidylinositol 3-kinase (PI3K) complex are critically involved in modulating this pathway [18–20].

The autophagic process is typically divided into distinct stages, including initiation, nucleation, elongation, lysosome fusion, and autophagosome degradation [17]. Each step is characterized by specific molecular events and regulatory mechanisms that ensure the efficient turnover of cellular components and adaptation to stress conditions [20,21]. Understanding these stages in detail is crucial for elucidating the role of autophagy in health and disease, as well as for identifying potential therapeutic targets in pathological contexts.

2.1. Molecular Machinery and Signaling Pathways

2.1.1. Initiation

Autophagy initiation begins with the formation of the autophagosome, requiring the synthesis of an isolation membrane, or "omegasome", which originates from the ER. This membrane develops into the phagophore, a cup-based structure composed of a single membrane. While the ER is the primary source, other organelles like the Golgi apparatus, endosomes, mitochondria, and plasma membrane also contribute to its formation [21]. mTORC1 regulates this stage, especially under nutrient deprivation. mTORC1 exists in two functionally distinct complexes: the rapamycin-sensitive mTORC1 that regulates cell size, and mTORC2 that is involved in modulating actin cytoskeleton organization. When nutrients are plentiful, mTORC1 localizes to the lysosome, where it is activated by the Rheb subunit, suppressing autophagy. Rapamycin, an mTORC1 inhibitor, induces autophagy even in nutrient-rich conditions [22,23]. mTORC1's regulation of autophagy initiation involves its interaction with the ULK1 complex, which consists of ULK1, ATG13, ATG101, and FIP200. Under nutrient-rich conditions, mTORC1 phosphorylates ULK1 and ATG13, inhibiting the ULK1 complex and autophagy. Under nutrient deprivation, mTORC1 is inhibited, releasing the ULK1 complex to activate autophagy through AMPK's phosphorylation of Rheb and RAPTOR. The activated ULK1 complex then facilitates the formation of the phagophore by phosphorylating Beclin-1 within the PI3K complex, triggering autophagic pathway initiation [23–26].

2.1.2. Nucleation and Elongation

Autophagosome nucleation is triggered by the Class III PI3K complex, composed of VPS34, Beclin-1 (ATG6), ATG14L, and p150 (VPS15) [27]. Beclin-1, located on the ER membrane, modulates this complex by binding to UVRAG or members of BCL2 family members, activating or inhibiting autophagy. ULK1, when activated, phosphorylates Beclin-1 and AMBRA1, promoting the PI3K complex recruitment to the ER and facilitating omegasome formation, the initial structure for the phagophore [24,28,29]. The activated PI3K in the ER produces phosphatidylinositol 3-phosphate (PIP3) on the omegasome membrane, recruiting WIPI proteins that attract other ATG proteins crucial for autophagy. ATG9, the only transmembrane ATG protein, is essential for lipid transport to the phagophore. The phagophore expands via two ubiquitin-like conjugation systems: the ATG12-ATG5-ATG16L system and LC3-II (ATG8). LC3 is conjugated with phosphatidylethanolamine, forming LC3-II, which becomes inserted into the expanding phagophore membrane and serves as an autophagosome marker, facilitating selective autophagy by interacting with autophagic cargo receptors [24,30,31].

2.1.3. Selective Autophagy

Although autophagy is generally non-selective, evidence suggests substrate selectivity, as exemplified by LC3-II's interaction with SQSTM1/p62. This adaptor protein binds ubiquitinated proteins, facilitating their capture and delivery to autophagosomes through LC3-II in a process termed LC3-associated phagocytosis. In addition, chaperone-mediated autophagy provides additional selectivity mechanisms, underscoring the dynamic adaptability of autophagy to several cellular needs [25,30,32,33].

2.1.4. Fusion with Lysosomes and Degradation

Upon completion, the autophagosome fuses with endosomes via the HOPS complex and then with lysosomes to form an autolysosome. The Rab7 GTPase protein, activated by UVRAG, regulates this process, with SNARE proteins mediating membrane fusion. Proteins LAMP1 and LAMP2 stabilize the fusion process, facilitating material transport. The lysosomal enzymes then degrade the autophagosome's contents, with permeases excreting the breakdown products into the cytosol for recycling [23,24,34].

This intricate autophagic process showcases its significance in cellular regulation, with each stage offering potential therapeutic intervention points in cancer treatment. As a multifaceted process, autophagy integrates several signaling pathways, underscoring its role in cellular adaptation and survival under stress (Figure 1).

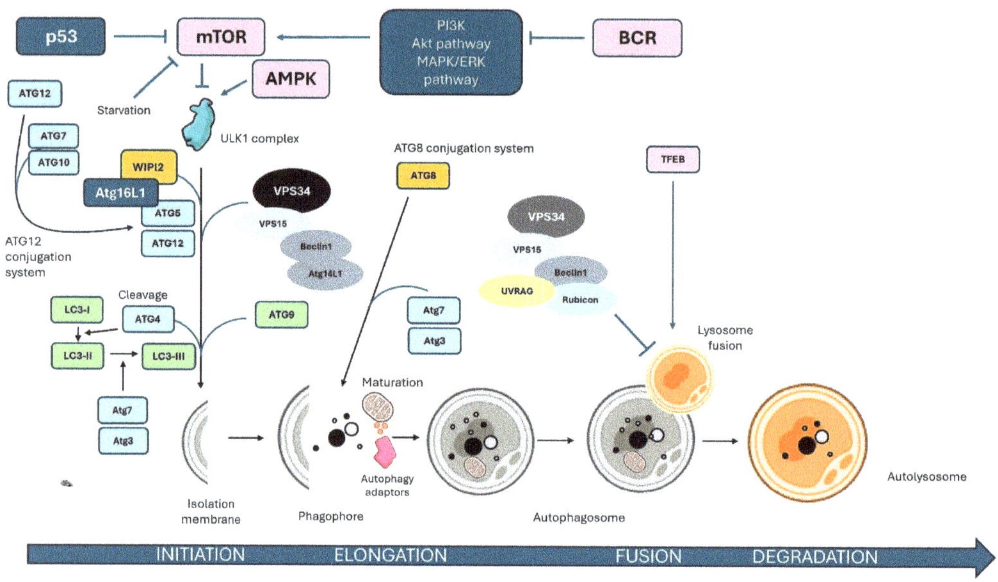

Figure 1. Autophagy pathway.

2.2. Types of Autophagy

Autophagy encompasses two main mechanisms: microautophagy and macroautophagy. Whereas microautophagy is a non-selective process where cellular components are directly engulfed through membrane invaginations of the lysosome or vacuole, macroautophagy (commonly referred to as autophagy) involves recycling damaged or dysfunctional organelles within an autophagosome that later fuses with the lysosome to degrade its contents [31,35]. On the other hand, autophagy can be classified as selective or non-selective. Whereas non-selective autophagy degrades cellular materials without prior recognition, primarily maintaining basic cellular functions, selective autophagy is a specific chaperone-mediated process that targets harmful cellular elements such as damaged proteins, toxic aggregates, or invasive pathogens for lysosomal degradation [36,37].

3. Autophagy Regulatory Drugs

In recent years, there has been a significant focus on drugs targeting the autophagy pathway, largely due to the role of autophagy in cellular homeostasis, cancer, and other diseases. Autophagy modulators are classified broadly as autophagy inducers and autophagy inhibitors, each with different mechanisms and clinical potential.

3.1. Autophagy Inducers

Autophagy inducers have shown promise in cancer and neurodegenerative diseases, where promoting the clearance of damaged cellular components can be beneficial. Key drugs include rapamycin, resveratrol, and spermidine.

- Rapamycin: Rapamycin is a well-characterized mTORC1 inhibitor that blocks the mTOR signaling pathway, a central regulator of autophagy. By inhibiting mTORC1, rapamycin induces autophagy initiation and has demonstrated efficacy in promoting autophagic cell death in cancer cells, particularly in those resistant to apoptosis [38–40]. Beyond its anticancer properties, rapamycin has shown therapeutic potential in other age-related diseases, emphasizing its broader clinical applications [41].
  Limitations: Rapamycin's inhibition of mTORC1 can lead to side effects, including suppression of T-cell proliferation [42,43], which is critical for immune responses against pathogens. Additionally, Rapamycin's inhibition produces thrombocytopenia, hyperlipidemia, insulin resistance and hyperglycemia [42–45]. These facts limit its long-term use and application as a preventive tool. Strategies to overcome these side effects include intermittent dosing, selective inhibition of mTORC1 (without affecting mTORC2) and combination therapies with metformin [45,46].
  Resveratrol: Resveratrol is a natural polyphenol found in plants, including knotweed and berries. Chemically, it is a stilbene derivative composed of two phenyl rings connected by an ethylene bridge. This unique chemical structure underpins its biological activities, particularly its ability to scavenge ROS and regulate signaling pathways involved in cellular stress responses [46,47]. Resveratrol, commonly found in dietary sources such as grapes and red wine, has been shown to activate autophagy through the inhibition of the mTOR pathway and the activation of AMPK, which further suppresses mTOR signaling [48]. Additionally, Resveratrol exhibits significant anti-tumor properties by inducing both apoptosis and autophagy, especially in cancers characterized by high oxidative stress [49].
  Limitations: Resveratrol may impair glucose metabolism, potentially leading to insulin resistance and hyperglycemia. As Rapamycin, it may suppress immune responses by affecting T-cell proliferation and cytokine production, increasing susceptibility to infections or impairing wound healing [50]. Prolonged inhibition of mTORC1 has also been linked to liver inflammation and gastrointestinal discomfort or diarrhea, although these effects are generally mild [51]. Mitigation strategies to minimize side effects include intermittent dosing, targeted delivery (such as CNS-specific formulations), and combination therapies with agents that counteract metabolic dysregulation (e.g., metformin) [52].
- Spermidine: Spermidine is an endogenous polyamine that enhances autophagy by inhibiting acetyltransferases and promoting the deacetylation of ATG proteins, which are essential for autophagy initiation. It has demonstrated anti-aging, anticancer, and geroprotective effects, reducing oxidative stress and lowering the incidence of cardiovascular and neurodegenerative diseases [53–55]. Studies show that spermidine levels increase during fasting or caloric restriction across species, and blocking its synthesis impairs fasting-induced autophagy and negates the lifespan- and healthspan-extending effects of these interventions. Spermidine mediates these effects through autophagy induction and hypusination of the translation regulator eIF5A, positioning the polyamine–hypusination axis as a conserved metabolic hub for longevity and health benefits [56,57].
  Limitations: Spermidine's interaction with mTORC1 can disrupt nutrient sensing and energy metabolism, potentially leading to imbalances in amino acid homeostasis and energy utilization, particularly during nutrient deprivation [58]. In some contexts,

spermidine may also impair immune cell proliferation and function, increasing susceptibility to infections or reducing the body's ability to respond to stressors. While beneficial in cancer therapy [59,60], spermidine-induced inhibition of mTORC1 can suppress normal cell proliferation and growth, potentially affecting healthy tissues. Moreover, spermidine has been shown to enhance apoptosis via mitochondrial pathways, which is advantageous for targeting cancer cells but could harm normal cells if not carefully controlled. Given that excessive polyamine accumulation has been linked to genomic instability and neurodegeneration due to deregulated protein degradation and nutrient sensing pathways, dosing and long-term use of spermidine need to be considered carefully. Mitigation strategies to reduce spermidine-associated risks include controlled dosing, tissue-specific delivery systems, and combination therapies with agents that counteract its adverse effects (e.g., metabolic regulators).

3.2. Autophagy Inhibitors

Even though autophagy supports cell survival under stress conditions, excessive autophagy can lead to autophagic cell death. Inhibitors of autophagy are, therefore, relevant in treating cancers that exploit autophagy for survival.

Chloroquine (CQ) and Hydroxychloroquine (HCQ): Both chloroquine and hydroxychloroquine are lysosomotropic agents that disrupt lysosomal acidification, thereby inhibiting the fusion of autophagosomes with lysosomes [61]. By blocking the final stages of autophagy, these agents induce cell death in cancer cells that rely on autophagy for survival. CQ and HCQ have been extensively studied in clinical trials and have demonstrated significant potential, particularly when used in combination with other cancer therapies, highlighting their promise as adjunctive treatments in oncology [62–64].

Bafilomycin A1: An inhibitor of vacuolar H+-ATPase, Bafilomycin A1 prevents lysosomal acidification in a manner like CQ [65]. It has shown significant anti-tumor properties, particularly in cancers that are highly dependent on autophagy [66,67]. Due to its ability to effectively block autophagic flux, Bafilomycin A1 has become an invaluable tool in research for studying the autophagy pathway and its implications in cancer biology.

3-Methyladenine (3-MA): 3-MA is a well-established inhibitor of autophagy that acts by blocking class III phosphoinositide 3-kinase (PI3K), a key regulator in the early stages of autophagosome formation. By inhibiting this kinase, 3-MA prevents the initiation of autophagy, thereby reducing the formation of autophagosomes [68]. Although its use in clinical applications is limited due to potential off-target effects and the incomplete inhibition of autophagy, 3-MA remains an indispensable tool in experimental research [69]. It is widely used to investigate autophagy's roles in cellular processes like survival, stress response, and disease progression, enabling researchers to explore its contribution to homeostasis and its involvement in diseases such as cancer, neurodegeneration, and infection [70–72].

Therefore, modulating autophagy in cancer therapy requires a deep understanding of the cellular and molecular context of each tumor. Developing effective strategies will depend on how we predict and manipulate the balance between the cytoprotective and cytotoxic effects of autophagy in cancer cells.

4. Oxidative Stress and ROS

Cell metabolism involves anabolic and catabolic pathways that maintain energy balance. In multicellular organisms, oxygen is the main substrate for aerobic respiration, producing adenosine triphosphate (ATP) [73,74]. Under physiological and resting conditions, most of the oxygen consumed by cells is reduced to water via cytochrome oxidase activity, but 1–2% generate ROS through electron transfer events or reduction/oxidation (redox) reactions within the mitochondria [75].

ROS were first identified as free radicals in skeletal muscle with harmful effects on cells [76]. These specific oxygen-containing molecules are highly reactive and unstable, classified into non-radical and free radicals based on unpaired electrons (Table 1) [77]. Recent research highlights their dual nature [78,79]. While they function as pleiotropic physiological molecules at the baseline cell homeostatic state, involved in signaling pathways, immune defense and cell differentiation, elevated ROS levels cause cellular damage and contribute to disease development [77,80].

Table 1. Reactive species classification.

Classification	Definition	Species	Abbreviations
Free Radicals	At least one unpaired electron, making them highly reactive.	Superoxide Hydroxyl radical Peroxyl radical Alkoxyl radical Nitric oxide *	O_2^- HO· ROO· RO· NO·
Non-radicals	Reactive species without unpaired electrons but, still, participating in oxidative reactions. They can form radicals under certain conditions.	Hydrogen peroxide Singlet oxygen Hypochlorous acid * Ozone Organic hydroperoxides	H_2O_2 $^1O_2$ HOCl O_3 ROOH

The term reactive oxygen species (ROS) is frequently employed to refer to reactive oxygen-containing molecules, as well as reactive nitrogen or chlorine species. * These chemical species are examples of reactive nitrogen and chlorine species.

Cells maintain ROS homeostasis by tightly regulated biological mechanisms through a balance between ROS production and scavenging mechanisms. Disruption of this balance, typically due to elevated ROS levels, results in oxidative stress, a state characterized by the disturbance of cellular redox homeostasis [81,82]. Understanding the complex interplay between ROS, oxidative stress, antioxidants and cellular metabolism is crucial for developing targeted interventions in several diseases associated with redox imbalance such as cancer [83,84].

4.1. Sources of ROS in Cells

ROS are well-known to be produced from two primary sources: endogenous and exogenous factors like radiation, pollutants, cigarette smoke, and nutrition [85]. Endogenously, ROS are mainly produced by mitochondria and nicotinamide adenine dinucleotide phosphate (NADPH) oxidases (NOXs), with other enzymes such as endoplasmic reticulum (ER) oxidases, peroxisomes, superoxide dismutases (SODs), xanthine oxidoreductase, nitric oxide synthases (NOSs), lipoxygenases, prostaglandin synthases, cyclooxygenases and cytochrome P450 also contributing to their production [80,86,87].

The electron transport chain (ETC) in mitochondria is crucial for ATP production through oxidative phosphorylation. Electrons from metabolic substrates are transferred through protein complexes in the inner mitochondrial membrane (complexes I-IV), reducing oxygen to water and generating a proton gradient that drives ATP synthesis via the ATP synthase (complex V) [88]. Normally, ROS production in the ETC is low and regulated, serving as signaling messengers for processes like metabolism, apoptosis, and stress adaptation. However, complexes I and III are major ROS sources, leaking electrons that generate superoxide anion radical (O_2^-) and hydrogen peroxide (H_2O_2) [89–91]. When ETC function is impaired, this electron leak can overwhelm antioxidant defenses, causing mitochondrial dysfunction, macromolecular damage, and disrupting signaling pathways linked to disease, or triggering immune responses as danger-associated molecular patterns (DAMPs) [92,93].

On the other hand, NOXs are a family of enzymes in the plasma membrane that play a key role in cytoplasmic ROS production. In humans, the NOX family includes seven members (NOX1-NOX5, DUOX1 and DUOX2), which primarily produce ROS, unlike other cellular sources where ROS are by-products [94]. NOXs catalyze electron transfer from NADPH to oxygen, generating O_2^- that can form other ROS like H_2O_2 or hydroxyl radicals (-OH). NOX-derived ROS are involved in host defense (e.g., NOS2 in phagocytes killing pathogens) [95], signaling pathways (e.g., NOX4 regulating vascular tone [96], and thyroid hormone biosynthesis (DUOX-produced H_2O_2) [97]. Dysregulation of NOXs leads to excessive ROS, contributing to oxidative stress and damage in various diseases, including cardiovascular, chronic inflammatory diseases, blood disorders, and tumors [98].

The ER and peroxisomes are key cellular compartments for ROS production. In the ER, H_2O_2 is generated during oxidative protein folding by enzymes like protein disulfide isomerase and oxidoreductin-1. In peroxisomes, H_2O_2 is produced during fatty acid β-oxidation, amino acid catabolism, and purine metabolism, and can be neutralized by CATs. However, excessive ROS levels can overwhelm antioxidant defenses, contributing to lipid peroxidation and oxidative stress [99,100].

Last, exogenous ROS from sources like radiation, pollutants, toxins, or therapeutic drugs can amplify endogenous ROS production by damaging organelles and activating ROS-producing enzymes like NOXs [101]. These ROS regulate signaling pathways but can cause oxidative damage to DNA, lipids, and proteins when levels exceed antioxidant defenses [102]. This interaction contributes to diseases such as hematological malignancies, solid tumors, and neurodegenerative and cardiovascular disorders, emphasizing the importance of maintaining redox balance to prevent pathological outcomes [103].

4.2. Antioxidant Defense Systems

Cells maintain redox homeostasis by balancing ROS production and antioxidant defenses. ROS production is initially limited by mitochondria during OXPHOS, with NOXs and other oxidases suppressed in a preventive phase. When ROS levels rise, cells activate antioxidant systems to neutralize potential damage [81]. Key defense mechanisms, including autophagy, counteract ROS through a dynamic interplay of oxidants, antioxidants, and cellular responses [104,105].

Antioxidant defense components are categorized based on their synthesis, nature, or function and can be divided into first-line and second-line defenses. The system is regulated by cellular mechanisms to cope with chronic oxidative stress [106]. Enzymatic components like SODs, catalases (CATs) and glutathione peroxidases (GPx) provide rapid first-line defense by neutralizing ROS. Non-enzymatic components like reduced glutathione (GSH), and peroxiredoxin/thioredoxin (TRX) system also contribute to defense. Second-line defenses include ubiquinol (Coenzyme Q10) and exogenous antioxidants, such as vitamins, minerals, flavonoids, and carotenoids, which further support ROS neutralization [107] (Table 2).

Finally, despite preventive and detoxification measures, oxidative damage can occur due to prolonged exposure to ROS. Hence, cells have evolved an adaptive third-line defense response to restore redox balance by upregulating antioxidant defenses, repairing oxidatively damaged molecules, and removing defective cellular components. Key mechanisms of this cellular response include: (1) activation of antioxidant enzymes; (2) nuclear factor erythroid 2-related factor2 (Nrf2); (3) autophagy; (4) mitophagy; (5) non-enzymatic defense; and (6) metabolic reprogramming. For instance, stress signals dissociate Nrf2 from its inhibitory complex (Kelch-like ECH-associated protein 1, Keap1), allowing its translocation to the nucleus and activation of target genes encoding antioxidant enzymes such as SODs, CATs or GPxs, while also promoting the catabolic process to degrade damaged organelles, misfolded proteins and other toxic aggregates by inducing expression of ATGs (e.g., p62/SQSTM1). Furthermore, impaired autophagy leads to p62 accumulation, which competes with Nrf2 for binding KEAP1, enhancing Nrf2 activation [108]. This cross-regulation is critical for protecting cells from oxidative stress, and emerging evidence highlights the potential of targeting the Nrf2–autophagy axis in therapeutic interventions for neurodegenerative diseases, cardiovascular disorders, and cancer [11,109–111].

Table 2. Antioxidant defense systems.

Classification	Antioxidant	Characteristics
First-line	Superoxide dismutase (SOD)	Endogenous; enzymatic. Degradation of superoxide anions to more stable ROS: $O_2^- \rightarrow H_2O_2$ Three isoforms: cytoplasmic Cu/Zn-SOD (SOD1); mitochondrial Mn-SOD (SOD2), and EC-SOD (SOD3).
	Catalase (CAT)	Endogenous; enzymatic. Abundant in peroxisomes, it is absent in mitochondria of mammalian cells. Degradation of hydrogen peroxide $O_2^- \rightarrow H_2O_2 \rightarrow H_2O + O_2$
	Glutathione peroxidase (GPX)	Endogenous; enzymatic. Mainly expressed in the mitochondria and sometimes in the cytosol. Degradation of hydrogen peroxide, with glutathione as substrate: $O_2^- \rightarrow H_2O_2 \rightarrow H_2O + O_2$ GSH $\rightarrow$ GSSG Its activity may depend on its cofactor selenium, so it is known as selenocysteine peroxidase.
Second-line	Thioredoxin (TRX) system	Endogenous; first- or second-line defense depending on the author. Antioxidant proteins that facilitate reduction in proteins by cysteine thiol-disulfide exchange.
	Glutathione (GSH)	Endogenous; non-enzymatic first- or second-line defense depending on the author. Cofactor for GPx; directly neutralizes free radicals and ROS.
	Coenzyme Q10	Endogenous ubiquinone or exogenous from diet; non-enzymatic. Participates in the ETC and neutralizes free radicals within mitochondria.
	Carotenoids	Exogenous; non-enzymatic. Efficient quench of singlet oxygen and upregulation of antioxidant enzyme activity.
	Flavonoids	Exogenous; non-enzymatic. Direct free radical scavengers and metal-chelating properties.
	Vitamin C	Exogenous; non-enzymatic. Ascorbate enters cells from plasma by co-transporters, being particularly effective at scavenging superoxide radicals where SOD activity is lower.
Third-line	Nrf2 Autophagy Mitophagy	Endogenous adaptive response. It involves all mechanisms that upregulate antioxidant systems to remove free radicals left during the previous lines of defense.

4.3. *Redox Signaling*

Redox signaling and oxidative stress are closely related but distinct, with ROS playing a key role in determining cellular fate depending on their concentration and context (Figure 2). Redox signaling involves low to moderate ROS levels that regulate biological processes, while oxidative stress occurs when ROS levels surpass the cell's antioxidant capacity, leading to cellular damage, disrupted signaling, and disease [112].

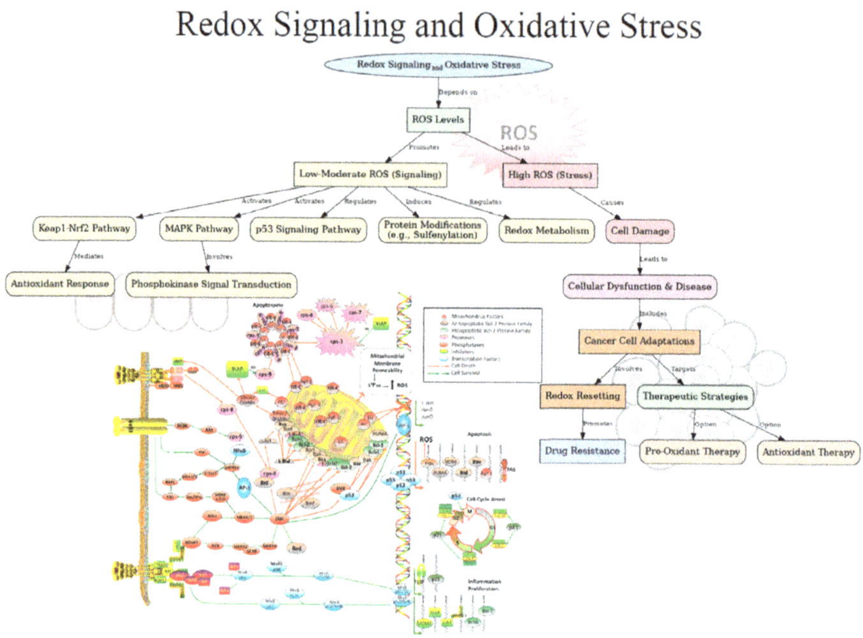

Figure 2. Redox signaling and oxidative stress.

Spatial and temporal regulation is central to redox signaling. ROS are transiently produced to enable dynamic responses, localized to specific cellular compartments such as mitochondria, the ER, or the plasma membrane, ensuring precise outcomes. Key targets are redox-sensitive residues, particularly cysteines and methionines, whose reversible modifications regulate protein activity [112,113]. ROS like O_2^-, H_2O_2, and OH^- are essential for oxidative stress and activating signaling cascades [80]. These signals are propagated through complex communication networks, influencing processes like mitogen-activated protein kinase (MAPK) cascades and p53 signaling, leading to responses such as cell cycle arrest, senescence, or apoptosis [114]. Thus, redox signaling plays a key role in regulating cellular processes, including antioxidant response, phosphokinase signal transduction and redox metabolism [114,115]. Understanding redox chemistry involves considering reaction kinetics. Redox signaling requires an oxidant (electrophile) reacting with a reductant (nucleophile). Unlike conventional second messengers like cyclic adenosine monophosphate (cAMP), redox signaling uses molecules with greater potential for non-specific reactions. There are two main types of redox reactions: oxidation, where the oxidant accepts electrons, and leaving the reducing agent in a more oxidized state. The oxidant may take one electron (a free radical reaction) or two, leading to the oxidation of target proteins. Two-electron oxidations predominate in redox signaling, as free radicals are more likely to trigger further reactions. These reactions can alter protein function, gene expression, or post-translational modifications [115,116]. The second type involves the formation of a covalent bond between the reductant and oxidant, where atoms share electrons instead of fully losing or gaining them [115]. However, as it will be discussed in more detail in subsequent sections, dysregulated redox reactions and ROS production play crucial roles in blood and solid cancers, where ROS act as second messengers regulating cell proliferation, death, and chemoresistance [117–119].

Upon therapy, some tumor cells undergo redox resetting, acquiring a new balance with higher ROS levels and stronger antioxidant systems. This enables cancer cells to resist anticancer drugs through mechanisms like increased drug efflux, altered drug metabolism, mutated targets, activated pro-survival pathways, and reduced cell death [115]. Understanding these mechanisms offers promising strategies to overcome drug resistance and improve treatment outcomes [120]. Furthermore, during metastasis, cancer cells face significant oxidative stress as they migrate through diverse environments. To survive, they undergo reversible metabolic changes that enhance oxidative stress resistance. However, oxidative stress can also induce ferroptosis, limiting the survival of metastasizing cells [112,121]. Given the role of ROS in cancer, therapeutic strategies often target redox status. Pro-oxidant therapies aim to increase oxidative stress in cancer cells, while antioxidant therapies seek to reduce it. Natural substances from plants have chemopreventive potential by modifying redox status [122–124]. Therefore, redox reactions and oxidative stress are central to cancer biology, affecting tumor development, progression, and response to treatment.

5. Crosstalk Between Autophagy and Oxidative Stress

Autophagy and oxidative stress are tightly regulated processes significantly influence cancer onset and tumor progression [125–127] (Figure 3). Their interplay can suppress or promote tumor growth, depending on the context [128]. In early tumorigenesis, autophagy acts as a tumor suppressor mechanism by degrading oncogenic molecules, damaged organelles, and misfolded or polyubiquitinated proteins [129,130]. It also helps reduce oxidative stress and cytoplasmic debris [131–133], which have been related to genomic instability and the accumulation of oncogenic mutations [129,130,134]. However, in later stages with established tumors and during cancer progression, autophagy influences tumor metabolism, supporting cell survival by sustaining energy needs for DNA repair, adapting to the microenvironment [135], and modulating ROS production, metabolic reprogramming, immune evasion, metastasis, and resistance to treatments [136].

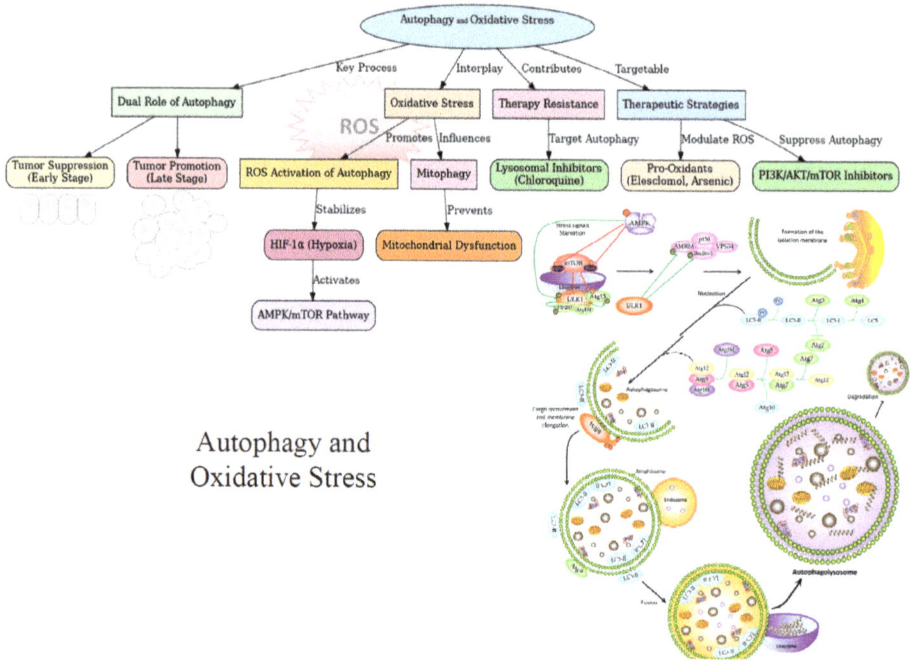

Figure 3. Autophagy and oxidative stress in hematological malignancies.

5.1. ROS as Inducers of Autophagy

Multiple studies have suggested that the crosstalk between autophagy and oxidative stress is mediated by redox-sensitive proteins, which contain specific amino acid residues particularly susceptible to oxidation or reduction [137,138]. These proteins modulate the intracellular redox environment, often shifting it towards a more oxidizing state [139]. During starvation, exposure to H_2O_2 triggers the efficient extrusion of GSH via the MRP1 drug efflux pump. This process activates AMPK through S-glutathionylation of specific reactive cysteine residues (Cys299 and Cys304) in α and β subunits, which phosphorylates and activates key autophagy proteins, including ULK1 [140], mTORC1, and PIK3C3/VPS34 [141–144]. Since S-glutathionylation can induce autophagy without other stimuli, thiol redox homeostasis appears crucial for regulating autophagy. In addition to AMPK, several proteins involved in the autophagy initiation, such as the ubiquitin-like systems ATG7-ATG3 [143,145] and ATG7-ATG10 [143], Beclin-1 [140], PI3K [140], members of Rab GTPase [146,147], PTEN (Cys124 and Cys71) [148] and SQSTM1/p62 [140], are modulated by oxidation of specific cysteine residues. In support of the hypothesis suggesting the regulation of autophagy-related proteins through the oxidation of cysteine residues, it has previously been demonstrated that the H_2O_2-mediated oxidation of cysteine residues in ATG4, ATG3, and ATG7 proteins is essential for inhibiting their hydrolyzing activity on LC3-II, facilitating proper autophagosome elongation [143,144]. H_2O_2 inactivates ATG4B by oxidizing Cys81 near the catalytic site [143,149] and reduces the interaction between ATG3 and ATG7 with LC3, preventing LC3 lipidation and autophagy initiation [143]. In addition, mutations affecting Cys292 and Cys361 residues in the *ATG4B* locus have been linked to increased autophagy flux, likely by altering the protein's redox sensitivity [150,151]. Furthermore, under oxidative stress, AKT forms disulfide bonds between Cys297 and Cys311, leading to its dephosphorylation and inactivation, which reduces mTORC1 activity and induces autophagy [152]. Similarly, ROS increase AMPK phosphorylation and activity, thus leading to the induction of autophagy through the inhibition of mTORC1 activity and PI3K-AKT signaling [153]. Furthermore, ROS oxidize ATM, promoting the formation of intramolecular disulfide bonds at Cys-2991. This oxidation activates ATM independently of the DNA damage response pathway and induces TSC2-mTOR signaling pathway, thereby promoting autophagy initiation [154]. ROS can also activate p53, which induces the transcription of sestrin proteins that promote autophagy initiation through AMPK activation and mTORC1 inhibition via the assembly of TSC1 and TSC2 [153]. Finally, it has been reported that H_2O_2 induces the translocation of TFEB from the cytoplasm to the nucleus. This translocation triggers autophagy and lysosomal biogenesis as a defensive response against oxidative damage [155]. Although the translocation mechanism is not fully understood, it is believed to be directly induced by ROS, which oxidize specific cysteine residues in TFEB, TFE, and MITF, leading to enhanced expression of genes implicated in the autophagy-lysosome pathway [156], thus linking redox signaling with autophagic regulation.

In addition to the post-transcriptional regulation of autophagy by oxidative stress, it has been reported the existence of redox-independent relationship between autophagy and antioxidant response, primarily mediated by the p62/Keap1/Nrf2 pathway [131,140]. Furthermore, it has been shown to selectively target oxidized and damaged biomaterials for lysosomal degradation [157], reducing oxidative stress and promoting cell survival.

5.2. *Autophagy as Regulator of Oxidative Stress*

Autophagy regulates oxidative stress by clearing damaged organelles [137], oxidized proteins [158], and protein aggregates [159], as well as by reducing ROS levels through different pathways, including the regulation of TFEB [156]. It is well known that autophagy plays a key role in maintaining cellular homeostasis by selectively targeting specific organelles for degradation, including mitochondria (mitophagy), peroxisomes (peroxiphagy), the ER (reticulophagy) and lysosomes (lysophagy) [132,137]. Once formed, the autophagosome can engulf these organelles or harmful protein aggregates, which are then degraded by lysosomal enzymes [160]. This process is vital for preventing ROS accumulation particularly from dysfunctional mitochondria [161,162], peroxisomes [143,163] and lysosomes [132,156]. It also helps maintain the balance between ROS production and scavenging [164,165], facilitating the recycling of their components for energy production and biosynthesis [160,166]. ROS from mitochondria are mainly involved in oxidative phosphorylation reactions within the inner mitochondrial membrane. These ROS are regulated by classical scavengers, including SOD family proteins and the GSH redox system, which sequentially convert O_2^- into H_2O_2, and then reduce it to O_2 and H_2O [167]. When mitochondria are dysfunctional, ROS accumulate leading to cellular damage [168] and activating autophagy. Conformational changes in the mitochondrial membrane trigger autophagy activation through Parkin-dependent ubiquitination [169] and the BNIP3-NIX-FUNDC1 mitochondrial adaptor pathways. When Parkin is phosphorylated by PTEN-induced putative kinase 1 (PINK1), it ubiquitinates outer membrane proteins (VDAC1, Mfn1 and Mfn2) [158,170], as well as other proteins such as fission protein (FIS) and its adaptor (TBC1D15), and mitochondrial translocases (TOMM20 and TOMM70) [170]. Once ubiquitinated and tagged for proteasomal degradation, these proteins bind to autophagy cargo receptors (SQSTM1, NDP52 and optineurin) [158], promoting mitochondrial engulfment by the autophagosome. This process is also activated by Rab signaling proteins, including RABGEF1, RAB5 and RAB7A [171,172], and autophagy receptors such as p62, TAX1BP1, and CALCOCO2 [170]. Furthermore, the BNIP3-NIX-FUNDC1 mitochondrial adaptor pathway promotes mitochondrial attachment to the autophagosome. This step is positively controlled by ULK1 and Src [173,174] and involves the recruitment of WIPI proteins (WIPI1,

WIPI2 and WIPI3) to facilitate the recruitment of downstream proteins of the autophagy machinery [175].

On the other hand, the engulfment of peroxisomes plays a key role in modulating oxidative stress. These organelles are involved in lipid metabolism, ketogenesis, and the metabolism of cholesterol and isoprenoids [176]. They contain acyl-CoA (ACOX) and D-amino oxidases, which generate intracellular H_2O_2 [177], as well as xanthine oxidases and small ETCs in their membranes that produce anion superoxide (O_2^-) [178]. When peroxisomes are defective or damaged, they cause an elevation in intracellular ROS levels, activating ATM through the oxidation of specific cysteine residues, including Cys2991. This oxidation results in the formation of multiple intracellular disulfide bonds, promoting ATM dimerization [179]. Once activated, ATM promotes AMPK and ULK1 activation while inhibiting mTORC1 to induce autophagy. Additionally, ATM phosphorylates PEX5 at Ser141 and promotes its mono-ubiquitination at K209 [180], facilitating its recognition by p62 and NRB1. These adaptor proteins, in association with LC3, guide the autophagosome to the damaged peroxisomes [181]. Another peroxisomal protein recognized by p62 and NRB1 after undergoing oxidative modifications is PEX14, which is implicated in the timely removal of dysfunctional peroxisomes. H_2O_2-induced phosphorylation of PEX14 at Ser232 inhibits the peroxisomal import of CAT in vivo and disrupts the interaction of CAT with the PEX14-PEX5 complex in vitro [182].

Regarding reticulophagy and lysophagy, there is solid evidence suggesting that they help in eliminating damaged ER and lysosomes. Reticulophagy is activated during ER stress and helps in maintaining ER homeostasis by degrading damaged ER components, which can be triggered by oxidative stress through the unfolded protein response (UPR) [183]. Additionally, reticulophagy indirectly influences oxidative stress by preserving mitochondrial function, as intact mitochondria are observed during excessive ER-phagy [184]. Reticulophagy helps in reducing ER stress-induced ROS production, which can otherwise damage mitochondria [185]. In addition, ER stress activates the Nrf2 transcription factor, which enhances the expression of antioxidant response genes, thus protecting mitochondria from oxidative damage [185]. One key mechanism involves the PERK pathway, where the ER stress sensor PERK phosphorylates and activates NRF2, causing it to dissociate from its repressor KEAP1 and translocate to the nucleus [186,187]. Recent studies have demonstrated that PERK activation stimulates NRF2 expression via the transcription factor ATF4, suggesting that NRF2 has a central role in preventing oxidative damage [186]. A noncanonical pathway also involves the autophagy receptor p62/SQSTM1, which binds and degrades KEAP1, thus facilitating NRF2 activation. Once activated, NRF2 induces the expression of antioxidant genes such as *NQO1* and *HMOX1/HO-1*, which help in neutralizing ROS and protect mitochondria from oxidative damage [188]. Furthermore, NRF2 activation promotes components of the UPR, including XBP1 and ATF6α, contributing to ER integrity and protein homeostasis [189,190]. By coordinating these protective responses, NRF2 activation helps maintain redox balance, reduce mitochondrial oxidative damage, and support cell survival during stress [188]. Besides these mechanisms, reticulophagy supports mitochondrial quality control by maintaining ER function, which is essential for protein folding [191–194], lipid synthesis [195], and mitochondrial membrane integrity [196,197]. It also regulates mitophagy by providing membrane sources for autophagosome formation and influences mitochondrial energy metabolism by regulating lipid homeostasis [198] and calcium signaling between the ER and mitochondria [197,199], affecting ATP production. Likewise, reticulophagy impacts mitochondrial dynamics, including fission and fusion [185], by modulating the structure of the ER, which is essential for mitochondrial network formation and cellular stress adaptation. Reticulophagy also controls oxidative stress by influencing lipid metabolism [200] and lipid droplets (LDs) homeostasis, which store excess lipids. LDs play a protective role by preventing lipotoxicity and the toxic effects of unesterified lipids [201–203]. Conversely, changes such as the accumulation of free fatty acids, cholesterol and ceramide lead to lysosomal membrane permeabilization and lipid-ROS production [184,198]. The ER and mitochondria are connected through structures known as mitochondria-associated membranes [204–206], which are crucial for lipid synthesis and exchange [207,208], particularly involving phospholipids like phosphatidylcholine, phosphatidylethanolamine, diacylglycerol, and cholesterol [209]. Disruptions in lipid metabolism at these sites can destabilize lysosomal membranes, leading to lipotoxicity [210,211], accumulation of lipid hydroperoxides, and increased membrane permeability [212,213]. This destabilization facilitates the release of ROS and damaging contents from ribosomes and lysosomes, such as cathepsins, exacerbating oxidative stress [214].

Similarly to reticulophagy, ribophagy, and lysophagy, the selective autophagy of damaged ribosomes and lysosomes can mitigate oxidative stress [215]. Given that these processes are faster compared than the autophagy of entire organelles, it has been proposed that they are selective mechanisms [200,216–218]. Among these specific autophagic processes, lysophagy has gained significant attention as it supports mitochondrial quality control by maintaining lysosomal function, which is critical for mitophagy, and reducing ROS production [212,219]. Recent studies have suggested that ubiquitination plays a key role in the regulation of both lysophagy and ribophagy [216,220]. Ubiquitin-based modifications are commonly involved in the selective elimination of cellular structures, suggesting they could dictate which ribosomal and lysosomal components are targeted for degradation. Upon lysosomal damage, extensive ubiquitination of lysosomal proteins occurs [221], involving both K63-linked and K48-linked ubiquitin chains that serve as recruitment platforms for autophagy receptors, enabling the identification of damaged organelles [222,223]. This ubiquitination cascade relies on E1 ubiquitin-activating enzymes, E2 ubiquitin-conjugating enzymes like UBE2QL1, and E3 ubiquitin ligases such as TRIM16 and SCF FBXO27 [222]. UBE2QL1 is particularly critical, as its depletion reduces ubiquitination and disrupts lysophagy [224]. Temporal dynamic studies have revealed that K63 chain formation occurs within 30–60 min of damage, while K48 chains peak after 2–3 h [222]. These ubiquitin chains recruit autophagy receptors, such as p62/SQSTM1, TAX1BP1, and Optineurin, which link damaged lysosomes to the autophagy machinery [225]. Additionally, ubiquitination facilitates the recruitment of the AAA-ATPase VCP/p97 and the TRIM16-Galectin-3 complex, which, along with factors like ATG16L1 and ULK1, drive local phagophore formation [222,223]. This orchestrated process ensures the efficient removal of damaged lysosomes, maintaining cellular homeostasis.

In ribophagy, the Ubp3-Bre5 complex interacts and controls the ubiquitination of ATG19 [226], a receptor in the cytoplasm-to-vacuole targeting pathway [227]. ATG5-ATG19 autophagy interaction motifs (AIM) interaction competes with the ATG8-ATG19 AIM interaction [228], suggesting a regulatory mechanism involving ubiquitination and deubiquitination activities. In addition, it is also supported by the fact that decreased levels of the ubiquitin ligase Rsp5, along with the deletion of Ubp3, impair ribosome turnover, although other cytoplasmic proteins are still degraded by autophagy [229]. These findings underscore the importance of both ubiquitination and deubiquitination in regulating ribophagy and suggest the importance of understanding the precise mechanisms behind these processes and its regulation.

Finally, it is important to highlight the role of lipophagy in cellular lipid metabolism and homeostasis, particularly under oxidative stress conditions [230]. High glucose levels, for example, can activate lipophagy to alleviate lipid accumulation by promoting LD breakdown and enhancing mitochondrial β-oxidation, with oxidative and ER stress pathways acting as key regulators [231]. ROS also triggers lipophagy through the activation of transcription factors like TFEB via lysosomal calcium release, creating a feedback mechanism to mitigate oxidative damage [232]. However, prolonged oxidative stress can impair lipophagy [183,209], as seen in endothelial cells exposed to oxidized low-density lipoprotein (ox-LDL), where reduced lipophagic activity leads to lipid accumulation and cellular damage [233]. Interestingly, exposure to ox-LDL also induces oxidative stress in liver, increasing LD enriched with cholesteryl ester hydroperoxidases and deregulating genes like *SREBP1*, *FASN* and *DGAT1* [234]. These findings underscore the critical role of lipophagy in lipid homeostasis [231] and its dysfunction under oxidative stress, contributing to diseases like atherosclerosis and non-alcoholic fatty liver disease (NAFLD) [230,234]. Furthermore, lysosomes are central to this process, as impaired lysosomal function exacerbates oxidative stress and metabolic dysfunctions, highlighting the interplay between lysosomal activity, ROS production, and lipophagy in cellular health.

Although the information above links mitophagy, reticulophagy, ribophagy, lysophagy, lipophagy and oxidative stress, further research is needed to fully understand their roles in maintaining cellular redox balance and their contributions to diseases such as NAFLD, neurodegenerative diseases, and cancer.

6. The Role of Autophagy and Oxidative Stress in Hematological Malignancies

Autophagy and oxidative stress play crucial roles in the development, progression, and treatment of hematological malignancies. Disruption in autophagy and oxidative imbalance during hematopoiesis can lead to malignant transformation and increased cell proliferation [21] and it may have different biological effects depending on the specific tumor type, genetic context, and stage of development [235]. The complex interplay between autophagy and oxidative stress significantly impacts malignant cell survival, drug resistance, and therapeutic outcomes.

6.1. Autophagy and ROS as Modulators of Tumor Survival, Treatment and Disease Progression

In the early stages of hematological cancers, autophagy serves as a survival mechanism that helps cancer cells cope with metabolic stress caused by rapid proliferation, nutrient deprivation, or hypoxia. This adaptive response allows tumor cells to maintain viability under harsh conditions and contributes to their persistence and potential relapse. Autophagy enables cancer cells to recycle intracellular components, providing energy and essential building blocks during metabolic stress. This process is particularly important in apoptosis-defective cells, allowing them to survive prolonged nutrient and oxygen deprivation [59,236]. In leukemic cells, hypoxia-induced autophagy has been shown to support the survival of leukemia stem cells (LSCs), contributing to chemoresistance and disease progression [237]. Additionally, autophagy facilitates tumor dormancy by enabling residual cancer cells to endure metabolic deprivation. These dormant cells can later re-enter the cell cycle and drive relapse when conditions become favorable [238,239]. The ability of autophagy to maintain cellular homeostasis under stress resembles a "hibernation-like" state that enhances long-term survival [236,238]. While autophagy supports cancer cell survival, its suppression in early tumor stages can lead to increased genomic instability, inflammation, and necrotic cell death, promoting tumorigenesis [236,237].

On the other hand, in advanced stages, autophagy becomes a pro-survival mechanism that sustains malignant growth and resistance to therapy [236,240]. Therapeutically, inhibiting autophagy may improve treatment outcomes in hematological cancers by sensitizing cancer cells to stress-induced death, particularly in apoptosis-defective tumors [236,240]. However, the paradoxical role of autophagy as both a tumor suppressor and promoter complicates therapeutic strategies. Careful timing and context-specific targeting are critical to avoid unintended consequences. Clinical trials are currently investigating the efficacy of therapies targeting autophagy and oxidative stress in combination with traditional treatments to enhance patient outcomes. Strategies aimed at oxidative stress focus on two key approaches: mitigating ROS-induced damage to healthy tissues or leveraging elevated ROS levels to selectively target cancer cells. Increasing evidence highlights the potential of combination therapies that concurrently modulate autophagy and oxidative stress, offering a promising avenue for more effective cancer treatments. For example, combining autophagy inhibitors with pro-oxidants has shown synergistic effects in preclinical models, as the inhibition of autophagy sensitizes cancer cells to ROS-induced death [18]. Additionally, targeting upstream regulators of autophagy and oxidative stress, such as the PI3K/AKT/mTOR axis, offers a promising avenue for integrated therapeutic strategies.

6.2. ROS and Autophagy in Hematological Malignancies

6.2.1. Leukemias

Chronic Lymphocytic Leukemia

In CLL, oxidative stress levels are higher compared with normal B cells. The main source of ROS in CLL cells is mitochondria, which also has an increased mitochondrial mass. Mitochondrial ROS, specifically superoxide and hydrogen peroxide, are products of mitochondrial respiration and play a role in B-cell receptor (BCR) signaling by modulating cellular metabolism. This process involves oxidative phosphorylation and highlights the differences between naïve B cells and anergic B cells [241]. Higher levels of ROS produce genomic instability and DNA damage which affects disease progression. Mitochondrial DNA mutations (mtDNA) can increase the nitric oxide (NO) levels, which have an influence on mitochondrial biogenesis [242]. Inhibition of NOS, the enzymes that produce NO and oxidative stress, can modify this process. It is demonstrated that L-NAME, an inhibitor of NOS, induces apoptosis in CLL cells by the reduction in the NO production affecting the oxidative stress pathways and the mitochondrial biogenesis [242,243].

Additionally, PI3K/AKT signaling pathways play a key role for cell proliferation and survival. It is overexpressed in CLL cells due to the inhibition of the SH1P phosphatase, which usually inhibits this pathway. Restoring the SHIP1 activity could be a potential target for CLL by limiting this pathway and promoting cell death [244]. Higher levels of phosphorylated STAT3 in Ser727 (pSTAT3Ser727) in mitochondria is another significant mechanism for the CLL. Overexpression of STAT3 improves the antioxidant defenses of the CLL cells, improving their survival. So, it could be a potential target therapy to reduce malignant B cells in CLL [245]. In conclusion, these processes highlight the role of the mitochondrial function in the PI3K/AKT signalization and the antioxidant defense mechanism in CLL, suggesting several therapeutics targets in future treatments.

The transcription factor Nrf2 (the nuclear factor erythroid 2-related factor 2) presents higher levels by oxidative stress and toxic aggressions. Nrf2 function is the regulation of the expression of numerous proteins that play a role in the antioxidant response, improving the CLL cell survival. The increased mitochondrial mass and the production of mitochondrial ROS activates this signalization pathway in CLL cells [246]. Under normal conditions, Keap1 negatively regulates Nrf2, promoting its degradation through the ubiquitin-proteasome pathway. However, under pathological conditions, such as oxidative stress, Keap1 modified in its cysteine reactive residues, these modifications produce conformational changes in the Keap1 protein, releasing Nrf2. Once released, Nrf2 is translocated to the nucleus and activates the antioxidant and cytoprotective gene transcription [247]. Nrf2 promotes the expression of the catalytic and modulates antioxidant subunits, GCL (Glutamate-Cysteine Ligase) subunits, which enhances the expression of GSH. Furthermore, GSH positively regulates the heme oxygenase-1, which also positively regulates the mitochondrial transcription factor A, stimulating mitochondrial biogenesis. This process reduces the ROS damage and compensates for reduced mitochondrial energy production [248].

Sánchez-Lopez et al. (2020) showed that the activation of p-62-Nrf2 pathway, dependent on NF-kB plays a key role in the survival and drug resistance in CLL cells with high levels of ROR 1, a tyrosine kinase receptor associated with a poor prognosis [249]. The activation of NF-kB by microenvironmental factors such as BAFF (B-cells activation factor), increases ROS production. Furthermore, the signaling adaptor p62 (SQSTM1) is involved in the union of NF-kB with Nrf2. Consequently, higher levels of p62 promote the sequestration of Keap1, protecting the CLL cells by reducing ROS cell effects. In addition, in higher expression of ROR1 CLL cells, the activation of NF-kB through the BAFF signalization improves the autophagy flux, producing an accumulation of p62. To summarize, this process is involved in cell survival and drug resistance, by the reduction in the oxidative stress induced by ROS levels [249].

The autophagy process implications in the disease vary depending on the patient's stage. In early Binet stage patients, the BECN1 and ATG5 expressions are higher, and LC3-II has shown a similar tendency. These are associated with the del(13q) and the negativity of CD38 biomarker, associating the autophagy process to a better prognosis. Additionally, survival analysis showed that high expression of ATG5 correlated with a longer survival without treatment [250,251]. SLAMF1 is also associated with the prognosis of the disease. Low levels of this gene correlate with aggressive forms of CLL and reduce autophagy. The expression of SLAMF1 depends on the ROS levels within the cell, and a low expression of SLAMF1 negatively regulates ROS, reducing their levels. It also depends on the MAP Kinases that regulate cellular signaling, and by the BCL2 complex phosphorylation, which releases Beclin-1. In conclusion, reduced SLAMF1 levels diminish the formation of autophagy complexes and produce resistance to certain therapies such as fludarabine and ABT-737 [252].

On the other hand, the overexpression of the PI3K components, including the *PIK3C3*, *PIK3R4*, and *BECN* genes, is associated with a poorer prognosis. Additionally, it was verified that these three genes can be independent prognosis markers [253]. Smith et al. (2019) investigated the viability of CLL with autophagy inhibition using VPS34-IN1. They observed that inhibition produces lower levels of LC3B-II mediated for BCR but did not produce effects on BCR signalization. Their study concluded that autophagy has a protector effect in CLL patients, and its inhibition could be a potential therapy [254]. Recently, Chen et al. (2024) showed the role of USF2 in CLL. The overexpression of this gene promotes cell proliferation and inhibits apoptosis, which is related to a poorer prognosis in CLL. Their study revealed that USF2 can act as an autophagy enhancer, since its overexpression produces an increase in the LC3II/LC3I ratio and Beclin-1 expression [255].

Therapeutic implications: In CLL, targeting mitochondrial metabolism offers a promising therapeutic approach, as drugs that disrupt mitochondrial function or increase mitochondrial ROS selectively induce cytotoxicity in CLL cells, sparing normal cells. For instance, PK11195, which targets mitochondrial F1F0-ATPase, increases superoxide production and triggers apoptosis in CLL cells. Additionally, inhibiting antioxidant defenses by targeting pathways such as Nrf2 or STAT3 could reduce the antioxidant capacity of CLL cells, rendering them more susceptible to oxidative damage. Furthermore, combination therapies that pair ROS-inducing agents with inhibitors of autophagy or antioxidant pathways (like p62-Nrf2 and USF2) may enhance therapeutic efficacy and help overcome drug resistance, offering a more effective treatment strategy for CLL.

Acute Lymphoid Leukemia

Acute lymphocytic leukemia (ALL) is characterized by the abnormal clonal proliferation of naive or mature T to B lymphocyte cells, leading to their infiltration into bone marrow, peripheral blood, and sometimes other organs and tissues. This disease exhibits significant clinical heterogeneity and diverse biological features. ALL predominantly affects children more than adults, with B-lymphocyte lineage being the most involved subtype [256].

The most common genetic alteration in patients with ALL, occurring in 20–40% of cases, is BCR/ABL translocation [257]. This gene fusion plays a crucial role in cellular growth and the reduction in apoptosis by the transcription of BCR/ABL protein with tyrosine kinase activity [258]. Studies have shown that the BCR/ABL protein can increase intracellular ROS levels through the activation of the NOX complex [259]. Additionally, BCR/ABL can further elevate ROS by activating other pathways, such as the PI3K/AKT/mTOR signaling pathway. Malignant cells with this mutation often develop mechanisms to resist the DNA damage caused by elevated ROS levels [260]. Additional studies analyzed the interaction between the PI3K/AKT pathway and IL-7 in the production of ROS. These studies also demonstrated that the use of ROS eliminators inhibited the viability of T-ALL cells, and in some cases, it induced the death of malignant cells [261]. On the other hand, Lim et al. (2020) discovered that IL-7 signaling in the JAK/STAT pathway enhances cell growth and increases ROS levels in malignant cells. B-ALL cells are dependent on high levels of ROS for survival [262]. NOTCH1, a membrane receptor with an essential function in the proliferation, differentiation, and activation of T-cells, is the least regulated pathway in T-ALL [263]. Patients that carry this mutation have higher levels of ROS due to the regulation of c-Myc that activates the PI3K/Akt/mTOR pathway [264] and the upregulation of CK2 (casein kinase 2) caused by the downregulation of the function of the PTEN protein. The inhibition of CK2 and normal levels of ROS cause the death of T-ALL cells without producing any damage to normal T-cells [265]. Ping et al. (2022) show that the levels of creatine, albumin, or C-reactive protein, indicators of cellular stress levels, could be independent prognostic factors for overall survival (OS) in T-ALL [266].

Kantner et al. (2013) found in murine models that the fusion gene ETV6/RUNX1 (TEL/AML1), the most common chromosomal aberration in the pediatric form of ALL, which occurs in 25% of children with B-ALL, generates a preleukemic clone and induces elevated levels of ROS. These increased ROS levels result in genetic instability and DNA strand breaks, leading to the transformation of preleukemic clones into malignant cells [267]. Polak et al. (2019) discovered another critical function of the aberration ETV6/RUNX1, showing that it regulates autophagy levels in leukemic cells even in the absence of cellular stress. Specifically, ETV6/RUNX1 induces the activation of Vps34, a key component of the central regulatory complex for autophagy. In this context, autophagy promotes the survival and proliferation of leukemic cells. Importantly, the inhibition of Vps34 and autophagy pharmacologically was shown to reduce the survival and proliferation of these cells [268]. Building on this, Bwanika et al. (2024) corroborated the findings of Polak et al. by reporting elevated levels of Vps34 and autophagy in patients with the ETV6/RUNX1 fusion gene. Additionally, they identified the upregulation of ATG14, a protein closely linked to autophagy. These findings emphasize the role of ETV6/RUNX1 in enhancing autophagy and supporting cell survival [256]. Collectively, these studies demonstrate a connection between the ETV6/RUNX1 fusion gene, autophagy, and cellular stress. However, it is necessary to conduct more research in these fields to explore the interplay between these processes and their therapeutics implications.

In B-ALL, resistance to glucocorticoids is the principal treatment for the disease. It is associated with an increased activation of the MAPK pathway, which leads to a poor prognosis. The MEK1/2 inhibitor, selumetinib, enhances the effectiveness of GC and reduces the activation of pERK1/2, also affecting the mTOR pathway [269]. Additionally, selumetinib increases the level of LC3-II, a marker crucial for autophagy [270,271]. In pediatric patients, leukemic cells show low expression of ATGs such as *ATG7*. Additional studies indicated that the deletion of this key gene in murine models resulted in an increased proliferation of leukemic cells [271]. Furthermore, activating autophagy with rapamycin has been shown to improve survival in mice with B-ALL [271]. These findings suggest that targeting autophagy could be a promising therapeutic approach.

In T-ALL, research in Jurkat cells models of the disease, have shown that certain therapies, such as timosaponin A III, can activate autophagy and apoptosis, suggesting that autophagy could be a potential therapy for T-ALL [272]. Another study discovered that the JAK/STAT pathway is frequently mutated in T-ALL, proposing TG101209 inhibitor of JAK2 can suppress the autophagy and the cell proliferation through the modulation of JAK/STAT pathway [273]. Other drugs, like MK-2206, and CQ inhibit the autophagy and protect the malignant cells for the apoptosis [264,274]. In the case of FAPP2, its overexpression in T-ALL is involved in the activation of PI3K/AKT/mTOR pathway contributing to leukemic cell proliferation and survival. The negative regulation of FAPP2 induce the autophagy and trigger the inhibition of the malignant cell proliferation, suggesting that the modulation of the expression of this gene could be a potential therapeutic strategy, due to the autophagy induce by its negative regulation produce a leukemic cell death and help to control the T-ALL progression [264]. Therefore, new therapies with autophagy present challenges and require further investigation, but in general, autophagy suppression represents a potentially interesting therapeutic approach.

Therapeutic implications: Targeting oxidative stress in ALL offers promising strategies for treatment. In T-ALL, ROS eliminators, such as NOX inhibitors or CK2 targeting, can induce apoptosis in malignant cells while sparing normal cells. Combining ROS modulation with inhibitors of critical pathways like PI3K/AKT/mTOR may enhance therapeutic efficacy. In parallel, modulating autophagy provides additional therapeutic potential. Inhibiting autophagy, for example with VPS34 inhibitors, disrupts survival mechanisms in leukemic cells, while activating autophagy with agents like rapamycin can improve outcomes, particularly in B-ALL with low ATG expression. Furthermore, pathway-specific inhibitors targeting PI3K/AKT/mTOR or JAK/STAT pathways can suppress both ROS production and autophagy, reducing leukemic cell viability. Additionally, MEK inhibitors like selumetinib have shown potential in enhancing GC sensitivity while modulating autophagic flux, offering new avenues for therapeutic intervention.

Chronic Myeloid Leukemia

Chronic myeloid leukemia (CML) is a malignant myeloproliferative neoplasm characterized by the uncontrolled cell proliferation of myeloid cells in different stages of maturation. The disease progression is heterogeneous, and the patients can present one of three clinical phases: the chronic phase, the accelerated phase and the blast crisis. The chronic phase is the initial stage, defined by less than 10% of blast in bone marrow or peripheral blood. The accelerated phase is an intermediate stage, in which the blast represents between 10 and 19%. Finally, the blast crisis is the most advanced progression, and it is characterized by more than 20% of blast, which could be of myeloid, lymphoid or undifferentiated origin [275].

CML patients have a reciprocal translocation between the long arm of chromosome 9 and the long arm of chromosome 22, resulting in the Philadelphia chromosome (t(9;22)(q34;q11)), which creates the hybrid gene BCR/ABL. This gene encodes a tyrosine kinase with a key function in the transformation of the leukemic HSC, promoting abnormal cellular proliferation, protein synthesis and antiapoptotic signals [276,277]. Nowicki et al. (2004) demonstrated the importance of the aberration BCR/ABL in CML. Their study has shown that the double-strand breaks in the patients with this aberration occur by the increase in ROS levels induced by the gene fusion. Furthermore, the HSC stimulation for growth factors or the BCR/ABL kinase results in higher levels of ROS in comparison than the normal cells [278]. The reason for this is that the Philadelphia chromosome inhibits two detoxifying enzymes, the CAT and Glrx1, contributing to the oxidative stress [279]. Similar to ALL, this aberration can activate the PI3K/mTOR pathway, increasing the intracellular ROS levels [260]. The activation of this pathway induces the activation of ATF5, a transcription factor that regulates mTORC1, depending on Fox4, a factor involved in cell survival and metabolism. This suggests that the BCR/ABL gene increases the expression of mTORC1, contributing to the inhibition of autophagy [280]. On the other hand, studies demonstrated that the inhibitor of BCR/ABL used in the treatment against CML, imatinib, inhibits the expression of microRNA-30a in CML cells producing an increase in autophagic flux and higher levels of the proteins Beclin-1 and ATG5 [281]. In addition, Colecchia et al. (2015) found that MAPK15 (also known as ERK8) plays a crucial role in autophagy induced by BCR/ABL in CML. MAPK15 regulates the interaction between the protein fusion BCR/ABL and the autophagy vesicles, facilitating autophagy activation. It also interacts with the LC3 family proteins depending on LIR (LC3-Interacting region), which is essential for autophagy. The inhibition of MAPK15 reduces cell proliferation and the tumor development produced by the Philadelphia chromosome, presenting MAPK15 as a therapeutic target in CML [282].

Another study in murine models suggests that BCR/ABL kinase activity regulates autophagy by phosphorylating Beclin-1 at tyrosine residues 233 and 352 in CML. This phosphorylation disrupts the interaction between key autophagy regulators, including UVRAG, VPS15, ATG14, VPS34, RUBICON, and Beclin-1. The result is the inhibition of autophagy, which impacts cancer cell survival and proliferation. This mechanism highlights the role of BCR/ABL in manipulating cellular processes to promote leukemia cell survival [269].

Therapeutic implications: In CML, high ROS levels are crucial for cell survival but also contribute to DNA damage. Therapeutic strategies that modulate ROS levels or enhance antioxidant defenses could disrupt this balance, potentially sensitizing CML cells to treatment. Additionally, modulating autophagy presents a promising approach. Inhibiting autophagy in CML cells, for example, by targeting Vps34 or MAPK15, impairs autophagic flux and reduces leukemic cell viability. On the other hand, inducing autophagy in combination with tyrosine kinase inhibitors (TKIs) like imatinib may improve therapeutic outcomes by promoting apoptosis in resistant CML cells. Furthermore, combining TKIs with agents that target oxidative stress or autophagy-related pathways holds promise for improving outcomes in resistant or advanced-phase CML.

Acute Myeloid Leukemia

Acute myeloid leukemia (AML) is a hematological malignancy defined by an abnormal growth of myeloid blast or progranulocytes that do not mature properly. The disease has an unfavorable or poor prognosis. In 2024, the estimated new cases are 20,800 (1% of all new cancer diagnoses) and the median age of diagnosis is 69 years. The prognosis is poor with a general survival rate after 5 years lower than 50% in young patients with LMA and lower than 20% in older patients [264].

In AML the ROS levels are essential to predict the prognosis of the patients. There are multiple mechanisms to increase the ROS levels. The mutation in FLT3, affecting 30% of AML patients, is associated with a poor prognosis due to a shorter OS [283].

Stanicka et al. (2015) demonstrated that AML patients carrying this mutation had increased the levels of ROS due to the NOX, specifically NOX4 and p22phox. These molecules act as pro-survival signals [284]. Earlier, Hole et al. (2013) concluded that AML blast with NOX produces higher levels of ROS than the normal blast. They discovered that the ROS produced by NOX2 are associated with dysfunction in p38 MAPK and that inhibiting this molecule improved cell proliferation. Additionally, extracellular ROS contributed to the proliferation of AML cells [285]. More recently, this research group demonstrated that NOX2 enhanced glucose uptake and the glycolysis process through reprogramming cell metabolism. It is produced by the activation of a key enzyme of the glycolysis process, PFKFB3, generating NADPH and biosynthetic precursors in AML [286].

FLT3-ITD (FLT3 tyrosine kinase receptor) triggers downstream pathways such as STAT5, PI3K/AKT, and RAS/MAPK, which are linked to the higher levels of ROS in AML patients [287]. In contrast with other types of leukemias, these higher levels of ROS are cytoplasmic because the FLT3 mutation occurs in the cytoplasmic membrane [283]. Proteins such as Jab1 and TRX, which are involved in cell growth, can be activated by the higher levels of ROS produced by the FLT3 mutation, suggesting that ROS/Jab1/TRX could be a therapeutic target in AML [288]. Rasool et al. (2007) investigated the *NRAS* and *BCL2* genes and the ROS levels in the leukemic cell. Their study in murine models concluded that mutations in NRAS produce higher levels of ROS, increasing cellular stress. Furthermore, the double mutants NRAS and BCL2 produced more ROS levels and had a significant impact on the AML blast [289]. Other authors showed in murine models that autophagy is essential for leukemic initiator cells in the bone marrow but not for the differentiated leukemic blast, as it prevents cellular stress. The accumulation of ROS and mitochondria are closely linked to the maintenance of leukemic initiator cells. When comparing normal and leukemic initiator cells, the latter is shown to have a higher number of mitochondria than the former. In contrast, in peripheral blood, autophagy improves the survival of leukemic cells regardless of their differentiation stage [290]. Additionally, autophagy is closely correlated with glycolysis. Increasing glycolysis levels can suppress autophagy flux producing poorer disease prognosis. Studies show that the inhibition or deletion of the gene ATG5 reduces the levels of autophagy and increases AML cell proliferation by inducing higher levels of glycolysis [291]. Other studies show that the inhibition of ATG3 produces the same effect in tumor progression, showing the importance of autophagy in the disease [292]. Wang et al. (2019) discovered that patients with mutated NPM1 have an increased expression of PKM2, a glycolytic enzyme that increases the phosphorylation levels of Beclin-1, a key molecule in autophagy. They observed that the higher levels of PKM2 are associated with poorer prognosis in AML patients [293]. On the other hand, in de novo AML patients, the basal autophagy flux is lower, and the expression of *ATG7* and *LC3* genes is reduced, showing a strong correlation with autophagy levels. Therefore, a reduction in the autophagy pathway could produce the initiation of leukemogenesis [294].

Patients with *FLT3* mutation are associated with higher levels of basal autophagy, contributing to drug resistance. Elevated autophagy levels are associated with higher expressions of phospho-FLT3, phospho-BKT, and ATF4 in resistant AML cells [295]. Heydt et al. (2017) show in mice that the transcription factor ATF4 depends on FLT3-ITD activity, and the inhibition of ATF4 inhibits the proliferation of AML, increasing survival, mimicking the effects of autophagy inhibition [296]. Recently, Shang et al. (2019) investigated the implication of circular RNA in autophagy in therapy resistance cells. Their study revealed that circPAN3 has an important function in the acquired resistance in AML. circPAN3, which is expressed in resistant AML cells, enhances autophagy levels by the regulation of the AMPK/mTOR pathway, making circPAN3 a new therapy target in relapsed AML [297]. In conclusion, autophagy plays a heterogeneous role in AML. While higher levels of autophagy may improve prognosis due to the inhibition of glycolysis, it may also lead to a worse prognosis due to the resistance of AML cell therapy.

Therapeutic implications: Targeting ROS-producing pathways, such as NOX enzymes or FLT3 signaling, offers a promising strategy to reduce oxidative stress and impair leukemic cell survival. Additionally, the ROS/Jab1/TRX axis has emerged as a potential therapeutic target for disrupting pro-survival signaling in AML cells. Targeting this pathway could enhance the vulnerability of tumor cells to treatment by inhibiting their oxidative defense mechanisms and promoting cell death, offering new avenues for therapy in resistant AML cases. In addition, inhibiting key autophagy regulators, such as ATG5 and ATG7, has shown potential in reducing leukemic cell proliferation by increasing metabolic stress, thereby impairing their survival mechanisms. Emerging therapeutic targets also include circPAN3, which regulates autophagy through the AMPK/mTOR pathway. This circular RNA is implicated in therapy resistance, particularly in relapsed AML, suggesting that targeting circPAN3 could enhance treatment efficacy and overcome resistance in these patients.

6.2.2. Lymphomas

Lymphoma encompasses a diverse group of over 90 subtypes of hematological malignancies, traditionally categorized into Hodgkin lymphoma (HL) and non-Hodgkin lymphoma (NHL). In 2019, these diseases accounted for 4.7% of all newly diagnosed cancer cases in the United States. Known risk factors include genetic predisposition, infectious agents, and inflammatory conditions [298].

Hodgkin Lymphoma

HL is the most frequent lymphoma, and the prognosis is generally favorable when using chemotherapy and radiotherapy, as approximately 90% of patients can be cured. HL is usually diagnosed in young adults, around 35 years old. However, whereas chemotherapy is ineffective in some patients, in others, it produces toxic effects and a decrease in life expectancy [299]. Lymphoma is characterized by the presence of abnormal B-cells, Reed–Sternberg (RS) cells, which are big and multinucleated malignant cells, and a high density of immune effector cells in the tumoral microenvironment [300]. The origin of this type of cell is unknown, although Epstein–Barr virus (EBV) could be implicated in their development [301].

Oxidative stress in HL affects RS cells and the surrounding microenvironment. Bur et al. (2014) discovered oxidative stress damage in mononuclear cells of peripheral blood in non-treated HL patients caused by an increase in ROS levels in mitochondria. RS cells suffer from oxidative stress damage in DNA, specifically in advanced stages of HL, which is characterized by an increased expression of 8-OHdG, an oxidative stress marker. This damage produces genomic instability and reduces DNA repair enzymes. However, in aggressive forms of HL, RS cells and the microenvironment produce increased levels of antioxidant enzymes in mitochondria such as Mn-SOD and PrxV. This suggests an adaptive mechanism against oxidative stress in the cells [302]. Later, Marini et al. (2022) validated the presence of oxidative stress in peripheral blood mononuclear cells of untreated patients. Their study proposes that the decoupling of oxidative phosphorylation and the redox stress causes more damage to lymphocytes than to monocytes. The metabolic response in both types of cells involves an increased activity of hexose-6-phosphate dehydrogenase, producing an increase in glucose flux through the ER [303]. These studies suggest that chemotherapy based on increased ROS levels could be failed for the presence of antioxidants in RS and peripheral blood cells. Other studies on the senescence of HL cells revealed that certain senescence pathways are upregulated by oxidative stress. Specifically, oxidative stress increases the expression of p16 INK4a and p21Cip1 producing the inhibition of the cellular cycle in RS cells. Moreover, other biomarkers associated with senescence, such as H2AX and p53, show elevated expression in the Hodgkin lymphoma-derived L428 cell line under oxidative stress condition [304]. Ikeda et al. (2012) studied the HL cell lines L1236 and L428, which were found to have a tumorigenic potential. These cell lines can expel ROS maintaining low intracellular ROS levels. Their study proposed that the population with higher levels of aldehyde dehydrogenase (ALDH) and lower levels of ROS could be cancer initiator cells [305]. Additionally, ROS play a crucial role in the differentiation of the cell types implicated in HL. Immature HL cells reduce ROS levels through the action of HIF-1α, a protein that regulates the cellular response to hypoxic conditions. The stabilization of H1F-1α inhibits the differentiation of the HL cells treated with H_2O_2, a ROS that often stimulates cell differentiation. This inhibition is mediated by the protein HO-1, whose primary function is to eliminate ROS [306].

The autophagy process is also involved in the senescence. Some studies have shown that the high expression of p62 in RS cells could indicate a poorer prognosis in patients with HL. The function of p62 is the repair of the nuclear machinery of DNA but, when autophagy is inhibited, the accumulation of p62 inhibits RNF168 producing a reduction in the recruitment of DNA repair proteins. Moreover, this process produces an increase in the DNA damage produced by ROS and the degradation of certain DNA repair proteins [307]. Additionally, EBV appears to influence the autophagy flux levels in HL. In malignant cells, EBV protein LMP1 enhances the autophagy flux modulating stressful situations such as inanition conditions or chemotherapy treatment agents like doxorubicin (DOX). Murine models have shown that the inhibition of autophagy with CQ effectively eliminates HL cells that express LMP1. Interestingly, excessive autophagy can lead to cell death. In HL cell lines like L428 and KM-H2, LMP1 protects against apoptosis and increases the autophagy flux. Nevertheless, an excessive increase in autophagy could produce cell death. Therefore, autophagy acts as a double-edged sword in EBV-associated HL. It can protect tumor cells under certain conditions, but excessively high levels can result in their destruction, presenting autophagy as a promising therapeutic target [308].

Another study investigating the impact of microgravity on autophagy in HL patients found that exposure of human HL cells to time-averaged simulated microgravity (taSMG) for two days led to increased oxidative stress. This effect was attributed to the elevated expression of NOX family genes, while levels of ATPase and ATP synthase were reduced, resulting in lower intracellular ATP levels. Consequently, autophagy was activated via the AMPK/Akt/mTOR and MAPK pathways. However, this autophagy activation was inhibited when cells were treated with the ROS scavenger NAC. The findings suggest that autophagy activation driven by oxidative stress under taSMG conditions could hold potential as a novel anticancer strategy for HL patients [309]. Likewise, Wahyudianingsih et al. (2024) reviewed the role of autophagy in the chemotherapy of HL, and they reported that autophagy is activated in response to DNA damage caused by chemotherapy, which often induces apoptosis in tumor cells. However, in some cases other pathways such as autophagy or senescence could be activated instead of cell death, protecting tumor cells from dying. This process is regulated through the inhibition of mTORC1, ATR/Chk1 signaling, ULK1 phosphorylation, G endonuclease activation, and KU70 protein interaction. In line with previous findings, these results suggested that autophagy inhibition could constitute an efficient therapeutic strategy in HL patients [310].

Therapeutic implications: Inhibiting autophagy with agents such as CQ has demonstrated efficacy in eliminating EBV-positive HL cells by disrupting their adaptive stress responses. Chemotherapy-induced autophagy, on the other hand, can protect tumor cells from apoptosis, highlighting the need to target autophagy-related pathways such as mTORC1 or ATR/Chk1 to enhance treatment efficacy. Additionally, studies in simulated microgravity show increased oxidative stress in HL cells, driven by the upregulation of NOX genes and reduced ATP levels. This stress activates autophagy through the AMPK/Akt/mTOR pathways, suggesting that microgravity could be explored as a novel anticancer strategy for HL.

Non-Hodgkin Lymphoma

NHL is the most common hematological malignancy, and it is characterized by a proliferation of different B and T cells. It is differentiated from HL by the absence of RS cells and the histology markers CD15 and CD30. It is a very heterogeneous disease with more than 40 different subtypes [311]. Oxidative stress, which arises by an imbalance between pro-oxidant and antioxidant mechanisms, plays a crucial role in NHL. Wang et al. (2006) highlighted the importance of this pathway in NHL by the genotyping of 13 single nucleotide polymorphism (SNPs) in 10 genes of the oxidative stress pathway including *AKR1A1*, *AKR1C1*, *CYBA*, *GPX*, *MPO*, *NOS2A*, *NOS3*, *OGG1*, *PPARG* and *SOD2*. They concluded that the *NOS2A*, *SOD2* and *PPARG* genes could play a role in the oxidative stress and the risk of developing NHL [312]. Subsequently, Lan et al. (2007) analyzed 10 candidate genes from oxidative stress pathway (*AKR1A*, *AKR1C1*, *AKR1C3*, *CYBA*, *GPX1*, *MPO*, *NOS2A*, *NOS3*, *OGG1* and *SOD2*) in a cohort of female patients and identified 14 SNPs within the *NOX*, *AKR1A1* and *CYBA* genes significantly associated with the risk of developing NHL [313]. Likewise, Gustafson et al. (2014) studied polymorphisms in 28 genes of the oxidative stress pathway in NHL patients treated with anthracycline-based therapies. Their study identified that homozygous patients for the rs188312 SNP within the *NCF4* gene could be involved in the treatment outcomes because these patients showed a higher risk of hematological toxicity [314].

The autophagy process has been implicated in several types of NHL. For instance, chLym-1, a monoclonal anti-HLA-DR antibody, can activate the autophagy process in Raji cells, a cell line derived from an NHL subtype (Burkitt lymphoma). In treated patients, chLym-1 acts by inducing apoptosis through the activation of autophagy pathways such as Akt/mTOR and MEK/Erk [315]. In the case of mantle cell lymphoma (MCL), the association between TG2 and IL6 activates autophagy, promoting MCL cell survival. Moreover, the interaction with ATG5 produces a positive regulation of TG2/NFκB/IL6 signaling [316]. In primary effusion lymphoma (PEL), the anti-tumoral effects of CQ inhibited the autophagy process. This inhibition produced the accumulation of unfolded proteins, producing ER stress. These conditions induced apoptosis in PEL cells, suggesting that autophagy inhibition could be a potential therapy for PEL patients [317]. Considering these results, it seems that the role of autophagy in NHL is heterogeneous and varies according to the disease subtype.

Therapeutic implications: In NHL, autophagy acts as a double-edged sword in therapy; while it supports tumor cell survival under stress, its excessive activation can lead to cell death. Targeting autophagy pathways offers a promising strategy to enhance treatment efficacy or overcome drug resistance. Modulating oxidative stress pathways, such as reducing ROS levels or targeting antioxidant defenses, could also disrupt tumor survival mechanisms and increase the effectiveness of treatment. Additionally, manipulating autophagy by either inhibiting protective autophagy or inducing excessive autophagy could potentiate therapeutic responses and improve disease outcomes.

Diffuse Large B-Cell Lymphoma

Diffuse large B-cell lymphoma (DLBCL) is the most common type of lymphoma, accounting for approximately 30% of all cases. It is an aggressive form of B-cell lymphoma, with an average age of diagnosis around 70 years. The primary treatment typically involves chemotherapy, often combined with immunotherapy, including options such as chimeric antigen receptor T-cell (CAR-T) therapy for refractory or relapsed cases [318]. Nakamura et al. (2022) investigated oxidative stress as a prognosis factor in untreated patients with DLBCL. They showed that oxidative stress levels were significantly higher in patients compared to healthy controls. Derivatives of reactive oxygen metabolites correlated with several prognosis factors, including sIL-2r, a biomarker associated with the lymphoma activity, the international Prognostic Index that evaluates the risk of DLBCL and with elevated levels of lactate dehydrogenase that is linked with metabolic activity and tumor proliferation. The study concluded that oxidative stress may be associated with poorer prognosis, and that it plays an important role in the carcinogenesis of DLBCL patients [319]. Additional studies have consistently underscored the importance of the glutamine metabolism in DLBCL. In DLBCL, glutamine metabolism is upregulated, producing elevated levels of glutamine and lower levels of α-KG. Through the activity of malate dehydrogenase 1, α-KG is converted into 2-hydroxyglutarate, resulting in elevated levels of ROS in tumor cells. High ROS levels induce ferroptosis by activating lipid peroxidation and enhanced TP53 expression, which is associated with DNA damage. Furthermore, dimethyl-α-ketoglutarate inhibits tumor proliferation, suggesting that the regulation of glutamine metabolites could constitute a new therapy for DLBCL [320].

On the other hand, Zhao et al. (2025) studied the role of some oxidative stress-related genes in DLBCL. They identified 26 genes that were crucial for tumor proliferation processes such as DNA damage, lipid peroxidation, and the escape of the immune system. Notable genes included *CCND1, GPX3, ICAM1, IFNG, MT2A, NDRG1, NLRP3, PLAU, SQSTM1* and *TXN*. These researchers demonstrated that patients could be classified into two groups based on differences in immunity infiltration that were dependent on the levels of oxidative stress. The infiltration of tumor-killing cells, including CD4/CD8 T cells, dendritic cells, macrophages, and NK cells, differed significantly between groups. These differences were accompanied by markedly distinct levels of oxidative stress, which were likely responsible for the observed immune disparities [321]. Like HL, elevated levels of certain biomarkers, such as γH2AX and 8-OHdG, were associated with aggressive subtypes of DLBCL, particularly those positive for MYC/BCL2, including the Activated B-cell (ABC) subtype and high-grade B-cell lymphoma (HG-BCL). In these subtypes, the activation of DNA repair mechanisms and increased BCL-2 expression enable cells to withstand the oxidative stress induced by the oncogenic activity of MYC. Based on this observation, targeting DNA repair mechanisms and BCL2 inhibition could alleviate oxidative stress in malignant cells and enhance apoptosis without relying on conventional chemotherapy [322]. Prior to this study, Mai et al. (2016) investigated the role of oxidative stress in the two main subtypes of DLBCL: activated B-cell-like (ABC-DLBCL) and germinal center B-cell-like (GCB-DLBCL). ABC-DLBCL is more resistant to treatment, and the effectiveness of doxorubicin (DOX) in this subtype depends on its ability to generate reactive oxygen species (ROS) to kill tumor cells. In contrast, GCB-DLBCL is more sensitive to chemotherapy, where DOX primarily induces DNA damage through the activation of DNA repair mechanisms.

In the ABC-DLBCL subtype, activation of the STAT3 protein is a key feature. STAT3 regulates antioxidant mechanisms, including the expression of the SOD2 enzyme, which neutralizes ROS and contributes to the resistance of malignant B cells to DOX. However, when ROS levels exceed a critical threshold, STAT3's capacity to mitigate oxidative stress collapses, leading to cell death. This makes STAT3 a potential therapeutic target for DLBCL [323]. Additionally, evidence suggests that STAT3 plays a role in autophagy by suppressing oxidative stress-induced autophagy and protecting mitochondria from mitophagy [324]. Further studies have explored STAT3 inhibition in the context of antiretroviral therapy, which inhibits cellular proliferation and induces apoptosis, autophagy, and ferroptosis. These findings indicate that STAT3 inhibition is essential for regulating therapy, and combining antiretroviral therapy with autophagy inducers or STAT3 inhibitors could offer a novel treatment strategy for DLBCL [325].

Concerning autophagy, Li et al. (2019) investigated the role of *CUL4B*, a gene associated with autophagy and involved in multiple types of cancer, in the DLBCL. Their study showed that *CUL4B* is overexpressed in DLBCL and contributes to characteristics of aggressive tumors, such as a larger tumor size, metastasis and poorer prognosis. CUL4B regulates certain signalization pathways such as JNK that regulates several cellular processes including autophagy. Specifically, CUL4B positively regulates the activity of JNK, thereby promoting the autophagy process. Taking this into account, the inhibition of CUL4B could serve as a potential therapeutic target by inhibiting the JNK pathway, reducing the autophagy process, and ultimately reducing cell survival [326]. Other studies have developed a prognostic model based on the *ADD3, IGFBP3, TPM1, LYZ, AFDN, DNAJC10, GLIS3* and *CCDC102A* genes, which are involved in autophagy. This model integrates genomic prediction and immunological infiltration, offering a new therapeutic tool in personalized medicine, as they permit prediction of the survival probability and the drug resistance [327]. In addition, Mandhair et al. (2024) emphasized the pivotal role of ULK1, a key protein in the autophagy process, in germinal center B-cell-like diffuse large B-cell lymphoma (GCB-DLBCL). They found that ULK1 was overexpressed in patients with this disease subtype and influenced their response to treatment. Their findings suggest that suppressing ULK1 could represent a therapeutic strategy for GCB-DLBCL. Additionally, the study proposed that ATG biomarkers might serve as predictors of treatment response [328]. Another gene significantly influencing autophagy and DLBCL is *BECN1*, which encodes Beclin-1 protein. Autophagy activation associated with Beclin-1 contributes to improved prognoses by overcoming acquired resistance and enhancing therapeutic outcomes. Notably, venetoclax, which disrupts the Beclin-1/BCL2 interaction, has shown potential to induce autophagy and improve the efficacy of chemotherapy in treating DLBCL [329].

Therapeutic implications: Targeting oxidative stress presents a promising strategy for improving outcomes in DLBCL. Reducing ROS levels could alleviate DNA damage and inhibit tumor proliferation, while exploiting the heightened sensitivity of malignant B cells to elevated ROS could enhance cytotoxicity. In the ABC-DLBCL subtype, targeting antioxidant mechanisms like STAT3 or promoting excessive ROS accumulation may help overcome resistance to therapies like doxorubicin. For MYC/BCL2-positive subtypes, inhibiting DNA repair mechanisms or targeting BCL2 could enhance apoptosis by disrupting the oxidative stress balance. Therapeutic strategies such as combining STAT3 inhibitors with autophagy modulators or antiretroviral therapies have shown potential to induce apoptosis and ferroptosis in resistant DLBCL cases. Combination therapies that pair chemotherapy with agents modulating redox homeostasis and autophagy may improve therapeutic efficacy and reduce resistance, offering a more effective approach to treating DLBCL.

7. Therapeutic Potential

Autophagy and oxidative stress are intricately linked processes with significant implications for cancer therapy. Oxidative stress, driven by ROS, modulates autophagy through key signaling pathways such as AMPK, MAPK, Akt, and JNK, thereby influencing cancer cell survival, proliferation, and stress adaptation [330–334]. At low to moderate levels, ROS act as signaling molecules to activate these pathways, whereas excessive ROS levels induce autophagy as a protective mechanism [335]. Autophagy plays a dual role in cancer: it suppresses tumorigenesis by removing damaged organelles and mitigating oxidative damage [336], but it also enables tumor survival under conditions such as hypoxia, starvation, and therapeutic stress, contributing to drug resistance [337,338].

Therapeutic strategies targeting autophagy are promising but complex. General autophagy inhibition by agents such as CQ and HCQ has shown potential in overcoming resistance, although its efficacy varies with cancer type and treatment context [338,339]. In addition, selective types of autophagy, such as mitophagy and lysophagy, are emerging as precise tools for therapy, offering avenues to disrupt cancer-specific mechanisms [14,340]. ROS-inducing therapies, including chemotherapy and radiotherapy, exploit the dynamic interplay between oxidative stress and autophagy to improve treatment outcomes, although careful modulation is required to prevent resistance [341,342]. The dual role of autophagy and oxidative stress in cancer biology highlights their therapeutic potential as targets for innovative cancer therapies.

7.1. Autophagy Modulators

Targeting autophagy is a promising approach for cancer therapy. Below, we report key strategies organized by therapeutic focus:

7.1.1. Role of Autophagy Inhibitors

Autophagy inhibitors have emerged as important tools in cancer therapy, enhancing the efficacy of conventional treatments by sensitizing cancer cells. Agents like 3-methyladenine (3-MA), wortmannin, CQ, and HCQ have demonstrated promising effects in hematological malignancies and solid tumors affecting cancer cell viability, whereas wortmannin has shown to inhibit autophagy independently of nutrient availability and promote apoptosis by downregulating proliferative pathways (PI3K/Akt and NF-kappaB) [338,343,344].

Clinically approved CQ and HCQ, which block lysosomal fusion, not only enhance chemotherapy efficacy in leukemias and lymphomas [21,64] but also exhibit anticancer effects beyond autophagy suppression and promote drug sensitization in both solid tumors and hematological malignancies [21,64,345–348]. However, the relatively limited potency of these agents has driven the development of more potent analogs, such as EAD1, which has shown encouraging preclinical results in solid tumors [349,350]. These findings underscore the therapeutic potential of autophagy inhibitors while highlighting the need for further optimization to improve potency and specificity. In addition, autophagy modulation through targeted therapies offers new opportunities in cancer treatment. Tyrosine kinase inhibitors like imatinib, INNO-406, and dasatinib induce autophagic cell death in CML and ovarian cancer, demonstrating the utility of leveraging autophagy as a cell death mechanism [349]. mTOR inhibitors such as rapamycin and its analogs (temsirolimus, everolimus, and deforolimus) stimulate autophagy and exhibit anti-tumor activity in multiple hematological malignancies including AML, MCL, and MM [351–353], while AMPK activators like metformin [354] and AICAR [355] suppress proliferation and induce apoptosis through autophagy activation among other mechanisms [349,354,356,357]. Additionally, the modulation of pathways such as Akt, mTOR, and tyrosine kinases, as well as other key signaling pathways like Notch, Wnt, and Hedgehog, underscores the complexity and context-dependent roles of autophagy in hematological malignancies [358–360] and solid tumors [361,362]. These approaches highlight autophagy's dual potential to either inhibit tumor initiation or promote cancer progression, depending on the cancer type and therapeutic context, offering diverse strategies for cancer management.

7.1.2. ATGs and Proteins

ATGs and proteins play pivotal roles in cancer progression and therapy, acting as critical modulators of tumorigenesis and cellular survival. Mutations in ATGs, such as *ATG2B*, *ATG5*, *ATG7*, *ATG9B*, and *ATG12*, have been linked to frameshift mutations in leukemias [363] but also gastrointestinal and liver cancers [364], highlighting their significance in cancer biology. Similarly, Beclin-1, a key regulator of autophagosome formation, often shows allelic loss, reduced or increased expression [329,365] or inhibiting phosphorylation in hematological malignancies [365] and solid tumors, implicating its dysfunction in carcinogenesis [366].

Other players, such as p62 (SQSTM1), which activates tumor-promoting NFκB and Nrf2 pathways [367], and mitophagy receptors BNIP3 and BNIP3L (NIX), which protect against tumorigenesis by maintaining mitochondrial quality [368], further demonstrate the multifaceted role of autophagy in hematological malignancies [369–371] and its role in disease prognosis [371].

These findings underscore the intricate functions of autophagy-associated pathways in regulating tumor growth and survival. The diverse roles of these genes and proteins not only deepen our understanding of cancer biology but also reveal promising targets for therapeutic development, paving the way for novel interventions in cancer treatment.

7.1.3. Flavonoid-Based Autophagy Modulation

Flavonoids, a diverse group of plant-derived compounds, have received considerable attention for their anticancer potential, largely due to their ability to modulate autophagy. Compounds such as apigenin, quercetin, epigallocatechin gallate (EGCG), and curcumin exhibit potent biological activity in hematological malignancies despite challenges related to their limited oral bioavailability [372,373].

Clinical studies underline their therapeutic relevance. For example, a bioflavonoid mixture containing apigenin and EGCG (20 mg each) is currently being studied as a preventive measure against recurrence in hematological malignancies and solid tumors, highlighting its translational potential in both hematology and oncology areas [374]. In hematological malignancies, flavonoids have been found to interfere with different signaling pathways and molecules, demonstrating anticancer properties in leukemia and lymphoma cells [375,376]. In addition, it has been found that flavonoids induce cell cycle arrest, apoptosis, inhibition of fatty acid synthesis, oxidation, and metal chelation, and they have chemosensitization features [377,378]. These results suggest that the integration of flavonoids with traditional chemotherapy agents might constitute a promising therapeutic approach. In line with this hypothesis, it has been reported that the use of quercetin or flavonoid methyl esters in combination with specific mitogen-activated extracellular kinases (MEK) 1/2 inhibitors substantially enhanced leukemic cell death, confirming the clinical implications for the use of these compounds in combination with MEK 1/2 inhibitors as potential therapeutic agents for leukemia [376]. Additionally, it has been demonstrated that flavonoids such as quercetin, catechin, and brusatol reduce the risk of lymphoma [379] by inhibiting proliferation and inducing the apoptosis of tumor cells. Similar effects have been observed in ALL, AML, CLL, CML, and MM cell lines [372,373,380,381]. Importantly, they are also able to induce apoptosis and promote tumor regression in lymphoma and myeloma xenograft models acting synergistically with dexamethasone, venetoclax, or bortezomib [382–385]. However, other authors claim that caution should be taken with their use as flavonoids because it could inhibit the anticancer effects of bortezomib [386]. Curcumin, another prominent flavonoid, has demonstrated safety and efficacy in a range of hematological malignancies [387], further validating its clinical applicability [388]. Curcumin diminishes the viability and survival rate of leukemia, myeloma, and lymphoma cells by inducing cell cycle arrest and apoptosis, and it inhibits molecular pathways linked to tumor progression such as NFKB, STAT, Akt/PI3K, and MEK/ERK [387,389–391]. The use of Curcumin in a myeloma patient with a third relapse and in the absence of further anti-myeloma treatments, controlled the disease for 5 years with good quality of life [390]. In addition, it has been suggested that Curcumin enhances the efficacy of chemotherapy drugs by modulating drug resistance pathways [387] and might represent a viable alternative to corticosteroids in combination with immunomodulatory drugs or proteasome inhibitors [392]. Similarly, Silibinin shows promise as a therapeutic intervention for β-Talassemia, AML, anaplastic large cell lymphoma, and MM [393]. However, despite the large amount of information available, the mechanistic effects of flavonoids on autophagy are nuanced, as they can stimulate or inhibit autophagic pathways depending on the context. Compounds such as EGCG and quercetin play dual roles in regulating cellular processes such as cell survival, angiogenesis, and resistance to therapy. While some flavonoids, such as silibinin, induce toxic autophagic cell death, which contributes to their anti-tumor effects, others may promote tumor survival by activating protective autophagy, thereby complicating their therapeutic impact [394,395]. These findings suggest that the flavonoid-induced modulation of autophagy holds promise as a multilayered approach to cancer therapy, which requires further investigation to optimize its clinical benefits.

7.1.4. Targeting ROS via Autophagy

Keeping ROS levels low is essential for normal hematopoiesis and stem cell function, and impaired ROS homeostasis is a common signature of hematological malignancies, such as AML and CML [396]. In addition, chronic oxidative stress has been associated with BCR-ABL, FLT3-ITD, and RAS mutations; genomic instability and DNA damage; and disease relapse and poor prognosis in AML patients [397]. On the other hand, given that ROS play a central role in the regulation of autophagy, several chemotherapeutic agents have exploited this interplay to enhance their efficacy in cancer treatment [398]. For instance, arabinocytosine (Ara-C), a purine analog used as a first-line treatment in AML (also known as cytarabine), has been found to induce ROS production, which in turn can trigger autophagy in leukemic cells. Interestingly, enhanced autophagy has been observed in AraC-resistant U937 leukemia cells, suggesting a potential role of ROS-induced autophagy in cancer cell survival [399,400] and drug resistance [400]. In addition, Ara-C reduced the phosphorylation of mTOR and its downstream target p70S6 kinase in REH cells, which was associated with the downregulation of the mTOR activator Akt and the activation of extracellular signal-regulated kinase. These data suggested that the therapeutic efficiency of Ara-C in leukemic patients could be increased by the inhibition of the mTOR-dependent autophagic response [399,401]. Similarly, leukemic cells treated with anthracyclines exhibited increased ROS formation and enhanced autophagy, which promoted tumorigenesis and drug resistance [402]. However, in other cases, autophagy contributed to cytarabine's antineoplastic effects, particularly at low doses [403], which suggest a complex and dual effect of autophagy in blood cancers. While the precise mechanisms of this dual effect remain to be elucidated, it highlights the promise of targeting autophagic pathways in blood cancer treatments.

7.1.5. Antidepressants as Autophagy Modulators

Antidepressants have emerged as interesting modulators of autophagy in cancer, exhibiting both stimulatory and suppressive effects depending on the type and stage of the disease. Tricyclic and tetracyclic antidepressants (TCA/TeCAs) such as imipramine, desipramine, and amitriptyline have been investigated for their role in autophagy regulation. Maprotiline has shown the ability to induce autophagic programmed cell death in chemoresistant Burkitt lymphoma cells, highlighting its potential against resistant cancers [348]. Similarly, selective serotonin reuptake inhibitors (SSRIs) have shown anti-tumor activity through their effects on autophagy. For example, sertraline acts through both apoptotic and autophagic pathways and has potent effects in acute myeloid leukemia cells [404,405]. In addition, loss of the selective autophagy receptor p62 impaired murine myeloid leukemia progression and mitophagy, which suggested that antidepressants have potential in modulating autophagy and exhibiting anticancer effects in hematological malignancies [406]. On the other hand, Vortioxetine has been shown to induce apoptosis and autophagy in gastric cancer cells via the PI3K/AKT pathway, representing a novel therapeutic approach for this solid tumor. Likewise, paroxetine was found to block autophagic flux and cause mitochondrial fragmentation in lung cancer cells, illustrating a unique mechanism of action [348]. These examples highlight the potential of antidepressants, including TCAs, TeCAs, and SSRIs, as modulators of autophagy, offering innovative strategies for therapeutic intervention in hematological malignancies and solid tumors.

7.2. Selective Autophagy Processes as Therapeutic Targets

Mitophagy, the selective degradation of damaged mitochondria, is a therapeutic target in cancer treatment with several promising compounds. For example, BH3 mimetics targeting different BCL-2 family members have been found to be efficient at killing AML cells through the activation of the apoptosis pathway [407]. Interestingly, blockage of autophagy or specific targeting of MFN2 potentiates BH3-mimetic action in eliminating leukemic cells [407]. Likewise, there has been reported that splicing factor mutations (SRSF2P95H/+) are common in hematological malignancies (MDS and AML) and that the inhibition of splicing with glycogen synthase kinase 3 inhibitors impairs mitophagy and activates apoptosis in SRSF2P95H/+ mutated cells [408]. These results suggest that combining mitophagy inhibitors with anticancer agents could represent an effective approach to overcome drug resistance in cancer [409]. Some natural compounds have been shown to affect cancer cell death and exhibit anticancer properties by modulating mitophagy [410]. Notably, fluorizoline inhibits mitophagy by targeting PHB1/PHB2, disrupting mitochondrial energy production and demonstrating anti-tumor effects in hematological malignancies [411,412]. Additionally, fluorizoline upregulates pro-apoptotic factors such as NOXA and BIM, inhibits C-RAF activation, and increases p21 expression, thereby exhibiting activity against CLL, CML, and AML cells [411,412]. Importantly, fluorizoline shows anti-tumoral activity in CLL irrespective of *TP53* and *ATM* gene alterations or *IGHV* mutation status [411]. However, unlike ibrutinib, it failed to prevent leukemia development in a mouse model of aggressive CLL [413]. Moreover, while no studies to date have investigated its effects in hematological malignancies, nitazoxanide has been reported to promote ROS-mediated mitophagy in solid cancers and exhibits synergistic effects when combined with CQ, a well-established autophagy inhibitor [414].

Besides mitophagy, ER-phagy plays a critical role in cancer therapy as it is regulated by the ubiquitin–proteasome system and autophagy. Loperamide induces ER-phagy and potently inhibits the proliferation of leukemia cell lines and primary leukemia cells from AML and ALL patients in a dose-dependent manner [415]. In addition, it triggers DNA damage and induces apoptosis in leukemic cells [415]. Additionally, xenophagy, the autophagic degradation of intracellular pathogens, is another key therapeutic mechanism in hematological malignancies. Resveratrol has been demonstrated to have antiproliferative and pro-apoptotic effects in various leukemic cell lines by inducing autophagy through AMPK activation and JNK-mediated p62/SQSTM1 expression [416], and inhibiting PI3K phosphorylation and Akt/mTOR pathway, reducing cyclin D1, and upregulating Caspase-3 [417,418]. However, its use in clinical trials has shown unexpected results. A clinical trial using SRT501, a formulation of resveratrol, in MM patients was terminated due to adverse events, including renal failure [419]. Additionally, salinomycin exhibits potent inhibitory activity against AML and mixed lineage leukemia-rearranged (MLLr) cell lines and primary cells [420] and impairs colony formation and reduces leukemia repopulation ability in AML and MLLr models [420]. Finally, lipophagy, the selective degradation of lipid droplets, has also emerged as a valuable target in cancer therapy. Tripterine (celastrol), a novel HSP90 inhibitor, activates lypophagy and it has been shown to inhibit proliferation of leukemia cells, including acute promyelocytic leukemia (APL) HL-60 cells. It depletes Bcr-Abl and induces apoptosis in imatinib-resistant CML cells harboring T315I mutation [421]. Furthermore, celastrol induces cell apoptosis and inhibits the expression of the AML1-ETO/C-KIT oncoprotein in t(8;21) leukemia [422]. Notably, celastrol has also been suggested as an effective therapeutic agent in signal transduction therapy for the treatment of patients with MM. It induces cell cycle arrest at G1 phase and apoptosis in human myeloma U266 cells through the activation of caspase-3 and NF-κB pathways [423–425]. Finally, it has been demonstrated that celastrol has synergistic effects with other drugs. For instance, it enhances the cytotoxic effects of TNF, paclitaxel, and doxorubicin in leukemia cells [426].

Finally, lysophagy, the degradation of damaged lysosomes, is targeted by compounds such as loperamide and pimozide, which induce lysosomal membrane permeability, leading to apoptosis of cancer cells [415]. Pimozide also inhibits STAT5, exhibiting efficacy in models of AML driven by FLT3 mutations [427]. These findings illustrate the therapeutic promise of targeting specific forms of autophagy to treat different types of hematological malignancies.

7.3. *Antioxidant Therapies*

Antioxidant therapies based on oxidative stress in cancer exploit the susceptibility of cancer cells to elevated levels of ROS. Here are the main types and their mechanisms of action:

7.3.1. Pro-Oxidant Chemotherapeutic Agents

Pro-oxidant chemotherapeutic agents play a crucial role in the treatment of hematological malignancies by inducing oxidative stress to enhance their anticancer efficacy [428] and even help in designing individualized therapies for patients suffering from refractory diseases [429]. Cisplatin, for instance, exerts its effects by binding to the N7 position of guanine in DNA, interfering with repair mechanisms and preferentially targeting guanine over adenine [430]. This binding promotes the overproduction of ROS, reducing the antioxidant defenses of cancer cells, which in turn increases DNA damage and enhances cisplatin's overall anticancer activity [431,432]. These combined effects make cisplatin a potent pro-oxidant therapy for several cancers, including hematological malignancies. Cisplatin inhibits cell proliferation and induces apoptosis in APL cells by forming DNA adducts and by activating p53 and AP-1 transcription factors [433]. Similarly, anthracyclines such as doxorubicin targets DNA replication and repair by intercalating into replicating DNA and inhibiting topoisomerase II [434]. In addition to disrupting these processes, anthracyclines generate oxygen-derived free radicals through two mechanisms: a non-enzymatic pathway involving iron and an enzymatic pathway associated with the mitochondrial respiratory chain. Both pathways contribute to oxidative damage, thereby enhancing the therapeutic efficacy of anthracyclines [431]. These dual mechanisms highlight the potential of pro-oxidant chemotherapeutic agents in exploring oxidative stress to combat hematological malignancies [435]. However, despite the promise of pro-oxidative therapies, challenges remain in achieving the selective targeting of malignant cells while sparing normal hematopoietic cells. One potential strategy to address this issue could be combining pro-oxidant agents with other treatments to improve therapeutic outcomes.

7.3.2. Small Pro-Oxidant Molecules

Elesclomol (STA-4783), imexon, motexafin gadolinium (MGd), and buthionine sulfoximine (BSO) are pro-oxidant agents that exploit oxidative stress to promote cancer cell death. Elesclomol chelates copper ions and transports them into mitochondria, disrupting the mitochondrial respiratory chain and inducing apoptosis. Imexon and MGd enhance oxidative stress by inhibiting the antioxidant defenses of cancer cells, while BSO targets the glutamate-cysteine ligase complex, a key enzyme in GSH synthesis. By reducing GSH levels, BSO further increases cancer cell susceptibility to oxidative damage, highlighting the therapeutic potential of pro-oxidant strategies in cancer treatment [431]. In AML, elesclomol has shown a potent anti-leukemic effect at concentrations as low as 10 nM, which is well below the concentrations achieved in cancer patients [436]. In addition, imexon induced apoptosis in MM tumor cells [437] and has shown to have efficacy in clinical trials for MM [438] and refractory B-cell non-Hodgkin lymphoma [429]. Likewise, MdG induces oxidative stress by oxidizing intracellular metabolites, leading to the generation of ROS and apoptosis in malignant cells, including those from CLL, non-HL, and MM [439,440]. Interestingly, preclinical studies have reported that MGd is cytotoxic to various hematological malignancies. It has been shown to enhance the effects of rituximab in NHL and has induced complete remissions when combined with radioimmunotherapy in relapsed NHL patients [439]. Similarly, BSO synergistically enhances melphalan activity against MM [441], whereas elesclomol in combination with paclitaxel showed improved efficacy compared to paclitaxel alone, particularly in terms of progression-free survival in patients with metastatic solid tumors [442,443]. These results point out that parallel strategies need to be explored for hematological malignancies for all these pro-oxidant compounds.

7.3.3. Targeted Therapies

NOX inhibitors and GSH depletion are strategies that modulate oxidative stress to target cancer cells. NOX inhibitors reduce ROS production by targeting NOX enzymes overexpressed in certain cancers. For instance, NOX2 is critical for the self-renewal and differentiation of leukemia-initiating stem cells (LSCs) and its inhibition impairs core metabolism in LSCs, leading to reduced disease development in murine models of leukemia [444]. This suggests that NOX2 plays a significant role in maintaining the malignant phenotype of LSCs, making it a potential therapeutic target for hematological cancers. Likewise, several studies have reported that GSH depletion improves the therapeutic effects of drugs by increasing oxidative stress within cancer cells, making them more susceptible to treatment [445]. Together, these approaches highlight the therapeutic potential of manipulating oxidative stress pathways in the treatment of hematological malignancies.

7.4. Approaches Combining Oxidative Stress and Autophagy

Combination therapies targeting autophagy and oxidative stress in cancer have shown significant promise in preclinical studies, leveraging their intricate interplay to enhance therapeutic efficacy. Autophagy, by clearing dysfunctional mitochondria, reduces ROS accumulation and protects leukemia cells from oxidative stress [446]. Research by Sumitomo et al. revealed that leukemia-initiating cells lacking autophagy, due to the deletion of ATG5 or ATG7 in AML mouse models, exhibited increased mitochondrial activity and higher ROS levels [290]. This led to enhanced cell death, underscoring the essential role of autophagy in supporting leukemia-initiating cell survival [290]. Therefore, combining pro-oxidants with chemotherapy, such as nutrient deprivation paired with anticancer therapies, further increases ROS production and promotes apoptosis in cancer cells [134]. A recent study showed that caloric and nutrient restriction during chemotherapy for B-cell ALL reduced minimal residual disease (MRD) risk, suggesting improved treatment efficacy [447]. In addition, other studies have shown that combining pro-oxidants with chemotherapy, such as nutrient deprivation paired with cisplatin or methioninase (a methionine-depleting enzyme), further increases ROS production and promotes apoptosis in cancer cells [448–450]. Moreover, AML blasts—malignant cells with significant deficiencies in the arginine-recycling pathway—have been found to be sensitive to BCT-100, a pegylated human recombinant arginase. BCT-100 induces a rapid depletion of both extracellular and intracellular arginine levels, leading to the inhibition of AML blast proliferation and a reduction in AML engraftment [451]. Interestingly, BCT-100 acted synergistically in combination with cytarabine [451]. Additionally, targeting specific proteins and pathways, such as H_2O_2-activated AMPK or p62 oxidation, offers novel avenues for therapy [140]. Strategies that inhibit antioxidant enzymes like GPXs can help in predicting disease outcome and overcome drug resistance by increasing oxidative stress and sensitizing tumors to treatment [452]. These approaches demonstrate the potential of combining autophagy modulation with oxidative stress therapies, either by suppressing autophagy's pro-survival role or enhancing its tumor-suppressive effects, tailored to cancer type and genetic context [134,349].

8. Future Directions, Current Limitations, and Emerging Technologies and Approaches

8.1. Future Directions

Personalized approaches are crucial for advancing cancer therapies by tailoring autophagy and oxidative stress modulation to the unique characteristics and genetic profiles of individual tumors. Such customization could enhance therapeutic precision and improve patient outcomes. Combination therapies represent another promising avenue, focusing on the synergistic effects of pairing autophagy modulators with traditional chemotherapies or targeted therapies. These strategies may boost treatment efficacy by leveraging complementary mechanisms of action. Biomarker identification is vital for the prediction and monitoring of therapy responses. Discovering reliable biomarkers for autophagy and oxidative stress-based treatments could help refine patient selection and track therapeutic effectiveness more accurately. Novel drug discovery is also a key area of focus, aiming to identify new compounds capable of selectively modulating autophagy or oxidative stress pathways in cancer cells. These targeted interventions could minimize off-target effects and improve treatment specificity. Improved mechanistic knowledge is essential to deepen our understanding of the molecular interplay between autophagy, oxidative stress, and cancer progression. Such insights can uncover new therapeutic targets and inform the design of innovative treatments. Optimizing treatment timing is another critical consideration, as the therapeutic benefit of autophagy modulation may depend on its timing relative to cancer type and stage. Determining the ideal timing could enhance treatment efficacy and reduce resistance. Finally, exploring the tumor microenvironment is necessary to understand how autophagy and oxidative stress influence cancer progression and treatment response within this complex ecosystem. Investigating these dynamics could reveal novel strategies to disrupt tumor growth and improve therapeutic outcomes.

To realize the potential of autophagy modulation in cancer therapy while reducing risks and improving patient outcomes, future research directions should focus on overcoming these challenges.

8.2. Current Limitations in Research and Clinical Implications

8.2.1. Research Limitations

The regulation of autophagy constitutes a key obstacle to the development of targeted cancer therapies. The intricate link between autophagy and oxidative stress in cancer cells remains poorly understood, complicating the development of effective therapeutic strategies [129,453]. Additionally, autophagy can act as both a tumor suppressor and a tumor promoter depending on cancer type, stage, and genetic factors, further complicating the development of universal therapeutic guidelines [235,454]. The current lack of reliable biomarkers to predict which patients will benefit from autophagy modulation also hampers the ability to stratify patients and optimize treatment outcomes [235,453]. More advanced animal models are also needed to study the role of specific autophagy-associated genes in tumor progression and response to treatment, as current models often fail to replicate the complexity of human cancer [235].

8.2.2. Clinical Implications

Clinically, the balance between the inhibition of autophagy to target cancer cells and the minimization of toxicity to normal tissues remains a considerable challenge. In cancer treatment, it is critical to identify the therapeutic window that maximizes efficacy while minimizing side effects [453,454]. Increased autophagy during chemotherapy has been shown to contribute to drug resistance in cancer, leading to disease recurrence. Understanding this phenomenon is essential to overcome treatment failure and improve patient outcomes [129,235]. Tumor heterogeneity also complicates treatment, as the extent of autophagy dependency differs between cancer types and stages, making a one-size-fits-all approach difficult [235]. The complexity of combination therapies, particularly the integration of autophagy modulators with conventional or targeted therapies, also requires extensive research to determine the most effective treatment programs [235,453]. The development of selective inhibitors that specifically target autophagy in cancer cells without affecting normal cells is still a major challenge due to the risk of off-target effects [453,454].

Despite promising preclinical findings, robust clinical evidence supporting the efficacy of antioxidants in cancer therapy is limited. Many studies are underpowered or fail to address the complex interactions between antioxidants, cancer cells, and chemotherapy, highlighting the need for large-scale controlled trials to establish clear guidelines [455]. While antioxidants may improve the tolerability of chemotherapy by reducing side effects, careful evaluation of their interactions with chemotherapeutic agents is needed to avoid compromising treatment outcomes [456].

8.3. Emerging Technologies and Approaches

Emerging technologies and approaches in cancer therapies related to autophagy and oxidative stress encompass several key areas. Targeted autophagy modulation focuses on developing selective inhibitors that target autophagy in cancer cells while sparing normal tissues, reducing systemic toxicity and enhancing the efficacy of conventional treatments such as chemotherapy and radiotherapy [137]. Oxidative stress manipulation involves strategies to selectively increase ROS production in tumor cells or inhibit antioxidant pathways like those regulated by sirtuin 3 (Sirt3), thereby sensitizing cancer cells to ROS-induced cytotoxicity while minimizing effects on normal tissues [235]. Additionally, iron homeostasis targeting leverages the role of autophagy in regulating intracellular iron levels to disrupt tumor survival and proliferation [457].

Autophagy-based immunotherapies explore the modulation of autophagy in immune cells, such as dendritic cells and T lymphocytes, to improve anti-tumor immune responses [453]. Identifying autophagic biomarkers is another critical focus, with efforts aimed at discovering markers from human biopsy samples to stratify cancer subtypes and guide autophagy-inhibiting therapies [453]. Similarly, metabolic therapies target the interplay between autophagy and tumor metabolism, such as glutaminolysis, to exploit cancer cells' metabolic vulnerabilities, reduce resistance, and enhance treatment efficacy [453].

The integration of experimental methodologies and biocomputational techniques plays a pivotal role in advancing these therapeutic strategies. Experimental approaches include genetic modulation, biomarker identification, metabolic profiling, immunomodulation, and the use of nanoparticle delivery systems to enhance precision and reduce off-target effects [458,459]. In contrast, biocomputational techniques utilize machine learning, network analysis, and systems biology to predict drug responses, identify therapeutic targets, and optimize treatment strategies. High-throughput screening, pathway analysis, and pharmacogenomics further facilitate personalized medicine approaches, enabling the rational design of drug combinations that integrate autophagy inhibitors with chemotherapy or targeted therapies for maximum therapeutic benefit [460]. These multidisciplinary advancements are reshaping cancer treatment paradigms by exploiting the dynamic interplay between autophagy and oxidative stress.

9. Conclusions

Autophagy and oxidative stress are essential mechanisms for maintaining cellular homeostasis, and their intricate interplay plays a pivotal role in cancer biology by influencing tumor progression, metastasis, and therapy resistance. Over the last decade, numerous studies have demonstrated that autophagy can act as both a tumor suppressor and a protumorigenic mechanism, depending on the cancer type, stage, and microenvironment. In addition, autophagy promotes the survival of cancer cells under stress conditions such as hypoxia and nutrient deprivation.

This review highlights the dual role of autophagy and reactive oxygen species (ROS) in mediating cancer cell death and suppressing tumor progression in hematological malignancies. This interplay is tightly regulated by key signaling pathways, including PI3K/AKT/mTOR, AMPK, and HIF-1α, which maintain a balance between autophagic activity and ROS production. Notably, the dysregulation of autophagy can paradoxically exacerbate oxidative stress, establishing a feedback loop that promotes tumor survival and growth.

Understanding the crosstalk between autophagy and oxidative stress in tumorigenesis offers promising opportunities for targeted cancer therapies. Strategies such as autophagy inhibition, the amplification of ROS levels using pro-oxidant compounds, and the integration of these approaches with conventional treatments have shown potential to overcome therapeutic resistance and improve clinical outcomes. However, effective clinical translation requires a nuanced understanding of tumor-specific contexts and the dynamic nature of the autophagy–oxidative stress axis. This review underscores the need for continued research to refine therapeutic strategies and leverage this interplay for more effective and personalized cancer treatments.

Author Contributions: Conceptualization, A.J.C.-S., J.M.S.-M., F.J.R.-Z., and J.S.; methodology, A.J.C.-S., J.M.S.-M., M.C.-F., P.G.-M., E.M.P., C.G.-O., and J.S.; writing—original draft preparation, A.J.C.-S., J.M.S.-M., C.G.-O., M.C.-F., L.D.-B., F.J.R.-Z., J.F.G.-B., F.J.G.-V., F.G.-M., J.A.L.-L., P.S.-R., and J.S.; writing—review and editing, all authors; illustrations, F.J.R.-Z. and J.S.; supervision, F.J.R.-Z. and J.S.; project administration, J.S.; funding acquisition, J.S. All authors have read and agreed to the published version of the manuscript.

Funding: This work was partially supported by Instituto de Salud Carlos III—ISCIII (Spanish Government) co-funded by FEDER funds/European Regional Development Fund (ERDF)—a way to build Europe (PI20/01845). Additional support came from the Consejería de Transformación Económica, Industria, Conocimiento y Universidades and FEDER (PY20/01282).

Conflicts of Interest: The authors declare no conflicts of interest. The funders had no role in the writing of the manuscript or in the decision to publish the reviewed material.

References

1. Bray, F.; Laversanne, M.; Weiderpass, E.; Soerjomataram, I. The Ever-Increasing Importance of Cancer as a Leading Cause of Premature Death Worldwide. *Cancer* **2021**, *127*, 3029–3030. [CrossRef] [PubMed]
2. Pizzino, G.; Irrera, N.; Cucinotta, M.; Pallio, G.; Mannino, F.; Arcoraci, V.; Squadrito, F.; Altavilla, D.; Bitto, A. Oxidative Stress: Harms and Benefits for Human Health. *Oxid. Med. Cell. Longev.* **2017**, *2017*, 8416763. [CrossRef] [PubMed]
3. Klionsky, D.J.; Petroni, G.; Amaravadi, R.K.; Baehrecke, E.H.; Ballabio, A.; Boya, P.; Bravo-San Pedro, J.M.; Cadwell, K.; Cecconi, F.; Choi, A.M.K.; et al. Autophagy in Major Human Diseases. *EMBO J.* **2021**, *40*, e108863. [CrossRef] [PubMed]
4. Morselli, E.; Galluzzi, L.; Kepp, O.; Criollo, A.; Maiuri, M.C.; Tavernarakis, N.; Madeo, F.; Kroemer, G. Autophagy Mediates Pharmacological Lifespan Extension by Spermidine and Resveratrol. *Aging* **2009**, *1*, 961–970. [CrossRef]
5. Rubinsztein, D.C.; Mariño, G.; Kroemer, G. Autophagy and Aging. *Cell* **2011**, *146*, 682–695. [CrossRef]
6. Fernández, Á.F.; Sebti, S.; Wei, Y.; Zou, Z.; Shi, M.; McMillan, K.L.; He, C.; Ting, T.; Liu, Y.; Chiang, W.-C.; et al. Disruption of the Beclin 1-BCL2 Autophagy Regulatory Complex Promotes Longevity in Mice. *Nature* **2018**, *558*, 136–140. [CrossRef]
7. Leidal, A.M.; Levine, B.; Debnath, J. Autophagy and the Cell Biology of Age-Related Disease. *Nat. Cell Biol.* **2018**, *20*, 1338–1348. [CrossRef]
8. Guo, J.; Huang, X.; Dou, L.; Yan, M.; Shen, T.; Tang, W.; Li, J. Aging and Aging-Related Diseases: From Molecular Mechanisms to Interventions and Treatments. *Signal Transduct. Target. Ther.* **2022**, *7*, 391. [CrossRef]
9. Poetsch, A.R. The Genomics of Oxidative DNA Damage, Repair, and Resulting Mutagenesis. *Comput. Struct. Biotechnol. J.* **2020**, *18*, 207–219. [CrossRef]
10. Gómez-Virgilio, L.; Silva-Lucero, M.-D.-C.; Flores-Morelos, D.-S.; Gallardo-Nieto, J.; Lopez-Toledo, G.; Abarca-Fernandez, A.-M.; Zacapala-Gómez, A.-E.; Luna-Muñoz, J.; Montiel-Sosa, F.; Soto-Rojas, L.O.; et al. Autophagy: A Key Regulator of Homeostasis and Disease: An Overview of Molecular Mechanisms and Modulators. *Cells* **2022**, *11*, 2262. [CrossRef]
11. Ornatowski, W.; Lu, Q.; Yegambaram, M.; Garcia, A.E.; Zemskov, E.A.; Maltepe, E.; Fineman, J.R.; Wang, T.; Black, S.M. Complex Interplay between Autophagy and Oxidative Stress in the Development of Pulmonary Disease. *Redox Biol.* **2020**, *36*, 101679. [CrossRef] [PubMed]
12. Kopinski, P.K.; Singh, L.N.; Zhang, S.; Lott, M.T.; Wallace, D.C. Mitochondrial DNA Variation and Cancer. *Nat. Rev. Cancer* **2021**, *21*, 431–445. [CrossRef] [PubMed]
13. Sainero-Alcolado, L.; Liaño-Pons, J.; Ruiz-Pérez, M.V.; Arsenian-Henriksson, M. Targeting Mitochondrial Metabolism for Precision Medicine in Cancer. *Cell Death Differ.* **2022**, *29*, 1304–1317. [CrossRef] [PubMed]
14. Rakesh, R.; PriyaDharshini, L.C.; Sakthivel, K.M.; Rasmi, R.R. Role and Regulation of Autophagy in Cancer. *Biochim. Biophys. Acta Mol. Basis Dis.* **2022**, *1868*, 166400. [CrossRef]
15. Noguchi, M.; Hirata, N.; Tanaka, T.; Suizu, F.; Nakajima, H.; Chiorini, J.A. Autophagy as a Modulator of Cell Death Machinery. *Cell Death Dis.* **2020**, *11*, 517. [CrossRef]
16. Yu, L.; Chen, Y.; Tooze, S.A. Autophagy Pathway: Cellular and Molecular Mechanisms. *Autophagy* **2018**, *14*, 207–215. [CrossRef]
17. Mizushima, N.; Levine, B. Autophagy in Human Diseases. *N. Engl. J. Med.* **2020**, *383*, 1564–1576. [CrossRef]
18. Levine, B.; Kroemer, G. Biological Functions of Autophagy Genes: A Disease Perspective. *Cell* **2019**, *176*, 11–42. [CrossRef]
19. Silva, V.R.; Neves, S.P.; Santos, L.d.S.; Dias, R.B.; Bezerra, D.P. Challenges and Therapeutic Opportunities of Autophagy in Cancer Therapy. *Cancers* **2020**, *12*, 3461. [CrossRef]
20. Urbańska, K.; Orzechowski, A. The Secrets of Alternative Autophagy. *Cells* **2021**, *10*, 3241. [CrossRef]
21. García Ruiz, O.; Sánchez-Maldonado, J.M.; López-Nevot, M.Á.; García, P.; Macauda, A.; Hernández-Mohedo, F.; González-Sierra, P.A.; Martínez-Bueno, M.; Pérez, E.; Reyes-Zurita, F.J.; et al. Autophagy in Hematological Malignancies. *Cancers* **2022**, *14*, 5072. [CrossRef] [PubMed]
22. Mizushima, N. Autophagy: Process and Function. *Genes Dev.* **2007**, *21*, 2861–2873. [CrossRef] [PubMed]
23. Ravanan, P.; Srikumar, I.F.; Talwar, P. Autophagy: The Spotlight for Cellular Stress Responses. *Life Sci.* **2017**, *188*, 53–67. [CrossRef] [PubMed]
24. Dong, Z.; Liang, S.; Hu, J.; Jin, W.; Zhan, Q.; Zhao, K. Autophagy as a Target for Hematological Malignancy Therapy. *Blood Rev.* **2016**, *30*, 369–380. [CrossRef]
25. Hansen, M.; Rubinsztein, D.C.; Walker, D.W. Autophagy as a Promoter of Longevity: Insights from Model Organisms. *Nat. Rev. Mol. Cell Biol.* **2018**, *19*, 579–593. [CrossRef]
26. Noda, T. Regulation of Autophagy through TORC1 and mTORC1. *Biomolecules* **2017**, *7*, 52. [CrossRef]
27. Yang, Z.; Klionsky, D.J. Mammalian Autophagy: Core Molecular Machinery and Signaling Regulation. *Curr. Opin. Cell Biol.* **2010**, *22*, 124–131. [CrossRef]
28. Devereaux, K.; Dall'Armi, C.; Alcazar-Roman, A.; Ogasawara, Y.; Zhou, X.; Wang, F.; Yamamoto, A.; De Camilli, P.; Di Paolo, G. Regulation of Mammalian Autophagy by Class II and III PI 3-Kinases through PI3P Synthesis. *PLoS ONE* **2013**, *8*, e76405. [CrossRef]

29. Müller, A.J.; Proikas-Cezanne, T. Function of Human WIPI Proteins in Autophagosomal Rejuvenation of Endomembranes? *FEBS Lett.* **2015**, *589*, 1546–1551. [CrossRef]
30. Djavaheri-Mergny, M.; Giuriato, S.; Tschan, M.P.; Humbert, M. Therapeutic Modulation of Autophagy in Leukaemia and Lymphoma. *Cells* **2019**, *8*, 103. [CrossRef]
31. Glick, D.; Barth, S.; Macleod, K.F. Autophagy: Cellular and Molecular Mechanisms. *J. Pathol.* **2010**, *221*, 3–12. [CrossRef] [PubMed]
32. Cuervo, A.M.; Wong, E. Chaperone-Mediated Autophagy: Roles in Disease and Aging. *Cell Res.* **2014**, *24*, 92–104. [CrossRef] [PubMed]
33. Riffelmacher, T.; Simon, A.-K. Mechanistic Roles of Autophagy in Hematopoietic Differentiation. *FEBS J.* **2017**, *284*, 1008–1020. [CrossRef] [PubMed]
34. McEwan, D.G.; Popovic, D.; Gubas, A.; Terawaki, S.; Suzuki, H.; Stadel, D.; Coxon, F.P.; Miranda de Stegmann, D.; Bhogaraju, S.; Maddi, K.; et al. PLEKHM1 Regulates Autophagosome-Lysosome Fusion through HOPS Complex and LC3/GABARAP Proteins. *Mol. Cell* **2015**, *57*, 39–54. [CrossRef]
35. Chun, Y.; Kim, J. Autophagy: An Essential Degradation Program for Cellular Homeostasis and Life. *Cells* **2018**, *7*, 278. [CrossRef]
36. Galluzzi, L.; Baehrecke, E.H.; Ballabio, A.; Boya, P.; Bravo-San Pedro, J.M.; Cecconi, F.; Choi, A.M.; Chu, C.T.; Codogno, P.; Colombo, M.I.; et al. Molecular Definitions of Autophagy and Related Processes. *EMBO J.* **2017**, *36*, 1811–1836. [CrossRef]
37. Kroemer, G.; Mariño, G.; Levine, B. Autophagy and the Integrated Stress Response. *Mol. Cell* **2010**, *40*, 280–293. [CrossRef]
38. Chen, G.; Zhang, Y.; Zhou, Y.; Luo, H.; Guan, H.; An, B. Targeting the mTOR Pathway in Hepatocellular Carcinoma: The Therapeutic Potential of Natural Products. *J. Inflamm. Res.* **2024**, *17*, 10421–10440. [CrossRef]
39. Wang, S.; Liu, G.; Yu, L.; Zhang, C.; Marcucci, F.; Jiang, Y. Fluorofenidone Enhances Cisplatin Efficacy in Non-Small Cell Lung Cancer: A Novel Approach to Inhibiting Cancer Progression. *Transl. Lung Cancer Res.* **2024**, *13*, 3175–3188. [CrossRef]
40. Wang, Y.; Pei, W.; Yang, Y.; Xia, C.; Zhang, Q.; Geng, Z.; Shi, X.; Wang, F. Inhibition of XIST Restrains Paclitaxel Resistance in Breast Cancer Cells by Targeting Hsa-Let-7d-5p/ATG16L1 through Regulation of Autophagy. *Cell. Signal.* **2024**, *127*, 111534. [CrossRef]
41. Alvers, A.L.; Wood, M.S.; Hu, D.; Kaywell, A.C.; Dunn, W.A., Jr.; Aris, J.P. Autophagy Is Required for Extension of Yeast Chronological Life Span by Rapamycin. *Autophagy* **2009**, *5*, 847–849. [CrossRef] [PubMed]
42. Li, J.; Kim, S.G.; Blenis, J. Rapamycin: One Drug, Many Effects. *Cell Metab.* **2014**, *19*, 373–379. [CrossRef] [PubMed]
43. Thomson, A.W.; Turnquist, H.R.; Raimondi, G. Immunoregulatory Functions of mTOR Inhibition. *Nat. Rev. Immunol.* **2009**, *9*, 324–337. [CrossRef] [PubMed]
44. Lamming, D.W.; Ye, L.; Sabatini, D.M.; Baur, J.A. Rapalogs and mTOR Inhibitors as Anti-Aging Therapeutics. *J. Clin. Investig.* **2013**, *123*, 980–989. [CrossRef]
45. Ballou, L.M.; Lin, R.Z. Rapamycin and mTOR Kinase Inhibitors. *J. Chem. Biol.* **2008**, *1*, 27–36. [CrossRef]
46. Shan, W.; Niu, W.; Lin, Q.; Shen, Y.; Shen, F.; Lou, K.; Zhang, Y. Bisphenol S Exposure Promotes Cell Apoptosis and Mitophagy in Murine Osteocytes by Regulating mtROS Signaling. *Microsc. Res. Tech.* **2023**, *86*, 481–493. [CrossRef]
47. Tellone, E.; Galtieri, A.; Russo, A.; Giardina, B.; Ficarra, S. Resveratrol: A Focus on Several Neurodegenerative Diseases. *Oxid. Med. Cell. Longev.* **2015**, *2015*, 392169. [CrossRef]
48. Wang, X.; Gao, M.; Lu, X.; Lei, Y.; Sun, J.; Ren, M.; Xu, T.; Lin, H. Resveratrol Alleviates Mono-2-Ethylhexyl Phthalate-Induced Mitophagy, Ferroptosis, and Immunological Dysfunction in Grass Carp Hepatocytes by Regulating the Nrf2 Pathway. *J. Environ. Manag.* **2024**, *371*, 123235. [CrossRef]
49. Li, J.; Fan, Y.; Zhang, Y.; Liu, Y.; Yu, Y.; Ma, M. Resveratrol Induces Autophagy and Apoptosis in Non-Small-Cell Lung Cancer Cells by Activating the NGFR-AMPK-mTOR Pathway. *Nutrients* **2022**, *14*, 2413. [CrossRef]
50. Liu, M.; Wilk, S.A.; Wang, A.; Zhou, L.; Wang, R.-H.; Ogawa, W.; Deng, C.; Dong, L.Q.; Liu, F. Resveratrol Inhibits mTOR Signaling by Promoting the Interaction between mTOR and DEPTOR. *J. Biol. Chem.* **2010**, *285*, 36387–36394. [CrossRef]
51. Soefje, S.A.; Karnad, A.; Brenner, A.J. Common Toxicities of Mammalian Target of Rapamycin Inhibitors. *Target. Oncol.* **2011**, *6*, 125–129. [CrossRef] [PubMed]
52. Ehinger, Y.; Zhang, Z.; Phamluong, K.; Soneja, D.; Shokat, K.M.; Ron, D. Brain-Specific Inhibition of mTORC1 Eliminates Side Effects Resulting from mTORC1 Blockade in the Periphery and Reduces Alcohol Intake in Mice. *Nat. Commun.* **2021**, *12*, 4407. [CrossRef] [PubMed]
53. Eisenberg, T.; Knauer, H.; Schauer, A.; Büttner, S.; Ruckenstuhl, C.; Carmona-Gutierrez, D.; Ring, J.; Schroeder, S.; Magnes, C.; Antonacci, L.; et al. Induction of Autophagy by Spermidine Promotes Longevity. *Nat. Cell Biol.* **2009**, *11*, 1305–1314. [CrossRef] [PubMed]
54. Kaminsky, C.J.; Mill, J.; Patel, V.; Pierce, D.; Haj, A.; Hess, A.S.; Li, L.; Raife, T. The Longevity Factor Spermidine Is Part of a Highly Heritable Complex Erythrocyte Phenotype Associated with Longevity. *Aging Cell* **2024**, *23*, e14311. [CrossRef]
55. Kriebs, A. Spermidine Controls Autophagy during Fasting. *Nat. Aging* **2024**, *4*, 1172. [CrossRef]
56. Hofer, S.J.; Daskalaki, I.; Abdellatif, M.; Stelzl, U.; Sedej, S.; Tavernarakis, N.; Kroemer, G.; Madeo, F. A Surge in Endogenous Spermidine Is Essential for Rapamycin-Induced Autophagy and Longevity. *Autophagy* **2024**, *20*, 2824–2826. [CrossRef]

57. Lubas, M.; Harder, L.M.; Kumsta, C.; Tiessen, I.; Hansen, M.; Andersen, J.S.; Lund, A.H.; Frankel, L.B. eIF5A Is Required for Autophagy by Mediating ATG3 Translation. *EMBO Rep.* **2018**, *19*, e46072. [CrossRef]
58. Hofer, S.J.; Daskalaki, I.; Bergmann, M.; Friščić, J.; Zimmermann, A.; Mueller, M.I.; Abdellatif, M.; Nicastro, R.; Masser, S.; Durand, S.; et al. Spermidine Is Essential for Fasting-Mediated Autophagy and Longevity. *Nat. Cell Biol.* **2024**, *26*, 1571–1584. [CrossRef]
59. Akinyele, O.; Wallace, H.M. Understanding the Polyamine and mTOR Pathway Interaction in Breast Cancer Cell Growth. *Med. Sci.* **2022**, *10*, 51. [CrossRef]
60. Chen, Y.; Zhuang, H.; Chen, X.; Shi, Z.; Wang, X. Spermidine-induced Growth Inhibition and Apoptosis via Autophagic Activation in Cervical Cancer. *Oncol. Rep.* **2018**, *39*, 2845–2854. [CrossRef]
61. Yang, Y.-P.; Hu, L.-F.; Zheng, H.-F.; Mao, C.-J.; Hu, W.-D.; Xiong, K.-P.; Wang, F.; Liu, C.-F. Application and Interpretation of Current Autophagy Inhibitors and Activators. *Acta Pharmacol. Sin.* **2013**, *34*, 625–635. [CrossRef] [PubMed]
62. Ferreira, P.M.; de Sousa, R.W.; de Oliveira Ferreira, J.R.; Militão, G.C.; Bezerra, D.P. Chloroquine and Hydroxychloroquine in Antitumor Therapies Based on Autophagy-Related Mechanisms. *Pharmacol. Res.* **2021**, *168*, 105582. [CrossRef] [PubMed]
63. Manic, G.; Obrist, F.; Kroemer, G.; Vitale, I.; Galluzzi, L. Chloroquine and Hydroxychloroquine for Cancer Therapy. *Mol. Cell. Oncol.* **2014**, *1*, e29911. [CrossRef] [PubMed]
64. Verbaanderd, C.; Maes, H.; Schaaf, M.B.; Sukhatme, V.P.; Pantziarka, P.; Sukhatme, V.; Agostinis, P.; Bouche, G. Repurposing Drugs in Oncology (ReDO)-Chloroquine and Hydroxychloroquine as Anti-Cancer Agents. *Ecancermedicalscience* **2017**, *11*, 781. [CrossRef] [PubMed]
65. Mauvezin, C.; Neufeld, T.P. Bafilomycin A1 Disrupts Autophagic Flux by Inhibiting Both V-ATPase-Dependent Acidification and Ca-P60A/SERCA-Dependent Autophagosome-Lysosome Fusion. *Autophagy* **2015**, *11*, 1437–1438. [CrossRef]
66. Jovanović Stojanov, S.; Kostić, A.; Ljujić, M.; Lupšić, E.; Schenone, S.; Pešić, M.; Dinić, J. Autophagy Inhibition Enhances Anti-Glioblastoma Effects of pyrazolo[3,4-*d*]pyrimidine Tyrosine Kinase Inhibitors. *Life* **2022**, *12*, 1503. [CrossRef]
67. Yan, Y.; Jiang, K.; Liu, P.; Zhang, X.; Dong, X.; Gao, J.; Liu, Q.; Barr, M.P.; Zhang, Q.; Hou, X.; et al. Bafilomycin A1 Induces Caspase-Independent Cell Death in Hepatocellular Carcinoma Cells via Targeting of Autophagy and MAPK Pathways. *Sci. Rep.* **2016**, *6*, 37052. [CrossRef]
68. Heckmann, B.L.; Yang, X.; Zhang, X.; Liu, J. The Autophagic Inhibitor 3-Methyladenine Potently Stimulates PKA-Dependent Lipolysis in Adipocytes. *Br. J. Pharmacol.* **2013**, *168*, 163–171. [CrossRef]
69. Wu, Y.-T.; Tan, H.-L.; Shui, G.; Bauvy, C.; Huang, Q.; Wenk, M.R.; Ong, C.-N.; Codogno, P.; Shen, H.-M. Dual Role of 3-Methyladenine in Modulation of Autophagy via Different Temporal Patterns of Inhibition on Class I and III Phosphoinositide 3-Kinase. *J. Biol. Chem.* **2010**, *285*, 10850–10861. [CrossRef]
70. Lin, Y.-C.; Kuo, H.-C.; Wang, J.-S.; Lin, W.-W. Regulation of Inflammatory Response by 3-Methyladenine Involves the Coordinative Actions on Akt and Glycogen Synthase Kinase 3β rather than Autophagy. *J. Immunol.* **2012**, *189*, 4154–4164. [CrossRef]
71. Slavin, S.A.; Leonard, A.; Grose, V.; Fazal, F.; Rahman, A. Autophagy Inhibitor 3-Methyladenine Protects against Endothelial Cell Barrier Dysfunction in Acute Lung Injury. *Am. J. Physiol. Lung Cell. Mol. Physiol.* **2018**, *314*, L388–L396. [CrossRef] [PubMed]
72. Wear, D.; Bhagirath, E.; Balachandar, A.; Vegh, C.; Pandey, S. Autophagy Inhibition via Hydroxychloroquine or 3-Methyladenine Enhances Chemotherapy-Induced Apoptosis in Neuro-Blastoma and Glioblastoma. *Int. J. Mol. Sci.* **2023**, *24*, 12052. [CrossRef] [PubMed]
73. Rigoulet, M.; Bouchez, C.L.; Paumard, P.; Ransac, S.; Cuvellier, S.; Duvezin-Caubet, S.; Mazat, J.P.; Devin, A. Cell Energy Metabolism: An Update. *Biochim. Biophys. Acta Bioenerg.* **2020**, *1861*, 148276. [CrossRef] [PubMed]
74. Walker, M.A.; Tian, R. NAD(H) in Mitochondrial Energy Transduction: Implications for Health and Disease. *Curr. Opin. Physiol.* **2018**, *3*, 101–109. [CrossRef]
75. Boveris, A.; Oshino, N.; Chance, B. The Cellular Production of Hydrogen Peroxide. *Biochem. J.* **1972**, *128*, 617–630. [CrossRef]
76. Commoner, B.; Townsend, J.; Pake, G.E. Free Radicals in Biological Materials. *Nature* **1954**, *174*, 689–691. [CrossRef]
77. Li, R.; Jia, Z.; Trush, M.A. Defining ROS in Biology and Medicine. *React. Oxyg. Species* **2016**, *1*, 9–21. [CrossRef]
78. Bardaweel, S.K.; Gul, M.; Alzweiri, M.; Ishaqat, A.; Al Salamat, H.A.; Bashatwah, R.M. Reactive Oxygen Species: The Dual Role in Physiological and Pathological Conditions of the Human Body. *Eurasian J. Med.* **2018**, *50*, 193–201. [CrossRef]
79. Panieri, E.; Santoro, M.M. ROS Homeostasis and Metabolism: A Dangerous Liason in Cancer Cells. *Cell Death Dis.* **2016**, *7*, e2253. [CrossRef]
80. Sies, H.; Jones, D.P. Reactive Oxygen Species (ROS) as Pleiotropic Physiological Signalling Agents. *Nat. Rev. Mol. Cell Biol.* **2020**, *21*, 363–383. [CrossRef]
81. He, L.; He, T.; Farrar, S.; Ji, L.; Liu, T.; Ma, X. Antioxidants Maintain Cellular Redox Homeostasis by Elimination of Reactive Oxygen Species. *Cell. Physiol. Biochem.* **2017**, *44*, 532–553. [CrossRef] [PubMed]
82. Ray, P.D.; Huang, B.-W.; Tsuji, Y. Reactive Oxygen Species (ROS) Homeostasis and Redox Regulation in Cellular Signaling. *Cell. Signal.* **2012**, *24*, 981–990. [CrossRef] [PubMed]

83. Krishnamurthy, H.K.; Pereira, M.; Rajavelu, I.; Jayaraman, V.; Krishna, K.; Wang, T.; Bei, K.; Rajasekaran, J.J. Oxidative Stress: Fundamentals and Advances in Quantification Techniques. *Front. Chem.* **2024**, *12*, 1470458. [CrossRef] [PubMed]
84. Hayes, J.D.; Dinkova-Kostova, A.T.; Tew, K.D. Oxidative Stress in Cancer. *Cancer Cell* **2020**, *38*, 167–197. [CrossRef]
85. Samet, J.M.; Wages, P.A. Oxidative Stress from Environmental Exposures. *Curr. Opin. Toxicol.* **2018**, *7*, 60–66. [CrossRef]
86. Checa, J.; Aran, J.M. Reactive Oxygen Species: Drivers of Physiological and Pathological Processes. *J. Inflamm. Res.* **2020**, *13*, 1057–1073. [CrossRef]
87. Auten, R.L.; Davis, J.M. Oxygen Toxicity and Reactive Oxygen Species: The Devil Is in the Details. *Pediatr. Res.* **2009**, *66*, 121–127. [CrossRef]
88. Sousa, J.S.; D'Imprima, E.; Vonck, J. Mitochondrial Respiratory Chain Complexes. *Subcell. Biochem.* **2018**, *87*, 167–227.
89. Zhang, B.; Pan, C.; Feng, C.; Yan, C.; Yu, Y.; Chen, Z.; Guo, C.; Wang, X. Role of Mitochondrial Reactive Oxygen Species in Homeostasis Regulation. *Redox Rep.* **2022**, *27*, 45–52. [CrossRef]
90. Sinenko, S.A.; Starkova, T.Y.; Kuzmin, A.A.; Tomilin, A.N. Physiological Signaling Functions of Reactive Oxygen Species in Stem Cells: From Flies to Man. *Front. Cell Dev. Biol.* **2021**, *9*, 714370. [CrossRef]
91. Sena, L.A.; Chandel, N.S. Physiological Roles of Mitochondrial Reactive Oxygen Species. *Mol. Cell* **2012**, *48*, 158–167. [CrossRef] [PubMed]
92. Zong, Y.; Li, H.; Liao, P.; Chen, L.; Pan, Y.; Zheng, Y.; Zhang, C.; Liu, D.; Zheng, M.; Gao, J. Mitochondrial Dysfunction: Mechanisms and Advances in Therapy. *Signal Transduct. Target. Ther.* **2024**, *9*, 124. [CrossRef] [PubMed]
93. Wang, L.; Yang, Z.; He, X.; Pu, S.; Yang, C.; Wu, Q.; Zhou, Z.; Cen, X.; Zhao, H. Mitochondrial Protein Dysfunction in Pathogenesis of Neurological Diseases. *Front. Mol. Neurosci.* **2022**, *15*, 974480. [CrossRef] [PubMed]
94. Vermot, A.; Petit-Härtlein, I.; Smith, S.M.E.; Fieschi, F. NADPH Oxidases (NOX): An Overview from Discovery, Molecular Mechanisms to Physiology and Pathology. *Antioxidants* **2021**, *10*, 890. [CrossRef]
95. Nauseef, W.M. The Phagocyte NOX2 NADPH Oxidase in Microbial Killing and Cell Signaling. *Curr. Opin. Immunol.* **2019**, *60*, 130–140. [CrossRef]
96. Manea, A. NADPH Oxidase-Derived Reactive Oxygen Species: Involvement in Vascular Physiology and Pathology. *Cell Tissue Res.* **2010**, *342*, 325–339. [CrossRef]
97. Szanto, I.; Pusztaszeri, M.; Mavromati, M. H_2O_2 Metabolism in Normal Thyroid Cells and in Thyroid Tumorigenesis: Focus on NADPH Oxidases. *Antioxidants* **2019**, *8*, 126. [CrossRef]
98. Eun, H.S.; Cho, S.Y.; Joo, J.S.; Kang, S.H.; Moon, H.S.; Lee, E.S.; Kim, S.H.; Lee, B.S. Gene Expression of NOX Family Members and Their Clinical Significance in Hepatocellular Carcinoma. *Sci. Rep.* **2017**, *7*, 11060. [CrossRef]
99. Snezhkina, A.V.; Kudryavtseva, A.V.; Kardymon, O.L.; Savvateeva, M.V.; Melnikova, N.V.; Krasnov, G.S.; Dmitriev, A.A. ROS Generation and Antioxidant Defense Systems in Normal and Malignant Cells. *Oxid. Med. Cell. Longev.* **2019**, *2019*, 6175804. [CrossRef]
100. Sandalio, L.M.; Rodríguez-Serrano, M.; Romero-Puertas, M.C.; del Río, L.A. Role of Peroxisomes as a Source of Reactive Oxygen Species (ROS) Signaling Molecules. *Subcell. Biochem.* **2013**, *69*, 231–255.
101. Lin, L.-S.; Wang, J.-F.; Song, J.; Liu, Y.; Zhu, G.; Dai, Y.; Shen, Z.; Tian, R.; Song, J.; Wang, Z.; et al. Cooperation of Endogenous and Exogenous Reactive Oxygen Species Induced by Zinc Peroxide Nanoparticles to Enhance Oxidative Stress-Based Cancer Therapy. *Theranostics* **2019**, *9*, 7200–7209. [CrossRef]
102. Srinivas, U.S.; Tan, B.W.Q.; Vellayappan, B.A.; Jeyasekharan, A.D. ROS and the DNA Damage Response in Cancer. *Redox Biol.* **2019**, *25*, 101084. [CrossRef] [PubMed]
103. Yang, S.; Lian, G. ROS and Diseases: Role in Metabolism and Energy Supply. *Mol. Cell. Biochem.* **2020**, *467*, 1–12. [CrossRef] [PubMed]
104. Adwas, A.A.; Elsayed, A.; Azab, A.E.; Quwaydir, F.A. Oxidative Stress and Antioxidant Mechanisms in Human Body. *J. Appl. Biotechnol. Bioeng.* **2019**, *6*, 43–47.
105. Birben, E.; Sahiner, U.M.; Sackesen, C.; Erzurum, S.; Kalayci, O. Oxidative Stress and Antioxidant Defense. *World Allergy Organ. J.* **2012**, *5*, 9–19. [CrossRef] [PubMed]
106. Jomova, K.; Alomar, S.Y.; Alwasel, S.H.; Nepovimova, E.; Kuca, K.; Valko, M. Several Lines of Antioxidant Defense against Oxidative Stress: Antioxidant Enzymes, Nanomaterials with Multiple Enzyme-Mimicking Activities, and Low-Molecular-Weight Antioxidants. *Arch. Toxicol.* **2024**, *98*, 1323–1367. [CrossRef]
107. de Almeida, A.J.P.O.; de Oliveira, J.C.P.L.; da Silva Pontes, L.V.; de Souza, J.F., Jr.; Gonçalves, T.A.F.; Dantas, S.H.; de Almeida Feitosa, M.S.; Silva, A.O.; de Medeiros, I.A. ROS: Basic Concepts, Sources, Cellular Signaling, and Its Implications in Aging Pathways. *Oxid. Med. Cell. Longev.* **2022**, *2022*, 1225578. [CrossRef]
108. Dodson, M.; Redmann, M.; Rajasekaran, N.S.; Darley-Usmar, V.; Zhang, J. KEAP1-NRF2 Signalling and Autophagy in Protection against Oxidative and Reductive Proteotoxicity. *Biochem. J.* **2015**, *469*, 347–355. [CrossRef]
109. Zhao, L.; Li, H.; Wang, Y.; Zheng, A.; Cao, L.; Liu, J. Autophagy Deficiency Leads to Impaired Antioxidant Defense via p62-FOXO1/3 Axis. *Oxid. Med. Cell. Longev.* **2019**, *2019*, 2526314. [CrossRef]

110. Shan, C.; Wang, Y.; Wang, Y. The Crosstalk between Autophagy and Nrf2 Signaling in Cancer: From Biology to Clinical Applications. *Int. J. Biol. Sci.* **2024**, *20*, 6181–6206. [CrossRef]
111. Underwood, B.R.; Imarisio, S.; Fleming, A.; Rose, C.; Krishna, G.; Heard, P.; Quick, M.; Korolchuk, V.I.; Renna, M.; Sarkar, S.; et al. Antioxidants Can Inhibit Basal Autophagy and Enhance Neurodegeneration in Models of Polyglutamine Disease. *Hum. Mol. Genet.* **2010**, *19*, 3413–3429. [CrossRef] [PubMed]
112. Loreto Palacio, P.; Godoy, J.R.; Aktas, O.; Hanschmann, E.-M. Changing Perspectives from Oxidative Stress to Redox Signaling-Extracellular Redox Control in Translational Medicine. *Antioxidants* **2022**, *11*, 1181. [CrossRef] [PubMed]
113. Schieber, M.; Chandel, N.S. ROS Function in Redox Signaling and Oxidative Stress. *Curr. Biol.* **2014**, *24*, R453–R462. [CrossRef] [PubMed]
114. Hong, Y.; Boiti, A.; Vallone, D.; Foulkes, N.S. Reactive Oxygen Species Signaling and Oxidative Stress: Transcriptional Regulation and Evolution. *Antioxidants* **2024**, *13*, 312. [CrossRef] [PubMed]
115. Forman, H.J.; Ursini, F.; Maiorino, M. An Overview of Mechanisms of Redox Signaling. *J. Mol. Cell. Cardiol.* **2014**, *73*, 2–9. [CrossRef]
116. Chen, N.; Du, N.; Shen, R.; He, T.; Xi, J.; Tan, J.; Bian, G.; Yang, Y.; Liu, T.; Tan, W.; et al. Redox Signaling-Driven Modulation of Microbial Biosynthesis and Biocatalysis. *Nat. Commun.* **2023**, *14*, 6800. [CrossRef]
117. Cook, J.A.; Gius, D.; Wink, D.A.; Krishna, M.C.; Russo, A.; Mitchell, J.B. Oxidative Stress, Redox, and the Tumor Microenvironment. *Semin. Radiat. Oncol.* **2004**, *14*, 259–266. [CrossRef]
118. Kim, E.-K.; Jang, M.; Song, M.-J.; Kim, D.; Kim, Y.; Jang, H.H. Redox-Mediated Mechanism of Chemoresistance in Cancer Cells. *Antioxidants* **2019**, *8*, 471. [CrossRef]
119. Li, Y.; Zhang, X.; Wang, Z.; Li, B.; Zhu, H. Modulation of Redox Homeostasis: A Strategy to Overcome Cancer Drug Resistance. *Front. Pharmacol.* **2023**, *14*, 1156538. [CrossRef]
120. Hegedűs, C.; Kovács, K.; Polgár, Z.; Regdon, Z.; Szabó, É.; Robaszkiewicz, A.; Forman, H.J.; Martner, A.; Virág, L. Redox Control of Cancer Cell Destruction. *Redox Biol.* **2018**, *16*, 59–74. [CrossRef]
121. Voltan, R.; Secchiero, P.; Casciano, F.; Milani, D.; Zauli, G.; Tisato, V. Redox Signaling and Oxidative Stress: Cross Talk with TNF-Related Apoptosis Inducing Ligand Activity. *Int. J. Biochem. Cell Biol.* **2016**, *81*, 364–374. [CrossRef] [PubMed]
122. Acharya, A.; Das, I.; Chandhok, D.; Saha, T. Redox Regulation in Cancer: A Double-Edged Sword with Therapeutic Potential. *Oxid. Med. Cell. Longev.* **2010**, *3*, 23–34. [CrossRef] [PubMed]
123. Tasdogan, A.; Ubellacker, J.M.; Morrison, S.J. Redox Regulation in Cancer Cells during Metastasis. *Cancer Discov.* **2021**, *11*, 2682–2692. [CrossRef] [PubMed]
124. Arfin, S.; Jha, N.K.; Jha, S.K.; Kesari, K.K.; Ruokolainen, J.; Roychoudhury, S.; Rathi, B.; Kumar, D. Oxidative Stress in Cancer Cell Metabolism. *Antioxidants* **2021**, *10*, 642. [CrossRef]
125. Guerra-Castellano, A.; Díaz-Quintana, A.; Pérez-Mejías, G.; Elena-Real, C.A.; González-Arzola, K.; García-Mauriño, S.M.; De la Rosa, M.A.; Díaz-Moreno, I. Oxidative Stress Is Tightly Regulated by Cytochrome c Phosphorylation and Respirasome Factors in Mitochondria. *Proc. Natl. Acad. Sci. USA* **2018**, *115*, 7955–7960. [CrossRef]
126. Chen, Y.; Klionsky, D.J. The Regulation of Autophagy—Unanswered Questions. *J. Cell Sci.* **2011**, *124*, 161–170. [CrossRef]
127. He, C.; Klionsky, D.J. Regulation Mechanisms and Signaling Pathways of Autophagy. *Annu. Rev. Genet.* **2009**, *43*, 67–93. [CrossRef]
128. Rahman, M.A.; Ahmed, K.R.; Haque, F.; Park, M.N.; Kim, B. Recent Advances in Cellular Signaling Interplay between Redox Metabolism and Autophagy Modulation in Cancer: An Overview of Molecular Mechanisms and Therapeutic Interventions. *Antioxidants* **2023**, *12*, 428. [CrossRef]
129. Taucher, E.; Mykoliuk, I.; Fediuk, M.; Smolle-Juettner, F.-M. Autophagy, Oxidative Stress and Cancer Development. *Cancers* **2022**, *14*, 1637. [CrossRef]
130. Hasan, A.; Rizvi, S.F.; Parveen, S.; Pathak, N.; Nazir, A.; Mir, S.S. Crosstalk between ROS and Autophagy in Tumorigenesis: Understanding the Multifaceted Paradox. *Front. Oncol.* **2022**, *12*, 852424. [CrossRef]
131. Filomeni, G.; De Zio, D.; Cecconi, F. Oxidative Stress and Autophagy: The Clash between Damage and Metabolic Needs. *Cell Death Differ.* **2015**, *22*, 377–388. [CrossRef] [PubMed]
132. Guo, H.; Bechtel-Walz, W. The Interplay of Autophagy and Oxidative Stress in the Kidney: What Do We Know? *Nephron* **2023**, *147*, 627–642. [CrossRef] [PubMed]
133. Mukhopadhyay, P.; Eid, N.; Abdelmegeed, M.A.; Sen, A. Interplay of Oxidative Stress, Inflammation, and Autophagy: Their Role in Tissue Injury of the Heart, Liver, and Kidney. *Oxid. Med. Cell. Longev.* **2018**, *2018*, 2090813. [CrossRef] [PubMed]
134. Antunes, F.; Erustes, A.G.; Costa, A.J.; Nascimento, A.C.; Bincoletto, C.; Ureshino, R.P.; Pereira, G.J.S.; Smaili, S.S. Autophagy and Intermittent Fasting: The Connection for Cancer Therapy? *Clinics* **2018**, *73*, e814s. [CrossRef]
135. Ciccarone, F.; Castelli, S.; Ciriolo, M.R. Oxidative Stress-Driven Autophagy acROSs Onset and Therapeutic Outcome in Hepatocellular Carcinoma. *Oxid. Med. Cell. Longev.* **2019**, *2019*, 6050123. [CrossRef]

136. Chen, Y.; McMillan-Ward, E.; Kong, J.; Israels, S.J.; Gibson, S.B. Oxidative Stress Induces Autophagic Cell Death Independent of Apoptosis in Transformed and Cancer Cells. *Cell Death Differ.* **2008**, *15*, 171–182. [CrossRef]
137. Yun, H.R.; Jo, Y.H.; Kim, J.; Shin, Y.; Kim, S.S.; Choi, T.G. Roles of Autophagy in Oxidative Stress. *Int. J. Mol. Sci.* **2020**, *21*, 3289. [CrossRef]
138. Scherz-Shouval, R.; Elazar, Z. Regulation of Autophagy by ROS: Physiology and Pathology. *Trends Biochem. Sci.* **2011**, *36*, 30–38. [CrossRef]
139. Li, L.; Tan, J.; Miao, Y.; Lei, P.; Zhang, Q. ROS and Autophagy: Interactions and Molecular Regulatory Mechanisms. *Cell. Mol. Neurobiol.* **2015**, *35*, 615–621. [CrossRef]
140. He, J.; Dong, L.; Luo, L.; Wang, K. Redox Regulation of Autophagy in Cancer: Mechanism, Prevention and Therapy. *Life* **2022**, *13*, 98. [CrossRef]
141. Wang, S.; Li, H.; Yuan, M.; Fan, H.; Cai, Z. Role of AMPK in Autophagy. *Front. Physiol.* **2022**, *13*, 1015500. [CrossRef]
142. Ge, Y.; Zhou, M.; Chen, C.; Wu, X.; Wang, X. Role of AMPK Mediated Pathways in Autophagy and Aging. *Biochimie* **2022**, *195*, 100–113. [CrossRef] [PubMed]
143. Ning, B.; Hang, S.; Zhang, W.; Mao, C.; Li, D. An Update on the Bridging Factors Connecting Autophagy and Nrf2 Antioxidant Pathway. *Front. Cell Dev. Biol.* **2023**, *11*, 1232241. [CrossRef] [PubMed]
144. Li, Y.; Chen, Y. AMPK and Autophagy. *Adv. Exp. Med. Biol.* **2019**, *1206*, 85–108. [PubMed]
145. Frudd, K.; Burgoyne, T.; Burgoyne, J.R. Oxidation of Atg3 and Atg7 Mediates Inhibition of Autophagy. *Nat. Commun.* **2018**, *9*, 95. [CrossRef]
146. Ao, X.; Zou, L.; Wu, Y. Regulation of Autophagy by the Rab GTPase Network. *Cell Death Differ.* **2014**, *21*, 348–358. [CrossRef]
147. Szatmári, Z.; Sass, M. The Autophagic Roles of Rab Small GTPases and Their Upstream Regulators: A Review. *Autophagy* **2014**, *10*, 1154–1166. [CrossRef]
148. Leslie, N.R.; Bennett, D.; Lindsay, Y.E.; Stewart, H.; Gray, A.; Downes, C.P. Redox Regulation of PI 3-Kinase Signalling via Inactivation of PTEN. *EMBO J.* **2003**, *22*, 5501–5510. [CrossRef]
149. Scherz-Shouval, R.; Shvets, E.; Fass, E.; Shorer, H.; Gil, L.; Elazar, Z. Reactive Oxygen Species Are Essential for Autophagy and Specifically Regulate the Activity of Atg4. *EMBO J.* **2007**, *26*, 1749–1760. [CrossRef]
150. Zheng, X.; Yang, Z.; Gu, Q.; Xia, F.; Fu, Y.; Liu, P.; Yin, X.-M.; Li, M. The Protease Activity of Human ATG4B Is Regulated by Reversible Oxidative Modification. *Autophagy* **2020**, *16*, 1838–1850. [CrossRef]
151. Park, N.Y.; Jo, D.S.; Cho, D.-H. Post-Translational Modifications of ATG4B in the Regulation of Autophagy. *Cells* **2022**, *11*, 1330. [CrossRef] [PubMed]
152. Murata, H.; Ihara, Y.; Nakamura, H.; Yodoi, J.; Sumikawa, K.; Kondo, T. Glutaredoxin Exerts an Antiapoptotic Effect by Regulating the Redox State of Akt. *J. Biol. Chem.* **2003**, *278*, 50226–50233. [CrossRef] [PubMed]
153. Zhao, Y.; Hu, X.; Liu, Y.; Dong, S.; Wen, Z.; He, W.; Zhang, S.; Huang, Q.; Shi, M. ROS Signaling under Metabolic Stress: Cross-Talk between AMPK and AKT Pathway. *Mol. Cancer* **2017**, *16*, 79. [CrossRef] [PubMed]
154. Xie, X.; Zhang, Y.; Wang, Z.; Wang, S.; Jiang, X.; Cui, H.; Zhou, T.; He, Z.; Feng, H.; Guo, Q.; et al. ATM at the Crossroads of Reactive Oxygen Species and Autophagy. *Int. J. Biol. Sci.* **2021**, *17*, 3080–3090. [CrossRef]
155. Sun, X.; Chang, R.; Tang, Y.; Luo, S.; Jiang, C.; Jia, H.; Xu, Q.; Dong, Z.; Liang, Y.; Loor, J.J.; et al. Transcription Factor EB (TFEB)-Mediated Autophagy Protects Bovine Mammary Epithelial Cells against H_2O_2-Induced Oxidative Damage In Vitro. *J. Anim. Sci. Biotechnol.* **2021**, *12*, 35. [CrossRef]
156. Wang, H.; Wang, N.; Xu, D.; Ma, Q.; Chen, Y.; Xu, S.; Xia, Q.; Zhang, Y.; Prehn, J.H.M.; Wang, G.; et al. Oxidation of Multiple MiT/TFE Transcription Factors Links Oxidative Stress to Transcriptional Control of Autophagy and Lysosome Biogenesis. *Autophagy* **2020**, *16*, 1683–1696. [CrossRef]
157. Murrow, L.; Debnath, J. Autophagy as a Stress-Response and Quality-Control Mechanism: Implications for Cell Injury and Human Disease. *Annu. Rev. Pathol.* **2013**, *8*, 105–137. [CrossRef]
158. Chang, K.-C.; Liu, P.-F.; Chang, C.-H.; Lin, Y.-C.; Chen, Y.-J.; Shu, C.-W. The Interplay of Autophagy and Oxidative Stress in the Pathogenesis and Therapy of Retinal Degenerative Diseases. *Cell Biosci.* **2022**, *12*, 1. [CrossRef]
159. Kaushik, S.; Cuervo, A.M. Chaperone-Mediated Autophagy: A Unique Way to Enter the Lysosome World. *Trends Cell Biol.* **2012**, *22*, 407–417. [CrossRef]
160. Singh, R.; Cuervo, A.M. Autophagy in the Cellular Energetic Balance. *Cell Metab.* **2011**, *13*, 495–504. [CrossRef]
161. Rambold, A.S.; Lippincott-Schwartz, J. Mechanisms of Mitochondria and Autophagy Crosstalk. *Cell Cycle* **2011**, *10*, 4032–4038. [CrossRef] [PubMed]
162. Roca-Agujetas, V.; de Dios, C.; Lestón, L.; Marí, M.; Morales, A.; Colell, A. Recent Insights into the Mitochondrial Role in Autophagy and Its Regulation by Oxidative Stress. *Oxid. Med. Cell. Longev.* **2019**, *2019*, 3809308. [CrossRef] [PubMed]
163. Li, H.; Lismont, C.; Revenco, I.; Hussein, M.A.F.; Costa, C.F.; Fransen, M. The Peroxisome-Autophagy Redox Connection: A Double-Edged Sword? *Front. Cell Dev. Biol.* **2021**, *9*, 814047. [CrossRef] [PubMed]

164. Dikic, I.; Elazar, Z. Mechanism and Medical Implications of Mammalian Autophagy. *Nat. Rev. Mol. Cell Biol.* **2018**, *19*, 349–364. [CrossRef]
165. Ohsumi, Y. Historical Landmarks of Autophagy Research. *Cell Res.* **2014**, *24*, 9–23. [CrossRef]
166. Salete-Granado, D.; Carbonell, C.; Puertas-Miranda, D.; Vega-Rodríguez, V.-J.; García-Macia, M.; Herrero, A.B.; Marcos, M. Autophagy, Oxidative Stress, and Alcoholic Liver Disease: A Systematic Review and Potential Clinical Applications. *Antioxidants* **2023**, *12*, 1425. [CrossRef]
167. Ribas, V.; García-Ruiz, C.; Fernández-Checa, J.C. Glutathione and Mitochondria. *Front. Pharmacol.* **2014**, *5*, 151. [CrossRef]
168. Yang, S.; Xia, C.; Li, S.; Du, L.; Zhang, L.; Zhou, R. Defective Mitophagy Driven by Dysregulation of Rheb and KIF5B Contributes to Mitochondrial Reactive Oxygen Species (ROS)-Induced Nod-like Receptor 3 (NLRP3) Dependent Proinflammatory Response and Aggravates Lipotoxicity. *Redox Biol.* **2014**, *3*, 63–71. [CrossRef]
169. Wang, Y.; Nartiss, Y.; Steipe, B.; McQuibban, G.A.; Kim, P.K. ROS-Induced Mitochondrial Depolarization Initiates PARK2/PARKIN-Dependent Mitochondrial Degradation by Autophagy. *Autophagy* **2012**, *8*, 1462–1476. [CrossRef]
170. Sarraf, S.A.; Raman, M.; Guarani-Pereira, V.; Sowa, M.E.; Huttlin, E.L.; Gygi, S.P.; Harper, J.W. Landscape of the PARKIN-Dependent Ubiquitylome in Response to Mitochondrial Depolarization. *Nature* **2013**, *496*, 372–376. [CrossRef]
171. Heo, J.-M.; Ordureau, A.; Paulo, J.A.; Rinehart, J.; Harper, J.W. The PINK1-PARKIN Mitochondrial Ubiquitylation Pathway Drives a Program of OPTN/NDP52 Recruitment and TBK1 Activation to Promote Mitophagy. *Mol. Cell* **2015**, *60*, 7–20. [CrossRef] [PubMed]
172. Eiyama, A.; Okamoto, K. PINK1/Parkin-Mediated Mitophagy in Mammalian Cells. *Curr. Opin. Cell Biol.* **2015**, *33*, 95–101. [CrossRef] [PubMed]
173. Bellot, G.; Garcia-Medina, R.; Gounon, P.; Chiche, J.; Roux, D.; Pouysségur, J.; Mazure, N.M. Hypoxia-Induced Autophagy Is Mediated through Hypoxia-Inducible Factor Induction of BNIP3 and BNIP3L via Their BH3 Domains. *Mol. Cell. Biol.* **2009**, *29*, 2570–2581. [CrossRef] [PubMed]
174. Sowter, H.M.; Ratcliffe, P.J.; Watson, P.; Greenberg, A.H.; Harris, A.L. HIF-1-Dependent Regulation of Hypoxic Induction of the Cell Death Factors BNIP3 and NIX in Human Tumors. *Cancer Res.* **2001**, *61*, 6669–6673.
175. Adriaenssens, E.; Schaar, S.; Cook, A.S.I.; Stuke, J.F.M.; Sawa-Makarska, J.; Nguyen, T.N.; Ren, X.; Schuschnig, M.; Romanov, J.; Khuu, G.; et al. Reconstitution of BNIP3/NIX-Mediated Autophagy Reveals Two Pathways and Hierarchical Flexibility of the Initiation Machinery. *bioRxiv* **2024**. [CrossRef]
176. Wanders, R.J.A.; Waterham, H.R. Biochemistry of Mammalian Peroxisomes Revisited. *Annu. Rev. Biochem.* **2006**, *75*, 295–332. [CrossRef]
177. Wei, Y.; Ni, L.; Pan, J.; Li, X.; Xu, B.; Deng, Y.; Yang, T.; Liu, W. The Roles of Oxidative Stress in Regulating Autophagy in Methylmercury-Induced Neurotoxicity. *Neuroscience* **2021**, *469*, 175–190. [CrossRef]
178. Sandalio, L.M.; Peláez-Vico, M.A.; Molina-Moya, E.; Romero-Puertas, M.C. Peroxisomes as Redox-Signaling Nodes in Intracellular Communication and Stress Responses. *Plant Physiol.* **2021**, *186*, 22–35. [CrossRef]
179. Ueno, S.; Sudo, T.; Hirasawa, A. ATM: Functions of ATM Kinase and Its Relevance to Hereditary Tumors. *Int. J. Mol. Sci.* **2022**, *23*, 523. [CrossRef]
180. Zhang, J.; Tripathi, D.N.; Jing, J.; Alexander, A.; Kim, J.; Powell, R.T.; Dere, R.; Tait-Mulder, J.; Lee, J.-H.; Paull, T.T.; et al. ATM Functions at the Peroxisome to Induce Pexophagy in Response to ROS. *Nat. Cell Biol.* **2015**, *17*, 1259–1269. [CrossRef]
181. Johansen, T.; Lamark, T. Selective Autophagy Mediated by Autophagic Adapter Proteins. *Autophagy* **2011**, *7*, 279–296. [CrossRef] [PubMed]
182. Okumoto, K.; El Shermely, M.; Natsui, M.; Kosako, H.; Natsuyama, R.; Marutani, T.; Fujiki, Y. The Peroxisome Counteracts Oxidative Stresses by Suppressing Catalase Import via Pex14 Phosphorylation. *eLife* **2020**, *9*, e55896. [CrossRef] [PubMed]
183. Guan, X.; Iyaswamy, A.; Sreenivasmurthy, S.G.; Su, C.; Zhu, Z.; Liu, J.; Kan, Y.; Cheung, K.-H.; Lu, J.; Tan, J.; et al. Mechanistic Insights into Selective Autophagy Subtypes in Alzheimer's Disease. *Int. J. Mol. Sci.* **2022**, *23*, 3609. [CrossRef] [PubMed]
184. Liu, S.; Yao, S.; Yang, H.; Liu, S.; Wang, Y. Autophagy: Regulator of Cell Death. *Cell Death Dis.* **2023**, *14*, 648. [CrossRef]
185. Zdanowicz, A.; Grosicka-Maciąg, E. The Interplay between Autophagy and Mitochondria in Cancer. *Int. J. Mol. Sci.* **2024**, *25*, 9143. [CrossRef]
186. Sarcinelli, C.; Dragic, H.; Piecyk, M.; Barbet, V.; Duret, C.; Barthelaix, A.; Ferraro-Peyret, C.; Fauvre, J.; Renno, T.; Chaveroux, C.; et al. ATF4-Dependent NRF2 Transcriptional Regulation Promotes Antioxidant Protection during Endoplasmic Reticulum Stress. *Cancers* **2020**, *12*, 569. [CrossRef]
187. Cantoni, O.; Zito, E.; Guidarelli, A.; Fiorani, M.; Ghezzi, P. Mitochondrial ROS, ER Stress, and Nrf2 Crosstalk in the Regulation of Mitochondrial Apoptosis Induced by Arsenite. *Antioxidants* **2022**, *11*, 1034. [CrossRef]
188. Dong, L.; Xu, M.; Li, Y.; Xu, W.; Wu, C.; Zheng, H.; Xiao, Z.; Sun, G.; Ding, L.; Li, X.; et al. SMURF1 Attenuates Endoplasmic Reticulum Stress by Promoting the Degradation of KEAP1 to Activate NRF2 Antioxidant Pathway. *Cell Death Dis.* **2023**, *14*, 361. [CrossRef]
189. He, F.; Ru, X.; Wen, T. NRF2, a Transcription Factor for Stress Response and beyond. *Int. J. Mol. Sci.* **2020**, *21*, 4777. [CrossRef]

190. Glover-Cutter, K.M.; Lin, S.; Blackwell, T.K. Integration of the Unfolded Protein and Oxidative Stress Responses through SKN-1/Nrf. *PLoS Genet.* **2013**, *9*, e1003701. [CrossRef]
191. Yang, M.; Luo, S.; Wang, X.; Li, C.; Yang, J.; Zhu, X.; Xiao, L.; Sun, L. ER-Phagy: A New Regulator of ER Homeostasis. *Front. Cell Dev. Biol.* **2021**, *9*, 684526. [CrossRef] [PubMed]
192. Bhat, T.A.; Chaudhary, A.K.; Kumar, S.; O'Malley, J.; Inigo, J.R.; Kumar, R.; Yadav, N.; Chandra, D. Endoplasmic Reticulum-Mediated Unfolded Protein Response and Mitochondrial Apoptosis in Cancer. *Biochim. Biophys. Acta Rev. Cancer* **2017**, *1867*, 58–66. [CrossRef] [PubMed]
193. Smith, M.D.; Wilkinson, S. CCPG1, an Unconventional Cargo Receptor for ER-Phagy, Maintains Pancreatic Acinar Cell Health. *Mol. Cell. Oncol.* **2018**, *5*, e1441631. [CrossRef] [PubMed]
194. Nakada, E.M.; Sun, R.; Fujii, U.; Martin, J.G. The Impact of Endoplasmic Reticulum-Associated Protein Modifications, Folding and Degradation on Lung Structure and Function. *Front. Physiol.* **2021**, *12*, 665622. [CrossRef]
195. Moncan, M.; Mnich, K.; Blomme, A.; Almanza, A.; Samali, A.; Gorman, A.M. Regulation of Lipid Metabolism by the Unfolded Protein Response. *J. Cell. Mol. Med.* **2021**, *25*, 1359–1370. [CrossRef]
196. Li, L.; Xu, J.; Chen, L.; Jiang, Z. Receptor-Mediated Reticulophagy: A Novel Promising Therapy Target for Diseases. *Acta Biochim. Biophys. Sin.* **2016**, *48*, 774–776. [CrossRef]
197. Malhotra, J.D.; Kaufman, R.J. ER Stress and Its Functional Link to Mitochondria: Role in Cell Survival and Death. *Cold Spring Harb. Perspect. Biol.* **2011**, *3*, a004424. [CrossRef]
198. Pang, L.; Liu, K.; Liu, D.; Lv, F.; Zang, Y.; Xie, F.; Yin, J.; Shi, Y.; Wang, Y.; Chen, D. Differential Effects of Reticulophagy and Mitophagy on Nonalcoholic Fatty Liver Disease. *Cell Death Dis.* **2018**, *9*, 90. [CrossRef]
199. Yang, M.; Li, C.; Yang, S.; Xiao, Y.; Xiong, X.; Chen, W.; Zhao, H.; Zhang, Q.; Han, Y.; Sun, L. Mitochondria-Associated ER Membranes—The Origin Site of Autophagy. *Front. Cell Dev. Biol.* **2020**, *8*, 595. [CrossRef]
200. Singh, R.; Kaushik, S.; Wang, Y.; Xiang, Y.; Novak, I.; Komatsu, M.; Tanaka, K.; Cuervo, A.M.; Czaja, M.J. Autophagy Regulates Lipid Metabolism. *Nature* **2009**, *458*, 1131–1135. [CrossRef]
201. Farese, R.V., Jr.; Walther, T.C. Lipid Droplets Finally Get a Little R-E-S-P-E-C-T. *Cell* **2009**, *139*, 855–860. [CrossRef] [PubMed]
202. Prinz, W.A.; Toulmay, A.; Balla, T. The Functional Universe of Membrane Contact Sites. *Nat. Rev. Mol. Cell Biol.* **2020**, *21*, 7–24. [CrossRef] [PubMed]
203. Zadoorian, A.; Du, X.; Yang, H. Lipid Droplet Biogenesis and Functions in Health and Disease. *Nat. Rev. Endocrinol.* **2023**, *19*, 443–459. [CrossRef] [PubMed]
204. Simmen, T.; Herrera-Cruz, M.S. Plastic Mitochondria-Endoplasmic Reticulum (ER) Contacts Use Chaperones and Tethers to Mould Their Structure and Signaling. *Curr. Opin. Cell Biol.* **2018**, *53*, 61–69. [CrossRef]
205. Giacomello, M.; Pellegrini, L. The Coming of Age of the mitochondria–ER Contact: A Matter of Thickness. *Cell Death Differ.* **2016**, *23*, 1417–1427. [CrossRef]
206. Wilson, E.L.; Metzakopian, E. ER-Mitochondria Contact Sites in Neurodegeneration: Genetic Screening Approaches to Investigate Novel Disease Mechanisms. *Cell Death Differ.* **2021**, *28*, 1804–1821. [CrossRef]
207. Szymański, J.; Janikiewicz, J.; Michalska, B.; Patalas-Krawczyk, P.; Perrone, M.; Ziółkowski, W.; Duszyński, J.; Pinton, P.; Dobrzyń, A.; Więckowski, M. Interaction of Mitochondria with the Endoplasmic Reticulum and Plasma Membrane in Calcium Homeostasis, Lipid Trafficking and Mitochondrial Structure. *Int. J. Mol. Sci.* **2017**, *18*, 1576. [CrossRef]
208. Xu, J.; Huang, X. Lipid Metabolism at Membrane Contacts: Dynamics and Functions beyond Lipid Homeostasis. *Front. Cell Dev. Biol.* **2020**, *8*, 615856. [CrossRef]
209. Chen, Z.; Shrestha, R.; Yang, X.; Wu, X.; Jia, J.; Chiba, H.; Hui, S.-P. Oxidative Stress and Lipid Dysregulation in Lipid Droplets: A Connection to Chronic Kidney Disease Revealed in Human Kidney Cells. *Antioxidants* **2022**, *11*, 1387. [CrossRef]
210. Obaseki, E.; Adebayo, D.; Bandyopadhyay, S.; Hariri, H. Lipid Droplets and Fatty Acid-Induced Lipotoxicity: In a Nutshell. *FEBS Lett.* **2024**, *598*, 1207–1214. [CrossRef]
211. Jaishy, B.; Abel, E.D. Lipids, Lysosomes, and Autophagy. *J. Lipid Res.* **2016**, *57*, 1619–1635. [CrossRef] [PubMed]
212. Kakuda, K.; Ikenaka, K.; Kuma, A.; Doi, J.; Aguirre, C.; Wang, N.; Ajiki, T.; Choong, C.-J.; Kimura, Y.; Badawy, S.M.M.; et al. Lysophagy Protects against Propagation of α-Synuclein Aggregation through Ruptured Lysosomal Vesicles. *Proc. Natl. Acad. Sci. USA* **2024**, *121*, e2312306120. [CrossRef] [PubMed]
213. Radulovic, M.; Stenmark, H. Lysophagy Prevents Neurotoxic Aggregate Transmission. *Proc. Natl. Acad. Sci. USA* **2024**, *121*, e2321181121. [CrossRef] [PubMed]
214. Oberle, C.; Huai, J.; Reinheckel, T.; Tacke, M.; Rassner, M.; Ekert, P.G.; Buellesbach, J.; Borner, C. Lysosomal Membrane Permeabilization and Cathepsin Release Is a Bax/Bak-Dependent, Amplifying Event of Apoptosis in Fibroblasts and Monocytes. *Cell Death Differ.* **2010**, *17*, 1167–1178. [CrossRef]
215. Ma, W.; Lu, Y.; Jin, X.; Lin, N.; Zhang, L.; Song, Y. Targeting Selective Autophagy and beyond: From Underlying Mechanisms to Potential Therapies. *J. Adv. Res.* **2024**, *65*, 297–327. [CrossRef]

216. Kraft, C.; Deplazes, A.; Sohrmann, M.; Peter, M. Mature Ribosomes Are Selectively Degraded upon Starvation by an Autophagy Pathway Requiring the Ubp3p/Bre5p Ubiquitin Protease. *Nat. Cell Biol.* **2008**, *10*, 602–610. [CrossRef]
217. Deegan, S.; Saveljeva, S.; Gorman, A.M.; Samali, A. Stress-Induced Self-Cannibalism: On the Regulation of Autophagy by Endoplasmic Reticulum Stress. *Cell. Mol. Life Sci.* **2013**, *70*, 2425–2441. [CrossRef]
218. Sica, V.; Galluzzi, L.; Bravo-San Pedro, J.M.; Izzo, V.; Maiuri, M.C.; Kroemer, G. Organelle-Specific Initiation of Autophagy. *Mol. Cell* **2015**, *59*, 522–539. [CrossRef]
219. Kubota, C.; Torii, S.; Hou, N.; Saito, N.; Yoshimoto, Y.; Imai, H.; Takeuchi, T. Constitutive Reactive Oxygen Species Generation from Autophagosome/lysosome in Neuronal Oxidative Toxicity. *J. Biol. Chem.* **2010**, *285*, 667–674. [CrossRef]
220. Kraft, C.; Peter, M.; Hofmann, K. Selective Autophagy: Ubiquitin-Mediated Recognition and beyond. *Nat. Cell Biol.* **2010**, *12*, 836–841. [CrossRef]
221. Chen, R.-H.; Chen, Y.-H.; Huang, T.-Y. Ubiquitin-Mediated Regulation of Autophagy. *J. Biomed. Sci.* **2019**, *26*, 80. [CrossRef] [PubMed]
222. Koerver, L.; Papadopoulos, C.; Liu, B.; Kravic, B.; Rota, G.; Brecht, L.; Veenendaal, T.; Polajnar, M.; Bluemke, A.; Ehrmann, M.; et al. The Ubiquitin-Conjugating Enzyme UBE2QL1 Coordinates Lysophagy in Response to Endolysosomal Damage. *EMBO Rep.* **2019**, *20*, e48014. [CrossRef] [PubMed]
223. Papadopoulos, C.; Meyer, H. Detection and Clearance of Damaged Lysosomes by the Endo-Lysosomal Damage Response and Lysophagy. *Curr. Biol.* **2017**, *27*, R1330–R1341. [CrossRef] [PubMed]
224. Kravic, B.; Behrends, C.; Meyer, H. Regulation of Lysosome Integrity and Lysophagy by the Ubiquitin-Conjugating Enzyme UBE2QL1. *Autophagy* **2020**, *16*, 179–180. [CrossRef]
225. Eapen, V.V.; Swarup, S.; Hoyer, M.J.; Paulo, J.A.; Harper, J.W. Quantitative Proteomics Reveals the Selectivity of Ubiquitin-Binding Autophagy Receptors in the Turnover of Damaged Lysosomes by Lysophagy. *eLife* **2021**, *10*, e72328. [CrossRef]
226. Baxter, B.K.; Abeliovich, H.; Zhang, X.; Stirling, A.G.; Burlingame, A.L.; Goldfarb, D.S. Atg19p Ubiquitination and the Cytoplasm to Vacuole Trafficking Pathway in Yeast. *J. Biol. Chem.* **2005**, *280*, 39067–39076. [CrossRef]
227. Scott, S.V.; Guan, J.; Hutchins, M.U.; Kim, J.; Klionsky, D.J. Cvt19 Is a Receptor for the Cytoplasm-to-Vacuole Targeting Pathway. *Mol. Cell* **2001**, *7*, 1131–1141. [CrossRef]
228. Fracchiolla, D.; Sawa-Makarska, J.; Zens, B.; de Ruiter, A.; Zaffagnini, G.; Brezovich, A.; Romanov, J.; Runggatscher, K.; Kraft, C.; Zagrovic, B.; et al. Mechanism of Cargo-Directed Atg8 Conjugation during Selective Autophagy. *eLife* **2016**, *5*, e18544. [CrossRef]
229. Kraft, C.; Peter, M. Is the Rsp5 Ubiquitin Ligase Involved in the Regulation of Ribophagy? *Autophagy* **2008**, *4*, 838–840. [CrossRef]
230. Zhao, T.; Wu, K.; Hogstrand, C.; Xu, Y.-H.; Chen, G.-H.; Wei, C.-C.; Luo, Z. Lipophagy Mediated Carbohydrate-Induced Changes of Lipid Metabolism via Oxidative Stress, Endoplasmic Reticulum (ER) Stress and ChREBP/PPARγ Pathways. *Cell. Mol. Life Sci.* **2020**, *77*, 1987–2003. [CrossRef]
231. Liu, K.; Czaja, M.J. Regulation of Lipid Stores and Metabolism by Lipophagy. *Cell Death Differ.* **2013**, *20*, 3–11. [CrossRef]
232. Zhang, X.; Cheng, X.; Yu, L.; Yang, J.; Calvo, R.; Patnaik, S.; Hu, X.; Gao, Q.; Yang, M.; Lawas, M.; et al. MCOLN1 Is a ROS Sensor in Lysosomes That Regulates Autophagy. *Nat. Commun.* **2016**, *7*, 12109. [CrossRef] [PubMed]
233. Zhang, C.-P.; Ding, X.-X.; Tian, T.; Li, B.-J.; Wang, C.-Y.; Jiang, S.-S.; Shao, J.-Q.; Yuan, Y.-L.; Tian, Y.; Zhang, M.; et al. Impaired Lipophagy in Endothelial Cells with Prolonged Exposure to Oxidized Low-Density Lipoprotein. *Mol. Med. Rep.* **2020**, *22*, 2665–2672. [CrossRef] [PubMed]
234. Sazaki, I.; Sakurai, T.; Yamahata, A.; Mogi, S.; Inoue, N.; Ishida, K.; Kikkai, A.; Takeshita, H.; Sakurai, A.; Takahashi, Y.; et al. Oxidized Low-Density Lipoproteins Trigger Hepatocellular Oxidative Stress with the Formation of Cholesteryl Ester Hydroperoxide-Enriched Lipid Droplets. *Int. J. Mol. Sci.* **2023**, *24*, 4281. [CrossRef] [PubMed]
235. Debnath, J.; Gammoh, N.; Ryan, K.M. Autophagy and Autophagy-Related Pathways in Cancer. *Nat. Rev. Mol. Cell Biol.* **2023**, *24*, 560–575. [CrossRef] [PubMed]
236. Salazar-Ramírez, K.; Molinares-Rodríguez, J.; Bolívar-González, S. Molecular Mechanisms of Autophagy and Its Role in Cancer Development. *Rev. Fac. Med. Univ. Nac. Colomb.* **2016**, *64*, 529. [CrossRef]
237. Nazio, F.; Bordi, M.; Cianfanelli, V.; Locatelli, F.; Cecconi, F. Autophagy and Cancer Stem Cells: Molecular Mechanisms and Therapeutic Applications. *Cell Death Differ.* **2019**, *26*, 690–702. [CrossRef]
238. Mathew, R.; Karantza-Wadsworth, V.; White, E. Role of Autophagy in Cancer. *Nat. Rev. Cancer* **2007**, *7*, 961–967. [CrossRef]
239. Alva, A.S.; Gultekin, S.H.; Baehrecke, E.H. Autophagy in Human Tumors: Cell Survival or Death? *Cell Death Differ.* **2004**, *11*, 1046–1048. [CrossRef]
240. Ahmadi-Dehlaghi, F.; Mohammadi, P.; Valipour, E.; Pournaghi, P.; Kiani, S.; Mansouri, K. Autophagy: A Challengeable Paradox in Cancer Treatment. *Cancer Med.* **2023**, *12*, 11542–11569. [CrossRef]
241. Jitschin, R.; Hofmann, A.D.; Bruns, H.; Giessl, A.; Bricks, J.; Berger, J.; Saul, D.; Eckart, M.J.; Mackensen, A.; Mougiakakos, D. Mitochondrial Metabolism Contributes to Oxidative Stress and Reveals Therapeutic Targets in Chronic Lymphocytic Leukemia. *Blood* **2014**, *123*, 2663–2672. [CrossRef] [PubMed]

242. Carew, J.S.; Nawrocki, S.T.; Xu, R.H.; Dunner, K.; McConkey, D.J.; Wierda, W.G.; Keating, M.J.; Huang, P. Increased Mitochondrial Biogenesis in Primary Leukemia Cells: The Role of Endogenous Nitric Oxide and Impact on Sensitivity to Fludarabine. *Leukemia* **2004**, *18*, 1934–1940. [CrossRef] [PubMed]
243. Levesque, M.C.; Ghosh, D.K.; Beasley, B.E.; Chen, Y.; Volkheimer, A.D.; O'Loughlin, C.W.; Gockerman, J.P.; Moore, J.O.; Weinberg, J.B. CLL Cell Apoptosis Induced by Nitric Oxide Synthase Inhibitors: Correlation with Lipid Solubility and NOS1 Dissociation Constant. *Leuk. Res.* **2008**, *32*, 1061–1070. [CrossRef] [PubMed]
244. Ecker, V.; Stumpf, M.; Brandmeier, L.; Neumayer, T.; Pfeuffer, L.; Engleitner, T.; Ringshausen, I.; Nelson, N.; Jücker, M.; Wanninger, S.; et al. Targeted PI3K/AKT-Hyperactivation Induces Cell Death in Chronic Lymphocytic Leukemia. *Nat. Commun.* **2021**, *12*, 3526. [CrossRef]
245. Capron, C.; Jondeau, K.; Casetti, L.; Jalbert, V.; Costa, C.; Verhoeyen, E.; Massé, J.M.; Coppo, P.; Béné, M.C.; Bourdoncle, P.; et al. Viability and Stress Protection of Chronic Lymphoid Leukemia Cells Involves Overactivation of Mitochondrial phospho-STAT3Ser727. *Cell Death Dis.* **2014**, *5*, e1451. [CrossRef]
246. Wu, R.P.; Hayashi, T.; Cottam, H.B.; Jin, G.; Yao, S.; Wu, C.C.N.; Rosenbach, M.D.; Corr, M.; Schwab, R.B.; Carson, D.A. Nrf2 Responses and the Therapeutic Selectivity of Electrophilic Compounds in Chronic Lymphocytic Leukemia. *Proc. Natl. Acad. Sci. USA* **2010**, *107*, 7479–7484. [CrossRef]
247. Ngo, V.; Duennwald, M.L. Nrf2 and Oxidative Stress: A General Overview of Mechanisms and Implications in Human Disease. *Antioxidants* **2022**, *11*, 2345. [CrossRef]
248. Ryoo, I.-G.; Kwak, M.-K. Regulatory Crosstalk between the Oxidative Stress-Related Transcription Factor Nfe2l2/Nrf2 and Mitochondria. *Toxicol. Appl. Pharmacol.* **2018**, *359*, 24–33. [CrossRef]
249. Sanchez-Lopez, E.; Ghia, E.M.; Antonucci, L.; Sharma, N.; Rassenti, L.Z.; Xu, J.; Sun, B.; Kipps, T.J.; Karin, M. NF-κB-p62-NRF2 Survival Signaling Is Associated with High ROR1 Expression in Chronic Lymphocytic Leukemia. *Cell Death Differ.* **2020**, *27*, 2206–2216. [CrossRef]
250. Arroyo, D.S.; Rodriguez, C.M.; Bussi, C.; Manzone-Rodriguez, C.; Sastre, D.; Heller, V.; Stanganelli, C.; Slavutsky, I.; Iribarren, P. Increased Expression of Autophagy Protein LC3 in Two Patients with Progressing Chronic Lymphocytic Leukemia. *Front. Endocrinol.* **2020**, *11*, 321. [CrossRef]
251. Kong, Y.-L.; Huang, Y.; Wu, J.-Z.; Cao, X.; Liang, J.-H.; Xia, Y.; Wu, W.; Cao, L.; Zhu, H.-Y.; Wang, L.; et al. Expression of Autophagy Related Genes in Chronic Lymphocytic Leukemia Is Associated with Disease Course. *Leuk. Res.* **2018**, *66*, 8–14. [CrossRef] [PubMed]
252. Bologna, C.; Buonincontri, R.; Serra, S.; Vaisitti, T.; Audrito, V.; Brusa, D.; Pagnani, A.; Coscia, M.; D'Arena, G.; Mereu, E.; et al. SLAMF1 Regulation of Chemotaxis and Autophagy Determines CLL Patient Response. *J. Clin. Investig.* **2016**, *126*, 181–194. [CrossRef] [PubMed]
253. Kristensen, L.; Kristensen, T.; Abildgaard, N.; Thomassen, M.; Frederiksen, M.; Mourits-Andersen, T.; Møller, M.B. High Expression of PI3K Core Complex Genes Is Associated with Poor Prognosis in Chronic Lymphocytic Leukemia. *Leuk. Res.* **2015**, *39*, 555–560. [CrossRef]
254. Smith, L.D.; Minton, A.R.; Blunt, M.D.; Karydis, L.I.; Dutton, D.A.; Rogers-Broadway, K.-R.; Dobson, R.; Liu, R.; Norster, F.; Hogg, E.; et al. BCR Signaling Contributes to Autophagy Regulation in Chronic Lymphocytic Leukemia. *Leukemia* **2020**, *34*, 640–644. [CrossRef] [PubMed]
255. Chen, B.; Zhao, Y.; Xu, S.; Jiang, F.; Nie, Y.; Tang, A.; Zhou, Q. USF2 Promotes Autophagy and Proliferation in Chronic Lymphocytic Leukemia by Inhibiting STUB1-Induced NFAT5 Ubiquitination. *Ann. Hematol.* **2024**, *103*, 533–544. [CrossRef] [PubMed]
256. Bwanika, H.C.; Leo, I.R.; Struyf, N.; Talanti, A.; Aswad, L.; Konnur, A.; Björklund, A.-C.; Heyman, M.; Rassidakis, G.; Erkers, T.; et al. Targeting Autophagy as a Therapeutic Strategy in Pediatric Acute Lymphoblastic Leukemia. *Sci. Rep.* **2024**, *14*, 4000. [CrossRef]
257. Juric, D.; Lacayo, N.J.; Ramsey, M.C.; Racevskis, J.; Wiernik, P.H.; Rowe, J.M.; Goldstone, A.H.; O'Dwyer, P.J.; Paietta, E.; Sikic, B.I. Differential Gene Expression Patterns and Interaction Networks in BCR-ABL-Positive and -Negative Adult Acute Lymphoblastic Leukemias. *J. Clin. Oncol.* **2007**, *25*, 1341–1349. [CrossRef]
258. Parada, Y.; Banerji, L.; Glassford, J.; Lea, N.C.; Collado, M.; Rivas, C.; Lewis, J.L.; Gordon, M.Y.; Thomas, N.S.; Lam, E.W. BCR-ABL and Interleukin 3 Promote Haematopoietic Cell Proliferation and Survival through Modulation of Cyclin D2 and p27Kip1 Expression. *J. Biol. Chem.* **2001**, *276*, 23572–23580. [CrossRef]
259. Irwin, M.E.; Rivera-Del Valle, N.; Chandra, J. Redox Control of Leukemia: From Molecular Mechanisms to Therapeutic Opportunities. *Antioxid. Redox Signal.* **2013**, *18*, 1349–1383. [CrossRef]
260. Kim, J.H.; Chu, S.C.; Gramlich, J.L.; Pride, Y.B.; Babendreier, E.; Chauhan, D.; Salgia, R.; Podar, K.; Griffin, J.D.; Sattler, M. Activation of the PI3K/mTOR Pathway by BCR-ABL Contributes to Increased Production of Reactive Oxygen Species. *Blood* **2005**, *105*, 1717–1723. [CrossRef]

261. Silva, A.; Gírio, A.; Cebola, I.; Santos, C.I.; Antunes, F.; Barata, J.T. Intracellular Reactive Oxygen Species Are Essential for PI3K/Akt/mTOR-Dependent IL-7-Mediated Viability of T-Cell Acute Lymphoblastic Leukemia Cells. *Leukemia* **2011**, *25*, 960–967. [CrossRef] [PubMed]
262. Lim, M.; Batista, C.R.; de Oliveira, B.R.; Creighton, R.; Ferguson, J.; Clemmer, K.; Knight, D.; Iansavitchous, J.; Mahmood, D.; Avino, M.; et al. Janus Kinase Mutations in Mice Lacking PU.1 and Spi-B Drive B Cell Leukemia through Reactive Oxygen Species-Induced DNA Damage. *Mol. Cell. Biol.* **2020**, *40*, 1–19. [CrossRef] [PubMed]
263. Weng, A.P.; Ferrando, A.A.; Lee, W.; Morris, J.P., 4th; Silverman, L.B.; Sanchez-Irizarry, C.; Blacklow, S.C.; Look, A.T.; Aster, J.C. Activating Mutations of NOTCH1 in Human T Cell Acute Lymphoblastic Leukemia. *Science* **2004**, *306*, 269–271. [CrossRef] [PubMed]
264. Hounjet, J.; Habets, R.; Schaaf, M.B.; Hendrickx, T.C.; Barbeau, L.M.O.; Yahyanejad, S.; Rouschop, K.M.; Groot, A.J.; Vooijs, M. The Anti-Malarial Drug Chloroquine Sensitizes Oncogenic NOTCH1 Driven Human T-ALL to γ-Secretase Inhibition. *Oncogene* **2019**, *38*, 5457–5468. [CrossRef] [PubMed]
265. Silva, A.; Yunes, J.A.; Cardoso, B.A.; Martins, L.R.; Jotta, P.Y.; Abecasis, M.; Nowill, A.E.; Leslie, N.R.; Cardoso, A.A.; Barata, J.T. PTEN Posttranslational Inactivation and Hyperactivation of the PI3K/Akt Pathway Sustain Primary T Cell Leukemia Viability. *J. Clin. Investig.* **2008**, *118*, 3762–3774. [CrossRef]
266. Ping, L.; Gao, Y.; He, Y.; Wang, X.; Bai, B.; Huang, C.; Huang, H. Systematic Oxidative Stress Indexes Associated with the Prognosis in Patients with T Lymphoblastic Lymphoma/leukemia. *Oxid. Med. Cell. Longev.* **2022**, *2022*, 2679154. [CrossRef]
267. Kantner, H.-P.; Warsch, W.; Delogu, A.; Bauer, E.; Esterbauer, H.; Casanova, E.; Sexl, V.; Stoiber, D. ETV6/RUNX1 Induces Reactive Oxygen Species and Drives the Accumulation of DNA Damage in B Cells. *Neoplasia* **2013**, *15*, 1292–1300. [CrossRef]
268. Polak, R.; Bierings, M.B.; van der Leije, C.S.; Sanders, M.A.; Roovers, O.; Marchante, J.R.M.; Boer, J.M.; Cornelissen, J.J.; Pieters, R.; den Boer, M.L.; et al. Autophagy Inhibition as a Potential Future Targeted Therapy for ETV6-RUNX1-Driven B-Cell Precursor Acute Lymphoblastic Leukemia. *Haematologica* **2019**, *104*, 738–748. [CrossRef]
269. Yu, C.; Gorantla, S.P.; Müller-Rudorf, A.; Müller, T.A.; Kreutmair, S.; Albers, C.; Jakob, L.; Lippert, L.J.; Yue, Z.; Engelhardt, M.; et al. Phosphorylation of BECLIN-1 by BCR-ABL Suppresses Autophagy in Chronic Myeloid Leukemia. *Haematologica* **2020**, *105*, 1285–1293. [CrossRef]
270. George, A.A.; Paz, H.; Fei, F.; Kirzner, J.; Kim, Y.-M.; Heisterkamp, N.; Abdel-Azim, H. Phosphoflow-Based Evaluation of Mek Inhibitors as Small-Molecule Therapeutics for B-Cell Precursor Acute Lymphoblastic Leukemia. *PLoS ONE* **2015**, *10*, e0137917. [CrossRef]
271. Polak, A.; Kiliszek, P.; Sewastianik, T.; Szydłowski, M.; Jabłońska, E.; Białopiotrowicz, E.; Górniak, P.; Markowicz, S.; Nowak, E.; Grygorowicz, M.A.; et al. MEK Inhibition Sensitizes Precursor B-Cell Acute Lymphoblastic Leukemia (B-ALL) Cells to Dexamethasone through Modulation of mTOR Activity and Stimulation of Autophagy. *PLoS ONE* **2016**, *11*, e0155893. [CrossRef]
272. Wang, H.; Dong, R.; Fan, W.-W.; Zheng, X.-C.; Li, A.-M.; Wang, W.-D. Timosaponin A-III Induces Autophagy of T-cell Acute Lymphoblastic Leukemia Jurkat Cells via Inhibition of the PI3K/Akt/mTOR Pathway. *Oncol. Rep.* **2019**, *41*, 2937–2944. [CrossRef] [PubMed]
273. Cheng, Z.; Yi, Y.; Xie, S.; Yu, H.; Peng, H.; Zhang, G. The Effect of the JAK2 Inhibitor TG101209 against T Cell Acute Lymphoblastic Leukemia (T-ALL) Is Mediated by Inhibition of JAK-STAT Signaling and Activation of the Crosstalk between Apoptosis and Autophagy Signaling. *Oncotarget* **2017**, *8*, 106753–106763. [CrossRef] [PubMed]
274. Simioni, C.; Neri, L.M.; Tabellini, G.; Ricci, F.; Bressanin, D.; Chiarini, F.; Evangelisti, C.; Cani, A.; Tazzari, P.L.; Melchionda, F.; et al. Cytotoxic Activity of the Novel Akt Inhibitor, MK-2206, in T-Cell Acute Lymphoblastic Leukemia. *Leukemia* **2012**, *26*, 2336–2342. [CrossRef] [PubMed]
275. Minciacchi, V.R.; Kumar, R.; Krause, D.S. Chronic Myeloid Leukemia: A Model Disease of the Past, Present and Future. *Cells* **2021**, *10*, 117. [CrossRef]
276. Pascu Vînturiș, E.G.; Găman, A.M. Assessment of Oxidative Stress in Patients with Chronic Myeloid Leukemia Depending on Associated Comorbidities. *Curr. Health Sci. J.* **2020**, *46*, 23–30.
277. Rowley, J.D. Letter: A New Consistent Chromosomal Abnormality in Chronic Myelogenous Leukaemia Identified by Quinacrine Fluorescence and Giemsa Staining. *Nature* **1973**, *243*, 290–293. [CrossRef]
278. Nowicki, M.O.; Falinski, R.; Koptyra, M.; Slupianek, A.; Stoklosa, T.; Gloc, E.; Nieborowska-Skorska, M.; Blasiak, J.; Skorski, T. BCR/ABL Oncogenic Kinase Promotes Unfaithful Repair of the Reactive Oxygen Species-Dependent DNA Double-Strand Breaks. *Blood* **2004**, *104*, 3746–3753. [CrossRef]
279. Bourgeais, J.; Ishac, N.; Medrzycki, M.; Brachet-Botineau, M.; Desbourdes, L.; Gouilleux-Gruart, V.; Pecnard, E.; Rouleux-Bonnin, F.; Gyan, E.; Domenech, J.; et al. Oncogenic STAT5 Signaling Promotes Oxidative Stress in Chronic Myeloid Leukemia Cells by Repressing Antioxidant Defenses. *Oncotarget* **2017**, *8*, 41876–41889. [CrossRef]
280. Sheng, Z.; Ma, L.; Sun, J.E.; Zhu, L.J.; Green, M.R. BCR-ABL Suppresses Autophagy through ATF5-Mediated Regulation of mTOR Transcription. *Blood* **2011**, *118*, 2840–2848. [CrossRef]

281. Carayol, N.; Vakana, E.; Sassano, A.; Kaur, S.; Goussetis, D.J.; Glaser, H.; Druker, B.J.; Donato, N.J.; Altman, J.K.; Barr, S.; et al. Critical Roles for mTORC2- and Rapamycin-Insensitive mTORC1-Complexes in Growth and Survival of BCR-ABL-Expressing Leukemic Cells. *Proc. Natl. Acad. Sci. USA* **2010**, *107*, 12469–12474. [CrossRef] [PubMed]
282. Colecchia, D.; Rossi, M.; Sasdelli, F.; Sanzone, S.; Strambi, A.; Chiariello, M. MAPK15 Mediates BCR-ABL1-Induced Autophagy and Regulates Oncogene-Dependent Cell Proliferation and Tumor Formation. *Autophagy* **2015**, *11*, 1790–1802. [CrossRef] [PubMed]
283. Chen, Y.; Zou, Z.; Găman, M.-A.; Xu, L.; Li, J. NADPH Oxidase Mediated Oxidative Stress Signaling in FLT3-ITD Acute Myeloid Leukemia. *Cell Death Discov.* **2023**, *9*, 208. [CrossRef] [PubMed]
284. Stanicka, J.; Russell, E.G.; Woolley, J.F.; Cotter, T.G. NADPH Oxidase-Generated Hydrogen Peroxide Induces DNA Damage in Mutant FLT3-Expressing Leukemia Cells. *J. Biol. Chem.* **2015**, *290*, 9348–9361. [CrossRef]
285. Hole, P.S.; Zabkiewicz, J.; Munje, C.; Newton, Z.; Pearn, L.; White, P.; Marquez, N.; Hills, R.K.; Burnett, A.K.; Tonks, A.; et al. Overproduction of NOX-Derived ROS in AML Promotes Proliferation and Is Associated with Defective Oxidative Stress Signaling. *Blood* **2013**, *122*, 3322–3330. [CrossRef]
286. Robinson, A.J.; Hopkins, G.L.; Rastogi, N.; Hodges, M.; Doyle, M.; Davies, S.; Hole, P.S.; Omidvar, N.; Darley, R.L.; Tonks, A. Reactive Oxygen Species Drive Proliferation in Acute Myeloid Leukemia via the Glycolytic Regulator PFKFB3. *Cancer Res.* **2020**, *80*, 937–949. [CrossRef]
287. Sallmyr, A.; Fan, J.; Datta, K.; Kim, K.-T.; Grosu, D.; Shapiro, P.; Small, D.; Rassool, F. Internal Tandem Duplication of FLT3 (FLT3/ITD) Induces Increased ROS Production, DNA Damage, and Misrepair: Implications for Poor Prognosis in AML. *Blood* **2008**, *111*, 3173–3182. [CrossRef]
288. Zhou, F.; Pan, Y.; Wei, Y.; Zhang, R.; Bai, G.; Shen, Q.; Meng, S.; Le, X.-F.; Andreeff, M.; Claret, F.X. Jab1/Csn5-Thioredoxin Signaling in Relapsed Acute Monocytic Leukemia under Oxidative Stress. *Clin. Cancer Res.* **2017**, *23*, 4450–4461. [CrossRef]
289. Rassool, F.V.; Gaymes, T.J.; Omidvar, N.; Brady, N.; Beurlet, S.; Pla, M.; Reboul, M.; Lea, N.; Chomienne, C.; Thomas, N.S.B.; et al. Reactive Oxygen Species, DNA Damage, and Error-Prone Repair: A Model for Genomic Instability with Progression in Myeloid Leukemia? *Cancer Res.* **2007**, *67*, 8762–8771. [CrossRef]
290. Sumitomo, Y.; Koya, J.; Nakazaki, K.; Kataoka, K.; Tsuruta-Kishino, T.; Morita, K.; Sato, T.; Kurokawa, M. Cytoprotective Autophagy Maintains Leukemia-Initiating Cells in Murine Myeloid Leukemia. *Blood* **2016**, *128*, 1614–1624. [CrossRef]
291. Watson, A.S.; Riffelmacher, T.; Stranks, A.; Williams, O.; De Boer, J.; Cain, K.; MacFarlane, M.; McGouran, J.; Kessler, B.; Khandwala, S.; et al. Autophagy Limits Proliferation and Glycolytic Metabolism in Acute Myeloid Leukemia. *Cell Death Discov.* **2015**, *1*, 15008. [CrossRef]
292. Baker, F.; Polat, I.H.; Abou-El-Ardat, K.; Alshamleh, I.; Thoelken, M.; Hymon, D.; Gubas, A.; Koschade, S.E.; Vischedyk, J.B.; Kaulich, M.; et al. Metabolic Rewiring Is Essential for AML Cell Survival to Overcome Autophagy Inhibition by Loss of ATG3. *Cancers* **2021**, *13*, 6142. [CrossRef] [PubMed]
293. Wang, L.; Yang, L.; Yang, Z.; Tang, Y.; Tao, Y.; Zhan, Q.; Lei, L.; Jing, Y.; Jiang, X.; Jin, H.; et al. Glycolytic Enzyme PKM2 Mediates Autophagic Activation to Promote Cell Survival in NPM1-Mutated Leukemia. *Int. J. Biol. Sci.* **2019**, *15*, 882–894. [CrossRef] [PubMed]
294. Mohamadimaram, M.; Allahbakhshian Farsani, M.; Mirzaeian, A.; Shahsavan, S.; Hajifathali, A.; Parkhihdeh, S.; Mohammadi, M.H. Evaluation of ATG7 and Light Chain 3 (LC3) Autophagy Genes Expression in AML Patients. *Iran. J. Pharm. Res.* **2019**, *18*, 1060–1066. [PubMed]
295. Zhang, W.; Yu, G.; Zhang, H.; Basyal, M.; Ly, C.; Yuan, B.; Ruvolo, V.; Piya, S.; Bhattacharya, S.; Zhang, Q.; et al. Concomitant Targeting of FLT3 and BTK Overcomes FLT3 Inhibitor Resistance in Acute Myeloid Leukemia through the Inhibition of Autophagy. *Haematologica* **2023**, *108*, 1500–1514. [CrossRef] [PubMed]
296. Heydt, Q.; Larrue, C.; Saland, E.; Bertoli, S.; Sarry, J.-E.; Besson, A.; Manenti, S.; Joffre, C.; Mansat-De Mas, V. Oncogenic FLT3-ITD Supports Autophagy via ATF4 in Acute Myeloid Leukemia. *Oncogene* **2018**, *37*, 787–797. [CrossRef]
297. Shang, J.; Chen, W.-M.; Liu, S.; Wang, Z.-H.; Wei, T.-N.; Chen, Z.-Z.; Wu, W.-B. CircPAN3 Contributes to Drug Resistance in Acute Myeloid Leukemia through Regulation of Autophagy. *Leuk. Res.* **2019**, *85*, 106198. [CrossRef]
298. Lewis, W.D.; Lilly, S.; Jones, K.L. Lymphoma: Diagnosis and Treatment. *Am. Fam. Physician* **2020**, *101*, 34–41.
299. Brice, P.; de Kerviler, E.; Friedberg, J.W. Classical Hodgkin Lymphoma. *Lancet* **2021**, *398*, 1518–1527. [CrossRef]
300. Connors, J.M.; Cozen, W.; Steidl, C.; Carbone, A.; Hoppe, R.T.; Flechtner, H.-H.; Bartlett, N.L. Hodgkin Lymphoma. *Nat. Rev. Dis. Primers* **2020**, *6*, 61. [CrossRef]
301. Piris, M.A.; Medeiros, L.J.; Chang, K.-C. Hodgkin Lymphoma: A Review of Pathological Features and Recent Advances in Pathogenesis. *Pathology* **2020**, *52*, 154–165. [CrossRef]
302. Bur, H.; Haapasaari, K.-M.; Turpeenniemi-Hujanen, T.; Kuittinen, O.; Auvinen, P.; Marin, K.; Koivunen, P.; Sormunen, R.; Soini, Y.; Karihtala, P. Oxidative Stress Markers and Mitochondrial Antioxidant Enzyme Expression Are Increased in Aggressive Hodgkin Lymphomas. *Histopathology* **2014**, *65*, 319–327. [CrossRef] [PubMed]

303. Marini, C.; Cossu, V.; Bauckneht, M.; Carta, S.; Lanfranchi, F.; D'Amico, F.; Ravera, S.; Orengo, A.M.; Ghiggi, C.; Ballerini, F.; et al. Mitochondrial Generated Redox Stress Differently Affects the Endoplasmic Reticulum of Circulating Lymphocytes and Monocytes in Treatment-Naïve Hodgkin's Lymphoma. *Antioxidants* **2022**, *11*, 762. [CrossRef] [PubMed]
304. Gopas, J.; Stern, E.; Zurgil, U.; Ozer, J.; Ben-Ari, A.; Shubinsky, G.; Braiman, A.; Sinay, R.; Ezratty, J.; Dronov, V.; et al. Reed-Sternberg Cells in Hodgkin's Lymphoma Present Features of Cellular Senescence. *Cell Death Dis.* **2016**, *7*, e2457. [CrossRef] [PubMed]
305. Ikeda, J.-I.; Mamat, S.; Tian, T.; Wang, Y.; Luo, W.; Rahadiani, N.; Aozasa, K.; Morii, E. Reactive Oxygen Species and Aldehyde Dehydrogenase Activity in Hodgkin Lymphoma Cells. *Lab. Investig.* **2012**, *92*, 606–614. [CrossRef] [PubMed]
306. Nakashima, M.; Watanabe, M.; Nakano, K.; Uchimaru, K.; Horie, R. Differentiation of Hodgkin Lymphoma Cells by Reactive Oxygen Species and Regulation by Heme Oxygenase-1 through HIF-1α. *Cancer Sci.* **2021**, *112*, 2542–2555. [CrossRef]
307. Kyriazopoulou, L.; Karpathiou, G.; Hatzimichael, E.; Peoc'h, M.; Papoudou-Bai, A.; Kanavaros, P. Autophagy and Cellular Senescence in Classical Hodgkin Lymphoma. *Pathol. Res. Pract.* **2022**, *236*, 153964. [CrossRef]
308. Lin, H.-C.; Chang, Y.; Chen, R.-Y.; Hung, L.-Y.; Chen, P.C.-H.; Chen, Y.-P.; Medeiros, L.J.; Chiang, P.-M.; Chang, K.-C. Epstein-Barr Virus Latent Membrane Protein-1 Upregulates Autophagy and Promotes Viability in Hodgkin Lymphoma: Implications for Targeted Therapy. *Cancer Sci.* **2021**, *112*, 1589–1602. [CrossRef]
309. Jeong, A.J.; Kim, Y.J.; Lim, M.H.; Lee, H.; Noh, K.; Kim, B.-H.; Chung, J.W.; Cho, C.-H.; Kim, S.; Ye, S.-K. Microgravity Induces Autophagy via Mitochondrial Dysfunction in Human Hodgkin's Lymphoma Cells. *Sci. Rep.* **2018**, *8*, 14646. [CrossRef]
310. Wahyudianingsih, R.; Sanjaya, A.; Jonathan, T.; Pranggono, E.H.; Achmad, D.; Hernowo, B.S. Chemotherapy's Effects on Autophagy in the Treatment of Hodgkin's Lymphoma: A Scoping Review. *Discov. Oncol.* **2024**, *15*, 269. [CrossRef]
311. Thandra, K.C.; Barsouk, A.; Saginala, K.; Padala, S.A.; Barsouk, A.; Rawla, P. Epidemiology of Non-Hodgkin's Lymphoma. *Med. Sci.* **2021**, *9*, 5. [CrossRef] [PubMed]
312. Wang, S.S.; Davis, S.; Cerhan, J.R.; Hartge, P.; Severson, R.K.; Cozen, W.; Lan, Q.; Welch, R.; Chanock, S.J.; Rothman, N. Polymorphisms in Oxidative Stress Genes and Risk for Non-Hodgkin Lymphoma. *Carcinogenesis* **2006**, *27*, 1828–1834. [CrossRef]
313. Lan, Q.; Zheng, T.; Shen, M.; Zhang, Y.; Wang, S.S.; Zahm, S.H.; Holford, T.R.; Leaderer, B.; Boyle, P.; Chanock, S. Genetic Polymorphisms in the Oxidative Stress Pathway and Susceptibility to Non-Hodgkin Lymphoma. *Hum. Genet.* **2007**, *121*, 161–168. [CrossRef] [PubMed]
314. Gustafson, H.L.; Yao, S.; Goldman, B.H.; Lee, K.; Spier, C.M.; LeBlanc, M.L.; Rimsza, L.M.; Cerhan, J.R.; Habermann, T.M.; Link, B.K.; et al. Genetic Polymorphisms in Oxidative Stress-Related Genes Are Associated with Outcomes Following Treatment for Aggressive B-Cell Non-Hodgkin Lymphoma. *Am. J. Hematol.* **2014**, *89*, 639–645. [CrossRef]
315. Fan, J.; Zeng, X.; Li, Y.; Wang, S.; Wang, Z.; Sun, Y.; Gao, H.; Zhang, G.; Feng, M.; Ju, D. Autophagy Plays a Critical Role in ChLym-1-Induced Cytotoxicity of Non-Hodgkin's Lymphoma Cells. *PLoS ONE* **2013**, *8*, e72478. [CrossRef]
316. Zhang, H.; Chen, Z.; Miranda, R.N.; Medeiros, L.J.; McCarty, N. TG2 and NF-κB Signaling Coordinates the Survival of Mantle Cell Lymphoma Cells via IL6-Mediated Autophagy. *Cancer Res.* **2016**, *76*, 6410–6423. [CrossRef] [PubMed]
317. Masud Alam, M.; Kariya, R.; Kawaguchi, A.; Matsuda, K.; Kudo, E.; Okada, S. Inhibition of Autophagy by Chloroquine Induces Apoptosis in Primary Effusion Lymphoma In Vitro and In Vivo through Induction of Endoplasmic Reticulum Stress. *Apoptosis* **2016**, *21*, 1191–1201. [CrossRef]
318. Sukswai, N.; Lyapichev, K.; Khoury, J.D.; Medeiros, L.J. Diffuse Large B-Cell Lymphoma Variants: An Update. *Pathology* **2020**, *52*, 53–67. [CrossRef]
319. Nakamura, H.; Hara, T.; Mabuchi, R.; Matsumoto, T.; Nakamura, N.; Ninomiya, S.; Kitagawa, J.; Kanemura, N.; Kito, Y.; Takami, T.; et al. Clinical Significance of Oxidative Stress for Untreated Patients with Diffuse Large B-Cell Lymphoma. *Mol. Clin. Oncol.* **2022**, *16*, 4. [CrossRef]
320. Cai, Y.; Lv, L.; Lu, T.; Ding, M.; Yu, Z.; Chen, X.; Zhou, X.; Wang, X. α-KG Inhibits Tumor Growth of Diffuse Large B-Cell Lymphoma by Inducing ROS and TP53-Mediated Ferroptosis. *Cell Death Discov.* **2023**, *9*, 182. [CrossRef]
321. Zhao, K.; Wen, Q.; Li, Q.; Li, P.; Liu, T.; Zhu, F.; Tan, Q.; Zhang, L. Identification of Oxidative Stress-Related Hub Genes for Predicting Prognosis in Diffuse Large B-Cell Lymphoma. *Gene* **2025**, *935*, 149077. [CrossRef] [PubMed]
322. Rossi, A.; Orecchioni, S.; Falvo, P.; Tabanelli, V.; Baiardi, E.; Agostinelli, C.; Melle, F.; Motta, G.; Calleri, A.; Fiori, S.; et al. Dual Targeting of the DNA Damage Response Pathway and BCL-2 in Diffuse Large B-Cell Lymphoma. *Leukemia* **2022**, *36*, 197–209. [CrossRef] [PubMed]
323. Mai, Y.; Yu, J.J.; Bartholdy, B.; Xu-Monette, Z.Y.; Knapp, E.E.; Yuan, F.; Chen, H.; Ding, B.B.; Yao, Z.; Das, B.; et al. An Oxidative Stress-Based Mechanism of Doxorubicin Cytotoxicity Suggests New Therapeutic Strategies in ABC-DLBCL. *Blood* **2016**, *128*, 2797–2807. [CrossRef] [PubMed]
324. You, L.; Wang, Z.; Li, H.; Shou, J.; Jing, Z.; Xie, J.; Sui, X.; Pan, H.; Han, W. The Role of STAT3 in Autophagy. *Autophagy* **2015**, *11*, 729–739. [CrossRef]
325. Chen, Y.; Wang, F.; Wu, P.; Gong, S.; Gao, J.; Tao, H.; Shen, Q.; Wang, S.; Zhou, Z.; Jia, Y. Artesunate Induces Apoptosis, Autophagy and Ferroptosis in Diffuse Large B Cell Lymphoma Cells by Impairing STAT3 Signaling. *Cell. Signal.* **2021**, *88*, 110167. [CrossRef]

326. Li, Y.; Zhou, X.; Zhang, Y.; Yang, J.; Xu, Y.; Zhao, Y.; Wang, X. CUL4B Regulates Autophagy via JNK Signaling in Diffuse Large B-Cell Lymphoma. *Cell Cycle* **2019**, *18*, 379–394. [CrossRef]
327. Xiong, D.; Wei, X.; Huang, W.; Zheng, J.; Feng, R. Prediction Significance of Autophagy-Related Genes in Survival Probability and Drug Resistance in Diffuse Large B-Cell Lymphoma. *Aging* **2024**, *16*, 1049–1076. [CrossRef]
328. Mandhair, H.K.; Radpour, R.; Westerhuis, M.; Banz, Y.; Humbert, M.; Arambasic, M.; Dengjel, J.; Davies, A.; Tschan, M.P.; Novak, U. Analysis of Autophagy in DLBCL Reveals Subtype-Specific Differences and the Preferential Targeting of ULK1 Inhibition in GCB-DLBCL Provides a Rationale as a New Therapeutic Approach. *Leukemia* **2024**, *38*, 424–429. [CrossRef]
329. Salwa, A.; Ferraresi, A.; Secomandi, E.; Vallino, L.; Moia, R.; Patriarca, A.; Garavaglia, B.; Gaidano, G.; Isidoro, C. High BECN1 Expression Negatively Correlates with BCL2 Expression and Predicts Better Prognosis in Diffuse Large B-Cell Lymphoma: Role of Autophagy. *Cells* **2023**, *12*, 1924. [CrossRef]
330. Gorrini, C.; Harris, I.S.; Mak, T.W. Modulation of Oxidative Stress as an Anticancer Strategy. *Nat. Rev. Drug Discov.* **2013**, *12*, 931–947. [CrossRef]
331. Hart, P.C.; Mao, M.; de Abreu, A.L.P.; Ansenberger-Fricano, K.; Ekoue, D.N.; Ganini, D.; Kajdacsy-Balla, A.; Diamond, A.M.; Minshall, R.D.; Consolaro, M.E.L.; et al. MnSOD Upregulation Sustains the Warburg Effect via Mitochondrial ROS and AMPK-Dependent Signalling in Cancer. *Nat. Commun.* **2015**, *6*, 6053. [CrossRef] [PubMed]
332. Ito, K.; Hirao, A.; Arai, F.; Takubo, K.; Matsuoka, S.; Miyamoto, K.; Ohmura, M.; Naka, K.; Hosokawa, K.; Ikeda, Y.; et al. Reactive Oxygen Species Act through p38 MAPK to Limit the Lifespan of Hematopoietic Stem Cells. *Nat. Med.* **2006**, *12*, 446–451. [CrossRef] [PubMed]
333. Tang, H.-W.; Liao, H.-M.; Peng, W.-H.; Lin, H.-R.; Chen, C.-H.; Chen, G.-C. Atg9 Interacts with dTRAF2/TRAF6 to Regulate Oxidative Stress-Induced JNK Activation and Autophagy Induction. *Dev. Cell* **2013**, *27*, 489–503. [CrossRef] [PubMed]
334. Tsugawa, H.; Suzuki, H.; Saya, H.; Hatakeyama, M.; Hirayama, T.; Hirata, K.; Nagano, O.; Matsuzaki, J.; Hibi, T. Reactive Oxygen Species-Induced Autophagic Degradation of Helicobacter Pylori CagA Is Specifically Suppressed in Cancer Stem-like Cells. *Cell Host Microbe* **2012**, *12*, 764–777. [CrossRef]
335. Green, D.R.; Galluzzi, L.; Kroemer, G. Mitochondria and the Autophagy-Inflammation-Cell Death Axis in Organismal Aging. *Science* **2011**, *333*, 1109–1112. [CrossRef]
336. White, E. Deconvoluting the Context-Dependent Role for Autophagy in Cancer. *Nat. Rev. Cancer* **2012**, *12*, 401–410. [CrossRef]
337. Cheng, Y.; Ren, X.; Hait, W.N.; Yang, J.-M. Therapeutic Targeting of Autophagy in Disease: Biology and Pharmacology. *Pharmacol. Rev.* **2013**, *65*, 1162–1197. [CrossRef]
338. Levy, J.M.M.; Thorburn, A. Targeting Autophagy during Cancer Therapy to Improve Clinical Outcomes. *Pharmacol. Ther.* **2011**, *131*, 130–141. [CrossRef]
339. Mariño, G.; Niso-Santano, M.; Baehrecke, E.H.; Kroemer, G. Self-Consumption: The Interplay of Autophagy and Apoptosis. *Nat. Rev. Mol. Cell Biol.* **2014**, *15*, 81–94. [CrossRef]
340. Scrivo, A.; Bourdenx, M.; Pampliega, O.; Cuervo, A.M. Selective Autophagy as a Potential Therapeutic Target for Neurodegenerative Disorders. *Lancet Neurol.* **2018**, *17*, 802–815. [CrossRef]
341. Filomeni, G.; Desideri, E.; Cardaci, S.; Rotilio, G.; Ciriolo, M.R. Under the ROS: Thiol Network Is the Principal Suspect for Autophagy Commitment. *Autophagy* **2010**, *6*, 999–1005. [CrossRef] [PubMed]
342. Ivanova, D.; Bakalova, R.; Lazarova, D.; Gadjeva, V.; Zhelev, Z. The Impact of Reactive Oxygen Species on Anticancer Therapeutic Strategies. *Adv. Clin. Exp. Med.* **2013**, *22*, 899–908. [PubMed]
343. Amaravadi, R.K.; Lippincott-Schwartz, J.; Yin, X.-M.; Weiss, W.A.; Takebe, N.; Timmer, W.; DiPaola, R.S.; Lotze, M.T.; White, E. Principles and Current Strategies for Targeting Autophagy for Cancer Treatment. *Clin. Cancer Res.* **2011**, *17*, 654–666. [CrossRef]
344. Wu, Q.; Chen, Y.; Cui, G.; Cheng, Y. Wortmannin Inhibits K562 Leukemic Cells by Regulating PI3k/Akt Channel In Vitro. *J. Huazhong Univ. Sci. Technolog. Med. Sci.* **2009**, *29*, 451–456. [CrossRef] [PubMed]
345. Eng, C.H.; Wang, Z.; Tkach, D.; Toral-Barza, L.; Ugwonali, S.; Liu, S.; Fitzgerald, S.L.; George, E.; Frias, E.; Cochran, N.; et al. Macroautophagy Is Dispensable for Growth of KRAS Mutant Tumors and Chloroquine Efficacy. *Proc. Natl. Acad. Sci. USA* **2016**, *113*, 182–187. [CrossRef] [PubMed]
346. Maes, H.; Kuchnio, A.; Peric, A.; Moens, S.; Nys, K.; De Bock, K.; Quaegebeur, A.; Schoors, S.; Georgiadou, M.; Wouters, J.; et al. Tumor Vessel Normalization by Chloroquine Independent of Autophagy. *Cancer Cell* **2014**, *26*, 190–206. [CrossRef]
347. Maycotte, P.; Aryal, S.; Cummings, C.T.; Thorburn, J.; Morgan, M.J.; Thorburn, A. Chloroquine Sensitizes Breast Cancer Cells to Chemotherapy Independent of Autophagy. *Autophagy* **2012**, *8*, 200–212. [CrossRef]
348. Yang, Z.J.; Chee, C.E.; Huang, S.; Sinicrope, F. Autophagy Modulation for Cancer Therapy. *Cancer Biol. Ther.* **2011**, *11*, 169–176. [CrossRef]
349. Li, X.; Xu, H.-L.; Liu, Y.-X.; An, N.; Zhao, S.; Bao, J.-K. Autophagy Modulation as a Target for Anticancer Drug Discovery. *Acta Pharmacol. Sin.* **2013**, *34*, 612–624. [CrossRef]
350. Nordstrøm, L.U.; Sironi, J.; Aranda, E.; Maisonet, J.; Perez-Soler, R.; Wu, P.; Schwartz, E.L. Discovery of Autophagy Inhibitors with Antiproliferative Activity in Lung and Pancreatic Cancer Cells. *ACS Med. Chem. Lett.* **2015**, *6*, 134–139. [CrossRef]

351. Feng, Y.; Chen, X.; Cassady, K.; Zou, Z.; Yang, S.; Wang, Z.; Zhang, X. The Role of mTOR Inhibitors in Hematologic Disease: From Bench to Bedside. *Front. Oncol.* **2020**, *10*, 611690. [CrossRef] [PubMed]
352. Younes, A.; Samad, N. Utility of mTOR Inhibition in Hematologic Malignancies. *Oncologist* **2011**, *16*, 730–741. [CrossRef] [PubMed]
353. Raje, N.; Kumar, S.; Hideshima, T.; Ishitsuka, K.; Chauhan, D.; Mitsiades, C.; Podar, K.; Le Gouill, S.; Richardson, P.; Munshi, N.C.; et al. Combination of the mTOR Inhibitor Rapamycin and CC-5013 Has Synergistic Activity in Multiple Myeloma. *Blood* **2004**, *104*, 4188–4193. [CrossRef]
354. Cunha, A.D., Jr.; Pericole, F.V.; Carvalheira, J.B.C. Metformin and Blood Cancers. *Clinics* **2018**, *73*, e412s. [CrossRef] [PubMed]
355. Kozako, T.; Aikawa, A.; Ohsugi, T.; Honda, S.-I. AICAR Induces AMPK-Independent Cell Death in Adult T-Cell Leukemia/lymphoma and Has Anti-Tumor Activity. *Blood* **2023**, *142*, 7146. [CrossRef]
356. Lim, J.; Murthy, A. Targeting Autophagy to Treat Cancer: Challenges and Opportunities. *Front. Pharmacol.* **2020**, *11*, 590344. [CrossRef]
357. Zhang, Y.; Zhou, F.; Guan, J.; Zhou, L.; Chen, B. Action Mechanism of Metformin and Its Application in Hematological Malignancy Treatments: A Review. *Biomolecules* **2023**, *13*, 250. [CrossRef]
358. Gu, Y.; Masiero, M.; Banham, A.H. Notch Signaling: Its Roles and Therapeutic Potential in Hematological Malignancies. *Oncotarget* **2016**, *7*, 29804–29823. [CrossRef]
359. Varnum-Finney, B.; Xu, L.; Brashem-Stein, C.; Nourigat, C.; Flowers, D.; Bakkour, S.; Pear, W.S.; Bernstein, I.D. Pluripotent, Cytokine-Dependent, Hematopoietic Stem Cells Are Immortalized by Constitutive Notch1 Signaling. *Nat. Med.* **2000**, *6*, 1278–1281. [CrossRef]
360. Shi, Q.; Xue, C.; Zeng, Y.; Yuan, X.; Chu, Q.; Jiang, S.; Wang, J.; Zhang, Y.; Zhu, D.; Li, L. Notch Signaling Pathway in Cancer: From Mechanistic Insights to Targeted Therapies. *Signal Transduct. Target. Ther.* **2024**, *9*, 128. [CrossRef]
361. Nam, H.J. Autophagy Modulators in Cancer: Focus on Cancer Treatment. *Life* **2021**, *11*, 839. [CrossRef] [PubMed]
362. Rahman, M.A.; Saha, S.K.; Rahman, M.S.; Uddin, M.J.; Uddin, M.S.; Pang, M.-G.; Rhim, H.; Cho, S.-G. Molecular Insights into Therapeutic Potential of Autophagy Modulation by Natural Products for Cancer Stem Cells. *Front. Cell Dev. Biol.* **2020**, *8*, 283. [CrossRef] [PubMed]
363. Auberger, P.; Puissant, A. Autophagy, a Key Mechanism of Oncogenesis and Resistance in Leukemia. *Blood* **2017**, *129*, 547–552. [CrossRef] [PubMed]
364. Kang, M.R.; Kim, M.S.; Oh, J.E.; Kim, Y.R.; Song, S.Y.; Kim, S.S.; Ahn, C.H.; Yoo, N.J.; Lee, S.H. Frameshift Mutations of Autophagy-Related Genes ATG2B, ATG5, ATG9B and ATG12 in Gastric and Colorectal Cancers with Microsatellite Instability. *J. Pathol.* **2009**, *217*, 702–706. [CrossRef]
365. Zare-Abdollahi, D.; Safari, S.; Movafagh, A.; Ghadiani, M.; Tabarraee, M.; Riazi-Isfahani, S.; Gorji, S.; Keyvan, L.; Gachkar, L. Expression Analysis of BECN1 in Acute Myeloid Leukemia: Association with Distinct Cytogenetic and Molecular Abnormalities. *Int. J. Lab. Hematol.* **2016**, *38*, 125–132. [CrossRef]
366. Zhou, Y.; Rucker, E.B., 3rd; Zhou, B.P. Autophagy Regulation in the Development and Treatment of Breast Cancer. *Acta Biochim. Biophys. Sin.* **2016**, *48*, 60–74. [CrossRef]
367. Zhang, X.; Dai, M.; Li, S.; Li, M.; Cheng, B.; Ma, T.; Zhou, Z. The Emerging Potential Role of p62 in Cancer Treatment by Regulating Metabolism. *Trends Endocrinol. Metab.* **2023**, *34*, 474–488. [CrossRef]
368. Li, Y.; Zheng, W.; Lu, Y.; Zheng, Y.; Pan, L.; Wu, X.; Yuan, Y.; Shen, Z.; Ma, S.; Zhang, X.; et al. BNIP3L/NIX-Mediated Mitophagy: Molecular Mechanisms and Implications for Human Disease. *Cell Death Dis.* **2021**, *13*, 14. [CrossRef]
369. Trocoli, A.; Bensadoun, P.; Richard, E.; Labrunie, G.; Merhi, F.; Schläfli, A.M.; Brigger, D.; Souquere, S.; Pierron, G.; Pasquet, J.-M.; et al. p62/SQSTM1 Upregulation Constitutes a Survival Mechanism That Occurs during Granulocytic Differentiation of Acute Myeloid Leukemia Cells. *Cell Death Differ.* **2014**, *21*, 1852–1861. [CrossRef]
370. Fang, J.; Barker, B.; Bolanos, L.; Liu, X.; Jerez, A.; Makishima, H.; Rao, D.S.; Mulloy, J.C.; Maciejewski, J.P.; Cancelas, J.A.; et al. SQSTM1/p62 Is a Necessary Cofactor in MDS/AML with Deletion of Mir-146a. *Blood* **2013**, *122*, 747. [CrossRef]
371. Lazarini, M.; Machado-Neto, J.A.; Duarte, A.d.S.S.; Pericole, F.V.; Vieira, K.P.; Niemann, F.S.; Alvarez, M.; Traina, F.; Saad, S.T.O. BNIP3L in Myelodysplastic Syndromes and Acute Myeloid Leukemia: Impact on Disease Outcome and Cellular Response to Decitabine. *Haematologica* **2016**, *101*, e445–e448. [CrossRef] [PubMed]
372. Della Via, F.I.; Alvarez, M.C.; Basting, R.T.; Saad, S.T.O. The Effects of Green Tea Catechins in Hematological Malignancies. *Pharmaceuticals* **2023**, *16*, 1021. [CrossRef] [PubMed]
373. Lotfi, N.; Yousefi, Z.; Golabi, M.; Khalilian, P.; Ghezelbash, B.; Montazeri, M.; Shams, M.H.; Baghbadorani, P.Z.; Eskandari, N. The Potential Anti-Cancer Effects of Quercetin on Blood, Prostate and Lung Cancers: An Update. *Front. Immunol.* **2023**, *14*, 1077531. [CrossRef] [PubMed]
374. Yan, X.; Qi, M.; Li, P.; Zhan, Y.; Shao, H. Apigenin in Cancer Therapy: Anti-Cancer Effects and Mechanisms of Action. *Cell Biosci.* **2017**, *7*, 50. [CrossRef]

375. Monasterio, A.; Urdaci, M.C.; Pinchuk, I.V.; López-Moratalla, N.; Martínez-Irujo, J.J. Flavonoids Induce Apoptosis in Human Leukemia U937 Cells through Caspase- and Caspase-Calpain-Dependent Pathways. *Nutr. Cancer* **2004**, *50*, 90–100. [CrossRef]
376. Rubio, S.; León, F.; Quintana, J.; Cutler, S.; Estévez, F. Cell Death Triggered by Synthetic Flavonoids in Human Leukemia Cells Is Amplified by the Inhibition of Extracellular Signal-Regulated Kinase Signaling. *Eur. J. Med. Chem.* **2012**, *55*, 284–296. [CrossRef]
377. Spagnuolo, C.; Russo, M.; Bilotto, S.; Tedesco, I.; Laratta, B.; Russo, G.L. Dietary Polyphenols in Cancer Prevention: The Example of the Flavonoid Quercetin in Leukemia. *Ann. N. Y. Acad. Sci.* **2012**, *1259*, 95–103. [CrossRef]
378. Huseynova, N.; Çetinkaya, M.; Baran, Z.; Khalilov, R.; Mammadova, A.; Baran, Y. Flavonoids as Chemosensitizers in Leukemias. *Adv. Exp. Med. Biol.* **2024**, 1–30. [CrossRef]
379. Frankenfeld, C.L.; Cerhan, J.R.; Cozen, W.; Davis, S.; Schenk, M.; Morton, L.M.; Hartge, P.; Ward, M.H. Dietary Flavonoid Intake and Non-Hodgkin Lymphoma Risk. *Am. J. Clin. Nutr.* **2008**, *87*, 1439–1445. [CrossRef]
380. Maso, V.; Calgarotto, A.K.; Franchi, G.C., Jr.; Nowill, A.E.; Filho, P.L.; Vassallo, J.; Saad, S.T.O. Multitarget Effects of Quercetin in Leukemia. *Cancer Prev. Res.* **2014**, *7*, 1240–1250. [CrossRef]
381. Wei, J.; Chai, Q.; Qin, Y.; Li, L.; Guo, C.; Lu, Z.; Liu, H. Hyperoside Induces Ferroptosis in Chronic Myeloid Leukemia Cells by Targeting NRF2. *Mol. Med.* **2024**, *30*, 224. [CrossRef] [PubMed]
382. Szmyra, M.M.; Haingartner, S.; Jantscher, S.; Pansy, K.; Uhl, B.; Greinix, H.T.; Neumeister, P.; Bernhart, E.; Beham-Schmid, C.; Dengler, M.A.; et al. The Flavonoid Brusatol Induces Apoptosis in Aggressive Lymphoma Cells and Exhibits Synergistic Effect with Venetoclax. *Blood* **2022**, *140*, 4945–4946. [CrossRef]
383. Ding, K.; Jiang, W.; Jia, H.; Lei, M. Synergistically Anti-Multiple Myeloma Effects: Flavonoid, Non-Flavonoid Polyphenols, and Bortezomib. *Biomolecules* **2022**, *12*, 1647. [CrossRef] [PubMed]
384. He, D.; Guo, X.; Zhang, E.; Zi, F.; Chen, J.; Chen, Q.; Lin, X.; Yang, L.; Li, Y.; Wu, W.; et al. Quercetin Induces Cell Apoptosis of Myeloma and Displays a Synergistic Effect with Dexamethasone In Vitro and In Vivo Xenograft Models. *Oncotarget* **2016**, *7*, 45489–45499. [CrossRef] [PubMed]
385. Kawakatsu, R.; Tadagaki, K.; Yamasaki, K.; Kuwahara, Y.; Nakada, S.; Yoshida, T. The Combination of Venetoclax and Quercetin Exerts a Cytotoxic Effect on Acute Myeloid Leukemia. *Sci. Rep.* **2024**, *14*, 26418. [CrossRef]
386. Liu, F.-T.; Agrawal, S.G.; Movasaghi, Z.; Wyatt, P.B.; Rehman, I.U.; Gribben, J.G.; Newland, A.C.; Jia, L. Dietary Flavonoids Inhibit the Anticancer Effects of the Proteasome Inhibitor Bortezomib. *Blood* **2008**, *112*, 3835–3846. [CrossRef]
387. Entezari, M.; Tayari, A.; Paskeh, M.D.A.; Kheirabad, S.K.; Naeemi, S.; Taheriazam, A.; Dehghani, H.; Salimimoghadam, S.; Hashemi, M.; Mirzaei, S.; et al. Curcumin in Treatment of Hematological Cancers: Promises and Challenges. *J. Tradit. Complement. Med.* **2024**, *14*, 121–134. [CrossRef]
388. Talib, W.H.; Alsalahat, I.; Daoud, S.; Abutayeh, R.F.; Mahmod, A.I. Plant-Derived Natural Products in Cancer Research: Extraction, Mechanism of Action, and Drug Formulation. *Molecules* **2020**, *25*, 5319. [CrossRef]
389. Rafiq, S.; Raza, M.H.; Younas, M.; Naeem, F.; Adeeb, R.; Iqbal, J.; Anwar, P.; Sajid, U.; Manzoor, H.M. Molecular Targets of Curcumin and Future Therapeutic Role in Leukemia. *J. Biosci. Med.* **2018**, *06*, 33–50. [CrossRef]
390. Zaidi, A.; Lai, M.; Cavenagh, J. Long-Term Stabilisation of Myeloma with Curcumin. *BMJ Case Rep.* **2017**, *2017*, bcr2016218148. [CrossRef]
391. Flores-López, L.A.; De la Mora-De la Mora, I.; Malagón-Reyes, C.M.; García-Torres, I.; Martínez-Pérez, Y.; López-Herrera, G.; Hernández-Alcántara, G.; León-Avila, G.; López-Velázquez, G.; Olaya-Vargas, A.; et al. Selective Inhibition of Deamidated Triosephosphate Isomerase by Disulfiram, Curcumin, and Sodium Dichloroacetate: Synergistic Therapeutic Strategies for T-Cell Acute Lymphoblastic Leukemia in Jurkat Cells. *Biomolecules* **2024**, *14*, 1295. [CrossRef] [PubMed]
392. Ramakrishna, R.; Diamond, T.H.; Alexander, W.; Manoharan, A.; Golombick, T. Use of Curcumin in Multiple Myeloma Patients Intolerant of Steroid Therapy. *Clin. Case Rep.* **2020**, *8*, 739–744. [CrossRef] [PubMed]
393. Zou, H.; Zhu, X.-X.; Zhang, G.-B.; Ma, Y.; Wu, Y.; Huang, D.-S. Silibinin: An Old Drug for Hematological Disorders. *Oncotarget* **2017**, *8*, 89307–89314. [CrossRef] [PubMed]
394. Kiruthiga, C.; Devi, K.P.; Nabavi, S.M.; Bishayee, A. Autophagy: A Potential Therapeutic Target of Polyphenols in Hepatocellular Carcinoma. *Cancers* **2020**, *12*, 562. [CrossRef] [PubMed]
395. Liu, Y.; Gong, W.; Yang, Z.Y.; Zhou, X.S.; Gong, C.; Zhang, T.R.; Wei, X.; Ma, D.; Ye, F.; Gao, Q.L. Quercetin Induces Protective Autophagy and Apoptosis through ER Stress via the P-STAT3/Bcl-2 Axis in Ovarian Cancer. *Apoptosis* **2017**, *22*, 544–557. [CrossRef]
396. Romo-González, M.; Ijurko, C.; Hernández-Hernández, Á. Reactive Oxygen Species and Metabolism in Leukemia: A Dangerous Liaison. *Front. Immunol.* **2022**, *13*, 889875. [CrossRef]
397. Hole, P.S.; Darley, R.L.; Tonks, A. Do Reactive Oxygen Species Play a Role in Myeloid Leukemias? *Blood* **2011**, *117*, 5816–5826. [CrossRef]
398. Trombetti, S.; Cesaro, E.; Catapano, R.; Sessa, R.; Lo Bianco, A.; Izzo, P.; Grosso, M. Oxidative Stress and ROS-Mediated Signaling in Leukemia: Novel Promising Perspectives to Eradicate Chemoresistant Cells in Myeloid Leukemia. *Int. J. Mol. Sci.* **2021**, *22*, 2470. [CrossRef]

399. Bosnjak, M.; Ristic, B.; Arsikin, K.; Mircic, A.; Suzin-Zivkovic, V.; Perovic, V.; Bogdanovic, A.; Paunovic, V.; Markovic, I.; Bumbasirevic, V.; et al. Inhibition of mTOR-Dependent Autophagy Sensitizes Leukemic Cells to Cytarabine-Induced Apoptotic Death. *PLoS ONE* **2014**, *9*, e94374. [CrossRef]
400. Zhang, H.; Kang, J.; Liu, L.; Chen, L.; Ren, S.; Tao, Y. MicroRNA-143 Sensitizes Acute Myeloid Leukemia Cells to Cytarabine via Targeting ATG7- and ATG2B-Dependent Autophagy. *Aging* **2020**, *12*, 20111–20126. [CrossRef]
401. Visser, N.; Lourens, H.J.; Huls, G.; Bremer, E.; Wiersma, V.R. Inhibition of Autophagy Does Not Re-Sensitize Acute Myeloid Leukemia Cells Resistant to Cytarabine. *Int. J. Mol. Sci.* **2021**, *22*, 2337. [CrossRef] [PubMed]
402. Jin, S.; Wei, J.; You, L.; Liu, H.; Qian, W. Autophagy Regulation and Its Dual Role in Blood Cancers: A Novel Target for Therapeutic Development (Review). *Oncol. Rep.* **2018**, *39*, 2473–2481. [CrossRef] [PubMed]
403. Chen, L.; Guo, P.; Zhang, Y.; Li, X.; Jia, P.; Tong, J.; Li, J. Autophagy Is an Important Event for Low-Dose Cytarabine Treatment in Acute Myeloid Leukemia Cells. *Leuk. Res.* **2017**, *60*, 44–52. [CrossRef] [PubMed]
404. Xia, D.; Zhang, Y.-T.; Xu, G.-P.; Yan, W.-W.; Pan, X.-R.; Tong, J.-H. Sertraline Exerts Its Antitumor Functions through Both Apoptosis and Autophagy Pathways in Acute Myeloid Leukemia Cells. *Leuk. Lymphoma* **2017**, *58*, 1–10. [CrossRef]
405. Duarte, D.; Vale, N. Antidepressant Drug Sertraline against Human Cancer Cells. *Biomolecules* **2022**, *12*, 1513. [CrossRef]
406. Nguyen, T.D.; Shaid, S.; Vakhrusheva, O.; Koschade, S.E.; Klann, K.; Thölken, M.; Baker, F.; Zhang, J.; Oellerich, T.; Sürün, D.; et al. Loss of the Selective Autophagy Receptor p62 Impairs Murine Myeloid Leukemia Progression and Mitophagy. *Blood* **2019**, *133*, 168–179. [CrossRef]
407. Glytsou, C.; Chen, X.; Zacharioudakis, E.; Al-Santli, W.; Zhou, H.; Nadorp, B.; Lee, S.; Lasry, A.; Sun, Z.; Papaioannou, D.; et al. Mitophagy Promotes Resistance to BH3 Mimetics in Acute Myeloid Leukemia. *Cancer Discov.* **2023**, *13*, 1656–1677. [CrossRef]
408. Liu, X.; Devadiga, S.A.; Stanley, R.F.; Morrow, R.M.; Janssen, K.A.; Quesnel-Vallières, M.; Pomp, O.; Moverley, A.A.; Li, C.; Skuli, N.; et al. A Mitochondrial Surveillance Mechanism Activated by SRSF2 Mutations in Hematologic Malignancies. *J. Clin. Investig.* **2024**, *134*, e175619. [CrossRef]
409. Tang, Y.; Wang, L.; Qin, J.; Lu, Y.; Shen, H.-M.; Chen, H.-B. Targeting Mitophagy to Promote Apoptosis Is a Potential Therapeutic Strategy for Cancer. *Autophagy* **2023**, *19*, 1031–1033. [CrossRef]
410. Cao, M.; Tang, Y.; Luo, Y.; Gu, F.; Zhu, Y.; Liu, X.; Yan, C.; Hu, W.; Wang, S.; Chao, X.; et al. Natural Compounds Modulating Mitophagy: Implications for Cancer Therapy. *Cancer Lett.* **2024**, *582*, 216590. [CrossRef]
411. Cosialls, A.M.; Pomares, H.; Iglesias-Serret, D.; Saura-Esteller, J.; Núñez-Vázquez, S.; González-Gironès, D.M.; de la Banda, E.; Preciado, S.; Albericio, F.; Lavilla, R.; et al. The Prohibitin-Binding Compound Fluorizoline Induces Apoptosis in Chronic Lymphocytic Leukemia Cells through the Upregulation of NOXA and Synergizes with Ibrutinib, 5-Aminoimidazole-4-Carboxamide Riboside or Venetoclax. *Haematologica* **2017**, *102*, 1587–1593. [CrossRef] [PubMed]
412. Núñez-Vázquez, S.; Saura-Esteller, J.; Sánchez-Vera, I.; Guilbaud, E.; Cosialls, A.M.; Pons, G.; Ricci, J.-E.; Iglesias-Serret, D.; Marchetti, S.; Gil, J. The Prohibitin-Binding Compound Fluorizoline Inhibits Mitophagy in Cancer Cells. *Oncogenesis* **2021**, *10*, 64. [CrossRef] [PubMed]
413. Wierz, M.; Pierson, S.; Chouha, N.; Désaubry, L.; François, J.-H.; Berchem, G.; Paggetti, J.; Moussay, E. The Prohibitin-Binding Compound Fluorizoline Induces Apoptosis in Chronic Lymphocytic Leukemia Cells Ex Vivo but Fails to Prevent Leukemia Development in a Murine Model. *Haematologica* **2018**, *103*, e154–e157. [CrossRef] [PubMed]
414. Sun, H.; Ou, T.; Hu, J.; Yang, Z.; Lei, Q.; Li, Y.; Wang, G.; Li, Y.; Wu, K.; Wang, S.; et al. Nitazoxanide Impairs Mitophagy Flux through ROS-Mediated Mitophagy Initiation and Lysosomal Dysfunction in Bladder Cancer. *Biochem. Pharmacol.* **2021**, *190*, 114588. [CrossRef]
415. He, X.; Zhu, L.; Li, S.; Chen, Z.; Zhao, X. Loperamide, an Antidiarrheal Agent, Induces Apoptosis and DNA Damage in Leukemia Cells. *Oncol. Lett.* **2018**, *15*, 765–774. [CrossRef]
416. Puissant, A.; Robert, G.; Fenouille, N.; Luciano, F.; Cassuto, J.-P.; Raynaud, S.; Auberger, P. Resveratrol Promotes Autophagic Cell Death in Chronic Myelogenous Leukemia Cells via JNK-Mediated p62/SQSTM1 Expression and AMPK Activation. *Cancer Res.* **2010**, *70*, 1042–1052. [CrossRef]
417. Sui, T.; Ma, L.; Bai, X.; Li, Q.; Xu, X. Resveratrol Inhibits the Phosphatidylinositide 3-Kinase/protein Kinase B/mammalian Target of Rapamycin Signaling Pathway in the Human Chronic Myeloid Leukemia K562 Cell Line. *Oncol. Lett.* **2014**, *7*, 2093–2098. [CrossRef]
418. Yao, Y.; Zhu, J.; Qin, S.; Zhou, Z.; Zeng, Q.; Long, R.; Mao, Z.; Dong, X.; Zhao, R.; Zhang, R.; et al. Resveratrol Induces Autophagy Impeding BAFF-Stimulated B-Cell Proliferation and Survival by Inhibiting the Akt/mTOR Pathway. *Biochem. Pharmacol.* **2022**, *202*, 115139. [CrossRef]
419. Berman, A.Y.; Motechin, R.A.; Wiesenfeld, M.Y.; Holz, M.K. The Therapeutic Potential of Resveratrol: A Review of Clinical Trials. *NPJ Precis. Oncol.* **2017**, *1*, 35. [CrossRef]
420. Roulston, G.D.R.; Burt, C.L.; Kettyle, L.M.J.; Matchett, K.B.; Keenan, H.L.; Mulgrew, N.M.; Ramsey, J.M.; Dougan, C.; McKiernan, J.; Grishagin, I.V.; et al. Low-Dose Salinomycin Induces Anti-Leukemic Responses in AML and MLL. *Oncotarget* **2016**, *7*, 73448–73461. [CrossRef]

421. Lu, Z.; Jin, Y.; Qiu, L.; Lai, Y.; Pan, J. Celastrol, a Novel HSP90 Inhibitor, Depletes Bcr-Abl and Induces Apoptosis in Imatinib-Resistant Chronic Myelogenous Leukemia Cells Harboring T315I Mutation. *Cancer Lett.* **2010**, *290*, 182–191. [CrossRef] [PubMed]
422. Yu, X.; Ruan, X.; Zhang, J.; Zhao, Q. Celastrol Induces Cell Apoptosis and Inhibits the Expression of the AML1-ETO/C-KIT Oncoprotein in t (8;21) Leukemia. *Molecules* **2016**, *21*, 574. [CrossRef] [PubMed]
423. Tozawa, K.; Sagawa, M.; Kizaki, M. Quinone Methide Tripterine, Celastrol, Induces Apoptosis in Human Myeloma Cells via NF-κB Pathway. *Int. J. Oncol.* **2011**, *39*, 1117–1122.
424. Kannaiyan, R.; Hay, H.S.; Rajendran, P.; Li, F.; Shanmugam, M.K.; Vali, S.; Abbasi, T.; Kapoor, S.; Sharma, A.; Kumar, A.P.; et al. Celastrol Inhibits Proliferation and Induces Chemosensitization through down-Regulation of NF-κB and STAT3 Regulated Gene Products in Multiple Myeloma Cells. *Br. J. Pharmacol.* **2011**, *164*, 1506–1521. [CrossRef] [PubMed]
425. Ni, H.; Zhao, W.; Kong, X.; Li, H.; Ouyang, J. NF-Kappa B Modulation Is Involved in Celastrol Induced Human Multiple Myeloma Cell Apoptosis. *PLoS ONE* **2014**, *9*, e95846. [CrossRef] [PubMed]
426. Peng, B.; Xu, L.; Cao, F.; Wei, T.; Yang, C.; Uzan, G.; Zhang, D. HSP90 Inhibitor, Celastrol, Arrests Human Monocytic Leukemia Cell U937 at G0/G1 in Thiol-Containing Agents Reversible Way. *Mol. Cancer* **2010**, *9*, 79. [CrossRef]
427. Nelson, E.A.; Walker, S.R.; Xiang, M.; Weisberg, E.; Bar-Natan, M.; Barrett, R.; Liu, S.; Kharbanda, S.; Christie, A.L.; Nicolais, M.; et al. The STAT5 Inhibitor Pimozide Displays Efficacy in Models of Acute Myelogenous Leukemia Driven by FLT3 Mutations. *Genes Cancer* **2012**, *3*, 503–511. [CrossRef]
428. Allegra, A.; Tonacci, A.; Giordano, L.; Musolino, C.; Gangemi, S. Targeting Redox Regulation as a Therapeutic Opportunity against Acute Leukemia: Pro-Oxidant Strategy or Antioxidant Approach? *Antioxidants* **2022**, *11*, 1696. [CrossRef]
429. Barr, P.M.; Miller, T.P.; Friedberg, J.W.; Peterson, D.R.; Baran, A.M.; Herr, M.; Spier, C.M.; Cui, H.; Roe, D.J.; Persky, D.O.; et al. Phase 2 Study of Imexon, a Prooxidant Molecule, in Relapsed and Refractory B-Cell Non-Hodgkin Lymphoma. *Blood* **2014**, *124*, 1259–1265. [CrossRef]
430. Baik, M.-H.; Friesner, R.A.; Lippard, S.J. Theoretical Study of Cisplatin Binding to Purine Bases: Why Does Cisplatin Prefer Guanine over Adenine? *J. Am. Chem. Soc.* **2003**, *125*, 14082–14092. [CrossRef]
431. Marioli-Sapsakou, G.-K.; Kourti, M. Targeting Production of Reactive Oxygen Species as an Anticancer Strategy. *Anticancer Res.* **2021**, *41*, 5881–5902. [CrossRef] [PubMed]
432. Dasari, S.; Njiki, S.; Mbemi, A.; Yedjou, C.G.; Tchounwou, P.B. Pharmacological Effects of Cisplatin Combination with Natural Products in Cancer Chemotherapy. *Int. J. Mol. Sci.* **2022**, *23*, 1532. [CrossRef] [PubMed]
433. Kumar, S.; Tchounwou, P.B. Molecular Mechanisms of Cisplatin Cytotoxicity in Acute Promyelocytic Leukemia Cells. *Oncotarget* **2015**, *6*, 40734–40746. [CrossRef] [PubMed]
434. Bilardi, R.A.; Kimura, K.-I.; Phillips, D.R.; Cutts, S.M. Processing of Anthracycline-DNA Adducts via DNA Replication and Interstrand Crosslink Repair Pathways. *Biochem. Pharmacol.* **2012**, *83*, 1241–1250. [CrossRef]
435. Sochacka-Ćwikła, A.; Mączyński, M.; Regiec, A. FDA-Approved Drugs for Hematological Malignancies-the Last Decade Review. *Cancers* **2021**, *14*, 87. [CrossRef]
436. Chow, S.; Nagai, M.; He, S.; Blackman, R.K.; Barsoum, J.; Vukovic, V.; Hedley, D. Antileukemic Effects of the Novel Agent Elesclomol. *Blood* **2009**, *114*, 2736. [CrossRef]
437. Evens, A.M.; Prachand, S.; Shi, B.; Paniaqua, M.; Gordon, L.I.; Gartenhaus, R.B. Imexon-Induced Apoptosis in Multiple Myeloma Tumor Cells Is Caspase-8 Dependent. *Clin. Cancer Res.* **2004**, *10*, 1481–1491. [CrossRef]
438. van Nieuwenhuijzen, N.; Frunt, R.; May, A.M.; Minnema, M.C. Therapeutic Outcome of Early-Phase Clinical Trials in Multiple Myeloma: A Meta-Analysis. *Blood Cancer J.* **2021**, *11*, 44. [CrossRef]
439. Evens, A.M.; Balasubramanian, L.; Gordon, L.I. Motexafin Gadolinium Induces Oxidative Stress and Apoptosis in Hematologic Malignancies. *Curr. Treat. Options Oncol.* **2005**, *6*, 289–296. [CrossRef]
440. Evens, A.M. Motexafin Gadolinium: A Redox-Active Tumor Selective Agent for the Treatment of Cancer. *Curr. Opin. Oncol.* **2004**, *16*, 576–580. [CrossRef]
441. Tagde, A.; Singh, H.; Kang, M.H.; Reynolds, C.P. The Glutathione Synthesis Inhibitor Buthionine Sulfoximine Synergistically Enhanced Melphalan Activity against Preclinical Models of Multiple Myeloma. *Blood Cancer J.* **2014**, *4*, e229. [CrossRef] [PubMed]
442. O'Day, S.J.; Eggermont, A.M.M.; Chiarion-Sileni, V.; Kefford, R.; Grob, J.J.; Mortier, L.; Robert, C.; Schachter, J.; Testori, A.; Mackiewicz, J.; et al. Final Results of Phase III SYMMETRY Study: Randomized, Double-Blind Trial of Elesclomol plus Paclitaxel versus Paclitaxel Alone as Treatment for Chemotherapy-Naive Patients with Advanced Melanoma. *J. Clin. Oncol.* **2013**, *31*, 1211–1218. [CrossRef] [PubMed]
443. Lawson, D.H.; Gonzalez, R.; Weber, R.W.; Hutchins, L.F.; Anderson, C.M.; Williams, K.N.; Kong, S.; Jacobson, E.; O'Day, S.J. 2-Year Overall Survival (OS) Results of a Phase II Trial of Elesclomol (formerly STA-4783) and Paclitaxel in Stage IV Metastatic Melanoma (MM). *J. Clin. Oncol.* **2008**, *26*, 20023. [CrossRef]
444. Adane, B.; Ye, H.; Khan, N.; Pei, S.; Minhajuddin, M.; Stevens, B.M.; Jones, C.L.; D'Alessandro, A.; Reisz, J.A.; Zaberezhnyy, V.; et al. The Hematopoietic Oxidase NOX2 Regulates Self-Renewal of Leukemic Stem Cells. *Cell Rep.* **2019**, *27*, 238–254.e6. [CrossRef]

445. Cheng, X.; Xu, H.-D.; Ran, H.-H.; Liang, G.; Wu, F.-G. Glutathione-Depleting Nanomedicines for Synergistic Cancer Therapy. *ACS Nano* **2021**, *15*, 8039–8068. [CrossRef]
446. Chen, Y.; Chen, J.; Zou, Z.; Xu, L.; Li, J. Crosstalk between Autophagy and Metabolism: Implications for Cell Survival in Acute Myeloid Leukemia. *Cell Death Discov.* **2024**, *10*, 46. [CrossRef]
447. Orgel, E.; Framson, C.; Buxton, R.; Kim, J.; Li, G.; Tucci, J.; Freyer, D.R.; Sun, W.; Oberley, M.J.; Dieli-Conwright, C.; et al. Caloric and Nutrient Restriction to Augment Chemotherapy Efficacy for Acute Lymphoblastic Leukemia: The IDEAL Trial. *Blood Adv.* **2021**, *5*, 1853–1861. [CrossRef]
448. Kubota, Y.; Han, Q.; Aoki, Y.; Masaki, N.; Obara, K.; Hamada, K.; Hozumi, C.; Wong, A.C.W.; Bouvet, M.; Tsunoda, T.; et al. Synergy of Combining Methionine Restriction and Chemotherapy: The Disruptive next Generation of Cancer Treatment. *Cancer Diagn. Progn.* **2023**, *3*, 272–281. [CrossRef]
449. Abo Qoura, L.; Balakin, K.V.; Hoffman, R.M.; Pokrovsky, V.S. The Potential of Methioninase for Cancer Treatment. *Biochim. Biophys. Acta Rev. Cancer* **2024**, *1879*, 189122. [CrossRef]
450. Sedillo, J.C.; Cryns, V.L. Targeting the Methionine Addiction of Cancer. *Am. J. Cancer Res.* **2022**, *12*, 2249–2276.
451. Mussai, F.; Egan, S.; Higginbotham-Jones, J.; Perry, T.; Beggs, A.; Odintsova, E.; Loke, J.; Pratt, G.; U, K.P.; Lo, A.; et al. Arginine Dependence of Acute Myeloid Leukemia Blast Proliferation: A Novel Therapeutic Target. *Blood* **2015**, *125*, 2386–2396. [CrossRef] [PubMed]
452. Wei, J.; Xie, Q.; Liu, X.; Wan, C.; Wu, W.; Fang, K.; Yao, Y.; Cheng, P.; Deng, D.; Liu, Z. Identification the Prognostic Value of Glutathione Peroxidases Expression Levels in Acute Myeloid Leukemia. *Ann. Transl. Med.* **2020**, *8*, 678. [CrossRef] [PubMed]
453. Dong, L.; He, J.; Luo, L.; Wang, K. Targeting the Interplay of Autophagy and ROS for Cancer Therapy: An Updated Overview on Phytochemicals. *Pharmaceuticals* **2023**, *16*, 92. [CrossRef] [PubMed]
454. White, E.; DiPaola, R.S. The Double-Edged Sword of Autophagy Modulation in Cancer. *Clin. Cancer Res.* **2009**, *15*, 5308–5316. [CrossRef]
455. Luo, M.; Zhou, L.; Huang, Z.; Li, B.; Nice, E.C.; Xu, J.; Huang, C. Antioxidant Therapy in Cancer: Rationale and Progress. *Antioxidants* **2022**, *11*, 1128. [CrossRef]
456. Singh, K.; Bhori, M.; Kasu, Y.A.; Bhat, G.; Marar, T. Antioxidants as Precision Weapons in War against Cancer Chemotherapy Induced Toxicity—Exploring the Armoury of Obscurity. *Saudi Pharm. J.* **2018**, *26*, 177–190. [CrossRef]
457. Kongara, S.; Karantza, V. The Interplay between Autophagy and ROS in Tumorigenesis. *Front. Oncol.* **2012**, *2*, 171. [CrossRef]
458. Choi, K.S. Autophagy and Cancer. *Exp. Mol. Med.* **2012**, *44*, 109–120. [CrossRef]
459. Pluta, R. Editorial: Targeting Autophagy in Cancer Therapy: Focus on Small-Molecule Modulators and New Strategies. *Front. Pharmacol.* **2023**, *14*, 1145255. [CrossRef]
460. Klemm, J.D.; Singer, D.S.; Mesirov, J.P. Transforming Cancer Research through Informatics. *Cancer Discov.* **2024**, *14*, 1779–1782. [CrossRef]

antioxidants

MDPI

Review

Roles of Oxidative Stress and Autophagy in Alcohol-Mediated Brain Damage

Leon Ruiter-Lopez [1,*], Mohammed A. S. Khan [2], Xin Wang [2] and Byoung-Joon Song [1,*]

[1] Section of Molecular Pharmacology and Toxicology, National Institute on Alcohol Abuse and Alcoholism, Bethesda, MD 20892, USA
[2] Department of Neurosurgery, Brigham and Women's Hospital, Harvard Medical School, Boston, MA 02115, USA; mkhan5@bwh.harvard.edu (M.A.S.K.); xwang2@bwh.harvard.edu (X.W.)
* Correspondence: leon.ruiterlopez@nih.gov (L.R.-L.); bj.song@nih.gov (B.-J.S.); Tel.: +1-(301)-496-3985 (B.-J.S.)

Abstract: Excessive alcohol consumption significantly impacts human health, particularly the brain, due to its susceptibility to oxidative stress, which contributes to neurodegenerative conditions. Alcohol metabolism in the brain occurs primarily via catalase, followed by CYP2E1 pathways. Excess alcohol metabolized by CYP2E1 generates reactive oxygen/nitrogen species (ROS/RNS), leading to cell injury via altering many different pathways. Elevated oxidative stress impairs autophagic processes, increasing post-translational modifications and further exacerbating mitochondrial dysfunction and ER stress, leading to cell death. The literature highlights that alcohol-induced oxidative stress disrupts autophagy and mitophagy, contributing to neuronal damage. Key mechanisms include mitochondrial dysfunction, ER stress, epigenetics, and the accumulation of oxidatively modified proteins, which lead to neuroinflammation and impaired cellular quality control. These processes are exacerbated by chronic alcohol exposure, resulting in the suppression of protective pathways like NRF2-mediated antioxidant responses and increased susceptibility to neurodegenerative changes in the brain. Alcohol-mediated neurotoxicity involves complex interactions between alcohol metabolism, oxidative stress, and autophagy regulation, which are influenced by various factors such as drinking patterns, nutritional status, and genetic/environmental factors, highlighting the need for further molecular studies to unravel these mechanisms and develop targeted interventions.

Keywords: autophagy; ethanol; alcohol metabolism; brain; oxidative stress; mitophagy; neurotoxicity; neurodegeneration; antioxidants

1. Introduction

Excessive alcohol (ethanol) consumption causes severe consequences for human health, usually negatively affecting multiple organ systems and contributing to a variety of diseases. According to the National Institute on Alcohol Abuse and Alcoholism (NIAAA), excessive alcohol intake causes more than 200 diseases and accounts for a significant global burden of disease, with millions of individuals affected annually by alcohol-related morbidities and mortalities. In the United States alone, approximately 28.9 million people aged 12 and older reported alcohol use disorder (AUD) in 2023, with annual economic burdens of more than USD 250 billion [1].

Because of its high water solubility, ethanol is distributed to virtually all organs, including the digestive organs, liver, brain, etc., and negatively affects them after heavy drinking. The brain is particularly vulnerable to the toxic effects of alcohol, partly due to having very low levels of antioxidants and antioxidative enzymes and high levels of lipids compared to those in the peripheral tissues such as the liver. Chronic alcohol consumption is associated with various neurodegenerative conditions, including alcohol-related nervous system damage or neurodegeneration, including dementia, Wernicke–Korsakoff syndrome, and fetal alcohol spectrum disorders (FASD) [2–5]. For example, FASD, a condition resulting from fetal and/or prenatal alcohol exposure, leads to severe developmental and cognitive impairments [6–8]. In fact, neuronal cells in gestational periods are much more vulnerable to ethanol-mediated neurotoxicity than adult tissues, eventually leading to FASD [9].

Although the mechanisms underlying alcohol-induced neurodegeneration vary by pattern of alcohol intake such as frequency and amount, nutritional states, gender, genetic makeup, and age, they share several common pathways of toxicity. Key mechanisms include the production of reactive oxygen species (ROS) and reactive nitrogen species (RNS); accumulation of cytotoxic acetaldehyde and other reactive lipid aldehydes, such as 4-hydroxynonenal (4-HNE), malondialdehyde (MDA), and acrolein; induction of endoplasmic reticulum (ER) stress with accumulated misfolded proteins; and impaired lysosomal autophagy or mitophagy upon alcohol exposure [10–12]. In addition, alcohol intake alters various signaling pathways including activation of the cell death pathway, elevated inflammation, and mitochondrial dysfunction with depletion of energy supply [13]. Among these, oxidative stress seems to play a central role in initiating inflammation and exacerbating cellular damage, since intake of antioxidants or nutritional support with a balanced diet usually reduces the degree of alcohol-related organ damage in experimental models [14–17].

Oxidative stress arises from an imbalance between the production of ROS and the cell's ability to detoxify these reactive molecules [18]. In the context of alcohol metabolism, elevated ROS levels can suppress the function of subcellular organelles, including mitochondria and ER, which results in oxidative modification and inactivation of components in the mitochondrial electron transport chain (ETC), such as complex I (ubiquinone-dependent NADH-oxidoreductase). This modification and inactivation of the ETC produces more electron leakage and ROS, further causing mitochondrial dysfunction and an impaired energy supply, ER stress with elevated levels of misfolded proteins, and eventual cell death. In addition, in the presence of high alcohol concentrations, the ethanol-inducible cytochrome P450-2E1 (CYP2E1) and its isozymes, present in the ER and mitochondria [19,20], also participate in the production of ROS, which causes oxidative modifications to cellular macromolecules, including the proteins, lipids, and DNA. These changes lead to protein post-translational modifications (PTMs), lipid peroxidation products, and DNA-adducts, all of which can potentially contribute to tissue damage, mutagenesis, or carcinogenesis if not treated properly [21]. One notable consequence of oxidative stress is the bi-directional regulations of the lysosomal autophagic pathways [22,23]. Some reports showed that ethanol can activate autophagy, a highly conserved process to remove the damaged proteins or subcellular organelles, while others demonstrated that ethanol can also impair autophagic process through elevated oxidative stress, depending on the patterns of alcohol intake (e.g., chronic versus acute alcohol exposure), cellular contexts, nutritional status, redox balance states, etc. Since autophagy generally serves a protective function by mitigating oxidative damage, its dysregulation can have opposing effects, leading to increased inflammation and cell/tissue injury. In this review, we summarize the current evidence available regarding the involvement of the autophagic pathways in alcohol-related neurotoxicity and their relationship with oxidative stress.

2. Materials and Methods

A literature search was conducted on the impact of alcohol exposure on autophagy and oxidative stress in the brain. Investigators LRL and BJS performed the literature search. We searched PubMed until Nov 21, 2024, using the following search terms: "autophagy" and "oxidative stress" or "redox" or "reactive oxygen species" or "cellular stress" or "antioxidants" and "Wernicke-Korsakoff*" or "behavioral*" or "cognitive*" or "neuro degeneration" or "brain*" and "alcohol*" or "ethanol*." All articles were in English. The search strategy was supplemented with references found through the snowball technique to obtain information from relevant papers available.

Articles discussing autophagy and oxidative stress in response to alcohol consumption in the brain were selected. Papers with mouse models, cell lines, and human samples were considered. However, studies that did not directly evaluate the effects of alcohol on the brain in respect to the mechanisms of autophagy pathways were excluded. Methodological details and molecular effects on autophagy and oxidative stress of each study were extracted, and the information was summarized in different tables.

3. Literature Review

3.1. Regulation of Autophagy and Lysosomal Protein Degradation

Proteostasis is a normal process to maintain the proper balance of many cellular proteins by regulating the rates of new protein synthesis, adequate protein folding/misfolding, and degradation of cellular proteins [24]. Due to the critical nature of these functions, abnormal proteostasis is frequently associated with many disease states such as alcohol-associated liver disease, immune disorders, cancer, and neurodegeneration [25–27]. In mammals, two main protein degradation systems exist to regulate protein homeostasis and maintain their functions and levels. The first one is the ubiquitin-dependent proteasome-dependent degradation system, which is involved in the degradation numerous proteins that are abnormally misfolded in the ER. The other major protein degradation system is autophagic lysosomal proteolysis, which is responsible for the degradation of damaged subcellular organelles and/or aggregated proteins. Thus, disrupted proteostasis often results in accumulation of abnormally misfolded or aggregated proteins, which are potentially toxic to the cells, leading to cell death and various disease states, including alcohol-mediated brain injury and neurodegeneration [27,28].

Autophagy is a highly conserved cellular procedure that removes damaged subcellular organelles and proteins to be re-utilized for promoting cellular homeostasis and survival, especially during insufficient energy supply like fasting [29] or disease states that lead to autophagic flux and autophagic degradation, depending on the nature of disease [30–33]. Autophagy is usually very low in normal physiological states. However, it can be activated or induced under stressful conditions such as decreased energy supply, hypoxia, ischemia/reperfusion, and viral infections to overcome unfavorable conditions [34], for an excellent review of the autophagy processes, factors, and underlying mechanisms, while it can be suppressed by high levels of oxidative stress and long-term alcohol intake. In fact, autophagy can be regulated by many factors, including oxidative stress, which can cause oxidative DNA damage, alter gene/epigenetic expression, and promote PTMs (Figure 1). Changes in oxidative protein modifications and expression, or single nucleotide polymorphisms of the specific autophagy-related proteins (ATGs) and many associated genes [35], respectively (a few of which are exemplified in Figure 1), can result in different rates of mitophagy, ER stress, and autophagy.

It is also known that specific types of autophagy exist in different cell compartments for the proper disposal of cellular debris, aggregated proteins, and damaged subcellular organelles, such as mitochondria (mitophagy), ER (reticulophagy), peroxisomes (pexophagy) [36], and ribosomes (ribophagy) [37], although we only briefly described the functions of mitophagy and reticulophagy in this review. Thus, abnormal changes in the ubiquitin-dependent proteasomal activities and the lysosomal autophagy are frequently associated with many disease states, including alcohol- or nonalcohol-associated chronic liver diseases, cancer, and aging-related neurodegenerative disorders. Alcohol-associated neuronal injury and behavioral and cognitive impairments [38–40] are also known to result from elevated oxidative stress and abnormal regulations of autophagy. For instance, it is known that small amounts of ROS activate autophagy or mitophagy to prevent greater amounts from being produced in the mitochondria and thus providing protection from tissue injury. In contrast, large amounts of ROS (e.g., after chronic excessive alcohol intake) are known to impair autophagy process possibly through phosphorylation, Sirt1-dependent deacetylation, and other PTMs of many proteins involved in the autophagy machinery [34].

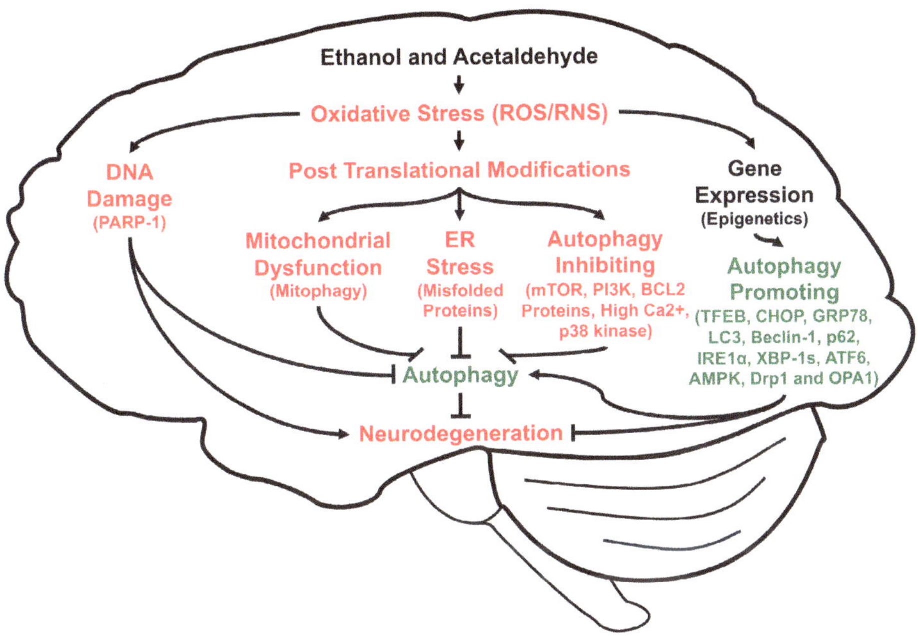

Figure 1. Schematic diagram of the multiple pathways to show how ethanol and acetaldehyde regulate autophagy through elevated oxidative stress, leading to alcohol-mediated neuronal injury and neurodegeneration. Lines with arrowheads indicate stimulation of the pathway while short perpendicular lines represent inhibition.

Autophagy also repairs DNA damage, which is elevated by oxidative stress or acetaldehyde [41]. In addition, DNA damage causes autophagy where PARP-1 is involved [42,43]. Thus, if autophagy is inhibited, DNA damage cannot be repaired, and the cells undergo apoptosis (instead of re-utilization of the cellular components via autophagy).

3.2. Increased Oxidative Stress in the Alcohol Metabolism in the Brain

The majority of consumed alcohol (ethanol) is known to be metabolized by oxidative and non-oxidative pathways in the liver as well as the stomach [44,45]. During the oxidative metabolism pathway, alcohol is oxidized by the cytosolic alcohol dehydrogenase (ADH) to acetaldehyde, which is further oxidized to acetate by the mitochondrial aldehyde dehydrogenase-2 (ALDH2) by using NAD^+ as a cofactor for both enzymes, resulting in a redox change. In addition, in the presence of a high ethanol concentration through chronic alcohol intake, CYP2E1 present in the endoplasmic reticulum and mitochondria [19,46–48] is induced and becomes involved in ethanol oxidation by using NADPH as a cofactor and produce a superoxide anion, which further leads to the production of other reactive oxygen and nitrogen species (ROS/RNS). During the non-oxidative pathway, ethanol is conjugated with various small molecules, such as fatty acids, to produce fatty acid ethyl esters (FAEEs) and phosphatidylethanol [49–51].

In general, the oxidative ethanol metabolism increasing the $NAD^+/NADH$ ratio and inducing CYP2E1 activity [52] is known to cause oxidative stress and tissue injury through activation of the cell death pathways and elevated production of the cytotoxic acetaldehyde and highly reactive lipid aldehydes such as 4-HNE, MDA, and acrolein-adducts [53]. This organ damage occurs in many peripheral tissues and the central nervous system (CNS). Recent studies also showed that non-oxidative ethanol metabolism is involved in tissue injury through elevated ER stress and cell death pathways in the peripheral tissues, including the adipocytes and liver [54].

Unlike the liver, the brain does not contain the classical oxidative ethanol metabolism pathway starting with the ADH, since all five ADH isozymes, including the major ethanol-metabolizing ADH-II, is absent or very low in the brain tissues [55]. In fact, other scientists reported that the majority of alcohol in the brain is known to be metabolized by catalase (~60%) and partially by CYP2E1 (~20%) and others, although the induction of CYP2E1 occurs after chronic alcohol intake [56–60]. However, it is important to consider the potential impacts of the elevated CYP2E1 on the oxidative cell and brain injury, since CYP2E1 was shown to be induced by 17.5 mM ethanol in primary neuronal cells [61], primary astrocytes [62], and rodent brains after chronic alcohol exposures [63–66].

In addition to these enzymes, ethanol is also known to be metabolized via the non-oxidative pathway to produce ethanol fatty acid esters, which are also known to cause neuroprotection [67,68] or mitochondrial dysfunction and neurotoxicity [49,50,69], depending on the moiety of the fatty acids and suppression of the oxidative ethanol metabolism enzymes [70]. For instance, FAEEs including docosahexaenoic acid (DHA) and eicosapentaenoic acid (EPA) were reported to prevent neurotoxicity or neurodegeneration in animal models of Alzheimer's disease [71], Parkinson's disease [67], and Huntington's disease [72]. On the other hand, ethyl oleate or ethyl palmitate produced through the non-oxidative ethanol metabolism could take place in various tissues, including the pancreas, heart, and brain, where the oxidative ethanol metabolism is weak and causes injury in those tissues [49]. In the latter cases, the amounts of FAEEs positively correlate with the levels of blood alcohol and may promote tissue injury by releasing the free fatty acids, which subsequently suppress the mitochondrial functions, leading to increased organ damage [69].

Finally, most of the ROS produced in the brain could result from the suppressed mitochondrial function and abnormal changes in mitochondrial fission and fusion, which are associated with many chronic disease states, including aging-related neurodegenerative diseases [73–76]. Excessive amounts of alcohol intake are also known to promote the mitochondrial dysfunction, leading to elevated electron leakage from the mitochondrial ETC to generate ROS and ultimately increased oxidative stress in the peripheral tissues and brain, as reported by many laboratories [77–79]. For instance, mitochondrial complexes I–III and IV subunit activities are suppressed by alcohol exposure in rodent models [80]. In addition, alcohol intake is known to alter the intracellular Ca^{2+} balance, cause changes in the mitochondrial Ca^{2+} levels, and alter the dynamics of mitochondrial fusion and fission, leading to mitochondrial dysfunction and neuroinflammation [81–83]. All these changes eventually result in elevated oxidative stress and subsequent neurotoxicity.

3.3. Effects of Increased Oxidative Stress on Autophagy and Neuronal Damage in Alcohol-Exposed Experimental Models and Individuals with AUD

3.3.1. Effects of Increased Oxidative Stress on Autophagy and Neuronal Damage

In general, the brain usually consumes oxygen at higher rates, possesses high lipid contents, and contains a much smaller amount of antioxidants, including reduced glutathione (GSH), and antioxidative enzymes such as superoxide dismutase (SOD) isozymes and catalase, as well as proteases, compared to those in the liver [84–86]. Consequently, various brain cells, including neurons and astroglial cells, are thought to be more sensitive to oxidative injury or cytotoxic agents acetaldehyde and lipid aldehydes, leading to mitochondrial dysfunction and ER stress with misfolded proteins, after exposure to chronic excessive alcohol and other neurotoxic agents compared to the liver hepatocytes. In addition, it is known that an injured liver can regenerate rapidly to fully recover its functions within a short period of time relative to the brain cells [87,88]. The oxidative ethanol metabolism via ethanol-induced CYP2E1, albeit a small amount and with less involvement in the cerebral oxidative ethanol metabolism than catalase, and can cause oxidative stress, neuroinflammation, impairment autophagy, and apoptosis of neuronal cells, leading to brain damage in specific regions, including the hippocampus, cerebellum, and brainstem [61,62,65]. Alcohol-mediated neuronal cell- and/or region-specific damage can result from the unequal distributions of pro-oxidant CYP2E1 [89] and antioxidant ALDH2 [90] in the brain. In addition, hydrogen peroxide (H_2O_2) can be generated during the turnover of neurotransmitters such as dopamine and serotonin, contributing to oxidative stress, if not properly managed [91]. Additionally, immune-cell-derived NADPH oxidase can contribute to produce oxidative stress in the brain, leading to ER stress, neuroinflammation, and neurodegeneration in the animal models [92,93] and people with AUD [94]. Furthermore, acetaldehyde generated from oxidative ethanol metabolism, mitochondrial dysfunction, and ER stress can produce additional levels of ROS, Ca^{2+} imbalance, and mitochondrial dynamic changes in the brain, contributing to inhibition of autophagy/mitophagy accompanied by increased neuroinflammation and neurodegeneration in ethanol-exposed cells in rodents [41,95].

Alcohol-mediated oxidative stress is known to cause neurotoxicity and altered autophagy responses possibly through multiple mechanisms as described below. Alcohol-induced changes in autophagic responses seem to be dependent on the different embryonic stages, frequency and patterns of ethanol exposure such as acute and chronic alcohol intake, which causes oxidative stress, various experimental models, nutritional status of the host cells/animals, etc. However, because of the often conflicting results, we have listed many recent reports on the effects of acute and chronic alcohol intake on autophagy regulation in rodent models in Tables 1 and 2, respectively. In continuation, we have also described the recent reports on the effects of alcohol exposure on autophagy in various brain cell culture models, including neurons, microglia, and astrocytes in Table 3. To provide clinical relevance of these experimental results, we also describe a summary of the effects of ethanol on autophagic flux in the brains of people with AUD (Table 4).

Table 1. Autophagy in acute alcohol exposure in animal models.

First Author, Year	Models and Methods	Summary of Effects
Alimov et al., 2013. [96]	C57BL/6 mice were injected subcutaneously with saline or ethanol (2.5 g/kg, 20% solution in saline) twice at 0 h and 2 h	Injection of ethanol induced neuroapoptosis on postnatal day 4 (PD4). However, little effect was observed in the brain of PD12 mice. Expression of genes that regulate UPR and autophagy was significantly higher on PD12 than PD4.
Chen et al., 2012. [97]	C57BL/6 mice were injected subcutaneously with saline or ethanol (2.5 g/kg, 20% solution in saline) twice at 0 and 2 h	Ethanol increased oxidative stress and neuronal death. By activating autophagy through the mTOR pathway with agents like rapamycin, some of the ethanol-mediated effects were attenuated.
Boschen et al., 2023. [98]	Pregnant C57BL/6J mice were exposed to a single dose of 2.9 g/kg ethanol, as an FASD model	Ethanol exposure during neurulation disrupts gene expression in the rostroventral neural tube. This affects pathways involved in metabolism, cell cycle, and organogenesis. Such deficits can contribute to developmental malformations in the brain and craniofacial structures.
Uguz et al., 2024. [99]	Wistar albino female rats (weighing between 250 and 350 g and 8–12 weeks old) were exposed to ethanol (18% *v*/*v*) via oral gavage. The total volume prepared was 2 mL, and the total dose administered was 1 g/kg body weight. Ethanol gavage was administered twice per week during the second and third weeks of pregnancy.	Acute alcohol exposure during pregnancy disrupted gene expression in the neural tube. This also affected developmental pathways, further contributing to craniofacial and brain malformations.
Montesinos et al., 2018. [100]	Thirty-day-old female C57BL/6 wild-type (WT) and TLR4 knockout (TLR4-KO) mice were exposed to morning doses of either saline or 25% (*v*/*v*) ethanol (3 g/kg) on two consecutive days with 2-day gaps without injections for 2 weeks Rapamycin to inhibit the mTOR pathway	Exposure to alcohol impaired autophagy mechanisms by increasing the activity of autophagy inhibitor mTOR, lowering LC3-II levels and accumulating p62. Inhibition of mTOR by rapamycin restored levels of excitatory scaffolding synaptic proteins (PSD-95 or SHANK3), p62, and partly re-established the LC3-II levels. Deletion of TLR4 ameliorated autophagy dysfunctions and decreased the frequency and size of the synaptic connections in ethanol-exposed mice.

Table 1. *Cont.*

First Author, Year	Models and Methods	Summary of Effects
Pascual et al., 2021. [101]	C57BL/6 adolescent female and male mice (PND30) were treated with ethanol (3 g/kg) on two consecutive days at 48 h intervals over 2 weeks	Ethanol treatment decreased the density and morphology of dendritic spines. These effects are associated with learning and memory impairments, and changes in the levels of both phosphorylation and miRNAs of the transcription factor CREB were observed. Rapamycin administration, inhibiting mTOR/autophagy dysfunctions, prior to ethanol administration restored ethanol-induced changes in both plasticity and behavior dysfunctions in adolescent mice.
Luo, 2014. [9] (REVIEW)	FASD Model, PD4 vs PD12	Acute ethanol exposure induced a protective autophagic response that helped alleviate oxidative stress and neuronal apoptosis in the developing brain.
Kurhaluk et al., 2020. [102] (REVIEW)		Acute alcohol exposure causes the depletion of the critical antioxidant GSH and a reduction in the GSH/GSSG redox state. The oxidative stress induced by acute ethanol intoxication led to structural and functional impairment in tissues that are indicated by the main marker of lysosomal activity. The plethora of melatonin effects can prevent lysosomal destruction in tissues during ethanol-induced intoxication by limiting the increased activity of lysosomal enzymes and resulting in oxidative stress.
Yang et al., 2015. [103] (REVIEW)		Acute alcohol exposure caused long-lasting effects on emotional and memory deficits, suggesting a functional and structural change in the hippocampus in mice. In PD7 mice, ethanol induced ER stress in the developing brain. In PD4 mice, ethanol induced wide-spread neuroapoptosis. In PD12 mice, ethanol induced little effect on the brain. Expression of pro-apoptotic genes, such as cleaved caspase-3, was much higher in PD4 than PD12. Expressed levels of genes that regulate UPR and autophagy, such as atg6, atg4, atg9, atg10, beclin1, bnip3, cebpb, ctsb, ctsd, ctss, grp78, ire1α, lamp, lc3 perk, pik3c3, and sqstm1, were significantly higher in PD12 than PD4.

Table 1. *Cont.*

First Author, Year	Models and Methods	Summary of Effects
		Ethanol exposures caused increased levels of autophagy markers, specifically LC3-II, and oxidative stress indicated by the upregulation of ER stress proteins (GRP78, ATF6, and CHOP) and phosphorylation of eIF2α, PERK, and IRE1α within 4 h in PD7.
Fujii et al., 2021. [104] (REVIEW)	FASD model, PD7 2.5 g/kg 20% saline twice s.c. injection	Ethanol and acetaldehyde impaired memory formation in hippocampal neurons by inducing ER stress.
	Rat hippocampal slices treated with ethanol or acetaldehyde in the absence or presence of integrated stress response inhibitor	Ethanol and acetaldehyde induced NMDAR activation and synthesis of 5α-reduced neurosteroids, leading to inhibition of long-term potentiation (LTP). This result was prevented by inhibiting integrated stress response (ISR) with ISRIB (ISR inhibitor) and stimulating the liver X receptor with agonist GW3965.
		These results suggest that ISR and ER stress responses exacerbate ethanol-mediated CNS damage, in contrast to the protective role of ISRIB.
De Ternay et al., 2019. [105] (REVIEW)	Acute ethanol exposure over 8 h for 4 days with CBD as a protective agent	Ethanol exposure led to oxidative stress, increasing neuronal degeneration in the hippocampus and entorhinal cortex. With co-administration of CBD, there was a significant reduction in cell death. CBD's antioxidant effects were comparable to tocopherol.

Table 2. Autophagy in chronic alcohol exposure in animal models.

First Author, Year	Models and Methods	Summary of Effects
Sumitomo et al., 2017. [106]	Ulk1-null mice were exposed to four cycles of chronic intermittent ethanol (CIE, 20% ethanol for 4 days followed by water for 7 days), followed by intraperitoneal (i.p.) injection of ethanol (2 g/kg/body weight, once daily, in 15% solution) for 4 days	Chronic intermittent ethanol exposure downregulated Ulk1-mediated autophagy in the prefrontal cortex, leading to p62 accumulation, impaired exploratory behavior, deficits in object recognition, and reduced voluntary ethanol consumption in these mice.

Table 2. *Cont.*

First Author, Year	Models and Methods	Summary of Effects
Davis-Anderson et al., 2018. [107]	Timed pregnant Sprague Dawley rats, as an FASD model	Chronic alcohol exposure during pregnancy altered the fetal brain proteome, which significantly impacted proteins involved in cellular growth, autophagy, oxidative stress, and mitochondrial dysfunction in the hippocampus, cortex, and cerebellum. These changes likely contribute to neurodevelopmental deficits associated with FASD.
Nasef et al., 2021. [108]	Seventy female Swiss albino mice aged 4–6 weeks, weighing 10–15 g, 15% alcohol solution for 55 days with or without simvastatin (10 mg/kg/day)	Chronic alcohol exposure induced neurodegeneration by promoting oxidative stress, inflammation, and protein aggregation. However, simvastatin treatment, especially when started early, mitigated the alcohol effects by improving the redox state, suppressing apoptosis, and promoting autophagy and neurogenesis.
Lu et al., 2020. [109]	Thirty-eight-week-old male Wistar rats were fed either an ethanol-containing liquid diet or an isocaloric pair-feeding control	Chronic ethanol exposure led to liver damage, increased inflammatory cytokines, and impaired autophagy. However, mice fed a diet containing fish oil had improved autophagic activity and were protected against ethanol-induced liver injury by inhibiting the Akt signaling pathway.
Hwang et al., 2017. [110]	Male (4~5 months old, 26–27 g) wild-type (WT) C57BL/6 mice and Park2 KO mice. Within 10 days, ethanol comprised 35.8% of the total calories consumed.	Ethanol exposure in Park2 KO mice exacerbated dopaminergic neurodegeneration by increasing reactive oxygen species, mitochondrial dysfunction, and pro-apoptotic protein expression while inhibiting autophagy and mitochondrial function through p38 kinase activation.
Uguz et al., 2024. [99]	Wistar albino female rats (weighing between 250 and 350 g and 8–12 weeks old) were exposed to ethanol (20% *v/v*) via oral gavage, at a total volume of 2 mL and a dose of 4.5 g/kg body weight for 4 weeks	Chronic alcohol exposure leads to increased oxidative stress, altered autophagy signaling in the hippocampus and cortex, and impaired learning ability in offspring. Sex differences were observed, with female mice outperforming males in learning tasks. The expressed levels of IBA1, LC3B, GAD65, and mGluR5 were higher in female rats with chronic alcohol exposure.

Table 2. *Cont.*

First Author, Year	Models and Methods	Summary of Effects
Pla et al., 2014. [111]	Male 7-week-old C57BL/6 WT and TLR4 knockout (KO, TLR4$^{-/-}$) mice weighing 18–20 g were maintained with water (WT and KO control) or water containing 10% (v/v) ethanol, and solid diet ad libitum for 4 months	Ethanol exposure downregulated p62 and other autophagic proteins while further impairing autophagy through inducing the formation of autophagic vacuoles with greater volume density. After alcohol exposure, inhibitor of mTOR, rapamycin administration partially reduced neuroinflammation. TLR4 is upstream in the mTOR activation cascade. Alcohol exposure caused little or no changes in mTOR phosphorylation and the autophagy pathway in TLR4-KO mice.
Bian et al., 2022. [39]	Female Kunming mice exposed to ethanol (4 g/kg/d) or saline for 28 days in the absence or presence of Puerarin (25, 50, or 100 mg/kg, ip)	Ethanol exposure caused cognitive impairment with elevation of p-mTOR/mTOR and suppressed autophagy marker proteins. The middle and high doses of Puerarin prevented these changes and improved cognitive function.
Chen et al., 2024. [112]	Young (3-month-old) and aged (23-month-old) male mice exposed to Gao's chronic+binge alcohol paradigm or chronic ethanol liquid diet for 4 weeks	Chronic alcohol exposure decreased in the levels of hippocampal transcription factor EB (TFEB), which regulates the expression of lysosomal autophagy-related genes, and spatial memory while increasing the levels of apoptotic cells and aggregated phosphorylated-Tau proteins in young mice but not in aged mice. Thus, natural aging has a greater impact on the rates of autophagic influx and spatial memory decline in mice than chronic alcohol exposure.
Luo et al., 2014. [9] (REVIEW)		Chronic ethanol exposure in mice activated mTOR signaling, leading to impaired autophagy and increased oxidative stress, which exacerbated neuronal vulnerability and neurodegeneration.

Table 2. *Cont.*

First Author, Year	Models and Methods	Summary of Effects
Kurhaluk et al., 2020. [102] (REVIEW)	Melatonin treatment	Ethanol exposure likely caused melatonin suppression, leading to desynchronosis (circadian disruption). The circadian timing system can also be related to an altered drinking behavior or ethanol response. Alcohol can alter the circadian rhythm and pace making functions of the suprachiasmatic nuclei. Chronic alcohol consumption also led to a depletion of the critical antioxidant GSH and reduction in the GSH/GSSG redox state. Alcohol exposure also elevated plasma endotoxin levels and activated the hepatic endotoxin signaling cascade. These alcohol-mediated changes could be mitigated by melatonin treatment.
Fujii et al., 2021. [104] (REVIEW)	Mice exposed to water containing 10% (*v*/*v*) ethanol for 5 months	Chronic ethanol exposure increased TLR4 signaling, which results in activation of caspase-1, NLRP3 inflammasomes, and production of IL-1β and IL-18 to induce pyroptosis (cell death).

Table 3. Autophagy in alcohol-exposed cell culture models—neurons, microglia, or astrocytes.

First Author, Year	Models and Methods	Summary of Effects
Wang et al., 2023. [113]	Mouse microglia BV-2 cells were treated with different doses of alcohol (0.5 mg/mL, 4 mg/mL, and 10 mg/mL) for 3 h or 12 h, respectively	Alcohol exposure in microglia BV-2 cells disrupted autophagy and promoted apoptosis.
Wu et al., 2012. [114]	HepG2 E47 cells which express CYP2E1 and HepG2 C34 cells which do not contain CYP2E1 were treated with 100 mM ethanol for 8 days. Some cells were also treated with 3-methyladenine (MA, 2.5 mM) or rapamycin (0.2 µg/mL) or Chlormethiazole (CMZ, a CYP2E1 inhibitor, 100 µM) or N-acetylcysteine (NAC, an ROS scavenger, 5 mM).	Ethanol treatment increased fat accumulation and oxidant stress but decreased autophagy in E47 HepG2 cells. These results suggest that ethanol-mediated oxidative stress inhibits autophagy.

Table 3. *Cont.*

First Author, Year	Models and Methods	Summary of Effects
Flores-Bellver et al., 2014. [115]	Human retinal pigment epithelial cell line ARPE-19; cells were treated for 24 h at different ethanol concentrations: 80, 200, 400, and 600 mM	Chronic ethanol exposure increased autophagy flux and mitochondrial fragmentation in ARPE-19 cells. Autophagy served as a protective factor in the cells by degrading damaged mitochondria and lowering lipid peroxidation products, such as 4-HNE, although the ethanol concentrations were unphysiologically high.
Bonet-Ponce et al., 2015. [116]	Human retinal pigment epithelial ARPE-19 cells were treated for 24 h with ethanol	Ethanol exposure induced mitochondrial fission and activated autophagy through Drp1 and OPA1 in ARPE-19 cells. Autophagy served a cytoprotective role by removing damaged mitochondria, while mitochondrial ROS drove the autophagic response.
Yan et al., 2022. [41]	Human neuroblastoma SH-SY5Y cells, acetaldehyde exposure	Acetaldehyde-induced cytotoxicity in SH-SY5Y cells triggered oxidative stress and excessive mitophagy. Increased levels of ATGs and mitochondrial degradation were observed after exposure.
Chen et al., 2012. [97]	Human neuroblastoma SH-SY5Y cells obtained from ATCC, 0.4% ethanol	Ethanol exposure caused decreased cell viability and increased oxidative stress, with the involvement of the mTOR pathway in mediating these effects.
You et al., 2024. [117]	Pheochromocytoma line 12 (PC12) cells	Ethanol exposure in PC12 neuronal cells induced mitochondrial fragmentation and dysfunction, activating autophagy during degeneration. PGC-1α-mediated mitochondrial biogenesis was crucial for neurite regrowth and cell survival, which allowed for recovery from this ethanol-induced damage.
Pla et al., 2016. [118]	Cultured astroglial cells, ethanol (50 mM) 0–24 h Cultured neuronal cells, ethanol (50 mM) 0–24 h	In astrocytes, ethanol induces overexpression of several autophagy markers (ATG12, LC3-II, CTSB, and lysosomal cathepsin B) induced via TLR4 pathways. An increased amount of lysosomes in the WT astrocytes created a basification of lysosomal pH and lowered phosphorylation levels of autophagy inhibitor mTOR, along with activation of complexes beclin-1 and ULK1.

Table 3. *Cont.*

First Author, Year	Models and Methods	Summary of Effects
Wang et al., 2023. [113]	Microglia BV-2 cells	Modest alcohol consumption activated autophagy. Chronic exposure induced organelle damage, oxidative stress, and affected autophagy function, leading to apoptosis.
Luo et al., 2014. [9] (REVIEW)	Cultured fetal cortical neurons	Ethanol exposure modulated autophagy through pathways involving mTOR and AMP-activated kinase (AMPK), resulting in oxidative stress and endoplasmic reticulum stress triggering neurotoxic effects.
Yang et al., 2015. [103] (REVIEW)	SH-SY5Y neuroblastoma cells and primary cerebellar granule neurons	Exacerbated ER stress (GRP78, CHOP, ATF4, ATF6, and phosphorylated PERK and EIF2a) was observed when ethanol was combined with tunicamycin or thapsigargin. Antioxidants such as GSH and NAC improved ethanol's stimulation of ER stress and cell death.
Fujii et al., 2021. [104] (REVIEW)	Microglia and monocytic cell line Neuronal cell line Neuroblastoma cell line with a phosphatase inhibitor (Salubrinal)	Mitochondrial ROS specifically induce NLRP3 but not NLRC4. Ethanol exposure caused Golgi fragmentation and disruption of protein transport between ER and Golgi. Ethanol was seen to cause compaction of the Golgi apparatus and interrupt normal neurite growth in developing neurons. Co-administration of Salubrinal with ethanol further exacerbated accumulation of amyloid beta.
Guo et al., 2023. [119] (REVIEW)	Microglia, human peripheral blood mononuclear cells, and the murine macrophage cell line J774	Ethanol may regulate the levels of specific miRNAs, subsequently controlling microglia activation. Ethanol exposure also increased oxidative stress, observed through elevated levels of mitochondrial ROS and inflammatory cytokines like IL-1β, with mitochondrial damage and ROS accumulation contributing to NLRP3 inflammasome activation, particularly in macrophages and microglia.

Table 3. *Cont.*

First Author, Year	Models and Methods	Summary of Effects
Aki et al., 2013. [120] (REVIEW)	Neuronal SH-SY5Y cells Various cell lines, ethanol exposure with rapamycin or wortmannin	Ethanol induced mitophagy by suppressing the mTOR pathway and increasing ROS generation, contributing to neuronal damage and stress. Autophagy reduced apoptosis caused by ethanol. The autophagy inducer rapamycin alleviates while the autophagy inhibitor wortmannin aggravates ethanol-induced apoptosis.

Table 4. Autophagy in humans with alcohol use disorder.

First Author, Year	Models and Methods	Summary of Effects
Kurhaluk et al., 2020. [102] (REVIEW)	Melatonin treatment	Chronic alcohol intoxication depleted the tissue resources of the pineal gland and leads to marked disturbances in its function. Chronic ethanol exposure also resulted in functional and structural changes in the nervous system that have been associated with learning and memory impairment. Alcohol administration significantly increased lipid and protein oxidation and decreased the activities of antioxidant enzymes.
De Ternay et al., 2019. [105] (REVIEW)	Cannabidiol (CBD)	CBD was protective against alcohol-related liver steatosis and brain damage (cognitive impairment) in individuals with AUD by reducing oxidative stress and stimulating autophagy.
Aki et al., 2013. [120] (REVIEW)		Chronic alcohol intake caused an increase in autophagy in the brain.

3.3.2. Effects of Increased Oxidative Stress on ER Stress and Neuronal Damage

Under increased oxidative and nitrosative stress, we expect that many oxidative PTMs, such as disulfide oxidation, mixed disulfide formation with glutathione, S-nitrosylation, nitration, phosphorylation, acetylation, and protein-adducts, including acetaldehyde-adducts [121–124], can take place. These oxidative PTMs can take place in virtually all subcellular organelles of the cytoplasm, ER, mitochondria, and nuclei, contributing to accumulation of oxidatively-modified and/or misfolded proteins, ER stress [125], mitochondrial dysfunction, and epigenetic regulations [126], respectively. Increased oxidative/nitrosative stress and subsequent PTMs also cause blood–brain barrier (BBB) destruction, neuroinflammation, and neurotoxicity [127–130]. For instance, daily ethanol exposures increased the levels of AGE-albumin [131], histone modifications [132], nitration or acrolein-adducts [133], phosphorylated Tau proteins [134], and amyloid beta accumulation with cognitive impairments [134–136].

Reticulophagy is a specific autophagy process where damaged ER with misfolded proteins is engulfed and then degraded by lysosomes. The damaged ER with many misfolded proteins under oxidative stress can result from inactivation of many ER chaperone proteins such as Hsp90, Grp78, and protein disulfide isomerase (PDI). Under normal conditions, these chaperone proteins are responsible for various modifications like glycosylation and disulfide formation for proper folding of their client proteins. However, these chaperone proteins can also be oxidatively modified, and their functions or activities become inhibited under oxidative stress conditions after exposure to alcohol or other neurotoxic agents. For instance, nitration of Hsp90 caused its inactivation, leading to death of motor neurons [137]. Phosphorylation of Grp78 became inactivated in the transformed cells, contributing to suppression of glycosylation with decreased binding with its client protein immunoglobulin heavy chains [138], ER stress with protein misfolding, and cellular damage [139,140]. In the case of alcohol exposure, PDI becomes oxidatively modified [141] and inactivated [142] (Moon KH et al. [122], unpublished results), possibly resulting in decreased binding with or misfolding of the substrate proteins, ultimately contributing to chronic liver disease or neurodegeneration, as extensively reviewed [143].

3.3.3. Effects of Increased Oxidative Stress on Mitophagy and Neuronal Damage

Special autophagy in mitochondria (mitophagy) is known to protect against oxidative stress, mitochondrial dysfunction, inflammation, and aging-related diseases since it not only removes damaged mitochondria but also regulates the rates of neuroinflammation and cognitive deficits [97,112,144–146]. Earlier reports showed that Parkin, an E3 ubiquitin ligase, is involved in removing damaged mitochondria [147], while PINK1 (PTEN-induced putative serine/threonine kinase 1) is stabilized on damaged mitochondria to stimulate Parkin, which regulates the cell quality control system by breaking down unneeded or damaged proteins [148]. Thus, PINK1-KO or Parkin-KO mice are thought to have impaired mitophagy compared to the wild-type (WT) mice, and these KO mice become more sensitive to mitochondrial dysfunction and tissue injury caused by alcohol [38,110,149] and other potentially other neurotoxic agents [150]. Additionally, Lin et al. recently showed that chronic alcohol exposure promoted impairment of both receptor-mediated and PINK1-related mitophagy in the medial prefrontal cortex, leading to elevated NLRP3-related neuroinflammation and cognitive decline in C57BL6/J mice through suppression of an antioxidant transcription factor nuclear factor erythroid 2-related factor 2 (NRf2) [40]. In this report, si-RNA mediated silencing of PINK1 or BNIP3 caused mitochondrial dysfunction and alcohol-induced neuroinflammation in BV2 microglial cells. However, treatment with RTA-408, an NRF2 activator, attenuated NLRP3-related neuroinflammation and mitophagy suppression, leading to improvement of alcohol-mediated cognitive dysfunction. These results indicate that alcohol-mediated oxidative stress plays an important role in suppressing mitophagy, which leads to NLRP3 neuroinflammation and cognitive impairment in mice.

In contrast, acetaldehyde induces mitophagic responses with elevated levels of PINK1, Parkin (a member of the E3 ubiquitin ligase, cell quality control system by breaking down unneeded or damaged proteins), resulting in mitochondrial dysfunction and decreased mitochondrial mass, and cytotoxicity in acetaldehyde-exposed SH-SY5Y cells. In this case, the levels of LC3-II, Beclin1, autophagy-related protein Atg5, and Atg16L1 were elevated, while p62 levels were decreased. However, treatment with an autophagy inhibitor such as chloroquine and 3-methyladenine (3-MA), or an antioxidant NAC, prevented decreased mitochondrial mass, suggesting a role of oxidative stress in acetaldehyde-mediated excessive mitophagy [41].

3.3.4. Effects of Increased Oxidative Stress on Neuroinflammation, NETosis, and Neuronal Damage

Excessive alcohol intake also causes neuroinflammation and NETosis in the brain through alterations of the functions of neutrophils. Neutrophils are white blood cells that play a pivotal role in innate and adaptive immunity, wound healing, the resolution of inflammation, and fight against infection from various pathogens [151,152]. The polymorphonuclear neutrophils (PMNs) are involved in several types of non-inflammatory events, e.g., senescence, apoptosis, and efferocytosis [153–155], as well as inflammatory processes, e.g., necroptosis, ferroptosis, and necrosis [156–158], including NETosis [159], while they defend the host against the inflammatory threat or infection. In many organs, especially in the brain, these types of cell death can contribute to secondary brain damage by causing a high-grade neuroinflammation.

Like other types of cell death, NETosis is also modulated by autophagy/mitophagy [154,155]. It also mediates a few molecular pathways through the oxidative stress, which activates signaling molecules such as NF-κB, NADPH oxidase, Protein Kinase C (PKC), cytokines (IL-1β, IL-8, and HMGB1), anti-neutrophilic cytoplasmic autoantibody (ANCA), all-trans-retinoic acid (ATRA), transient receptor potential channel M2 (TRPM2), etc. [160,161].

More importantly, autophagy regulates the formation of NETs/NETosis. During NETosis, autophagy can manipulate neutrophil cell death to resolve the inflammation in several organs by regulating neutrophil degranulation, differentiation, metabolism, and the formation of neutrophil extracellular traps (NETs) against the pathogens and dreadful stimuli. The active steps and sequence of events in the molecular pathways that occur during the coordination between the autophagy and induction of NETs/NETosis are very crucial in deciding the fate of the cells in which the mTOR/REDD1 (regulation in development and DNA damage response 1) pathway is the central regulator of autophagy in these granulocytes [162]. It has been shown that internal stimuli within the neutrophils activate the protein-arginine deiminase 4 (PAD4) enzyme, which is a common mediator in multiple signaling pathways, controlling the execution of the formation of NETs and occurrence of NETosis. In contrast, inhibition of the PAD4 enzyme significantly blocks the process of NETosis [163]. Alcohol can induce and inhibit autophagy/mitophagy, which modulates the formation of NETs and regulation of NETosis in various organs including the brain, depending on the severity of acute or chronic conditions, amounts of alcohol consumption, and host conditions. The autophagy process in neutrophils regulates not only neutrophil metabolism during granulopoiesis but also the formation of NETs and NETosis, which are closely associated with neuroinflammation and neuronal injury.

This section updates the advancement of the relationship between autophagy and not only intrinsic changes in neutrophil per se but also extrinsic regulation of the events, involving NETs formation/NETosis in response to acute and chronic alcohol consumption. For example, alcohol-exposed neutrophils produce several inflammatory danger molecules in their intracellular space as well as around their microenvironment in the brain. These pro-inflammatory environment prime neutrophils to form NETs/NETosis, which leads to autophagy-mediated generation of ROS and superoxide from NADPH oxidase activity, degranulation, and an increase in calcium levels to activate the PAD4 enzyme, influencing myeloperoxidase/elastase and histone citrullination activities for epigenetic regulation. Thus, understanding the molecular and cellular mechanisms involving the processes of autophagy and the formation of NETs/NETosis will identify potential targets to develop anti-alcohol drugs for clinical application and provide treatment options to patients with alcohol misuse.

3.3.5. Effects of Increased Oxidative Stress on Autophagy and Neuronal Damage by Regulating the Cell Signaling Pathways

As mentioned before, chronic or binge alcohol intake causes oxidative stress, leading to neuroinflammation and organ damage mainly through suppressing antioxidants and defensive enzymes with activation of pro-oxidant proteins and mitochondrial dysfunction possibly by oxidative PTMs. Alcohol-mediated oxidative stress can alter the activities of many protein kinases and phosphatases that are involved in the cell signaling pathways by the regulation of many proteins in ER stress, neuroinflammation, neurogenesis, and neurotoxicity [164–169]. For instance, the activities of mTOR kinase, AMPK/mTOR, PI3K/Akt/mTOR, mitogen activated protein kinases, PKC isoforms, and GSK-3β, known to be directly and indirectly involved in the regulation of autophagy-related proteins and genes, including ATG12, LC3-II, Beclin-1, p62, and Bcl-2 (Figure 1), are modulated by alcohol-mediated oxidative stress [101,170–176]. Furthermore, ethanol exposure can activate the TLR4-NF-κB-cytokines pathway, which can lead to impaired autophagy accompanied by elevated neuroinflammation and neuronal injury [101,111,118,135]. Although the underlying mechanisms by which ethanol-mediated oxidative stress can alter the rates of autophagy and neuronal injury are incompletely understood, the changes in autophagy responses seem to be dependent on the patterns of ethanol exposure such as the frequency, amount, and acute or chronic alcohol intake as well as nutritional status of the host cells/tissues.

3.4. Potential Therapeutic Agents Against Autophagy in Alcohol-Exposed Brains

Alcohol is eliminated from the brain much more slowly than from other organs, and alcohol accumulates in the largest amount in brain tissue compared to other organs [102]. Current medications for AUD are insufficiently effective, highlighting the need for novel highly effective therapies [177,178]. Autophagy plays an important role in neurodegenerative diseases [179], and modulating autophagy by melatonin or its precursor as a therapeutic strategy offers a promising potential against alcohol-related brain damage.

Since autophagy exhibits both a protective mechanism and a damage pathway related to programmed cell death [180], we and others have reported that autophagy can be a double-edged sword in the context of stroke-induced brain injury [180] and aging-related neurodegenerative diseases [179], as well as alcohol-mediated brain damage [181]. On one side, autophagy provides a protective mechanism against alcohol-induced brain damage, and ethanol treatment increased mTOR activity and decreased expression of several ATG genes including Atg12, Atg5, p62/SQSTM1, and LC3 [10]. In this case, autophagy enhancers/inducers likely enhance autophagic flux in alcohol-exposed brains by clearing damaged organelles or misfolded proteins. In contrast, we and others have reported that autophagy acts as a double-edged sword, contributing to brain damage, as seen in the context of stroke-induced brain injury [180,182] and alcohol-related brain damage [181]. Ethanol exposure enhances autophagy markers like Map1lc3-II (LC3-II) and Beclin-1 expression while decreasing SQSTM1 (p62) expression in the brain, liver, and neuroblastoma cells [97,183].

This dual nature of autophagy presents opportunities for targeted therapies. Enhancing autophagy with enhancers/inducers can protect against alcohol-induced brain damage, while inhibitors may mitigate harmful autophagy activation. In addition, targeting molecular pathways such as mTOR, AMPK, and PI3K/Akt/mTOR offers promising therapeutic strategies [102,170–176]. This review discusses potential therapeutic agents for modulating autophagy in alcohol-exposed brains, as exemplified in Tables 5–7.

Table 5. Autophagy enhancers/inducers/mitophagy activators.

Compound	Classification	Summary of Effects
Rapamycin	An mTOR Complex 1 (mTORC1) inhibitor	Rapamycin restores autophagic flux, preventing ethanol-induced cell death and vascular plasticity [32]. Rapamycin inhibits ethanol neonatal effect and normalizes NMDA receptor changes in the hippocampus, the prefrontal cortex, and the striatum of the brain of adult rats [184]. Rapamycin mitigates FASD-related behavioral deficits, improving spatial learning and reducing vulnerability to alcohol addiction [184]. Rapamycin also enhances LC3 lipidation and protects neurons from apoptosis. Inhibition of mTOR by rapamycin restores the levels of p62 and partly re-establishes the LC3-II levels in the prefrontal cortices of ethanol-treated mice [100]. Rapamycin restores mitophagy [97].
Spermidine	Upregulates the expression of autophagy promoting genes, (e.g., ATG5) Modulates the NMDA receptor	Spermidine can reverse the suppression of autophagy-promoting genes caused by oxidative damage and mitochondrial dysfunction. Spermidine facilitates the reinstatement of AUD-induced conditioned place preference/conditioned place preference, involving the polyamine binding site at the NMDA receptor [185].
Metformin	Autophagy enhancer	Metformin provides antioxidant, anti-inflammatory, and neuroprotective effects. Metformin promotes autophagy by increasing autophagosome formation, as evidenced by elevated LC3-II levels. Metformin increases autophagy in the brain by activating AMP-activated protein kinase (AMPK), which subsequently inhibits the mTOR signaling pathway, thereby triggering the process of autophagy [186]. Metformin decreases the expression of p62 in the brain, which is a marker of impaired autophagy, suggesting that metformin promotes autophagy by reducing p62 accumulation in brain tissues [187]. Metformin boosts mitophagy, protecting against alcohol-induced tissue injury [188].

Table 6. Autophagy inhibitors.

Compound	Classification	Summary of Effects
Bafilomycin A1 (BafA1)	Inhibitor of autophagosome and lysosome fusion It is a macrolide antibiotic that inhibits the later stages of autophagy	Bafilomycin A1 inhibits lysosomal acidification [189]. Ethanol exposure increases the p62 levels, while BafA1 potentiates ethanol-increased LC3 lipidation [97]. As the inhibitor of autophagy, ethanol exposure impeded the upregulation of LC3 II induced by BafA1 [40].
Piracetam	Nootropic drug Derived from neurotransmitter γ-aminobutyric acid	Piracetam prevents ethanol-induced memory loss by increasing hippocampus long-term potentiation (LPT) and inhibiting hippocampus neuronal apoptosis. Piracetam reduces ethanol-induced neuronal damage by regulation of autophagic action. In more detail, piracetam decreases ethanol-induced LC3-II and Beclin-1 expression, increases the phosphorylation of mTOR, and inhibits Akt phosphorylation [190].

Table 7. Selective modulators.

Compound	Classification	Summary of Effects
Erythropoietin (EPO)	Glycoprotein hormone	Intranasally administered EPO promotes remyelination and synapse formation in chronic alcohol-affected neocortex and hippocampus [191]. Exogenous recombinant human rhEPO, which enters the cerebrum of the brain through the intranasal route, activates the EPO receptor and the downstream ERKs and PI3K/AKT signaling and significantly suppresses autophagy-related degradation of NRf2 [191]. These results, thus, highlight autophagy-related Nrf2 activity as the key mechanism mediating the neuroprotective effects of EPO [191].
Wortmannin	Autophagy inhibitor	Wortmannin blocks the formation of autophagosomes and inhibits the PI3K/Akt pathway [192]. Wortmannin attenuates ethanol-promoted LC3 lipidation and LC3 puncta [97]. Wortmannin reverses increased phosphorylation of the PI3K-Akt-GSK3β-CREB pathway during alcohol withdrawal [193].
RTA-408 (omaveloxolone)	NrF2 activator	RTA-408 ameliorates chronic alcohol exposure-induced cognitive impairment by modulating mitophagy in the medial prefrontal cortex of C57BL/6J mice in vivo [40]. RTA-408 improves cognitive impairment in neonatal mice via reducing the apoptosis of hippocampal neurons and activating Nrf2 [194].

Table 7. *Cont.*

Compound	Classification	Summary of Effects
Cannabidiol (CBD)	Natural component of cannabis	CBD stimulates autophagy in vitro and in vivo, leading to alleviation of lipid accumulation [105]. CBD stimulates autophagy signaling transduction though crosstalk between the ERK1/2 and AKT kinases [195]. CBD's neuroprotective, immunomodulatory, and antioxidant properties could prevent or alleviate some alcohol-related brain damage [105].
Hydrogen disulfide (H_2S)	A gasotransmitter [196]	H_2S protects against ethanol-mediated oxidative stress, enhanced ER stress, neuronal damage, and neurotoxicity [125]. H_2S improves spatial memory impairment via increases in BDNF expression and hippocampal neurogenesis in early postnatal alcohol-exposed rat pups [197].

In addition, many other naturally occurring polyphenol flavonoids and NRF2 activator sulforaphane can prevent oxidative stress, leading to activation of autophagy and improvement of alcohol-associated liver injury, as extensively reviewed [198]. Since many small-molecule plant-derived polyphenols or flavonoids, like quercetin, luteolin, rutin, berberine, and curcumin, are known to have antioxidant effects and pass through the BBB [199–208], they can also be used for protecting against alcohol-mediated oxidative stress, impaired autophagy, and neurotoxicity.

4. Conclusions

In this review, we have briefly described various types of alcohol-mediated brain injury and neurodegeneration, literature search methods, alcohol metabolism in the brain, sources of oxidative stress, general properties and types of autophagy, and potential translational approaches against alcohol-mediated brain damage by regulating the rates of autophagy. However, as we emphasized, the rates of autophagy or mitophagy are differentially affected, depending on the pattern (binge or chronic) of alcohol intake, nutritional status, and other environmental and genetic factors, all of which affect various cell signaling pathways. Similar factors and underlying mechanisms for impaired autophagy and mitophagy with accumulation of damaged, aggregated proteins, and neuronal damage can be induced by various neurotoxic agents and aging-related neurodegenerative disease states [202–207]. A key distinction between alcohol-mediated brain damage and other neurodegenerative diseases could be the selective activation of CYP2E1 by alcohol, since CYP2E1 is not induced by aging-related neurodegeneration. Regardless of distinguished pathophysiological conditions, one common factor could be increased oxidative stress (Figure 1), which will negatively affect the downstream autophagic processes, leading to impaired autophagy and neurodegeneration. Due to the complexity of autophagy regulations, further molecular studies are warranted. For instance, we expect to see additional studies on oxidative PTMs of the individual proteins involved in the different steps of autophagy and their functional alterations. Based on the molecular mechanistic studies on alcohol-mediated autophagy regulations, additional therapeutic agents against alcohol-induced neurotoxicity as well as other brain diseases can be identified and developed for clinical usage in the future.

Author Contributions: Literature search, writing original draft, and revisions, L.R.-L.; writing and editing, M.A.S.K. and X.W.; conceptualization, writing original draft, and revisions, B.-J.S. All authors have read and agreed to the published version of the manuscript.

Funding: This work was partially supported by the Intramural Research Fund (to BJS; ZIA-AA000036-38) of the National Institute of Alcohol Abuse and Alcoholism (NIAAA). In addition, MASK and XW were supported by R21AA029925 and R21AA030087 grants, respectively, from the NIAAA.

Conflicts of Interest: All authors have declared no conflicts of interest.

Abbreviations

The following abbreviations are used in this manuscript:

AUD	Alcohol use disorder
FASD	Fetal alcohol spectrum disorders
ROS	Reactive oxygen species
4-HNE	4-hydroxynonenal
MDA	Malondialdehyde
ER	Endoplasmic reticulum
ETC	Electron transport chain
CYP2E1	Cytochrome P450-2E1
PTMs	Post-translational protein modifications
ATGs	Autophagy-related proteins
ADH	Alcohol dehydrogenase
ALDH2	Aldehyde dehydrogenase-2
FAEEs	Fatty acid ethyl esters
CNS	Central nervous system
DHA	Docosahexaenoic acid
EPA	Eicosapentaenoic acid
GSH	Glutathione, reduced
SOD	Superoxide dismutase
H_2O_2	Hydrogen peroxide
PD#	Postnatal day #
WT	Wild-type
KO	Knockout
PC12	Pheochromocytoma line 12 cells
AMPK	AMP-activated kinase
PKC	Protein Kinase C
CBD	Cannabidiol
BBB	Blood–brain barrier
PDI	Protein disulfide isomerase
PINK1	PTEN-induced putative serine/threonine kinase 1
NRf2	Nuclear factor erythroid 2-related factor 2
3-MA	3-methyladenine
PMNs	Polymorphonuclear neutrophils
ANCA	Anti-neutrophilic cytoplasmic autoantibody
ATRA	All-trans-retinoic acid
TRPM2	Transient receptor potential channel M2
REDD1	Regulated in development and DNA damage response 1
NETs	Neutrophil extracellular traps
PAD4	Protein-arginine deiminase 4
BafA1	Bafilomycin A1
EPO	Erythropoietin
H_2S	Hydrogen disulfide

References

1. Alcohol Use Disorder (AUD) in the United States: Age Groups and Demographic Characteristics. Available online: https://www.niaaa.nih.gov/alcohols-effects-health/alcohol-topics/alcohol-facts-and-statistics/alcohol-use-disorder-aud-united-states-age-groups-and-demographic-characteristics (accessed on 21 November 2024).
2. Medical Complications: Common Alcohol-Related Concerns. Available online: https://www.niaaa.nih.gov/health-professionals-communities/core-resource-on-alcohol/medical-complications-common-alcohol-related-concerns (accessed on 21 November 2024).
3. Eva, L.; Brehar, F.M.; Florian, I.A.; Covache-Busuioc, R.A.; Costin, H.P.; Dumitrascu, D.I.; Bratu, B.G.; Glavan, L.A.; Ciurea, A.V. Neuropsychiatric and Neuropsychological Aspects of Alcohol-Related Cognitive Disorders: An In-Depth Review of Wernicke's Encephalopathy and Korsakoff's Syndrome. *J. Clin. Med.* **2023**, *12*, 6101. [CrossRef] [PubMed]
4. Anton, P.E.; Rutt, L.N.; Kaufman, M.L.; Busquet, N.; Kovacs, E.J.; McCullough, R.L. Binge ethanol exposure in advanced age elevates neuroinflammation and early indicators of neurodegeneration and cognitive impairment in female mice. *Brain Behav. Immun.* **2024**, *116*, 303–316. [CrossRef] [PubMed]
5. Crews, F.T.; Coleman, L.G., Jr.; Macht, V.A.; Vetreno, R.P. Alcohol, HMGB1, and Innate Immune Signaling in the Brain. *Alcohol Res.* **2024**, *44*, 4. [CrossRef]
6. Popova, S.; Charness, M.E.; Burd, L.; Crawford, A.; Hoyme, H.E.; Mukherjee, R.A.S.; Riley, E.P.; Elliott, E.J. Fetal alcohol spectrum disorders. *Nat. Rev. Dis. Prim.* **2023**, *9*, 11. [CrossRef]
7. Mattson, S.N.; Bernes, G.A.; Doyle, L.R. Fetal Alcohol Spectrum Disorders: A Review of the Neurobehavioral Deficits Associated with Prenatal Alcohol Exposure. *Alcohol. Clin. Exp. Res.* **2019**, *43*, 1046–1062. [CrossRef] [PubMed]
8. Understanding Fetal Alcohol Spectrum Disorders. Available online: https://www.niaaa.nih.gov/publications/brochures-and-fact-sheets/understanding-fetal-alcohol-spectrum-disorders (accessed on 21 November 2024).
9. Luo, J. Autophagy and ethanol neurotoxicity. *Autophagy* **2014**, *10*, 2099–2108. [CrossRef]
10. Li, Y.; Wang, S.; Ni, H.M.; Huang, H.; Ding, W.X. Autophagy in alcohol-induced multiorgan injury: Mechanisms and potential therapeutic targets. *Biomed Res. Int.* **2014**, *2014*, 498491. [CrossRef]
11. Zhang, C.; Chen, H.; Rodriguez, Y.; Ma, X.; Swerdlow, R.H.; Zhang, J.; Ding, W.X. A perspective on autophagy and transcription factor EB in Alcohol-Associated Alzheimer's disease. *Biochem. Pharmacol.* **2023**, *213*, 115576. [CrossRef]
12. Wu, D.; Cederbaum, A.I. Alcohol, oxidative stress, and free radical damage. *Alcohol Res. Health* **2003**, *27*, 277–284.
13. Dlugos, C.A. ATF6 and caspase 12 expression in Purkinje neurons in acute slices from adult, ethanol-fed rats. *Brain Res.* **2014**, *1577*, 11–20. [CrossRef]
14. Comporti, M.; Signorini, C.; Leoncini, S.; Gardi, C.; Ciccoli, L.; Giardini, A.; Vecchio, D.; Arezzini, B. Ethanol-induced oxidative stress: Basic knowledge. *Genes Nutr.* **2010**, *5*, 101–109. [CrossRef]
15. Das, S.K.; Hiran, K.R.; Mukherjee, S.; Vasudevan, D.M. Oxidative stress is the primary event: Effects of ethanol consumption in brain. *Indian J. Clin. Biochem.* **2007**, *22*, 99–104. [CrossRef] [PubMed]
16. Zima, T.; Fialova, L.; Mestek, O.; Janebova, M.; Crkovska, J.; Malbohan, I.; Stipek, S.; Mikulikova, L.; Popov, P. Oxidative stress, metabolism of ethanol and alcohol-related diseases. *J. Biomed. Sci.* **2001**, *8*, 59–70. [CrossRef] [PubMed]
17. Hoek, J.B.; Pastorino, J.G. Ethanol, oxidative stress, and cytokine-induced liver cell injury. *Alcohol* **2002**, *27*, 63–68. [CrossRef] [PubMed]
18. Preiser, J.C. Oxidative stress. *JPEN J. Parenter. Enter. Nutr.* **2012**, *36*, 147–154. [CrossRef]
19. Gonzalez, H.C.; Misare, K.R.; Mendenhall, T.T.; Wolf, B.J.; Mulholland, P.J.; Gordon, K.L.; Hartman, J.H. Transgenic expression of human cytochrome P450 2E1 in C. elegans and rat PC-12 cells sensitizes to ethanol-induced locomotor and mitochondrial effects. *Biochem. Biophys. Res. Commun.* **2024**, *734*, 150735. [CrossRef]
20. Robin, M.A.; Sauvage, I.; Grandperret, T.; Descatoire, V.; Pessayre, D.; Fromenty, B. Ethanol increases mitochondrial cytochrome P450 2E1 in mouse liver and rat hepatocytes. *FEBS Lett.* **2005**, *579*, 6895–6902. [CrossRef]
21. LeFort, K.R.; Rungratanawanich, W.; Song, B.J. Contributing roles of mitochondrial dysfunction and hepatocyte apoptosis in liver diseases through oxidative stress, post-translational modifications, inflammation, and intestinal barrier dysfunction. *Cell. Mol. Life Sci.* **2024**, *81*, 34. [CrossRef]
22. Marchetti, B. Nrf2/Wnt resilience orchestrates rejuvenation of glia-neuron dialogue in Parkinson's disease. *Redox Biol.* **2020**, *36*, 101664. [CrossRef]
23. Li, H.; Lismont, C.; Revenco, I.; Hussein, M.A.F.; Costa, C.F.; Fransen, M. The Peroxisome-Autophagy Redox Connection: A Double-Edged Sword? *Front. Cell Dev. Biol.* **2021**, *9*, 814047. [CrossRef]
24. Thapa, R.; Ahmad Bhat, A.; Shahwan, M.; Ali, H.; PadmaPriya, G.; Bansal, P.; Rajotiya, S.; Barwal, A.; Siva Prasad, G.V.; Pramanik, A.; et al. Proteostasis disruption and senescence in Alzheimer's disease pathways to neurodegeneration. *Brain Res.* **2024**, *1845*, 149202. [CrossRef] [PubMed]
25. Ji, C. Advances and New Concepts in Alcohol-Induced Organelle Stress, Unfolded Protein Responses and Organ Damage. *Biomolecules* **2015**, *5*, 1099–1121. [CrossRef] [PubMed]

26. Allen, S.L.; Quinlan, J.I.; Dhaliwal, A.; Armstrong, M.J.; Elsharkawy, A.M.; Greig, C.A.; Lord, J.M.; Lavery, G.G.; Breen, L. Sarcopenia in chronic liver disease: Mechanisms and countermeasures. *Am. J. Physiol. Gastrointest. Liver Physiol.* **2021**, *320*, G241–G257. [CrossRef]
27. Pierson, S.R.; Kolling, L.J.; James, T.D.; Pushpavathi, S.G.; Marcinkiewcz, C.A. Serotonergic dysfunction may mediate the relationship between alcohol consumption and Alzheimer's disease. *Pharmacol. Res.* **2024**, *203*, 107171. [CrossRef]
28. Barmaki, H.; Nourazarian, A.; Khaki-Khatibi, F. Proteostasis and neurodegeneration: A closer look at autophagy in Alzheimer's disease. *Front. Aging Neurosci.* **2023**, *15*, 1281338. [CrossRef]
29. Yun, H.R.; Jo, Y.H.; Kim, J.; Shin, Y.; Kim, S.S.; Choi, T.G. Roles of Autophagy in Oxidative Stress. *Int. J. Mol. Sci.* **2020**, *21*, 3289. [CrossRef] [PubMed]
30. Palmer, J.E.; Wilson, N.; Son, S.M.; Obrocki, P.; Wrobel, L.; Rob, M.; Takla, M.; Korolchuk, V.I.; Rubinsztein, D.C. Autophagy, aging, and age-related neurodegeneration. *Neuron* **2025**, *113*, 29–48. [CrossRef]
31. Zhang, Z.; Yang, X.; Song, Y.Q.; Tu, J. Autophagy in Alzheimer's disease pathogenesis: Therapeutic potential and future perspectives. *Ageing Res. Rev.* **2021**, *72*, 101464. [CrossRef]
32. Girault, V.; Gilard, V.; Marguet, F.; Lesueur, C.; Hauchecorne, M.; Ramdani, Y.; Laquerriere, A.; Marret, S.; Jegou, S.; Gonzalez, B.J.; et al. Prenatal alcohol exposure impairs autophagy in neonatal brain cortical microvessels. *Cell Death Dis.* **2017**, *8*, e2610. [CrossRef]
33. Wang, L.; Cui, J. Palmitoylation promotes chaperone-mediated autophagic degradation of NLRP3 to modulate inflammation. *Autophagy* **2023**, *19*, 2821–2823. [CrossRef]
34. He, C.; Klionsky, D.J. Regulation mechanisms and signaling pathways of autophagy. *Annu. Rev. Genet.* **2009**, *43*, 67–93. [CrossRef] [PubMed]
35. Tamargo-Gomez, I.; Fernandez, A.F.; Marino, G. Pathogenic Single Nucleotide Polymorphisms on Autophagy-Related Genes. *Int. J. Mol. Sci.* **2020**, *21*, 8196. [CrossRef] [PubMed]
36. Wei, X.; Manandhar, L.; Kim, H.; Chhetri, A.; Hwang, J.; Jang, G.; Park, C.; Park, R. Pexophagy and Oxidative Stress: Focus on Peroxisomal Proteins and Reactive Oxygen Species (ROS) Signaling Pathways. *Antioxidants* **2025**, *14*, 126. [CrossRef] [PubMed]
37. Ye, M.; Chen, Y.; Liu, Z.; Wang, Y.; Yi, C. Detection of ribophagy in yeast and mammals. *Biophys. Rep.* **2024**, *10*, 82–101. [CrossRef]
38. Peng, H.; Qin, X.; Chen, S.; Ceylan, A.F.; Dong, M.; Lin, Z.; Ren, J. Parkin deficiency accentuates chronic alcohol intake-induced tissue injury and autophagy defects in brain, liver and skeletal muscle. *Acta Biochim. Biophys. Sin. (Shanghai)* **2020**, *52*, 665–674. [CrossRef]
39. Bian, H.; Wu, Y.; Cui, Z.; Zheng, H.; Li, Y.; Zou, D. Study on the autophagy-related mechanism of puerarin in improving the cognitive impairment induced by alcohol in female mice. *Brain Inj.* **2022**, *36*, 137–145. [CrossRef]
40. Lin, X.; Wang, H.; Zou, L.; Yang, B.; Chen, W.; Rong, X.; Zhang, X.; He, L.; Li, X.; Peng, Y. The NRF2 activator RTA-408 ameliorates chronic alcohol exposure-induced cognitive impairment and NLRP3 inflammasome activation by modulating impaired mitophagy initiation. *Free Radic. Biol. Med.* **2024**, *220*, 15–27. [CrossRef]
41. Yan, T.; Zhao, Y.; Jiang, Z.; Chen, J. Acetaldehyde Induces Cytotoxicity via Triggering Mitochondrial Dysfunction and Overactive Mitophagy. *Mol. Neurobiol.* **2022**, *59*, 3933–3946. [CrossRef]
42. Munoz-Gamez, J.A.; Rodriguez-Vargas, J.M.; Quiles-Perez, R.; Aguilar-Quesada, R.; Martin-Oliva, D.; de Murcia, G.; Menissier de Murcia, J.; Almendros, A.; Ruiz de Almodovar, M.; Oliver, F.J. PARP-1 is involved in autophagy induced by DNA damage. *Autophagy* **2009**, *5*, 61–74. [CrossRef]
43. Xu, X.; Sun, B.; Zhao, C. Poly (ADP-Ribose) polymerase 1 and parthanatos in neurological diseases: From pathogenesis to therapeutic opportunities. *Neurobiol. Dis.* **2023**, *187*, 106314. [CrossRef]
44. Lieber, C.S. Metabolism of alcohol. *Clin. Liver Dis.* **2005**, *9*, 1–35. [CrossRef] [PubMed]
45. Cederbaum, A.I. Alcohol metabolism. *Clin. Liver Dis.* **2012**, *16*, 667–685. [CrossRef]
46. Lieber, C.S. Microsomal ethanol-oxidizing system (MEOS): The first 30 years (1968–1998)—A review. *Alcohol. Clin. Exp. Res.* **1999**, *23*, 991–1007. [CrossRef]
47. Lu, Y.; Cederbaum, A.I. CYP2E1 and oxidative liver injury by alcohol. *Free Radic. Biol. Med.* **2008**, *44*, 723–738. [CrossRef]
48. Harjumaki, R.; Pridgeon, C.S.; Ingelman-Sundberg, M. CYP2E1 in Alcoholic and Non-Alcoholic Liver Injury. Roles of ROS, Reactive Intermediates and Lipid Overload. *Int. J. Mol. Sci.* **2021**, *22*, 8221. [CrossRef] [PubMed]
49. Laposata, E.A.; Lange, L.G. Presence of nonoxidative ethanol metabolism in human organs commonly damaged by ethanol abuse. *Science* **1986**, *231*, 497–499. [CrossRef]
50. Isenberg, K.E.; Bora, P.S.; Zhou, X.; Wu, X.; Moore, B.W.; Lange, L.G. Nonoxidative ethanol metabolism: Expression of fatty acid ethyl ester synthase-III in cultured neural cells. *Biochem. Biophys. Res. Commun.* **1992**, *185*, 938–943. [CrossRef] [PubMed]
51. Werner, J.; Saghir, M.; Fernandez-del Castillo, C.; Warshaw, A.L.; Laposata, M. Linkage of oxidative and nonoxidative ethanol metabolism in the pancreas and toxicity of nonoxidative ethanol metabolites for pancreatic acinar cells. *Surgery* **2001**, *129*, 736–744. [CrossRef]

52. Roy, T.S.; Sharma, V.; Seidler, F.J.; Slotkin, T.A. Quantitative morphological assessment reveals neuronal and glial deficits in hippocampus after a brief subtoxic exposure to chlorpyrifos in neonatal rats. *Brain Res. Dev. Brain Res.* **2005**, *155*, 71–80. [CrossRef]
53. Rungratanawanich, W.; Qu, Y.; Wang, X.; Essa, M.M.; Song, B.J. Advanced glycation end products (AGEs) and other adducts in aging-related diseases and alcohol-mediated tissue injury. *Exp. Mol. Med.* **2021**, *53*, 168–188. [CrossRef]
54. Park, S.H.; Seo, W.; Xu, M.J.; Mackowiak, B.; Lin, Y.; He, Y.; Fu, Y.; Hwang, S.; Kim, S.J.; Guan, Y.; et al. Ethanol and its Nonoxidative Metabolites Promote Acute Liver Injury by Inducing ER Stress, Adipocyte Death, and Lipolysis. *Cell. Mol. Gastroenterol. Hepatol.* **2023**, *15*, 281–306. [CrossRef]
55. Estonius, M.; Svensson, S.; Hoog, J.O. Alcohol dehydrogenase in human tissues: Localisation of transcripts coding for five classes of the enzyme. *FEBS Lett.* **1996**, *397*, 338–342. [CrossRef] [PubMed]
56. Zimatkin, S.M.; Deitrich, R.A. Ethanol metabolism in the brain. *Addict. Biol.* **1997**, *2*, 387–400. [CrossRef] [PubMed]
57. Vasiliou, V.; Ziegler, T.L.; Bludeau, P.; Petersen, D.R.; Gonzalez, F.J.; Deitrich, R.A. CYP2E1 and catalase influence ethanol sensitivity in the central nervous system. *Pharmacogenetics Genom.* **2006**, *16*, 51–58. [CrossRef]
58. Zimatkin, S.M.; Pronko, S.P.; Vasiliou, V.; Gonzalez, F.J.; Deitrich, R.A. Enzymatic mechanisms of ethanol oxidation in the brain. *Alcohol. Clin. Exp. Res.* **2006**, *30*, 1500–1505. [CrossRef] [PubMed]
59. Warner, M.; Gustafsson, J.A. Effect of ethanol on cytochrome P450 in the rat brain. *Proc. Natl. Acad. Sci. USA* **1994**, *91*, 1019–1023. [CrossRef]
60. Upadhya, S.C.; Tirumalai, P.S.; Boyd, M.R.; Mori, T.; Ravindranath, V. Cytochrome P4502E (CYP2E) in brain: Constitutive expression, induction by ethanol and localization by fluorescence in situ hybridization. *Arch. Biochem. Biophys.* **2000**, *373*, 23–34. [CrossRef]
61. Haorah, J.; Ramirez, S.H.; Floreani, N.; Gorantla, S.; Morsey, B.; Persidsky, Y. Mechanism of alcohol-induced oxidative stress and neuronal injury. *Free Radic. Biol. Med.* **2008**, *45*, 1542–1550. [CrossRef]
62. Montoliu, C.; Sancho-Tello, M.; Azorin, I.; Burgal, M.; Valles, S.; Renau-Piqueras, J.; Guerri, C. Ethanol increases cytochrome P4502E1 and induces oxidative stress in astrocytes. *J. Neurochem.* **1995**, *65*, 2561–2570. [CrossRef]
63. Montoliu, C.; Valles, S.; Renau-Piqueras, J.; Guerri, C. Ethanol-induced oxygen radical formation and lipid peroxidation in rat brain: Effect of chronic alcohol consumption. *J. Neurochem.* **1994**, *63*, 1855–1862. [CrossRef]
64. Tindberg, N.; Ingelman-Sundberg, M. Expression, catalytic activity, and inducibility of cytochrome P450 2E1 (CYP2E1) in the rat central nervous system. *J. Neurochem.* **1996**, *67*, 2066–2073. [CrossRef]
65. Zhong, Y.; Dong, G.; Luo, H.; Cao, J.; Wang, C.; Wu, J.; Feng, Y.Q.; Yue, J. Induction of brain CYP2E1 by chronic ethanol treatment and related oxidative stress in hippocampus, cerebellum, and brainstem. *Toxicology* **2012**, *302*, 275–284. [CrossRef] [PubMed]
66. Na, S.; Li, J.; Zhang, H.; Li, Y.; Yang, Z.; Zhong, Y.; Dong, G.; Yang, J.; Yue, J. The induction of cytochrome P450 2E1 by ethanol leads to the loss of synaptic proteins via PPARalpha down-regulation. *Toxicology* **2017**, *385*, 18–27. [CrossRef] [PubMed]
67. Luchtman, D.W.; Meng, Q.; Song, C. Ethyl-eicosapentaenoate (E-EPA) attenuates motor impairments and inflammation in the MPTP-probenecid mouse model of Parkinson's disease. *Behav. Brain Res.* **2012**, *226*, 386–396. [CrossRef] [PubMed]
68. Wen, M.; Ding, L.; Zhang, L.; Zhang, T.; Teruyoshi, Y.; Wang, Y.; Xue, C. Eicosapentaenoic Acid-Enriched Phosphatidylcholine Mitigated Abeta1-42-Induced Neurotoxicity via Autophagy-Inflammasome Pathway. *J. Agric. Food Chem.* **2019**, *67*, 13767–13774. [CrossRef]
69. Lange, L.G.; Sobel, B.E. Mitochondrial dysfunction induced by fatty acid ethyl esters, myocardial metabolites of ethanol. *J. Clin. Investig.* **1983**, *72*, 724–731. [CrossRef]
70. Zakhari, S. Overview: How is alcohol metabolized by the body? *Alcohol Res. Health* **2006**, *29*, 245–254. [PubMed]
71. Xu, Z.J.; Li, Q.; Ding, L.; Shi, H.H.; Xue, C.H.; Mao, X.Z.; Wang, Y.M.; Zhang, T.T. A comparative study of the effects of phosphatidylserine rich in DHA and EPA on Abeta-induced Alzheimer's disease using cell models. *Food Funct.* **2021**, *12*, 4411–4423. [CrossRef]
72. Puri, B.K.; Bydder, G.M.; Counsell, S.J.; Corridan, B.J.; Richardson, A.J.; Hajnal, J.V.; Appel, C.; McKee, H.M.; Vaddadi, K.S.; Horrobin, D.F. MRI and neuropsychological improvement in Huntington disease following ethyl-EPA treatment. *Neuroreport* **2002**, *13*, 123–126. [CrossRef]
73. Chaturvedi, R.K.; Flint Beal, M. Mitochondrial diseases of the brain. *Free Radic. Biol. Med.* **2013**, *63*, 1–29. [CrossRef]
74. Alrouji, M.; Al-Kuraishy, H.M.; Al-Gareeb, A.I.; Ashour, N.A.; Jabir, M.S.; Negm, W.A.; Batiha, G.E. Metformin role in Parkinson's disease: A double-sword effect. *Mol. Cell. Biochem.* **2024**, *479*, 975–991. [CrossRef] [PubMed]
75. Picca, A.; Faitg, J.; Auwerx, J.; Ferrucci, L.; D'Amico, D. Mitophagy in human health, ageing and disease. *Nat. Metab.* **2023**, *5*, 2047–2061. [CrossRef] [PubMed]
76. Madreiter-Sokolowski, C.T.; Hiden, U.; Krstic, J.; Panzitt, K.; Wagner, M.; Enzinger, C.; Khalil, M.; Abdellatif, M.; Malle, E.; Madl, T.; et al. Targeting organ-specific mitochondrial dysfunction to improve biological aging. *Pharmacol. Ther.* **2024**, *262*, 108710. [CrossRef] [PubMed]

77. Tapia-Rojas, C.; Carvajal, F.J.; Mira, R.G.; Arce, C.; Lerma-Cabrera, J.M.; Orellana, J.A.; Cerpa, W.; Quintanilla, R.A. Adolescent Binge Alcohol Exposure Affects the Brain Function Through Mitochondrial Impairment. *Mol. Neurobiol.* **2018**, *55*, 4473–4491. [CrossRef]
78. Leon, B.E.; Kang, S.; Franca-Solomon, G.; Shang, P.; Choi, D.S. Alcohol-Induced Neuroinflammatory Response and Mitochondrial Dysfunction on Aging and Alzheimer's Disease. *Front. Behav. Neurosci.* **2021**, *15*, 778456. [CrossRef]
79. Jamali, Z.; Salimi, A.; Garmabi, B.; Khezri, S.; Khaksari, M. Hesperidin Protects Alcohol-Induced Mitochondrial Abnormalities via the Inhibition of Oxidative Stress and MPT Pore Opening in Newborn Male Rats as a Fetal Alcohol Syndrome Model. *J. Stud. Alcohol Drugs* **2024**, *85*, 361–370. [CrossRef]
80. Karadayian, A.G.; Lombardi, P.; Bustamante, J.; Lores-Arnaiz, S. Alcohol hangover effects on brain cortex non-synaptic mitochondria and synaptosomes bioenergetics. *Alcohol* **2019**, *77*, 113–123. [CrossRef]
81. Mira, R.G.; Lira, M.; Quintanilla, R.A.; Cerpa, W. Alcohol consumption during adolescence alters the hippocampal response to traumatic brain injury. *Biochem. Biophys. Res. Commun.* **2020**, *528*, 514–519. [CrossRef]
82. Alvear, T.F.; Farias-Pasten, A.; Vergara, S.A.; Prieto-Villalobos, J.; Silva-Contreras, A.; Fuenzalida, F.A.; Quintanilla, R.A.; Orellana, J.A. Hemichannels contribute to mitochondrial Ca^{2+} and morphology alterations evoked by ethanol in astrocytes. *Front. Cell Dev. Biol.* **2024**, *12*, 1434381. [CrossRef]
83. Khatoon, R.; Fick, J.; Elesinnla, A.; Waddell, J.; Kristian, T. Sexual Dimorphism of Ethanol-Induced Mitochondrial Dynamics in Purkinje Cells. *Int. J. Mol. Sci.* **2024**, *25*, 13714. [CrossRef]
84. Dasuri, K.; Nguyen, A.; Zhang, L.; Fernandez-Kim, O.S.; Bruce-Keller, A.J.; Blalock, B.A.; Cabo, R.D.; Keller, J.N. Comparison of rat liver and brain proteasomes for oxidative stress-induced inactivation: Influence of ageing and dietary restriction. *Free Radic. Res.* **2009**, *43*, 28–36. [CrossRef]
85. Cobley, J.N.; Fiorello, M.L.; Bailey, D.M. 13 reasons why the brain is susceptible to oxidative stress. *Redox Biol.* **2018**, *15*, 490–503. [CrossRef] [PubMed]
86. Aoyama, K. Glutathione in the Brain. *Int. J. Mol. Sci.* **2021**, *22*, 5010. [CrossRef] [PubMed]
87. Gage, F.H.; Temple, S. Neural stem cells: Generating and regenerating the brain. *Neuron* **2013**, *80*, 588–601. [CrossRef] [PubMed]
88. Jessberger, S. Stem Cell-Mediated Regeneration of the Adult Brain. *Transfus. Med. Hemother.* **2016**, *43*, 321–326. [CrossRef]
89. Hansson, T.; Tindberg, N.; Ingelman-Sundberg, M.; Kohler, C. Regional distribution of ethanol-inducible cytochrome P450 IIE1 in the rat central nervous system. *Neuroscience* **1990**, *34*, 451–463. [CrossRef]
90. Zimatkin, S.M.; Rout, U.K.; Koivusalo, M.; Buhler, R.; Lindros, K.O. Regional distribution of low-Km mitochondrial aldehyde dehydrogenase in the rat central nervous system. *Alcohol. Clin. Exp. Res.* **1992**, *16*, 1162–1167. [CrossRef]
91. Sinet, P.M.; Heikkila, R.E.; Cohen, G. Hydrogen peroxide production by rat brain in vivo. *J. Neurochem.* **1980**, *34*, 1421–1428. [CrossRef]
92. Qin, L.; He, J.; Hanes, R.N.; Pluzarev, O.; Hong, J.S.; Crews, F.T. Increased systemic and brain cytokine production and neuroinflammation by endotoxin following ethanol treatment. *J. Neuroinflammation* **2008**, *5*, 10. [CrossRef]
93. Qin, L.; Crews, F.T. NADPH oxidase and reactive oxygen species contribute to alcohol-induced microglial activation and neurodegeneration. *J. Neuroinflammation* **2012**, *9*, 5. [CrossRef]
94. Qin, L.; Vetreno, R.P.; Crews, F.T. NADPH oxidase and endoplasmic reticulum stress is associated with neuronal degeneration in orbitofrontal cortex of individuals with alcohol use disorder. *Addict. Biol.* **2023**, *28*, e13262. [CrossRef]
95. Yan, T.; Zhao, Y. Acetaldehyde induces phosphorylation of dynamin-related protein 1 and mitochondrial dysfunction via elevating intracellular ROS and Ca^{2+} levels. *Redox Biol.* **2020**, *28*, 101381. [CrossRef] [PubMed]
96. Alimov, A.; Wang, H.; Liu, M.; Frank, J.A.; Xu, M.; Ou, X.; Luo, J. Expression of autophagy and UPR genes in the developing brain during ethanol-sensitive and resistant periods. *Metab. Brain Dis.* **2013**, *28*, 667–676. [CrossRef] [PubMed]
97. Chen, G.; Ke, Z.; Xu, M.; Liao, M.; Wang, X.; Qi, Y.; Zhang, T.; Frank, J.A.; Bower, K.A.; Shi, X.; et al. Autophagy is a protective response to ethanol neurotoxicity. *Autophagy* **2012**, *8*, 1577–1589. [CrossRef]
98. Boschen, K.E.; Steensen, M.C.; Simon, J.M.; Parnell, S.E. Short-term transcriptomic changes in the mouse neural tube induced by an acute alcohol exposure. *Alcohol* **2023**, *106*, 1–9. [CrossRef]
99. Uguz, A.C.; Okan, A.; Doganyigit, Z.; Yilmaz, S.; Ates, S.; Arikan Soylemez, E.S.; Karabulut, S.; Kumru, A.S.; Espino, J. Evaluation of TRPM2 Channel-Mediated Autophagic Signaling Pathway in Hippocampus and Cortex Tissues of Rat Offspring Following Prenatal Exposure to Elevated Alcohol Levels. *Environ. Toxicol.* **2024**, *40*, 222–244. [CrossRef]
100. Montesinos, J.; Pascual, M.; Millan-Esteban, D.; Guerri, C. Binge-like ethanol treatment in adolescence impairs autophagy and hinders synaptic maturation: Role of TLR4. *Neurosci. Lett.* **2018**, *682*, 85–91. [CrossRef]
101. Pascual, M.; Lopez-Hidalgo, R.; Montagud-Romero, S.; Urena-Peralta, J.R.; Rodriguez-Arias, M.; Guerri, C. Role of mTOR-regulated autophagy in spine pruning defects and memory impairments induced by binge-like ethanol treatment in adolescent mice. *Brain Pathol.* **2021**, *31*, 174–188. [CrossRef]
102. Kurhaluk, N.; Tkachenko, H. Melatonin and alcohol-related disorders. *Chronobiol. Int.* **2020**, *37*, 781–803. [CrossRef]
103. Yang, F.; Luo, J. Endoplasmic Reticulum Stress and Ethanol Neurotoxicity. *Biomolecules* **2015**, *5*, 2538–2553. [CrossRef]

104. Fujii, C.; Zorumski, C.F.; Izumi, Y. Ethanol, neurosteroids and cellular stress responses: Impact on central nervous system toxicity, inflammation and autophagy. *Neurosci. Biobehav. Rev.* **2021**, *124*, 168–178. [CrossRef] [PubMed]
105. De Ternay, J.; Naassila, M.; Nourredine, M.; Louvet, A.; Bailly, F.; Sescousse, G.; Maurage, P.; Cottencin, O.; Carrieri, P.M.; Rolland, B. Therapeutic Prospects of Cannabidiol for Alcohol Use Disorder and Alcohol-Related Damages on the Liver and the Brain. *Front. Pharmacol.* **2019**, *10*, 627. [CrossRef] [PubMed]
106. Sumitomo, A.; Ueta, K.; Mauchi, S.; Hirai, K.; Horike, K.; Hikida, T.; Sakurai, T.; Sawa, A.; Tomoda, T. Ulk1 protects against ethanol-induced neuronal stress and cognition-related behavioral deficits. *Neurosci. Res.* **2017**, *117*, 54–61. [CrossRef]
107. Davis-Anderson, K.L.; Wesseling, H.; Siebert, L.M.; Lunde-Young, E.R.; Naik, V.D.; Steen, H.; Ramadoss, J. Fetal regional brain protein signature in FASD rat model. *Reprod. Toxicol.* **2018**, *76*, 84–92. [CrossRef]
108. Nasef, N.A.; Keshk, W.A.; El-Meligy, S.M.; Allah, A.A.A.; Ibrahim, W.M. Modulatory effect of simvastatin on redox status, caspase-3 expression, p-protein kinase B (p-Akt), and brain-derived neurotrophic factor (BDNF) in an ethanol-induced neurodegeneration model. *Can. J. Physiol. Pharmacol.* **2021**, *99*, 478–489. [CrossRef]
109. Lu, N.S.; Chiu, W.C.; Chen, Y.L.; Peng, H.C.; Shirakawa, H.; Yang, S.C. Fish oil up-regulates hepatic autophagy in rats with chronic ethanol consumption. *J. Nutr. Biochem.* **2020**, *77*, 108314. [CrossRef]
110. Hwang, C.J.; Kim, Y.E.; Son, D.J.; Park, M.H.; Choi, D.Y.; Park, P.H.; Hellstrom, M.; Han, S.B.; Oh, K.W.; Park, E.K.; et al. Parkin deficiency exacerbate ethanol-induced dopaminergic neurodegeneration by P38 pathway dependent inhibition of autophagy and mitochondrial function. *Redox Biol.* **2017**, *11*, 456–468. [CrossRef]
111. Pla, A.; Pascual, M.; Renau-Piqueras, J.; Guerri, C. TLR4 mediates the impairment of ubiquitin-proteasome and autophagy-lysosome pathways induced by ethanol treatment in brain. *Cell Death Dis.* **2014**, *5*, e1066. [CrossRef]
112. Chen, H.; Hinz, K.; Zhang, C.; Rodriguez, Y.; Williams, S.N.; Niu, M.; Ma, X.; Chao, X.; Frazier, A.L.; McCarson, K.E.; et al. Late-Life Alcohol Exposure Does Not Exacerbate Age-Dependent Reductions in Mouse Spatial Memory and Brain TFEB Activity. *Biomolecules* **2024**, *14*, 1537. [CrossRef]
113. Wang, L.; Song, L.; Ma, J.; Wang, H.; Li, Y.; Huang, D. Alcohol induces apoptosis and autophagy in microglia BV-2 cells. *Food Chem. Toxicol.* **2023**, *177*, 113849. [CrossRef]
114. Wu, D.; Wang, X.; Zhou, R.; Yang, L.; Cederbaum, A.I. Alcohol steatosis and cytotoxicity: The role of cytochrome P4502E1 and autophagy. *Free Radic. Biol. Med.* **2012**, *53*, 1346–1357. [CrossRef]
115. Flores-Bellver, M.; Bonet-Ponce, L.; Barcia, J.M.; Garcia-Verdugo, J.M.; Martinez-Gil, N.; Saez-Atienzar, S.; Sancho-Pelluz, J.; Jordan, J.; Galindo, M.F.; Romero, F.J. Autophagy and mitochondrial alterations in human retinal pigment epithelial cells induced by ethanol: Implications of 4-hydroxy-nonenal. *Cell Death Dis.* **2014**, *5*, e1328. [CrossRef] [PubMed]
116. Bonet-Ponce, L.; Saez-Atienzar, S.; da Casa, C.; Flores-Bellver, M.; Barcia, J.M.; Sancho-Pelluz, J.; Romero, F.J.; Jordan, J.; Galindo, M.F. On the mechanism underlying ethanol-induced mitochondrial dynamic disruption and autophagy response. *Biochim. Biophys. Acta* **2015**, *1852*, 1400–1409. [CrossRef] [PubMed]
117. You, W.; Knoops, K.; Berendschot, T.; Benedikter, B.J.; Webers, C.A.B.; Reutelingsperger, C.P.M.; Gorgels, T. PGC-1a mediated mitochondrial biogenesis promotes recovery and survival of neuronal cells from cellular degeneration. *Cell Death Discov.* **2024**, *10*, 180. [CrossRef]
118. Pla, A.; Pascual, M.; Guerri, C. Autophagy Constitutes a Protective Mechanism against Ethanol Toxicity in Mouse Astrocytes and Neurons. *PLoS ONE* **2016**, *11*, e0153097. [CrossRef]
119. Guo, M.L.; Roodsari, S.K.; Cheng, Y.; Dempsey, R.E.; Hu, W. Microglia NLRP3 Inflammasome and Neuroimmune Signaling in Substance Use Disorders. *Biomolecules* **2023**, *13*, 922. [CrossRef]
120. Aki, T.; Funakoshi, T.; Unuma, K.; Uemura, K. Impairment of autophagy: From hereditary disorder to drug intoxication. *Toxicology* **2013**, *311*, 205–215. [CrossRef]
121. Cho, Y.E.; Song, B.J. Pomegranate prevents binge alcohol-induced gut leakiness and hepatic inflammation by suppressing oxidative and nitrative stress. *Redox Biol.* **2018**, *18*, 266–278. [CrossRef]
122. Song, B.J.; Abdelmegeed, M.A.; Henderson, L.E.; Yoo, S.H.; Wan, J.; Purohit, V.; Hardwick, J.P.; Moon, K.H. Increased nitroxidative stress promotes mitochondrial dysfunction in alcoholic and nonalcoholic fatty liver disease. *Oxidative Med. Cell. Longev.* **2013**, *2013*, 781050. [CrossRef]
123. Song, B.J.; Akbar, M.; Abdelmegeed, M.A.; Byun, K.; Lee, B.; Yoon, S.K.; Hardwick, J.P. Mitochondrial dysfunction and tissue injury by alcohol, high fat, nonalcoholic substances and pathological conditions through post-translational protein modifications. *Redox Biol.* **2014**, *3*, 109–123. [CrossRef] [PubMed]
124. Choi, Y.; Abdelmegeed, M.A.; Song, B.J. Preventive effects of indole-3-carbinol against alcohol-induced liver injury in mice via antioxidant, anti-inflammatory, and anti-apoptotic mechanisms: Role of gut-liver-adipose tissue axis. *J. Nutr. Biochem.* **2018**, *55*, 12–25. [CrossRef] [PubMed]
125. George, A.K.; Behera, J.; Kelly, K.E.; Zhai, Y.; Tyagi, N. Hydrogen sulfide, endoplasmic reticulum stress and alcohol mediated neurotoxicity. *Brain Res. Bull.* **2017**, *130*, 251–256. [CrossRef]

126. Rungratanawanich, W.; Ballway, J.W.; Wang, X.; Won, K.J.; Hardwick, J.P.; Song, B.J. Post-translational modifications of histone and non-histone proteins in epigenetic regulation and translational applications in alcohol-associated liver disease: Challenges and research opportunities. *Pharmacol. Ther.* **2023**, *251*, 108547. [CrossRef]
127. Novochadlo, M.; Goldim, M.P.; Bonfante, S.; Joaquim, L.; Mathias, K.; Metzker, K.; Machado, R.S.; Lanzzarin, E.; Bernades, G.; Bagio, E.; et al. Folic acid alleviates the blood brain barrier permeability and oxidative stress and prevents cognitive decline in sepsis-surviving rats. *Microvasc. Res.* **2021**, *137*, 104193. [CrossRef] [PubMed]
128. Sun, L.; Yang, L.; Xu, Y.W.; Liang, H.; Han, J.; Zhao, R.J.; Cheng, Y. Neuroprotection of hydroxysafflor yellow A in the transient focal ischemia: Inhibition of protein oxidation/nitration, 12/15-lipoxygenase and blood-brain barrier disruption. *Brain Res.* **2012**, *1473*, 227–235. [CrossRef]
129. Kim, Y.; Cho, A.Y.; Kim, H.C.; Ryu, D.; Jo, S.A.; Jung, Y.S. Effects of Natural Polyphenols on Oxidative Stress-Mediated Blood-Brain Barrier Dysfunction. *Antioxidants* **2022**, *11*, 197. [CrossRef]
130. Kim, S.; Jung, U.J.; Kim, S.R. Role of Oxidative Stress in Blood-Brain Barrier Disruption and Neurodegenerative Diseases. *Antioxidants* **2024**, *13*, 1462. [CrossRef]
131. Byun, K.; Bayarsaikhan, D.; Bayarsaikhan, E.; Son, M.; Oh, S.; Lee, J.; Son, H.I.; Won, M.H.; Kim, S.U.; Song, B.J.; et al. Microglial AGE-albumin is critical in promoting alcohol-induced neurodegeneration in rats and humans. *PLoS ONE* **2014**, *9*, e104699. [CrossRef]
132. Jarmasz, J.S.; Stirton, H.; Basalah, D.; Davie, J.R.; Clarren, S.K.; Astley, S.J.; Del Bigio, M.R. Global DNA Methylation and Histone Posttranslational Modifications in Human and Nonhuman Primate Brain in Association with Prenatal Alcohol Exposure. *Alcohol. Clin. Exp. Res.* **2019**, *43*, 1145–1162. [CrossRef]
133. Ray, B.; Rungratanawanich, W.; LeFort, K.R.; Chidambaram, S.B.; Song, B.J. Mitochondrial Aldehyde Dehydrogenase 2 (ALDH2) Protects against Binge Alcohol-Mediated Gut and Brain Injury. *Cells* **2024**, *13*, 927. [CrossRef]
134. Bailey, C.S.; Jagielo-Miller, J.E.; Keller, P.S.; Glaser, E.P.; Wilcox, A.L.; Prendergast, M.A. Ethanol sustains phosphorylated tau protein in the cultured neonatal rat hippocampus: Implications for fetal alcohol spectrum disorders. *Alcohol* **2022**, *103*, 45–54. [CrossRef] [PubMed]
135. Barnett, A.; David, E.; Rohlman, A.; Nikolova, V.D.; Moy, S.S.; Vetreno, R.P.; Coleman, L.G., Jr. Adolescent Binge Alcohol Enhances Early Alzheimer's Disease Pathology in Adulthood Through Proinflammatory Neuroimmune Activation. *Front. Pharmacol.* **2022**, *13*, 884170. [CrossRef] [PubMed]
136. D'Souza, Y.; Elharram, A.; Soon-Shiong, R.; Andrew, R.D.; Bennett, B.M. Characterization of Aldh2 (-/-) mice as an age-related model of cognitive impairment and Alzheimer's disease. *Mol. Brain* **2015**, *8*, 27. [CrossRef] [PubMed]
137. Franco, M.C.; Ye, Y.; Refakis, C.A.; Feldman, J.L.; Stokes, A.L.; Basso, M.; Melero Fernandez de Mera, R.M.; Sparrow, N.A.; Calingasan, N.Y.; Kiaei, M.; et al. Nitration of Hsp90 induces cell death. *Proc. Natl. Acad. Sci. USA* **2013**, *110*, E1102–E1111. [CrossRef]
138. Satoh, M.; Nakai, A.; Sokawa, Y.; Hirayoshi, K.; Nagata, K. Modulation of the phosphorylation of glucose-regulated protein, GRP78, by transformation and inhibition of glycosylation. *Exp. Cell Res.* **1993**, *205*, 76–83. [CrossRef]
139. Lugea, A.; Tischler, D.; Nguyen, J.; Gong, J.; Gukovsky, I.; French, S.W.; Gorelick, F.S.; Pandol, S.J. Adaptive unfolded protein response attenuates alcohol-induced pancreatic damage. *Gastroenterology* **2011**, *140*, 987–997. [CrossRef]
140. Wei, J.; Gu, X.; Wang, Y.; Wu, Y.; Yan, C. Two-dimensional separation system by on-line hyphenation of capillary isoelectric focusing with pressurized capillary electrochromatography for peptide and protein mapping. *Electrophoresis* **2011**, *32*, 230–237. [CrossRef]
141. Kim, B.J.; Hood, B.L.; Aragon, R.A.; Hardwick, J.P.; Conrads, T.P.; Veenstra, T.D.; Song, B.J. Increased oxidation and degradation of cytosolic proteins in alcohol-exposed mouse liver and hepatoma cells. *Proteomics* **2006**, *6*, 1250–1260. [CrossRef]
142. Carbone, D.L.; Doorn, J.A.; Kiebler, Z.; Petersen, D.R. Cysteine modification by lipid peroxidation products inhibits protein disulfide isomerase. *Chem. Res. Toxicol.* **2005**, *18*, 1324–1331. [CrossRef]
143. Imaoka, S. Chemical stress on protein disulfide isomerases and inhibition of their functions. *Int. Rev. Cell Mol. Biol.* **2011**, *290*, 121–166. [CrossRef]
144. Lemasters, J.J. Selective mitochondrial autophagy, or mitophagy, as a targeted defense against oxidative stress, mitochondrial dysfunction, and aging. *Rejuvenation Res.* **2005**, *8*, 3–5. [CrossRef] [PubMed]
145. Ding, W.X.; Yin, X.M. Mitophagy: Mechanisms, pathophysiological roles, and analysis. *Biol. Chem.* **2012**, *393*, 547–564. [CrossRef]
146. Ni, H.M.; Williams, J.A.; Ding, W.X. Mitochondrial dynamics and mitochondrial quality control. *Redox Biol.* **2015**, *4*, 6–13. [CrossRef] [PubMed]
147. Narendra, D.; Tanaka, A.; Suen, D.F.; Youle, R.J. Parkin is recruited selectively to impaired mitochondria and promotes their autophagy. *J. Cell Biol.* **2008**, *183*, 795–803. [CrossRef]
148. Narendra, D.P.; Jin, S.M.; Tanaka, A.; Suen, D.F.; Gautier, C.A.; Shen, J.; Cookson, M.R.; Youle, R.J. PINK1 is selectively stabilized on impaired mitochondria to activate Parkin. *PLoS Biol.* **2010**, *8*, e1000298. [CrossRef] [PubMed]

149. Paul, S.; Pickrell, A.M. Hidden phenotypes of PINK1/Parkin knockout mice. *Biochim. Biophys. Acta Gen. Subj.* **2021**, *1865*, 129871. [CrossRef]
150. Huo, S.; Zhang, X.; Xu, J.; Zhang, J.; Du, J.; Li, B.; Song, M.; Shao, B.; Li, Y.; Xu, F. Parkin-mediated mitophagy protects against aluminum trichloride-induced hippocampal apoptosis in mice via the mtROS-NLRP3 pathway. *Ecotoxicol. Environ. Saf.* **2023**, *264*, 115459. [CrossRef]
151. Rane, D.; Patil, T.; More, V.; Patra, S.S.; Bodhale, N.; Dandapat, J.; Sarkar, A. Neutrophils: Interplay between host defense, cellular metabolism and intracellular infection. *Cytokine* **2018**, *112*, 44–51. [CrossRef]
152. Awasthi, D.; Sarode, A. Neutrophils at the Crossroads: Unraveling the Multifaceted Role in the Tumor Microenvironment. *Int. J. Mol. Sci.* **2024**, *25*, 2929. [CrossRef]
153. Sun, J.K.; Wu, D.; Wong, G.C.; Lau, T.M.; Yang, M.; Hart, R.P.; Kwan, K.M.; Chan, H.Y.E.; Chow, H.M. Chronic alcohol metabolism results in DNA repair infidelity and cell cycle-induced senescence in neurons. *Aging Cell* **2023**, *22*, e13772. [CrossRef]
154. Huang, Y.; Flentke, G.R.; Rivera, O.C.; Saini, N.; Mooney, S.M.; Smith, S.M. Alcohol Exposure Induces Nucleolar Stress and Apoptosis in Mouse Neural Stem Cells and Late-Term Fetal Brain. *Cells* **2024**, *13*, 440. [CrossRef] [PubMed]
155. Bukong, T.N.; Cho, Y.; Iracheta-Vellve, A.; Saha, B.; Lowe, P.; Adejumo, A.; Furi, I.; Ambade, A.; Gyongyosi, B.; Catalano, D.; et al. Abnormal neutrophil traps and impaired efferocytosis contribute to liver injury and sepsis severity after binge alcohol use. *J. Hepatol.* **2018**, *69*, 1145–1154. [CrossRef] [PubMed]
156. Zhao, Y.; Zhang, R.; Wang, Z.; Chen, Z.; Wang, G.; Guan, S.; Lu, J. Melatonin Prevents against Ethanol-Induced Liver Injury by Mitigating Ferroptosis via Targeting Brain and Muscle ARNT-like 1 in Mice Liver and HepG2 Cells. *J. Agric. Food Chem.* **2022**, *70*, 12953–12967. [CrossRef]
157. Tamnanloo, F.; Chen, X.; Oliveira, M.M.; Tremblay, M.; Rose, C.F. Excessive intragastric alcohol administration exacerbates hepatic encephalopathy and provokes neuronal cell death in male rats with chronic liver disease. *J. Neurosci. Res.* **2024**, *102*, e25337. [CrossRef] [PubMed]
158. Thomson, A.D.; Pratt, O.E.; Jeyasingham, M.; Shaw, G.K. Alcohol and brain damage. *Hum. Toxicol.* **1988**, *7*, 455–463. [CrossRef]
159. Ortega-Ribera, M.; Zhuang, Y.; Babuta, M.; Brezani, V.; Joshi, R.S.; Zsengeller, Z.; Thevkar Nagesh, P.; Wang, Y.; Bronson, R.; Szabo, G. A Novel Multi-organ Male Model of Alcohol-induced Acute-on-chronic Liver Failure Reveals NET-mediated Hepatocellular Death, Which is Prevented by RIPK3 Inhibition. *Cell. Mol. Gastroenterol. Hepatol.* **2024**, *19*, 101446. [CrossRef]
160. Alfonso-Loeches, S.; Urena-Peralta, J.; Morillo-Bargues, M.J.; Gomez-Pinedo, U.; Guerri, C. Ethanol-Induced TLR4/NLRP3 Neuroinflammatory Response in Microglial Cells Promotes Leukocyte Infiltration Across the BBB. *Neurochem. Res.* **2016**, *41*, 193–209. [CrossRef]
161. Vorobjeva, N.; Dagil, Y.; Pashenkov, M.; Pinegin, B.; Chernyak, B. Protein kinase C isoforms mediate the formation of neutrophil extracellular traps. *Int. Immunopharmacol.* **2023**, *114*, 109448. [CrossRef]
162. Skendros, P.; Mitroulis, I.; Ritis, K. Autophagy in Neutrophils: From Granulopoiesis to Neutrophil Extracellular Traps. *Front. Cell Dev. Biol.* **2018**, *6*, 109. [CrossRef]
163. Tatsiy, O.; McDonald, P.P. Physiological Stimuli Induce PAD4-Dependent, ROS-Independent NETosis, With Early and Late Events Controlled by Discrete Signaling Pathways. *Front. Immunol.* **2018**, *9*, 2036. [CrossRef]
164. Kim, H.Y.; Huang, B.X.; Spector, A.A. Molecular and Signaling Mechanisms for Docosahexaenoic Acid-Derived Neurodevelopment and Neuroprotection. *Int. J. Mol. Sci.* **2022**, *23*, 4635. [CrossRef] [PubMed]
165. Yang, B.; Zhang, R.; Leong Bin Abdullah, M.F.I. The association between neuropsychiatric effects of substance use and occurrence of endoplasmic reticulum and unfolded protein response: A systematic review. *Toxicol. Lett.* **2024**, *391*, 71–85. [CrossRef] [PubMed]
166. Galan-Llario, M.; Rodriguez-Zapata, M.; Gramage, E.; Vicente-Rodriguez, M.; Fontan-Baselga, T.; Ovejero-Benito, M.C.; Perez-Garcia, C.; Carrasco, J.; Moreno-Herradon, M.; Sevillano, J.; et al. Receptor protein tyrosine phosphatase beta/zeta regulates loss of neurogenesis in the mouse hippocampus following adolescent acute ethanol exposure. *Neurotoxicology* **2023**, *94*, 98–107. [CrossRef]
167. Rodriguez-Zapata, M.; Galan-Llario, M.; Caneque-Rufo, H.; Sevillano, J.; Sanchez-Alonso, M.G.; Zapico, J.M.; Ferrer-Alcon, M.; Uribarri, M.; Pascual-Teresa, B.; Ramos-Alvarez, M.D.P.; et al. Implication of the PTN/RPTPbeta/zeta Signaling Pathway in Acute Ethanol Neuroinflammation in Both Sexes: A Comparative Study with LPS. *Biomedicines* **2023**, *11*, 1318. [CrossRef]
168. Galan-Llario, M.; Rodriguez-Zapata, M.; Fontan-Baselga, T.; Gramage, E.; Vicente-Rodriguez, M.; Zapico, J.M.; de Pascual-Teresa, B.; Lasek, A.W.; Herradon, G. Inhibition of RPTPbeta/zeta reduces chronic ethanol intake in adolescent mice and modulates ethanol effects on hippocampal neurogenesis and glial responses in a sex-dependent manner. *Neuropharmacology* **2023**, *227*, 109438. [CrossRef]
169. Wang, S.; Zhang, X.; Zhao, Y.; Lv, H.; Li, P.; Zhang, Z.; Qiao, X. BCI Improves Alcohol-Induced Cognitive and Emotional Impairments by Restoring pERK-BDNF. *J. Mol. Neurosci.* **2024**, *74*, 59. [CrossRef]
170. Huang, Y.; Flentke, G.R.; Smith, S.M. Alcohol induces p53-mediated apoptosis in neural crest by stimulating an AMPK-mediated suppression of TORC1, S6K, and ribosomal biogenesis. *Reprod. Toxicol.* **2024**, *130*, 108747. [CrossRef]

171. Liu, L.; Sun, T.; Xin, F.; Cui, W.; Guo, J.; Hu, J. Nerve Growth Factor Protects Against Alcohol-Induced Neurotoxicity in PC12 Cells via PI3K/Akt/mTOR Pathway. *Alcohol Alcohol.* **2017**, *52*, 12–18. [CrossRef]
172. Zyuz'kov, G.N.; Miroshnichenko, L.A.; Polyakova, T.Y.; Zhdanov, V.V.; Simanina, E.V.; Stavrova, L.A.; Churin, A.A.; Fomina, T.I. Role of MAPK ERK1/2 and p38 in the Regulation of Secretory Functions of Different Populations of Neuroglia in Ethanol-Induced Neurodegeneration. *Bull. Exp. Biol. Med.* **2021**, *171*, 699–703. [CrossRef]
173. Madaan, P.; Behl, T.; Sehgal, A.; Singh, S.; Sharma, N.; Yadav, S.; Kaur, S.; Bhatia, S.; Al-Harrasi, A.; Abdellatif, A.A.H.; et al. Exploring the Therapeutic Potential of Targeting Purinergic and Orexinergic Receptors in Alcoholic Neuropathy. *Neurotox. Res.* **2022**, *40*, 646–669. [CrossRef]
174. Behl, T.; Yadav, H.N.; Sharma, P.L. Alcoholic Neuropathy: Involvement of Multifaceted Signalling Mechanisms. *Curr. Mol. Pharmacol.* **2021**, *14*, 2–10. [CrossRef] [PubMed]
175. Zeng, T.; Zhang, C.L.; Song, F.Y.; Zhao, X.L.; Xie, K.Q. CMZ reversed chronic ethanol-induced disturbance of PPAR-alpha possibly by suppressing oxidative stress and PGC-1alpha acetylation, and activating the MAPK and GSK3beta pathway. *PLoS ONE* **2014**, *9*, e98658. [CrossRef]
176. Carabulea, A.L.; Janeski, J.D.; Naik, V.D.; Chen, K.; Mor, G.; Ramadoss, J. A multi-organ analysis of the role of mTOR in fetal alcohol spectrum disorders. *FASEB J.* **2023**, *37*, e22897. [CrossRef]
177. Rolland, B.; Paille, F.; Gillet, C.; Rigaud, A.; Moirand, R.; Dano, C.; Dematteis, M.; Mann, K.; Aubin, H.J. Pharmacotherapy for Alcohol Dependence: The 2015 Recommendations of the French Alcohol Society, Issued in Partnership with the European Federation of Addiction Societies. *CNS Neurosci. Ther.* **2016**, *22*, 25–37. [CrossRef]
178. Soyka, M.; Muller, C.A. Pharmacotherapy of alcoholism—An update on approved and off-label medications. *Expert. Opin. Pharmacother.* **2017**, *18*, 1187–1199. [CrossRef]
179. Luo, F.; Sandhu, A.F.; Rungratanawanich, W.; Williams, G.E.; Akbar, M.; Zhou, S.; Song, B.J.; Wang, X. Melatonin and Autophagy in Aging-Related Neurodegenerative Diseases. *Int. J. Mol. Sci.* **2020**, *21*, 7174. [CrossRef]
180. Zhou, H.; Wang, J.; Jiang, J.; Stavrovskaya, I.G.; Li, M.; Li, W.; Wu, Q.; Zhang, X.; Luo, C.; Zhou, S.; et al. N-acetyl-serotonin offers neuroprotection through inhibiting mitochondrial death pathways and autophagic activation in experimental models of ischemic injury. *J. Neurosci.* **2014**, *34*, 2967–2978. [CrossRef]
181. Li, C.; Li, J.; Xu, G.; Sun, H. Influence of Chronic Ethanol Consumption on Apoptosis and Autophagy Following Transient Focal Cerebral Ischemia in Male Mice. *Sci. Rep.* **2020**, *10*, 6164. [CrossRef]
182. Zhang, X.; Peng, B.; Zhang, S.; Wang, J.; Yuan, X.; Peled, S.; Chen, W.; Ding, J.; Li, W.; Zhang, A.; et al. The MT1 receptor as the target of ramelteon neuroprotection in ischemic stroke. *J. Pineal Res.* **2024**, *76*, e12925. [CrossRef]
183. Yang, Q.; Luo, C.; Zhang, X.; Liu, Y.; Wang, Z.; Cacciamani, P.; Shi, J.; Cui, Y.; Wang, C.; Sinha, B.; et al. Tartary buckwheat extract alleviates alcohol-induced acute and chronic liver injuries through the inhibition of oxidative stress and mitochondrial cell death pathway. *Am. J. Transl. Res.* **2020**, *12*, 70–89.
184. Lopatynska-Mazurek, M.; Antolak, A.; Grochecki, P.; Gibula-Tarlowska, E.; Bodzon-Kulakowska, A.; Listos, J.; Kedzierska, E.; Suder, P.; Silberring, J.; Kotlinska, J.H. Rapamycin Improves Spatial Learning Deficits, Vulnerability to Alcohol Addiction and Altered Expression of the GluN2B Subunit of the NMDA Receptor in Adult Rats Exposed to Ethanol during the Neonatal Period. *Biomolecules* **2021**, *11*, 650. [CrossRef]
185. Silva, A.A.; Henriques, G.d.M.; Nascimento-Rocha, V.; Dias-Júnior, B.C.; dos Anjos Santos, A.; Lima, A.J.O.; Marinho, E.A.V.; Rubin, M.A.; Mello, C.F. Spermidine prevents the reinstatement of alcohol conditioned place preference. *Addict. Neurosci.* **2023**, *9*, 100130. [CrossRef]
186. Gao, C.; Fang, L.; Zhang, H.; Zhang, W.S.; Li, X.O.; Du, S.Y. Metformin Induces Autophagy via the AMPK-mTOR Signaling Pathway in Human Hepatocellular Carcinoma Cells. *Cancer Manag. Res.* **2020**, *12*, 5803–5811. [CrossRef] [PubMed]
187. Chen, Y.; Zhao, S.; Fan, Z.; Li, Z.; Zhu, Y.; Shen, T.; Li, K.; Yan, Y.; Tian, J.; Liu, Z.; et al. Metformin attenuates plaque-associated tau pathology and reduces amyloid-beta burden in APP/PS1 mice. *Alzheimers Res. Ther.* **2021**, *13*, 40. [CrossRef]
188. Bergheim, I.; Guo, L.; Davis, M.A.; Lambert, J.C.; Beier, J.I.; Duveau, I.; Luyendyk, J.P.; Roth, R.A.; Arteel, G.E. Metformin prevents alcohol-induced liver injury in the mouse: Critical role of plasminogen activator inhibitor-1. *Gastroenterology* **2006**, *130*, 2099–2112. [CrossRef]
189. Redmann, M.; Benavides, G.A.; Berryhill, T.F.; Wani, W.Y.; Ouyang, X.; Johnson, M.S.; Ravi, S.; Barnes, S.; Darley-Usmar, V.M.; Zhang, J. Inhibition of autophagy with bafilomycin and chloroquine decreases mitochondrial quality and bioenergetic function in primary neurons. *Redox Biol.* **2017**, *11*, 73–81. [CrossRef]
190. Yang, Y.; Feng, J.; Xu, F.; Wang, J. Piracetam inhibits ethanol (EtOH)-induced memory deficit by mediating multiple pathways. *Brain Res.* **2017**, *1676*, 83–90. [CrossRef]
191. Nie, X.; Wang, W.; Wang, Q.; Zhu, D.; Song, H. Intranasal erythropoietin ameliorates neurological function impairments and neural pathology in mice with chronic alcoholism by regulating autophagy-related Nrf2 degradation. *Mol. Med. Rep.* **2019**, *19*, 1139–1149. [CrossRef]

192. Lin, J.; Huang, Z.; Wu, H.; Zhou, W.; Jin, P.; Wei, P.; Zhang, Y.; Zheng, F.; Zhang, J.; Xu, J.; et al. Inhibition of autophagy enhances the anticancer activity of silver nanoparticles. *Autophagy* **2014**, *10*, 2006–2020. [CrossRef]
193. Qiao, X.; Gai, H.; Su, R.; Deji, C.; Cui, J.; Lai, J.; Zhu, Y. PI3K-AKT-GSK3beta-CREB signaling pathway regulates anxiety-like behavior in rats following alcohol withdrawal. *J. Affect. Disord.* **2018**, *235*, 96–104. [CrossRef]
194. Sun, X.; Xie, Z.; Hu, B.; Zhang, B.; Ma, Y.; Pan, X.; Huang, H.; Wang, J.; Zhao, X.; Jie, Z.; et al. The Nrf2 activator RTA-408 attenuates osteoclastogenesis by inhibiting STING dependent NF-kappab signaling. *Redox Biol.* **2020**, *28*, 101309. [CrossRef] [PubMed]
195. Vrechi, T.A.M.; Leao, A.; Morais, I.B.M.; Abilio, V.C.; Zuardi, A.W.; Hallak, J.E.C.; Crippa, J.A.; Bincoletto, C.; Ureshino, R.P.; Smaili, S.S.; et al. Cannabidiol induces autophagy via ERK1/2 activation in neural cells. *Sci. Rep.* **2021**, *11*, 5434. [CrossRef]
196. Read, E.; Zhu, J.; Yang, G. Disrupted H(2)S Signaling by Cigarette Smoking and Alcohol Drinking: Evidence from Cellular, Animal, and Clinical Studies. *Antioxidants* **2021**, *10*, 49. [CrossRef]
197. Mohseni, F.; Bagheri, F.; Rafaiee, R.; Norozi, P.; Khaksari, M. Hydrogen sulfide improves spatial memory impairment via increases of BDNF expression and hippocampal neurogenesis following early postnatal alcohol exposure. *Physiol. Behav.* **2020**, *215*, 112784. [CrossRef] [PubMed]
198. Salete-Granado, D.; Carbonell, C.; Puertas-Miranda, D.; Vega-Rodriguez, V.J.; Garcia-Macia, M.; Herrero, A.B.; Marcos, M. Autophagy, Oxidative Stress, and Alcoholic Liver Disease: A Systematic Review and Potential Clinical Applications. *Antioxidants* **2023**, *12*, 1425. [CrossRef]
199. Stacchiotti, A.; Corsetti, G. Natural Compounds and Autophagy: Allies Against Neurodegeneration. *Front. Cell Dev. Biol.* **2020**, *8*, 555409. [CrossRef] [PubMed]
200. Brimson, J.M.; Prasanth, M.I.; Malar, D.S.; Thitilertdecha, P.; Kabra, A.; Tencomnao, T.; Prasansuklab, A. Plant Polyphenols for Aging Health: Implication from Their Autophagy Modulating Properties in Age-Associated Diseases. *Pharmaceuticals* **2021**, *14*, 982. [CrossRef]
201. Peng, C.; Ai, Q.; Zhao, F.; Li, H.; Sun, Y.; Tang, K.; Yang, Y.; Chen, N.; Liu, F. Quercetin attenuates cerebral ischemic injury by inhibiting ferroptosis via Nrf2/HO-1 signaling pathway. *Eur. J. Pharmacol.* **2024**, *963*, 176264. [CrossRef]
202. Liu, Y.L.; Guo, T.; Zhang, Y.J.; Tang, S.C.; Zhao, X.M.; He, H.Y.; Yu, C.L.; Deng, Y.H. Berberine Alleviates Ischemic Brain Injury by Enhancing Autophagic Flux via Facilitation of TFEB Nuclear Translocation. *Am. J. Chin. Med.* **2024**, *52*, 231–252. [CrossRef]
203. Singh, A.; Yadawa, A.K.; Rizvi, S.I. Curcumin protects against aging-related stress and dysfunction through autophagy activation in rat brain. *Mol. Biol. Rep.* **2024**, *51*, 694. [CrossRef]
204. Gu, L.; Wang, C.; Liu, J.; Zheng, M.; Tan, Y.; Du, Q.; Li, Q.; Yang, W.; Zhang, X. Unlocking the neuroprotective potential of Ziziphora clinopodioides flavonoids in combating neurodegenerative diseases and other brain injuries. *Biomed. Pharmacother.* **2025**, *182*, 117744. [CrossRef] [PubMed]
205. Liu, Y.; Liu, Q.; Shang, H.; Li, J.; Chai, H.; Wang, K.; Guo, Z.; Luo, T.; Liu, S.; Liu, Y.; et al. Potential application of natural compounds in ischaemic stroke: Focusing on the mechanisms underlying "lysosomocentric" dysfunction of the autophagy-lysosomal pathway. *Pharmacol. Ther.* **2024**, *263*, 108721. [CrossRef]
206. Zheng, Y.; Zhou, Z.; Liu, M.; Chen, Z. Targeting selective autophagy in CNS disorders by small-molecule compounds. *Pharmacol. Ther.* **2024**, *263*, 108729. [CrossRef] [PubMed]
207. Chandrasekaran, V.; Hediyal, T.A.; Anand, N.; Kendaganna, P.H.; Gorantla, V.R.; Mahalakshmi, A.M.; Ghanekar, R.K.; Yang, J.; Sakharkar, M.K.; Chidambaram, S.B. Polyphenols, Autophagy and Neurodegenerative Diseases: A Review. *Biomolecules* **2023**, *13*, 1196. [CrossRef] [PubMed]
208. LeFort, K.R.; Rungratanawanich, W.; Song, B.J. Melatonin Prevents Alcohol- and Metabolic Dysfunction- Associated Steatotic Liver Disease by Mitigating Gut Dysbiosis, Intestinal Barrier Dysfunction, and Endotoxemia. *Antioxidants* **2023**, *13*, 43. [CrossRef] [PubMed]

antioxidants

MDPI

Review

Dynamic Interplay Between Autophagy and Oxidative Stress in Stem Cells: Implications for Regenerative Medicine

Daniela Rossin *, Maria-Giulia Perrelli, Marco Lo Iacono , Raffaella Rastaldo † and Claudia Gi

Department of Clinical and Biological Sciences, University of Turin, 10043 Orbassano, Italy; mariagiulia.perrelli@unito.it (M.-G.P.); marco.loiacono@unito.it (M.L.I.); raffaella.rastaldo@unito.it (R.R.); claudia.giachino@unito.it (C.G.)

* Correspondence: d.rossin@unito.it

† These authors contributed equally to the work.

Abstract: The crosstalk between autophagy and oxidative stress is a cornerstone of stem cell biology. These processes are tightly interwoven, forming a regulatory network that impacts stem cell survival, self-renewal, and differentiation. Autophagy, a cellular recycling mechanism, ensures the removal of damaged organelles and proteins, thereby maintaining cellular integrity and metabolic balance. Oxidative stress, driven by the accumulation of reactive oxygen species (ROS), can act as both a signalling molecule and a source of cellular damage, depending on its levels and context. The interplay between autophagy and oxidative stress shapes stem cell fate by either promoting survival under stress conditions or triggering senescence and apoptosis when dysregulated. Recent evidence underscores the bidirectional relationship between these processes, where autophagy mitigates oxidative damage by degrading ROS-generating organelles, and oxidative stress can induce autophagy as a protective response. This crosstalk is critical not only for preserving stem cell function but also for addressing age-related decline and enhancing regenerative potential. Understanding the molecular mechanisms that govern this interplay offers novel insights into stem cell biology and therapeutic strategies. This review delves into the intricate molecular dynamics of autophagy and oxidative stress in stem cells, emphasizing their synergistic roles in health, disease, and regenerative medicine applications.

Keywords: ageing; antioxidant; autophagy; mitophagy; regenerative medicine; ROS; stem cell

1. Introduction

Stem cells are essential for maintaining tissue turnover and regeneration due to their ability to self-renew and differentiate in response to physiological stimuli or injury. A key aspect of adult stem cell regulation is quiescence, a reversible non-proliferative state that preserves genomic integrity and long-term replicative potential. This state is maintained by both intrinsic and extrinsic signals from the surrounding niche, acting as a protective mechanism against replicative and metabolic stress [1]. Regeneration refers to the ability of stem cells to exit quiescence, proliferate, and differentiate to replace damaged or lost cells, thereby sustaining tissue turnover and enabling effective responses to injury [2].

Ageing disrupts the regulatory circuits that maintain quiescence, leading to either aberrant exit from the non-proliferative state or a deep, unresponsive quiescence. These alterations result in reduced activation capacity, increased vulnerability to oxidative stress, and a progressive decline in regenerative potential [3–6]. Ageing further impairs the stem cell microenvironment and promotes molecular damage [6].

Within this delicate balance, two fundamental cellular processes, autophagy and oxidative stress, play a central role in determining stem cell vitality. Autophagy is a conserved mechanism responsible for removing damaged mitochondria, aggregated proteins, and dysfunctional organelles, thereby maintaining cellular homeostasis and preventing senescence [7]. In contrast, the accumulation of reactive oxygen species (ROS) leads to cellular damage, senescence, and programmed cell death [8,9]. These two processes are tightly interconnected: autophagy mitigates oxidative stress through mitophagy, while excessive ROS levels can, in turn, activate autophagy as an adaptive response [10,11].

Multiple studies underscore the significance of autophagy and oxidative stress in governing stem cell fate decisions, including self-renewal, differentiation, and senescence. For instance, autophagy has been shown to sustain the metabolic requirements of hematopoietic stem cells (HSCs) by eliminating damaged mitochondria and preventing the accumulation of ROS [12–18]. Subsequently, in mesenchymal stem cells (MSCs), oxidative stress has also been shown to induce autophagy, thereby supporting mitochondrial integrity as a cellular survival strategy [19–21]. Moderate levels of ROS have been implicated as signalling molecules that drive stem cell differentiation, while excessive ROS levels can lead to apoptosis or senescence [22,23].

Maintaining a functional balance between these mechanisms is crucial to preserving regenerative capacity and preventing ageing-related dysfunctions, including neurodegenerative and cardiovascular disorders [24–26]. Therefore, targeting the interplay between autophagy and oxidative stress represents a promising strategy to enhance regenerative therapies.

This review explores the molecular mechanisms underlying the crosstalk between autophagy and oxidative stress in stem cells, with a particular focus on their implications for quiescence, ageing, and tissue regeneration in the context of regenerative medicine.

2. Autophagy in Stem Cells

Autophagy is essential for maintaining stem cells by regulating mitochondrial content to meet the cell's metabolic demands. It prevents the build-up of damaged mitochondria and reduces ROS production. By protecting cells from metabolic stress, autophagy helps maintain genome stability and prevents stem cell death and senescence. Additionally, throughout its effect on epigenetic and metabolic programmes, autophagy exerts a role in determining cell fate, as well as regulating self-renewal, stem cell quiescence, activation, and differentiation. Dysregulated autophagy has been implicated in stem cell ageing, reduced regenerative capacity, and various diseases [27].

If not otherwise specified, the term autophagy in this review refers to macroautophagy, the most widespread and broadly characterized form of autophagy.

2.1. Molecular Pathways of Autophagy

The molecular pathways governing autophagy are complex and highly regulated. The autophagy programme is negatively regulated by the mechanistic target of rapamycin (mTOR) and positively regulated by AMP-activated protein kinase (AMPK). Autophagy begins with the formation of the phagophore, a double-membrane structure that engulfs cytoplasmic material for degradation. This process is regulated by a series of conserved autophagy-related (ATG) proteins and pathways that respond to cellular stress and metabolic cues [28].

2.1.1. Initiation and Regulation

The initiation of autophagy involves the formation of the Unc-51-like kinase 1/2 (ULK1/2) complex and Phosphatidylinositol 3-kinase (PI3K) protein complexes (Figure 1).

Under nutrient-rich conditions, mTOR directly inhibits autophagy by phosphorylating ULK1, thereby preventing AMPK activation. Conversely, during energy stress, AMPK activates autophagy by phosphorylating ULK1 on a different serine residue. At the same time, AMPK can directly phosphorylate a subunit of the mTOR complex, thus inhibiting it [28–30]. In stem cells, mTOR signalling plays a pivotal role in balancing self-renewal and differentiation, making its regulation critical for maintaining stem cell homeostasis [14,28,31–33]. However, the effects of mTOR signalling vary depending on the type of stem cells involved [34,35].

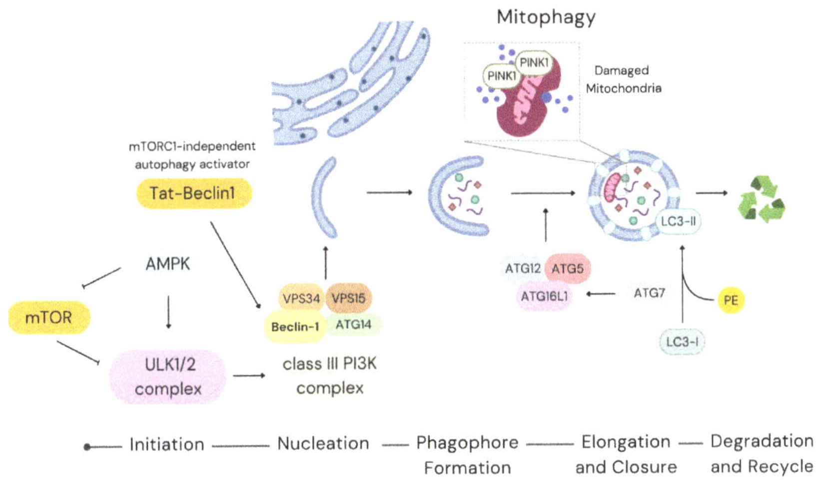

Figure 1. The phases of autophagy in stem cells. AMPK initiates the autophagic process by activation of the ULK1 complex and removing the inhibitory effect of mTOR. During nucleation, the activated ULK1/2 complex orchestrates the recruitment of the class III PI3K complex, which includes VPS34, VPS15, Beclin-1, and ATG14, with Tat-Beclin1 functioning as an mTORC1-independent autophagy inducer. The phagophore expands into the isolation membrane, which elongates and closes to form the autophagosome. This process is driven by two ubiquitin-like conjugation systems: one involving the ATG12–ATG5–ATG16L1 complex, and the other mediating the lipidation of LC3-I with phosphatidylethanolamine (PE) to generate LC3-II, a hallmark of autophagosome maturation. Both conjugation pathways critically depend on the E1-like enzyme ATG7.

2.1.2. Nucleation and Phagophore Formation

Following activation, the ULK1 complex recruits the class III PI3K complex, including VPS34, VPS15, Beclin-1 (Becn1), and ATG14 to initiate phagophore nucleation. The generation of phosphatidylinositol-3-phosphate (PIP3), mainly by VPS34 at the nucleation site, serves as a platform for recruiting additional ATG proteins, facilitating the assembly of the autophagosome membrane (Figure 1) [28,36]. The role of Becn1 in stem cell autophagy is particularly important, as its dysregulation has been linked to impaired self-renewal and differentiation capacity in neural stem cells (NSCs) [37]. The role of the VPS34 complex has also been pointed out in endothelial precursor cells (EPCs). Specifically, the role of autophagy in cardiac protection under conditions of oxygen and glucose deprivation was studied in EPCs, which were recruited from bone marrow in response to cardiac ischemic events. The authors highlighted that the slight activation of autophagy through rapamycin-mediated inhibition of mTOR did not increase the survival of bone marrow-derived EPCs against injury. Conversely, the VPS34 complex activator Tat-Beclin1 (mTORC1-independent autophagy activator) restored the autophagy process with a consequent decrease in apoptotic EPCs [38].

2.1.3. Elongation and Closure

The elongation and closure of the phagophore rely on two ubiquitin-like conjugation systems involving ATG12 and microtubule-associated protein 1A/1B-light chain 3 (LC3) (Figure 1). The ATG12-ATG5-ATG16L1 complex facilitates membrane expansion, while LC3 is conjugated to phosphatidylethanolamine (PE) to form LC3-II, which embeds into the autophagosome membrane [39]. LC3-II functions as a tag of autophagosome genesis and is crucial for cargo recognition and sequestration. In stem cells, LC3-mediated autophagy supports mitochondrial turnover, preventing ROS accumulation and preserving cellular function [40]. Recent findings underscored the importance of autophagy in the expansion and maturation of hematopoietic precursors [41].

ATG7 is an E1-like ligase, an essential protein in autophagosome biogenesis involved in Atg5-Atg12 and LC3-PE conjugation [42,43]. Using an in vitro model of embryonic stem cell (ESC) transition to epiblast-like cells (EpiLCs), it was recently demonstrated that dynamic changes in ATG7-dependent autophagy are essential for the naive-to-primed transition and germline specification [44].

Very recent experimental results confirmed that Atg7 is crucial for neurogenesis, though its influence can be exerted both on autophagy-dependent signalling pathways and through non-autophagic functions [45].

Stem cell viability is particularly dependent on the selective autophagic degradation of damaged mitochondria, known as mitophagy [46]. The PTEN-induced putative kinase 1 (PINK1)-Parkin pathway is a key regulator of mitophagy. Dysfunctional mitochondria show accumulated PINK1 on the outer mitochondrial membrane. This, in turn, recruits the E3 ubiquitin ligase Parkin to ubiquitinate mitochondrial proteins, marking the organelle for autophagic degradation [47]. Exploiting an innovative tool for investigating mitophagy, recent research demonstrated that PINK1 contributes to maintaining mitochondrial homeostasis and pluripotency in ESCs [48]. Stem cell mitophagy can also be mediated by two mitophagy receptor pathways, which involve BCL2-interacting protein 3 like/Nip3-like protein X (BNIP3L/NIX) and/or FUN14 domain containing 1 (FUNDC1) [49,50]. In mitophagy, damaged mitochondria, characterized by PINK1 accumulation, trigger their recognition and subsequent degradation. The final step involves autophagosome fusion with the lysosome, leading to the degradation and recycling of cellular components.

2.2. Transcriptional and Post-Transcriptional Regulation

Autophagy in stem cells is also regulated transcriptionally by factors such as Forkhead box O3 (FOXO3) and transcription factor EB (TFEB). Expression activation of Atg genes mediated by FOXO3 enhances the capability of stem cells to respond to stress and maintain homeostasis. Regulation of lysosomal biogenesis and autophagy mediated by TFEB functions through the activation of the transcription of genes involved in autophagosome formation and lysosomal function [51]. In neural stem and progenitor cells (NSPC), a network of Atg genes regulated by the transcription factor FOXO3 was identified while exploring the transcriptional programmes essential for cell function [52]. Further, it was found that FOXO3-mediated autophagy activation maintains redox balance during osteogenic differentiation [53] and protects HSCs from metabolic stress [54].

In a recent paper, the authors proposed a novel mechanism by which TFEB regulates the pluripotency of mouse embryonic stem cells (mESCs) through control of the pluripotency transcriptional network [55]. In another interesting paper, while trying to comprehend how quiescent long-term hematopoietic stem cells (LT-HSCs) perceive daily and stress-induced cues to transition into metabolically active progeny, the authors demonstrated that lysosomes, which function as advanced nutrient-sensing and signalling hubs, are modulated in a dual manner by TFEB and MYC to stabilize catabolic and anabolic activities essential for LT-HSC activation and lineage determination [56]. These findings establish TFEB-mediated lysosomal regulation as a key axis for orchestrating correct and synchronized stem cell fate decisions.

Post-transcriptional mechanisms, including non-coding RNAs such as microRNAs (miRNAs) and long non-coding RNAs (lncRNAs), further fine-tune autophagy.

For example, the expression of miR-145, miR-148a, and miR-185 was investigated in Wharton jelly multipotent stem cells (WJ-MSCs) from male and female donors in relation to the autophagic process and adipogenic/osteogenic differentiation potential. These miRNAs were chosen for their roles in regulating the stemness-related octamer-binding transcription factor 4 (OCT4) and DNMT1 gene expression and stem cell differentiation. Findings revealed a distinct regulatory mechanism involving the miR-148a/DNMT1/OCT4 autophagy pathway in male WJ-MSCs compared to female cells. However, no significant differences were observed in the expression of miR-145 and miR-185, which regulate differentiation [57]. Overall, these results highlight sex-based differences in WJ-MSC behaviour, offering insights into autophagy and stemness that could inform future clinical applications.

Further, lncRNAs can enhance autophagy by stabilizing the expression of key ATG proteins [58,59].

2.3. Autophagy and Stem Cell Ageing

Recent studies establish a strong connection between autophagy and stem cell ageing. Among others, the role of chaperone-mediated autophagy in ageing biology and stem cell rejuvenation has been reviewed in [60,61]. Ageing is associated with a decline in autophagic activity, causing the accumulation of damaged organelles and macromolecules. This contributes to stem cell exhaustion and a reduction in regenerative capacity. Enhancing autophagy through genetic or pharmacological means was shown to rejuvenate aged stem cells and improve their function.

The mechanisms underlying the decline of autophagy with age remain unclear and are the focus of ongoing research. Recent studies on aged muscle stem cells (MuSCs) and HSCs have shown that autophagy deteriorates with ageing, leading to impaired stem cell activity [13,62]. Both MuSCs and HSCs lose their regenerative potential with age, and old stem cells exhibit autophagy deficiencies, characterized by the autophagic vesicle enhancement, elevated intracellular p62 levels, increased LC3II expression, and the presence of ubiquitin-positive inclusions. However, treatment with rapamycin and spermidine restores autophagic function, mitigating autophagy-related deficiencies in both systems [13,62].

A previous study also highlighted that autophagy, particularly Atg7, is essential for meeting the bioenergetic demands required for the activation of quiescent MuSCs following injury, a process mediated by SIRT1 [63]. These findings confirm that autophagy is critical for preserving stemness in both MuSCs and HSCs, though the mechanisms appear to vary depending on the cellular niche.

In MSCs, instead, a dual role of autophagy has emerged in the context of ageing [64]. Under normal conditions, p62-dependent autophagy selectively degrades GATA4, a key regulator of the senescence-associated secretory phenotype (SASP), thereby suppressing senescence. However, when senescence-inducing stimuli arise, the interaction between GATA4 and p62 gradually declines, leading to the accumulation of GATA4, which subsequently activates the SASP transcriptionally [64].

2.4. Autophagy in Disease and Therapy

Dysregulated autophagy has been implicated in several stem cell-related diseases, like neurodegenerative diseases and cancers [65]. For instance, the expression of Presenilin 1

(PS1) progressively declines in the aged human brain, and PS1 mutations are the leading cause of early-onset familial Alzheimer's disease. While PS1-knockout and PS1 mutant neurons exhibit dominant autophagy-related phenotypes, it remains unclear whether autophagy in NSCs is significantly impaired by PS1 deficiency. Recently, authors utilized CRISPR/Cas9-based gene editing to produce human induced pluripotent stem cells (iPSCs) that were PS1-knockout in either heterozygosis or homozygosis, after which these cells differentiated into NSCs. In PS1-deficient NSCs, autophagosome formation as well as expression of mRNAs and proteins related to the autophagy–lysosome pathway (ALP), were reduced [66]. Mechanistically, inhibition of ERK/CREB signalling and activation of GSK3β played critical roles in suppressing TFEB expression in PS1-knockout NSCs [66]. These results indicate that PS1 deficiency leads to autophagy repression in human NSCs by downregulating ERK/CREB signalling, thus contributing to a major understanding of the role of PS1 in autophagy regulation.

Targeting autophagy pathways offers a promising therapeutic strategy for enhancing stem cell survival and function. Pharmacological activators of autophagy, such as rapamycin, have been explored for their ability to improve stem cell transplantation outcomes and tissue regeneration [36,67]. Transplantation of satellite cells, along with lineage-tracing approaches, revealed that hypercapnia disrupted satellite cell replication, activation, and myogenic potential. Sequencing analyses, performed both in bulk and at the single-cell level, revealed that hypercapnia altered autophagy, senescence, and other key cellular pathways [67]. In hypercapnic mice, rapamycin restored satellite cell autophagy flux, enhanced their activation and replication rates, and improved myogenic capability post-transplantation. These findings demonstrate that in hypercapnic mice treated with rapamycin, the functions of satellite cells were restored through AMPK activation and mTOR inhibition [67].

In another paper, authors faced the problem of stem cell transplantation after infarction, which is often impaired by the poor survival and engraftment of cells within the harsh microenvironment of the damaged heart. The study examined whether rapamycin-induced autophagy activation could enhance the survival of transplanted MSCs [68]. Rat bone marrow MSCs preconditioned with rapamycin exhibited reduced apoptosis and enhanced secretion of key factors, including hepatocyte growth factor (HGF), insulin-like growth factor-1 (IGF-1), stem cell factor (SCF), stromal cell-derived factor-1 (SDF-1), and vascular endothelial growth factor (VEGF). Moreover, rapamycin treatment significantly increased autophagic activity and lysosome production in MSCs. Following transplantation into a rat ischemia/reperfusion model, a few transplanted MSCs were observed to differentiate into cardiomyocytes (at least apparently) and endothelial cells in the damaged hearts [68]. These findings indicate that a low level of autophagy activation through rapamycin preconditioning sustains the engraftment and differentiation of transplanted cells, ultimately promoting myocardial repair and improving cardiac function.

Intriguingly, the regulation of autophagy can impact the regenerative potential of MSCs, both affecting MSC properties and through MSCs' capacity to modulate autophagy of cells in damaged tissues/organs [69]. For example, MSCs can modulate autophagy in immune cells related to injury-induced inflammation, diminishing their survival, proliferation, and function. As a consequence, this favours the clearance of inflammation. Furthermore, MSCs can modulate autophagy in endogenous progenitor cells, fostering their proliferation and differentiation. This contributes to the repair of altered tissue [69]. A greater clarification of the pathways through which MSCs regulate the autophagy of various types of target cells and how autophagy can impact MSCs' clinical potentialities will contribute to a broader perspective for the therapeutic application of MSCs in multiple pathologies.

In summary, dysregulated autophagy is a crucial element in the pathogenesis of various stem cell-related diseases. Modulating autophagy pathways presents a promising path for therapeutic treatments aimed at enhancing stem cell survival, improving transplantation outcomes, and promoting tissue regeneration.

3. Oxidative Stress in Stem Cells

Oxidative stress, characterized by an imbalance between ROS production and antioxidant defences, significantly impacts stem cell function. While moderate ROS levels serve as signalling molecules promoting stem cell differentiation, excessive ROS can lead to detrimental effects, including DNA damage, protein oxidation, and lipid peroxidation, ultimately impairing stem cell function [70].

ROS are chemically reactive molecules derived from oxygen, including superoxide anions ($O_2^{\bullet-}$), hydrogen peroxide (H_2O_2), and hydroxyl radicals ($^{\bullet}OH$). Electrons escaping from the electron transport chain react with molecular oxygen to form $O_2^{\bullet-}$, which are then converted to less reactive species via enzymatic and non-enzymatic antioxidant defences [71].

3.1. Sources and Regulation of ROS

The primary source of ROS in all cells, including stem cells, is the mitochondria, particularly during oxidative phosphorylation (OxPhos) [72,73]. About 0.1–0.2% of mitochondrial oxygen consumption produces ROS as byproducts of the respiratory chain [74]. The exact amount of ROS produced during mitochondrial respiration varies significantly based on cell type, environmental conditions, and mitochondrial activity [75]. Consequently, cells regulate ROS levels by modulating mitochondrial function and metabolic pathways. Precisely, ROS production can be reduced by drawing substrates away from OxPhos, as well as by boosting pathways that restore oxidized glutathione (GSH), like the pentose phosphate pathway.

ROS generated by OxPhos, and especially H_2O_2, are key regulators of stem and progenitor cell function in both physiological and pathological contexts. In quiescent HSCs, low H_2O_2 levels help maintain stemness, whereas increased H_2O_2 levels within HSCs or their niche promote survival, proliferative activity, differentiation, and cell migration [73]. Conversely, in pathological conditions such as ageing, atherosclerosis, heart failure, hypertension, and diabetes, excessive ROS levels contribute to an inflammatory and oxidative environment, triggering damage and apoptosis in stem and progenitor cells [73].

Another key ROS source in stem cells is the nicotinamide adenine dinucleotide phosphate oxidase (NOX) family, which contributes to redox balance together with the antioxidant systems [76,77]. Unlike mitochondrial ROS, NOXs intentionally produce ROS by transferring electrons from the nicotinamide adenine dinucleotide phosphate (NADPH) to O_2, thus generating superoxide ($O_2^{\bullet-}$) which can be converted to hydrogen peroxide (H_2O_2) by superoxide dismutase (SOD). A distinct NOX subcellular localization results in compartmentalized ROS production, enabling precise redox signalling regulation [78]. This redox equilibrium is closely linked to the regulation of stem cell fate, influencing self-renewal, proliferation, and differentiation, which are critical processes in embryonic development, adult tissue regeneration, and cell therapy applications [77]. Although cytochrome P450, xanthine oxidase (XO), and nitric oxide synthases (NOS) are minor ROS sources, they can influence redox balance [77].

3.2. Antioxidant Defence Mechanisms

Stem cells hold intrinsic antioxidant defence mechanisms which include both enzymatic systems such as SOD, catalase (CAT), and glutathione peroxidase (GPx), and non-enzymatic molecules like GSH, vitamins C and E, and flavonoids. These systems work synergistically to neutralize ROS and maintain redox balance [26,79–81].

HSCs are highly sensitive to intracellular redox balance, requiring minimal ROS levels and NOX expression to maintain quiescence [82]. Research indicates that quiescent, proliferative, and differentiated stem cells exhibit varying ROS levels due to metabolic differences. Maintaining low ROS levels, regulated by both internal and external factors, is crucial for stem cell self-renewal, migration, development, and cell cycle regulation [83–85]. However, elevated ROS levels drive HSCs out of quiescence, promoting differentiation at the expense of self-renewal. If left unchecked, this imbalance can deplete the HSC pool and contribute to disease development [86].

Conversely, MSCs have been shown to exhibit resistance to oxidative and nitrosative stress, at least in vitro, a capability linked to their constitutive expression of antioxidant enzymes like SOD1, SOD2, CAT, and GPx, as well as abundant levels of the antioxidant GSH [87]. Depleting GSH compromises their tolerance to oxidative stress. Additionally, MSCs constitutively express heat shock protein 70 (HSP70) and sirtuins (SIRT), especially SIRT1, 3, and 6 [88], which may further contribute to their resilience against oxidative and nitrosative damage. SIRT1 promotes MSC survival under H_2O_2-induced oxidative stress [89]. Similarly, SIRT6 has been implicated in reducing oxidative damage and basal ROS levels in MSCs by promoting the production of antioxidants, such as heme oxygenase-1 (HO-1) [90]. Overexpressing HO-1 has been shown to mitigate ROS accumulation and cellular senescence in SIRT6-deficient MSCs, highlighting its critical role in MSC survival under oxidative conditions [90].

Beyond their inherent antioxidant defences, MSCs can also adapt to redox stress. When treated with lipopolysaccharides (LPSs), MSCs produce oxidative and nitrosative free radicals, further demonstrating their dynamic response to environmental stressors [88].

3.3. Impacts of Oxidative Stress on Stem Cell Function

In stem cells, the equilibrium between self-renewal and differentiation is influenced by the redox balance regulation in coordination with metabolism [22]. Studies indicate that ROS amounts remain limited in niches where stem cells undergo self-renewal, while they increase as stem cells differentiate (Figure 2) [91,92]. In various stem cell types, both excessive and insufficient ROS levels can impair regenerative potential through the reduction in proliferation activity, differentiation potential, and self-renewal maintenance [90,93–96]. In particular, quiescent adult stem cells in their niches display ROS signalling suppression caused by antioxidant expression induced by high transcription factor levels, like nuclear factor erythroid 2–related factor 2 (Nrf2), while proliferating cells show activated growth factor kinase signalling and altered redox states consisting of ROS signalling activation caused by antioxidant reduction [97]. Therefore, maintaining ideal ROS levels is essential for appropriate stem cell function. However, primary neural progenitors with proliferative, self-renewing, and multipotency characteristics similar to NSCs unexpectedly maintained high ROS levels and exhibited strong responsiveness to ROS stimulation [93]. A ROS-driven increase in self-renewal and neurogenic capability was found to rely on the PI3K/AKT axis. Indeed, reduced intracellular ROS amounts in response to pharmacological and genetic interventions disrupted NSC and progenitor activity in vitro and in vivo [93]. AKT double-deficient HSCs display reduced ROS and remain quiescent, and restoring ROS pharmacologically rescues their differentiation capacity [94]. These results highlight AKT1 and AKT2 as essential regulators of HSC function and suggest that disrupted ROS homeostasis may contribute to impaired hematopoiesis. Notably, a modest rise in basal ROS levels has been shown to promote MSC proliferative and migratory activities through the triggering of ERK 1/2- and JNK-1/2-mediated signalling pathways [98–100].

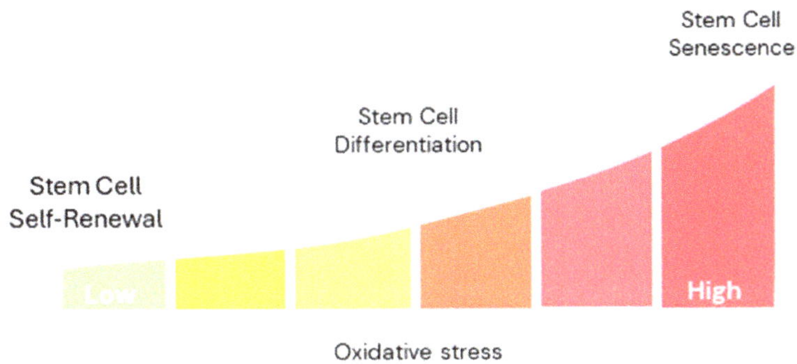

Figure 2. Oxidative stress gradient regulates stem cell fate. Low levels of oxidative stress promote stem cell self-renewal, while moderate levels drive differentiation. However, excessive oxidative stress leads to cellular damage and senescence, impairing stem cell function and regenerative potential. Maintaining an optimal oxidative balance is crucial for sustaining stem cell homeostasis and function.

3.3.1. ROS and Stem Cell Differentiation

Moderate levels of ROS act as secondary messengers in cellular signalling pathways, promoting stem cell differentiation. For example, ROS-mediated activation of the p38 MAPK (p38) and NF-κB pathways has driven MSC differentiation into osteoblasts [101]. The pluripotency markers of ESCs, including OCT4, NANOG, and sex-determining region Y-box 2 (SOX2), are downregulated in the presence of elevated ROS levels, promoting ESC differentiation toward mesodermal and endodermal lineages. Remarkably, this pluripotency can be restored through antioxidant treatment. These effects are regulated by several members of the mitogen-activated protein kinase (MAPK) family, which modulate numerous signalling pathways [102]. Moliner et al. demonstrated that the augmented differentiation of ESCs into neurons within spheres correlates with enhanced expression of genes linked to mitochondrial metabolism and ROS production [103]. In cortical clones, ROS are promptly generated in the culture condition, driving differentiation into both large pyramidal-like neurons and calretinin-expressing neurons [104]. Similarly, Le Belle et al. found that pharmacological inhibition of the NOS enzyme led to increased oxidative stress, which, in turn, stimulated neuroepithelial stem (NES) cell activity and self-renewal [93]. Moreover, ROS-driven neurogenesis relies on the activation of JNK signalling [105]. Spitkovsky et al. observed an increase in mitochondrial biogenesis during in vitro mESC cardiogenic differentiation. They also showed that complex III activity drives essential Ca^{2+} oscillations to initiate this differentiation, independent of ATP production [106].

Conversely, Chung and colleagues evidenced how the shift from anaerobic glycolysis to aerobic OxPhos was essential for proper mESC differentiation toward a functional cardiac phenotype [107,108].

3.3.2. Excessive ROS and Stem Cell Damage

On the other hand, excessive ROS disrupts this balance, leading to DNA damage, protein oxidation, and lipid peroxidation, ultimately impairing stem cell function and leading to stem cell senescence [109]. Jang and Sharkis demonstrated that mouse bone marrow-derived HSCs could be categorized into ROS^{high} and ROS^{low} cell groups based on the intensity of dichlorodihydrofluorescein (DCF) staining [82]. ROS^{high} HSCs showed a diminished capacity to generate long-term cells in vitro, as well as a reduced ability to sustain long-term engraftment upon transplantation compared to ROS^{low} HSCs. In NSCs, excessive ROS leads to oxidative DNA damage, triggering the activation of the p53 signalling pathway. This activation resulted in cell cycle arrest, senescence, or apoptosis, thereby impairing the regenerative capacity of NSCs, highlighting the sensitivity of these cells to oxidative stress [110]. However, minimal p53 signalling is key to these cells. In a recent paper, Navarro et al. investigated the p53 role in human brain development, using human iPSC-derived NSCs, along with brain organoids. They knocked down p53 in human iPSC-derived NES cells derived from iPSCs and observed that the knocked down cells suddenly developed centrosome amplification and genomic instability. Additionally, these cells exhibited diminished proliferative activity, downregulation of OxPhos-related genes, and increased glycolytic activity [111]. Furthermore, knocked-down NSCs differentiated into neurons at an accelerated rate, displaying characteristics of more mature neurons compared to controls. In brain organoid models of cortical neurogenesis, the loss of p53 led to a disorganized stem cell layer, a reduction in cortical progenitor cells and neurons, and a similar downregulation of OxPhos-related genes observed in NES cells [111]. Overall, these findings highlight a key role for p53 in ensuring genomic stability in NSCs, regulating neuronal differentiation, and maintaining proper structural organization and metabolic gene expression in neural progenitors within organoids.

Despite the significance of oxidative stress, its epigenetic effects on stem cells remain largely unexplored [112]. Epigenetic regulation appears to involve a complex interplay of multiple factors and coordinated signalling pathways. While an optimal stem cell model that accurately reflects epigenetic dynamics in the presence of ROS is still lacking, high-throughput sequencing could provide, in the future, valuable insights into the global epigenetic changes induced by ROS [112].

3.4. *Therapeutic Implications*

Understanding the dual role of ROS in stem cell biology is crucial for developing therapeutic approaches. To lower oxidative stress in stem cells, several strategies have been developed, including antioxidant therapies, metabolic reprogramming, activation of the Nrf2 pathway, and optimization of culture conditions.

Such approaches aim to maintain the delicate balance of ROS required for normal stem cell function and to prevent oxidative stress-induced impairments.

3.4.1. Antioxidant Therapies

Administration of exogenous antioxidants such as N-acetylcysteine (NAC), ascorbic acid 2-phosphate (AAP), edaravone, and atorvastatin has shown promise in reducing oxidative damage and enhancing stem cell viability [113–115]. NAC, a thiol-containing antioxidant and GSH precursor, attenuates oxidative stress by scavenging free radicals. Through a systematic analysis, the authors uncovered the synergistic protective mechanism of NAC and AAP on human MSCs (hMSCs) exposed to H_2O_2-induced oxidative stress. The combined NAC and AAP (NAC/AAP) treatment mitigates ROS production, preserves mitochondrial membrane potential, and reduces oxidative stress-induced mitochondrial fission and fragmentation [116]. However, it is interesting to note that the effects of NAC are concentration-dependent. For example, a study explored the effects and mechanisms of NAC on human dental follicle stem cells (hDFSC) which possess MSC characteristics [114]. These authors evaluated MSC properties and their role in alveolar bone regeneration when exposed to different NAC doses. Treatment with 5 mM NAC enhanced hDFSC proliferation, reduced senescence, and increased the expression of stem cell- and immune-related markers, resulting in the strongest osteogenic differentiation. Different doses also helped maintain stem cell features. The authors found that optimizing NAC concentration augments hDFSC characteristics, particularly osteogenesis, through PI3K/AKT/ROS signalling [114]. In another paper, the authors demonstrated that only ROS^{high,} and not ROS^{low}, HSCs became exhausted after the third transplantation [82]. Such impairments were linked to heightened activation of p38 and mTOR, which could be mitigated by treating the cells with an antioxidant, a p38 inhibitor, or rapamycin. Moreover, exposing mouse bone marrow-derived HSCs to high concentrations of buthionine sulfoximine, an inhibitor of GSH metabolism, significantly decreased HSC clonogenicity [94,117].

The treatment time windows of the antioxidant edaravone were evaluated in human umbilical cord mesenchymal stem cells (hUCMSCs) exposed to an LPS/H_2O_2 challenge. The therapeutic effects and underlying mechanisms of edaravone-treated hUCMSCs were then studied in vivo using a murine model of acute liver failure , where increased implanted stem cell numbers and improved hepatic function were evidenced [118].

Atorvastatin-treated MSCs derived from the bone marrow showed improved survival upon implant in a setting of renal ischemia–reperfusion injury, accompanied by injury amelioration outcomes [119]. Similarly, through activation of NOS, atorvastatin enhanced the efficacy of MSC treatment for swine myocardial infarction [120].

However, since different cell types showed different oxidative stress threshold susceptibility, further investigation is required to evaluate the dose-depentent effects of antioxidants and their cell type-specific actions before extensive clinical application.

3.4.2. Metabolic Reprogramming

Shifting stem cell metabolism from OxPhos to glycolysis can reduce mitochondrial ROS production. As mouse PSCs transition from the naïve to the primed pluripotent state, they naturally decrease their reliance on OxPhos and shift to high glycolytic activity. This occurs due to the elevated expression of glucose transporters, resulting in increased glucose uptake and glycolysis [121]. Research using genetically modified mouse models and progress in metabolomic analysis, particularly in HSCs, have enhanced our understanding of how metabolic signals regulate stem cell self-renewal. Multiple stem cell types primarily depend on anaerobic glycolysis, while their function is also influenced by bioenergetic signalling, the AKT–mTOR pathway, glutamine metabolism, and fatty acid metabolism [122]. Quiescent adult stem cells typically exhibit a preference for glycolysis, even under aerobic conditions, to minimize oxidative stress. This metabolic reprogramming is crucial for maintaining stem cell function and has been observed during processes such as neuronal differentiation [123]. The mechanisms underlying metabolic reprogramming during neuronal differentiation have remained unclear for a long time, until authors found that the passage from aerobic glycolysis in neural progenitor cells (NPCs) to OxPhos in mature neurons is defined by the downregulation of hexokinase (HK2) and lactate dehydrogenase (LDHA) proteins, along with a shift in pyruvate kinase splicing from PKM2 to PKM1. This shift coincides with a sharp decline in the amount of c-MYC and N-MYC, working as transcriptional activators of HK2 and LDHA [123]. Forcing the continuous expression of HK2 and LDHA along cell maturation determines neuronal cell death, highlighting the necessity of shutting down aerobic glycolysis for neuronal survival. Additionally, the metabolic regulators PGC-1α and ERRγ show a significant upregulation during differentiation, supporting the sustained transcriptional activation of metabolic and mitochondrial genes. Notably, these gene expression levels remain unmodified compared to NPCs, suggesting specific transcriptional regulation in proliferative versus post-mitotic differentiation states [123]. Furthermore, mitochondrial mass expands in proportion to neuronal growth, pointing to an as-yet unidentified mechanism that links mitochondrial biogenesis to cell size [123]. Recent research indicates that small non-coding RNAs, such as piRNAs, are involved in regulating this metabolic shift, further highlighting the complexity of metabolic control in stem cells [124].

3.4.3. Activation of Nrf2 Pathways

The Nrf2 pathway is a crucial regulator of cellular antioxidant responses. Pharmacological activation of Nrf2 upregulates the expression of antioxidant genes, protecting stem cells from oxidative stress and improving their regenerative capacity [125]. NAC has been shown to exert its protective effects, partially, through the activation of the Nrf2 pathway, leading to increased GSH synthesis and enhanced cellular defence mechanisms. However, to some extent, ROS production is necessary for various stem cell types to transition from quiescence to activation and differentiation. Therefore, Nrf2-mediated regulation of redox-related genes has to be precisely balanced to accommodate the functional needs of stem cells, depending on their dormant or active state. One example of Nrf's role in redox balance involves peroxiredoxins 1 and 6 (PRDX1/6), which play a key role in reducing intracellular H_2O_2. In human embryonic stem cells (hESCs), the maintenance of stemness requires ROS suppression, as PRDX1 deletion leads to ROS accumulation and diminished stem cell properties [126]. In contrast, dental pulp stem cells (DPSCs) require a reduction in PRDX6 levels to undergo osteogenic differentiation, as PRDX6 overexpression inhibits dental bone development [127]. These findings highlight how different stem cell niches necessitate distinct ROS levels based on their functional context, with Nrf2 and its redox targets playing a central role in mediating ROS-dependent shifts in stem cell status.

3.4.4. Improved Culture Conditions

Mimicking the hypoxic conditions of the stem cell niche by reducing oxygen levels in culture has long been shown to decrease ROS levels and to help maintain the stem cell undifferentiated state [128,129]. Further, culturing stem cells under low oxygen conditions enhances their therapeutic potential [130]. In the case of adipose-derived stem cells (ASCs), for instance, it was found that, compared to the hyperoxia group, cells in the physioxia group demonstrated enhanced proliferation, migration, and angiogenesis, along with reduced senescence and apoptosis [131]. The improved survival rate of ASCs cultured under physioxia was observed in both in vitro and in vivo ischemia models. Metabolic reprogramming analysis revealed a reduction in mitochondrial mass, an increase in intracellular pH alkalization, an enhanced glucose uptake, and glycogen synthesis [131]. These findings suggest that physioxia provides a more favourable environment for culturing ASCs for transplantation, as it preserves their native bioactivities while preventing hyperoxia-induced damage.

Pyruvate, a crucial byproduct of glycolysis, plays a crucial role in stem cell metabolism. Recently, hESC culture shows that higher exogenous pyruvate levels shift metabolism toward OxPhos and promote mesoderm and endoderm differentiation [132]. However, pyruvate production and its mitochondrial metabolism are crucial for mesoderm differentiation. TCA-cycle metabolites cannot replace their role [132]. Additional investigation revealed that pyruvate elevates the AMP/ATP ratio, activates AMPK, and regulates the mTOR pathway to promote mesoderm differentiation [132,133]. These results highlight that, besides its influence on hESC metabolism, exogenous pyruvate also modulates key signalling pathways in stem cell differentiation.

Beyond glucose metabolism, fatty acid metabolism is also essential for the terminal stages of hESC endodermal differentiation [134]. Increased fatty acid β-oxidation and decreased adipogenesis occur due to the AMPK-mediated phosphorylation of the adipogenic enzyme acetyl-CoA carboxylase [134]. As a result, inhibiting fatty acid synthesis through AMPK agonists exerts a crucial role in facilitating and regulating human endodermal differentiation. Recent research has identified the PI3K/AKT axis as a crucial metabolic signalling target for enhancing stem cell survival, offering new insights into optimizing long-term MSC culture [135]. Further, in bone marrow stem cells, the natural ginseng extract Rg1 activates the PI3K/AKT pathway, preventing MSC ageing and enhancing antioxidant capacity, thus making Rg1 a promising regenerative therapy [136].

In summary, oxidative stress exerts a complex role in stem cell biology, influencing both differentiation and survival. Maintaining ROS at optimal levels is essential for preserving stem cell function and developing effective therapeutic interventions.

4. Crosstalk Between Autophagy and Oxidative Stress

The interplay between autophagy and oxidative stress is a dynamic and tightly regulated process that significantly influences stem cell fate. Autophagy and oxidative stress are interdependent, with each modulating the other to maintain cellular homeostasis.

As reported, ROS-generating organelles such as mitochondria, as well as peroxisomes, organelles that undergo cellular pathways involved in lipid metabolism, can be degraded through autophagy. The process relies on the binding of ubiquitinated proteins to specific autophagy receptors (SQSTM1, NBR1, and NDP52). The autophagic process also withdraws unfolded proteins through specialized pathways like chaperone-mediated autophagy. Further, autophagy-dependent Nrf2 activation promotes expression of antioxidant genes to remove excess intracellular ROS.

On the other hand, a dual role of ROS is recognized in autophagy induction and inhibition. ROS trigger transcription factors like p53, HIF1A, and Nrf2 to induce the expression of Atg genes. In addition, ROS-mediated oxidation of Atg4 inhibits its LC3-PE deconjugation activity, resulting in the accumulation of autophagic LC3-II isoforms, which facilitate autophagosome formation. ROS directly oxidize cysteine residues on the α and β subunits of AMPK, triggering phosphorylation of the ULK1 complex and inhibition of PI3K-AKT-mTORC1 signalling pathway, both of which promote autophagy. In contrast, ROS can inactivate PTEN, which negatively affects the PI3K-AKT-mTORC1 pathway, ultimately suppressing autophagy. Moreover, the inhibition of autophagy is also mediated by oxidation of catalytic thiols on Atg3 and Atg7 by ROS, inhibiting LC3 lipidation [137,138].

In a feedback mechanism, autophagy helps reduce ROS levels and remove damaged organelles, including mitochondria, through mitophagy. Damaged mitochondria are selectively targeted for degradation by binding to LC3 and being enclosed within the autophagosome. The autophagosome then fuses with a lysosome, forming an autolysosome where the mitochondria are broken down and recycled [137].

In stem cells, this crosstalk is mediated through shared molecular pathways, including mitochondrial quality control, transcriptional regulators, and signalling molecules.

4.1. *Mitochondrial Quality Control*

Mitochondria are a predominant source of ROS within cells, and their dysfunction can exacerbate oxidative stress, leading to cellular damage and impaired stem cell function. Autophagy, particularly mitophagy, is crucial for maintaining mitochondrial quality by selectively removing damaged mitochondria that generate excessive ROS.

This quality control process is mediated by the PINK1-Parkin pathway, which tags defective mitochondria for degradation via ubiquitination. Additionally, other mediators such as BCL2 Interacting Protein 3 (BNIP3) and FUNDC1 regulate hypoxia-induced mitophagy, ensuring cellular adaptation to low oxygen environments [139]. Stem cells with impaired mitophagy exhibit elevated oxidative damage, resulting in diminished functionality and increased susceptibility to stress [49,140].

In HSCs and ESCs, a lower mitochondrial count is linked with decreased dependence on aerobic metabolism, leading to lower ROS production [121,141]. Additionally, mitophagy contributes to maintaining low ROS levels during somatic cell reprogramming into iPSCs via ATG proteins such as PINK1 and ATG3 [142–144]. Notably, the loss of PINK1-dependent mitophagy significantly reduces the speed and efficiency of iPSC reprogramming from mouse embryonic fibroblasts [143]. Consistent with this, iPSCs derived from Pink1-knockout mice exhibit decreased glycolytic metabolism and an increased tendency toward differentiation.

A recent study delved into the mechanisms of mitochondrial function maintenance in MuSCs [145]. In this research, the authors investigated mitophagy dynamics in MuSCs across different differentiation states of myogenesis and assessed the role of PINK1 in preserving their regenerative potential. Their findings reveal that quiescent MuSCs actively express mitophagy-related genes, show detectable mitophagy flux, and exhibit significant mitochondrial localization within autophagolysosomes, processes that suddenly decline upon activation [145]. In mice, genetic deletion of Pink1 disrupts Parkin recruitment to mitochondria and impairs mitophagy in quiescent MuSCs. This loss is associated with premature activation and commitment, leading to a decline in self-renewal and an ongoing loss of muscle regeneration, despite normal proliferation and differentiation capabilities. Additionally, authors found that the weakened fate decisions in Pink1-deficient MuSCs can be rescued by scavenging redundant mitochondrial ROS [145]. These results exemplify the critical contribution of mitophagy in MuSC regulation and establish PINK1 as a key mediator of mitochondrial integrity and stem cell fate.

Another recent research revealed that *O*-linked *N*-acetylglucosamine (O-GlcNAc) transferase (OGT) critically controls the stress response of HSCs by securing mitochondrial quality through PINK1-dependent mitophagy [146]. OGT is a unique enzyme that adds O-GlcNAc modifications to target proteins, playing a crucial role in regulating several cellular processes across different cell lineages. Nevertheless, its function in hematopoietic stem and progenitor cells (HSPCs) has remained unclear for a long time. The authors used Ogt conditional knockout mice to demonstrate that OGT is crucial for HSPC maintenance. They found that Ogt is particularly expressed in HSPCs, and its elimination causes a rapid loss of these cells, accompanied by increased ROS levels and apoptosis [146]. Notably, Ogt-deficient HSCs lose their quiescent state, fail to sustain themselves in vivo, and become highly susceptible to regeneration stress. Moreover, Ogt-deficient HSCs collect high amounts of faulty mitochondria because of impaired mitophagy, which is linked to reduced expression of the essential mitophagy regulator PINK1 via dysregulated H3K4me3 [146]. Importantly, excessive production of PINK1 re-establishes mitophagy and rescues the population of Ogt-deficient HSCs [146]. These findings underline the crucial role of OGT in maintaining HSC function and mitochondrial quality control.

Conversely, oxidative stress can also serve as a trigger for mitophagy, acting as a protective mechanism against mitochondrial dysfunction. Oxidative stress activates Nrf2, a transcription factor that upregulates the expression of Atg genes, including those required in mitophagy. This creates a feedback loop where ROS-induced mitophagy mitigates oxidative stress, thereby safeguarding stem cell viability and functionality. Moreover, the interdependence of autophagy and oxidative stress plays a pivotal role in maintaining stem cell homeostasis and preventing premature ageing [147].

Further research is needed, however, to uncover the molecular mechanisms underlying mitophagy-driven metabolic reprogramming and to explore its potential as a strategy for regulating stem cell quiescence and differentiation.

4.2. Transcriptional Regulation

Transcription factors such as FOXO3 and Nrf2 play pivotal roles in mediating the crosstalk between autophagy and oxidative stress. FOXO3 is activated under oxidative stress and induces the expression of genes implicated in both autophagy and antioxidant defence (Figure 3). This includes upregulation of LC3 and BNIP3, which are critical for autophagy initiation and selective mitochondrial clearance [148]. Recent studies suggest that FOXO3 also regulates the transcription of enzymes like CAT and SOD, directly enhancing antioxidant capacity to mitigate ROS-induced damage. Gomez-Puerto et al. demonstrate that FOXO3 activation drives the expression of genes involved in autophagy, like MAP1LC3B, GABARAPL1, and PARK2, in hMSCs, and Zhang et al. reveal that FOXO3 induces autophagy through a transcription-dependent mechanism, requiring FOXO1 [53,149]. Overexpression of FOXO3 leads to increased transcription of FOXO1 and promotes its nuclear-to-cytoplasmic translocation, resulting in enhanced autophagy. The findings suggest a coordinated role of FOXO3 and FOXO1 in regulating autophagy in response to oxidative stress [149]. These studies collectively elucidate the mechanisms by which FOXO3 activation under oxidative stress conditions promotes Atg gene expression, ensuring cellular adaptation and stress resistance. Altogether, they highlight that FOXO3 reduces ROS levels by activating autophagy, underscoring its role in maintaining redox balance under oxidative stress conditions.

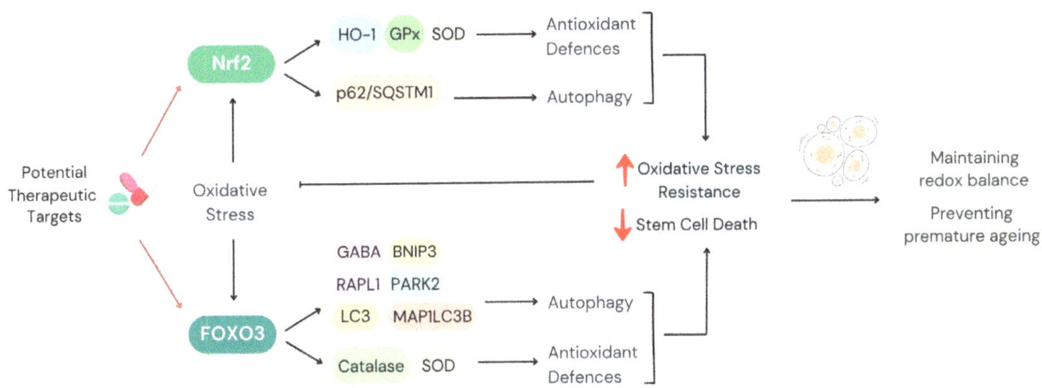

Figure 3. Redox balance triggered by FOXO3 and Nrf2 in stem cells. In response to oxidative stress, the transcription factors FOXO3 and Nrf2 are activated and orchestrate distinct yet complementary cryoprotective programmes. FOXO3 enhances the expression of different autophagy-related genes (e.g., LC3, BNIP3, MAP1LC3B, GABA, RAPL1, and PARK2) and antioxidant enzymes (e.g., catalase and SOD). Nrf2 upregulates antioxidant defences (e.g., HO-1, GPx, and SOD) and promotes autophagy via p62/SQSTM1. Together, the autophagy and antioxidant defences promote stem cell resistance to oxidative stress and limit cell death. This coordinated response preserves redox homeostasis and counteracts premature stem cell ageing. FOXO3 and Nrf2 thus represent promising therapeutic targets in age-related and oxidative stress-driven pathologies.

Similarly, Nrf2 coordinates the cellular response to oxidative stress by activating antioxidant response elements (AREs) in the promoters of genes coding for antioxidant enzymes, such as GPx and HO-1, as well as ATG proteins like p62/SQSTM1. Recent studies have elucidated the mechanisms by which, during oxidative stress stimuli, Nrf2 detaches from its inhibitor Keap1 and translocates to the cell nucleus to initiate transcriptional programmes that restore redox balance and promote autophagic degradation of damaged organelles [150].

In stem cells, the activation of these transcriptional programmes ensures adaptation to oxidative stress and maintenance of cellular homeostasis. FOXO3 activation has been shown to preserve HSC quiescence, while Nrf2 activation enhances MSC survival under oxidative conditions. For instance, FOXO3 plays a crucial role in preserving HSC quiescence under oxidative stress, acting as a prominent factor in the DNA damage response pathways of primitive hematopoietic cells, specifically in base excision repair, thereby protecting hematopoietic stem and progenitor cells from oxidative DNA damage during homeostasis [151]. Additionally, FOXO proteins, including FOXO3, exert critical roles in responding to physiological oxidative stress, not only mediating quiescence but also enhancing survival in the HSC niche. This function is crucial for maintaining the long-term regenerative potential of HSCs [152]. Furthermore, FOXO3 modulates ATM and oxidative stress, mediating distinct functions in regulating hematopoietic stem and progenitor cell fate [153]. These findings collectively underscore FOXO3′s pivotal role in maintaining HSC quiescence and protecting against oxidative stress, thereby ensuring the longevity and functionality of the hematopoietic system.

The differentiation of MSCs into osteoblasts necessitates a metabolic shift from glycolysis to enhanced mitochondrial respiration to meet the energy demands of this process. This metabolic transition leads to an increase in the production of endogenous ROS. Gomez-Puerto et al. investigated the role of FOXO3 in regulating ROS levels during osteogenic differentiation in hMSCs. Exposure to H_2O_2 triggered FOXO3 phosphorylation at Ser294 and its translocation to the nucleus, a process dependent on MAPK8/JNK activity. FOXO3 downregulation impaired osteoblastic differentiation and compromised the ability of hMSCs to regulate elevated ROS levels [53]. Additionally, they found that FOXO3 responds to increased ROS by inducing autophagy in hMSCs. Consistently, knockdown of ATG7 impaired autophagy, leading to disrupted ROS regulation and diminished osteoblast differentiation [53]. Collectively, these results support a model in which FOXO3 is essential for autophagy induction, thereby mitigating ROS accumulation resulting from heightened mitochondrial activity during osteoblast differentiation.

A few studies have investigated the role of Nrf2 activation in enhancing MSC survival under oxidative stress. One study demonstrated that transient overexpression of Nrf2 in MSCs safeguarded them from cell death activated by hypoxic and oxidative stress situations [154]. The activation of Nrf2 also augmented the activity of antioxidant enzymes like SOD and HO-1, contributing to increased cellular resilience [154]. Another recent research found that human umbilical cord-derived MSCs reduced high glucose-induced oxidative stress and prevented β-cell impairment through the activation of the Nrf2/HO-1 signalling axis [155]. A recent review emphasizes the crucial role of Nrf2 in maintaining MSC stemness, discussing how Nrf2 influences the self-renewal and differentiation of MSCs and contributes to their resilience under oxidative conditions [156]. These studies underscore the importance of Nrf2 activation in enhancing MSC survival under oxidative stress by upregulating antioxidant defences and maintaining cellular functions.

Emerging evidence highlights that these transcription factors do not act in isolation but form a tightly regulated network. Crosstalk between FOXO3 and Nrf2 allows for fine-tuning of autophagy and oxidative stress responses, ensuring optimal protection of stem cells from oxidative damage while maintaining their regenerative capacity [137]. This intricate regulatory interplay suggests that targeting FOXO3 and Nrf2 could be a promising therapeutic strategy to enhance stem cell resilience, particularly in the context of ageing and oxidative stress-related disorders.

4.3. *Drugs Regulating Oxidative Stress and Autophagy Balance in Stem Cells*

Several clinically used drugs modulate autophagy and oxidative stress, thereby interfering with key mechanisms that regulate stem cell viability and functions. Although originally developed for unrelated therapeutic purposes, many of these compounds exhibit pleiotropic effects on redox and mitochondrial homeostasis, ultimately impacting stem cell self-renewal, differentiation, and stress responsiveness either directly or indirectly.

Metformin, for instance, activates AMPK and inhibits mTOR phosphorylation, promoting autophagy and reducing mitochondrial ROS. In both in vitro and in vivo models, this has been associated with enhanced survival of NSCs and MSCs under oxidative stress conditions [157,158]. Statins likewise modulate redox signalling and have been implicated in the regulation of mitophagy and endoplasmic reticulum stress responses, particularly in vascular progenitor cells [159–161].

Interestingly, immunosuppressive drugs such as dexamethasone, widely used in clinical practice, in low dosage, have been shown to promote stem cell survival by inducing autophagy and fostering redox homeostasis [162,163].

Growing attention has been directed toward antioxidant compounds and natural polyphenols. Among natural compounds, resveratrol, a polyphenol well known in clinical treatments for its anti-inflammatory and immunomodulating properties, has been shown to modulate key cellular pathways involved in stem cell maintenance and function [164,165]. In mouse embryonic stem cells, resveratrol promotes pluripotency by activating AMPK/ULK1 and inhibiting mTORC1, thereby enhancing autophagy. This leads to upregulation of key pluripotency markers, improved mitochondrial function, and stabilization of the undifferentiated state under stress, supporting its potential as a tool to preserve stem cell identity in regenerative applications [166].

Melatonin, an endogenous hormone primarily secreted by the pineal gland, has emerged as a multifunctional modulator of autophagy and redox balance, playing a pivotal role in stem cell protection. In particular, it can exert a dual function: on one hand, it suppresses ROS production and activates antioxidant pathways such as Nrf2 and SOD2; on the other, it regulates autophagy in a context-dependent manner, thus promoting or suppressing autophagy by modulating the ERK/AKT/mTOR axis [167–172]. Indeed, in NSCs, melatonin promotes proliferation and differentiation under hypoxic conditions via ERK1/2 activation through the MT1 receptor [167], and counteracts toxin-induced excessive autophagy, such as that triggered by tri-ortho-cresyl phosphate, by restoring ERK1/2 signalling [173]. In pre-osteoblastic cells, it has been shown to suppress autophagy via ERK/AKT/mTOR pathway inhibition [171].

Similarly, melatonin exhibits potent antioxidant activity by reducing ROS production under both physiological and pathological conditions. In bone marrow-derived MSCs, it mitigates oxidative stress-induced apoptosis and enhances stem cell survival [172]. In NSCs, melatonin promotes proliferation and differentiation under hypoxia via ERK1/2 activation through the MT1 receptor [167]. Under inflammatory conditions, it upregulates SOX2 and HO-1 expression through PI3K/AKT-Nrf2 signalling, thereby supporting self-renewal while reducing apoptosis and aberrant differentiation [168–170].

Natural compounds such as icariin and curcumin have demonstrated protective effects in oxidative stress models by contextually modulating autophagy and redox responses. Icariin acts as a multitarget agent: it inhibits ROS-induced dysfunctional autophagy, enhances mitochondrial function, and activates PI3K/AKT/mTOR and MAPK/ERK pathways in EPCs and bone marrow MSCs [174,175], thereby reducing apoptosis and supporting cell survival, including in ischemic conditions [176].

Curcumin also exhibits a biphasic effect on autophagy. In NSCs, it reduces H_2O_2-induced ROS and malondialdehyde levels while inhibiting ERK1/2-mediated autophagy, thereby preserving cell viability [177,178]. Conversely, in adipose-derived stem cells, its protective effect is linked to autophagy induction and is abolished by 3-MA, indicating a cell-type- and microenvironment-dependent mechanism [179]. These findings highlight the importance of context-specific evaluation when considering curcumin for therapeutic applications.

4.4. Impact on Stem Cell Ageing and Regeneration

The balance between autophagy and oxidative stress is particularly critical in the context of ageing. A decline in autophagic activity with age causes the build-up of damaged mitochondria and increased ROS levels, contributing to stem cell exhaustion and impaired regenerative capacity. Recent studies emphasized that the disruption of this balance accelerates cellular senescence and reduces the therapeutic potential of stem cells. Pharmacological interventions that restore autophagy or reduce oxidative stress have emerged as promising strategies to combat stem cell ageing (Figure 4).

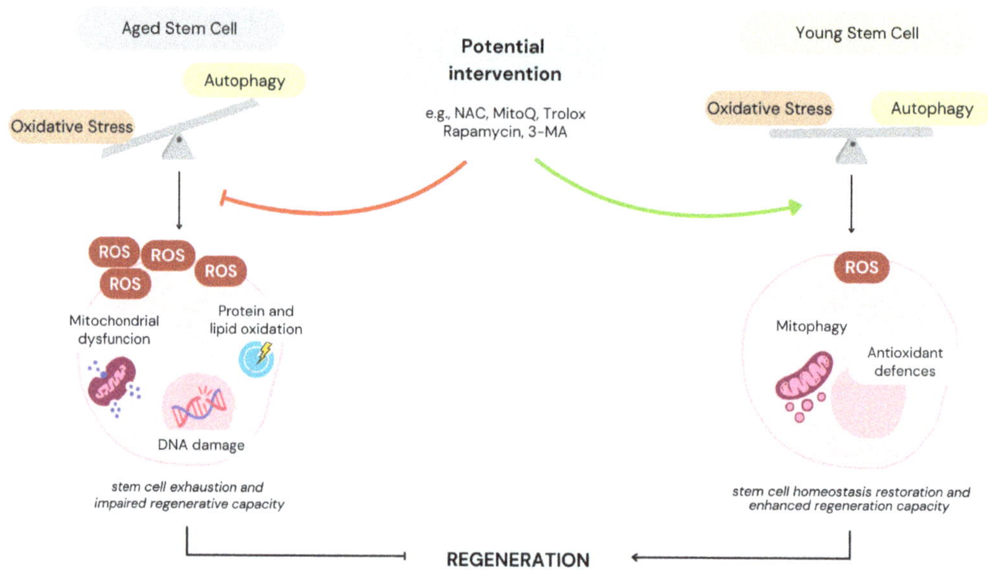

Figure 4. Pharmacological interventions targeting oxidative stress and autophagy to enhance tissue regenerative potential. Impaired autophagic activity and excessive oxidative stress in aged stem cells negatively impact their ability to regenerate. Elevated levels of ROS lead to mitochondrial dysfunction, as well as the oxidation of proteins and lipids, and DNA damage, ultimately resulting in stem cell senescence. In contrast, lower ROS levels combined with sufficient autophagic activity promote mitophagy and bolster antioxidant defences, which support stem cell renewal and differentiation, thereby enhancing tissue regeneration. Therapeutic agents such as NAC, MitoQ, Trolox, rapamycin, and 3-MA can help reduce oxidative stress and promote autophagy, ultimately restoring the homeostasis and regenerative capacity of stem cells.

For instance, activation of autophagy through compounds like rapamycin or resveratrol has been shown to rejuvenate aged HSCs through the improvement of mitochondrial functionality and reduction in ROS levels. These interventions not only restore self-renewal and differentiation potential but also enhance the overall longevity of stem cells [180–182]. HSC function declines with age, likely contributing to the weakened adaptive immune response seen in older individuals. Chen et al. discovered that mTOR activity is high in HSCs from aged mice compared to those from younger counterparts [180]. Inducing mTOR activation by conditionally deleting Tsc1 in young mice resulted in HSC characteristics resembling those of aged mice. These changes included increased expression of messenger RNA for the CDK inhibitors p16Ink4a, p19Arf, and p21Cip1, a decline in lymphopoiesis, and a reduced ability to regenerate the hematopoietic system [180]. In aged mice, treatment with rapamycin extended lifespan, restored HSC self-renewal and hematopoiesis, and improved vaccine response against a lethal influenza virus challenge [180]. These findings suggest that targeting mTOR signalling might be a promising therapeutic approach for counteracting age-related declines in HSC function. Further, it has been demonstrated that a three-week treatment with resveratrol increases both the frequency and total number of normal bone marrow HSC without affecting their competitive repopulation ability [181]. Furthermore, findings revealed that resveratrol enhances the multipotent progenitor capacity of bone marrow in vivo [181]. These results hold therapeutic potential for treating disorders related to HSCs and HSPCs, and may be valuable in bone marrow transplantation settings.

Similarly, mitochondrial-targeted antioxidants such as MitoQ and NAC have demonstrated efficacy in reducing oxidative damage and improving the survival of stem cells under stress conditions. These agents work by neutralizing ROS and supporting mitochondrial function, thereby maintaining the functional capacity of aged stem cells [183].

To investigate the role of ROS in vivo, Garcia-Prat et al. treated aged GFP-LC3 mice with intraperitoneal injections of the antioxidant factor Trolox, which enhanced autophagy and reduced senescence markers, such as p16Ink4a and senescence-associated β-galactosidase. Additionally, in vitro treatment with Trolox or p16Ink4a knockdown in MuSCs from aged and autophagy-deficient mice restored proliferation, delayed senescence, and improved regenerative potential [62]. More recently, in another in vivo study, the antioxidant icariin has been shown to promote the regeneration of pancreatic and germline stem cells, exert anti-inflammaging effects, and counteract age-related oxidative damage [184,185].

Additionally, the interplay between autophagy and oxidative stress has been related to the regulation of stem cell niche dynamics. Disrupted autophagy–oxidative stress balance can lead to an unfavourable niche environment, further impairing stem cell regeneration. Recent research underscores the role of Nrf2 and FOXO3 in modulating this balance to maintain a supportive microenvironment for stem cells. For example, Nrf2 activation has been shown to enhance the regenerative potential of mesenchymal stem cells in models of ageing and tissue repair [125].

The therapeutic implications of these findings extend to regenerative medicine, where targeting the autophagy–oxidative stress axis holds potential for improving the efficacy of stem cell-based therapies. Stem cell therapies have shown great potential as a therapeutic approach for several conditions associated with ischemic injury, such as ischemic stroke. However, a major challenge remains ensuring cell survival after transplantation. Recently, the effects of ischemia-induced oxidative stress were investigated by exposing human dental pulp stem cells (hDPSCs) and hMSCs to oxygen-glucose deprivation (OGD) [24]. This process led to excessive $O_2^{\bullet-}$ and H_2O_2 production, which upregulated Ambra1 and Becn1 expression, thereby enhancing autophagy in both hDPSCs and hMSCs. Pre-conditioning with ROS scavengers significantly suppressed Ambra1 and Becn1 expression, confirming the role of $O_2^{\bullet-}$ and H_2O_2 as upstream, unidirectional regulators of autophagy [24]. The involvement of ROS–p38–ERK1/2 signalling was further supported by the reversal of OGD-induced effects upon inhibition with SB202190 and PD98059, and by the observed activation of this pathway following SIRT3 depletion [24]. Global ROS inhibition with NAC, polyethylene glycol-SOD (PEG-SOD), or polyethylene glycol-CAT (PEG-CAT) further validated that elevated $O_2^{\bullet-}$ and H_2O_2 impair stem cell viability via excessive autophagy. Notably, blocking autophagy with 3-MA markedly improved hDPSC survival [24]. These findings deepen our understanding of post-transplantation cell loss in hDPSCs and hMSCs and may inform new strategies to mitigate oxidative stress-induced therapeutic failure.

By modulating critical pathways such as PINK1-Parkin-mediated mitophagy and Nrf2-driven antioxidant responses, it may be possible to extend the functional lifespan of stem cells and improve outcomes in ageing-related disorders and degenerative diseases [186]. These insights prepare for innovative therapeutic strategies aimed at restoring stem cell homeostasis and enhancing tissue regeneration in ageing individuals.

5. Conclusions and Future Directions

The insights gained from studying the interplay between autophagy and oxidative stress in stem cells have direct and promising implications for regenerative medicine.

Integrating targeted autophagy modulators with antioxidant-based strategies can enhance the effectiveness of stem cell therapies across a broad range of pathological conditions, including cardiovascular diseases, neurodegenerative disorders, and tissue injuries.

Despite substantial advances, critical aspects of the autophagy–oxidative stress crosstalk in stem cells remain incompletely understood. To fully exploit the therapeutic potential of redox–autophagy modulation in regenerative settings, several research directions should be prioritized. Among the most pressing challenges, a key priority is the need for in vivo studies employing conditional and lineage-specific deletion of autophagy-related genes (e.g., *Atg7* and *Atg5*) to clarify the intrinsic role of autophagy in the maintenance of adult stem cell compartments. Equally important is a deeper understanding of the tissue-specific dynamics of Nrf2 signalling and its interactions with other transcriptional regulators, which remain insufficiently characterized and currently limit the development of finely tuned redox-targeted therapies. Mitophagy also represents a critical yet under-investigated target, with only a limited number of selective pharmacological modulators currently available, in contrast to the broader toolkit developed for macroautophagy.

A deeper understanding of how these pathways integrate within distinct stem cell niches and pathological contexts will be essential to minimize off-target effects and support the safe clinical translation of modulatory strategies. Given the tight interconnection of the signalling pathways involved, therapeutic manipulation of this axis may carry the risk of unintended disruptions to stem cell homeostasis. Advancing our mechanistic understanding of this complex network will be key to developing effective and safe regenerative interventions.

Upcoming research should focus on elucidating the context-specific mechanisms of this interplay and identifying novel therapeutic targets to harness these pathways for regenerative medicine in clinical settings.

Author Contributions: Conceptualization, C.G. and R.R.; writing—original draft preparation, D.R.; writing—review and editing, R.R., C.G. and M.-G.P.; supervision, C.G. and R.R.; figure editing, D.R., M.-G.P. and M.L.I.; bibliographic searches, D.R., M.-G.P. and M.L.I. All authors have read and agreed to the published version of the manuscript.

Funding: This work was partially supported by local funds Rilo RASR_RILO_24_01 and GIAC_RILO_24_02.

Conflicts of Interest: The authors declare no conflicts of interest.

Abbreviations

The following abbreviations are used in this manuscript:

•OH	hydroxyl radicals
3-MA	3-methyladenine
AAP	ascorbic acid 2-phosphate
AKT	protein kinase B
ALA	α-lipoic acid
ALP	autophagy-lysosome pathway
Ambra1	activating molecule in BECN1-regulated autophagy protein 1
AMP	adenosine monophosphate

AMPK	AMP-activated protein kinase
AREs	antioxidant response elements
ASCs	adipose-derived stem cells
Atg	autophagy-related gene
ATG	autophagy-related protein
ATM	ataxia-telangiectasia mutated
ATP	adenosine triphosphate
Becn1	beclin-1
BMP4	bone morphogenetic protein 4
BNIP3	BCL2 Interacting Protein 3
BNIP3L	BCL2 Interacting Protein 3 like
CAT	catalase
CDK	cyclin-dependent Kinase
CDKIs	cyclin-dependent kinase inhibitors
c-MYC	cellular myelocytomatosis oncogene
CO_2	carbon dioxide
CREB	cAMP response element-binding protein
DCF	dichlorodihydrofluorescein
DNA	deoxyribonucleic acid
DNMT1	DNA (cytosine-5)-methyltransferase
DPSCs	dental pulp stem cells
EPCs	endothelial precursor cells
EpiLCs	epiblast-like cells
ERK	extracellular signal-regulated kinase
ERRγ	estrogen-related receptor gamma
ESC	embryonic stem cell
FOXO3	forkhead box O3
FPN1	ferroportin 1
FUNDC1	FUN14 domain containing 1
GABARAPL1	GABA type A receptor-associated protein like 1
GATA4	GATA Binding Protein 4
GFP	green fluorescent protein
GPx	glutathione peroxidase
GSH	glutathione
GSK3β	glycogen synthase kinase-3 beta
H_2O_2	hydrogen peroxide
H3K4me3	tri-methylation of lysine 4 of the H3 histone protein
hDFSC	human dental follicle stem cells
hDPSC	human dental pulp stem cells
hESCs	human embryonic stem cells
HGF	hepatocyte growth factor
HIF1A	hypoxia inducible factor 1 subunit alpha
HK2	hexokinase
hMSCs	human mesenchimal stem cells
HO-1	heme oxygenase-1
HSCs	hematopoietic stem cells
HSP70	heat shock protein 70
HSPCs	hematopoietic stem and progenitor cells
hUCMSCs	human umbilical cord mesenchymal stem cells
IGF-1	insulin-like growth factor-1
iPSCs	induced pluripotent stem cells
JNK-1/2	c-Jun N-terminal kinases-1/2
Keap1	kelch-like ECH-associated protein 1

LC3	microtubule-associated protein 1A/1B-light chain 3
LDHA	lactate dehydrogenase
lncRNAs	long non-coding RNAs
LPS	lipopolysaccharide
LT-HSCs	long-term hematopoietic stem cells
MAP1LC3B	microtubule-associated proteins 1A/1B light chain 3B
MAPK	mitogen-activated protein kinase
mESCs	mouse embryonic stem cells
miRNAs	microRNAs
MitoQ	mitoquinone mesylate
MSCs	mesenchymal stem cells
MT1	melatonin receptor type 1A
mTOR	mechanistic target of rapamycin
mTORC1	mechanistic target of rapamycin complex 1
MuSCs	muscle stem cells
NAC	N-acetylcysteine
NADPH	nicotinamide adenine dinucleotide phosphate
NANOG	homeobox protein NANOG
NBR1	neighbour of BRCA1 gene 1
NDP52	pulp nuclear dot protein 52
NES	neuroepithelial stem
NF-κB	nuclear factor kappa B
NIX	nip3-like protein X
N-MYC	neuroblastoma-derived v-myc avian myelocytomatosis viral-related oncogene
NOS	nitric oxide synthase
Notch	notch receptor
NOXs	NADPH oxidase enzymes
NPCs	neural progenitor cells
Nrf2	nuclear factor erythroid 2-related factor 2
NSCs	neural stem cells
NSPC	neural stem and progenitor cells
O_2	oxygen
$O_2^{\bullet-}$	superoxide anions
OCT4	octamer-binding transcription factor 4
OGD	oxygen-glucose deprivation
O-GlcNAc	*O*-linked N-acetylglucosamine
Ogt	*O*-GlcNAc transferase gene
OGT	*O*-GlcNAc transferase
OxPhos	oxidative phosphorylation
PARK2	parkin-2 gene
PE	phosphatidylethanolamine
PEG-CAT	polyethylene glycol-CAT
PEG-SOD	polyethylene glycol-SOD
PGC-1α	peroxisome proliferator-activated receptor-gamma coactivator 1-alpha
piRNAs	piwi-interacting RNAs
PI3K	phosphatidylinositol 3-kinase
PIP3	phosphatidylinositol-3-phosphate
PINK1	PTEN-induced putative kinase 1
PKM1	pyruvate kinase M1
PKM2	pyruvate kinase M2
PRDX1/6	peroxiredoxins 1 and 6
PS1	presenilin 1
RNA	ribonucleic acid
ROS	reactive oxygen species

SASP	senescence-associated secretory phenotype
SCF	stem cell factor
SDF-1	stromal cell-derived factor-1
SIRT	sirtuin
SOD	superoxide dismutase
SOX2	sex-determining region Y-box 2
SQSTM1	sequestosome 1
Tat-Beclin1	mTORC1-independent autophagy activator
TCA-cycle	tricarboxylic acid cycle
TFEB	transcription factor EB
TOR	target of rapamycin
Tsc1	tuberous sclerosis gene
ULK1/2	unc-51-like kinase ½
VEGF	vascular endothelial growth factor
VPS15	phosphoinositide-3-kinase regulatory subunit 4
VPS34	phosphatidylinositol-3-kinase class III
WJ-MSCs	Wharton jelly multipotent stem cells
XO	xanthine oxidase

References

1. Cheung, T.H.; Rando, T.A. Molecular Regulation of Stem Cell Quiescence. *Nat. Rev. Mol. Cell Biol.* **2013**, *14*, 329–340. [CrossRef]
2. Baraniak, P.R.; McDevitt, T.C. Stem Cell Paracrine Actions and Tissue Regeneration. *Regen. Med.* **2010**, *5*, 121–143. [CrossRef]
3. Cho, I.J.; Lui, P.P.W.; Obajdin, J.; Riccio, F.; Stroukov, W.; Willis, T.L.; Spagnoli, F.; Watt, F.M. Mechanisms, Hallmarks, and Implications of Stem Cell Quiescence. *Stem Cell Rep.* **2019**, *12*, 1190–1200. [CrossRef]
4. Mi, L.; Hu, J.; Li, N.; Gao, J.; Huo, R.; Peng, X.; Zhang, N.; Liu, Y.; Zhao, H.; Liu, R.; et al. The Mechanism of Stem Cell Aging. *Stem Cell Rev. Rep.* **2022**, *18*, 1281–1293. [CrossRef]
5. de Morree, A.; Rando, T.A. Regulation of Adult Stem Cell Quiescence and Its Functions in the Maintenance of Tissue Integrity. *Nat. Rev. Mol. Cell Biol.* **2023**, *24*, 334–354. [CrossRef]
6. Brunet, A.; Goodell, M.A.; Rando, T.A. Ageing and Rejuvenation of Tissue Stem Cells and Their Niches. *Nat. Rev. Mol. Cell Biol.* **2023**, *24*, 45–62. [CrossRef]
7. Lampert, M.A.; Gustafsson, Å.B. Mitochondria and Autophagy in Adult Stem Cells: Proliferate or Differentiate. *J. Muscle Res. Cell Motil.* **2020**, *41*, 355–362. [CrossRef]
8. Borodkina, A.V.; Shatrova, A.N.; Deryabin, P.I.; Griukova, A.A.; Abushik, P.A.; Antonov, S.M.; Nikolsky, N.N.; Burova, E.B. Calcium Alterations Signal Either to Senescence or to Autophagy Induction in Stem Cells upon Oxidative Stress. *Aging* **2016**, *8*, 3400–3418. [CrossRef]
9. Ma, Y.; Qi, M.; An, Y.; Zhang, L.; Yang, R.; Doro, D.H.; Liu, W.; Jin, Y. Autophagy Controls Mesenchymal Stem Cell Properties and Senescence during Bone Aging. *Aging Cell* **2018**, *17*, e12709. [CrossRef]
10. Murmu, N.; Shravage, B.V. Autophagy Slows the Aging of Germline Stem Cells in Drosophila through Modulation of E-Cadherin. *bioRxiv* **2022**, 2022.03.31.486570. [CrossRef]
11. Houri, K.; Mori, T.; Onodera, Y.; Tsujimoto, T.; Takehara, T.; Nakao, S.; Teramura, T.; Fukuda, K. MiR-142 Induces Accumulation of Reactive Oxygen Species (ROS) by Inhibiting Pexophagy in Aged Bone Marrow Mesenchymal Stem Cells. *Sci. Rep.* **2020**, *10*, 3735. [CrossRef]
12. Mortensen, M.; Soilleux, E.J.; Djordjevic, G.; Tripp, R.; Lutteropp, M.; Sadighi-Akha, E.; Stranks, A.J.; Glanville, J.; Knight, S.; Jacobsen, S.E.W.; et al. The Autophagy Protein Atg7 Is Essential for Hematopoietic Stem Cell Maintenance. *J. Exp. Med.* **2011**, *208*, 455–467. [CrossRef]
13. Ho, T.T.; Warr, M.R.; Adelman, E.R.; Lansinger, O.M.; Flach, J.; Verovskaya, E.V.; Figueroa, M.E.; Passegué, E. Autophagy Maintains the Metabolism and Function of Young and Old Stem Cells. *Nature* **2017**, *543*, 205–210. [CrossRef]
14. Borsa, M.; Obba, S.; Richter, F.C.; Zhang, H.; Riffelmacher, T.; Carrelha, J.; Alsaleh, G.; Jacobsen, S.E.W.; Simon, A.K. Autophagy Preserves Hematopoietic Stem Cells by Restraining MTORC1-Mediated Cellular Anabolism. *Autophagy* **2024**, *20*, 45–57. [CrossRef]
15. Chu, Y.; Yuan, X.; Tao, Y.; Yang, B.; Luo, J. Autophagy in Muscle Regeneration: Mechanisms, Targets, and Therapeutic Perspective. *Int. J. Mol. Sci.* **2024**, *25*, 11901. [CrossRef]
16. Dellorusso, P.V.; Proven, M.A.; Calero-Nieto, F.J.; Wang, X.; Mitchell, C.A.; Hartmann, F.; Amouzgar, M.; Favaro, P.; DeVilbiss, A.; Swann, J.W.; et al. Autophagy Counters Inflammation-Driven Glycolytic Impairment in Aging Hematopoietic Stem Cells. *Cell Stem Cell* **2024**, *31*, 1020–1037.e9. [CrossRef]

17. Fang, Y.; An, N.; Zhu, L.; Gu, Y.; Qian, J.; Jiang, G.; Zhao, R.; Wei, W.; Xu, L.; Zhang, G.; et al. Autophagy-Sirt3 Axis Decelerates Hematopoietic Aging. *Aging Cell* **2020**, *19*, e13232. [CrossRef]
18. Dong, S.; Wang, Q.; Kao, Y.R.; Diaz, A.; Tasset, I.; Kaushik, S.; Thiruthuvanathan, V.; Zintiridou, A.; Nieves, E.; Dzieciatkowska, M.; et al. Chaperone-Mediated Autophagy Sustains Haematopoietic Stem-Cell Function. *Nature* **2021**, *591*, 117–123. [CrossRef]
19. Ghanta, S.; Tsoyi, K.; Liu, X.; Nakahira, K.; Ith, B.; Coronata, A.A.; Fredenburgh, L.E.; Englert, J.A.; Piantadosi, C.A.; Choi, A.M.K.; et al. Mesenchymal Stromal Cells Deficient in Autophagy Proteins Are Susceptible to Oxidative Injury and Mitochondrial Dysfunction. *Am. J. Respir. Cell Mol. Biol.* **2017**, *56*, 300–309. [CrossRef]
20. Hu, C.; Zhao, L.; Wu, D.; Li, L. Modulating Autophagy in Mesenchymal Stem Cells Effectively Protects against Hypoxia- or Ischemia-Induced Injury. *Stem Cell Res. Ther.* **2019**, *10*, 120. [CrossRef]
21. Song, C.; Song, C.; Tong, F. Autophagy Induction Is a Survival Response against Oxidative Stress in Bone Marrow-Derived Mesenchymal Stromal Cells. *Cytotherapy* **2014**, *16*, 1361–1370. [CrossRef]
22. Bigarella, C.L.; Liang, R.; Ghaffari, S. Stem Cells and the Impact of ROS Signaling. *Development* **2014**, *141*, 4206–4218. [CrossRef]
23. Sinenko, S.A.; Starkova, T.Y.; Kuzmin, A.A.; Tomilin, A.N. Physiological Signaling Functions of Reactive Oxygen Species in Stem Cells: From Flies to Man. *Front. Cell Dev. Biol.* **2021**, *9*, 714370. [CrossRef]
24. Prakash, R.; Fauzia, E.; Siddiqui, A.J.; Yadav, S.K.; Kumari, N.; Shams, M.T.; Naeem, A.; Praharaj, P.P.; Khan, M.A.; Bhutia, S.K.; et al. Oxidative Stress-Induced Autophagy Compromises Stem Cell Viability. *Stem Cells* **2022**, *40*, 468–478. [CrossRef]
25. López-Otín, C.; Blasco, M.A.; Partridge, L.; Serrano, M.; Kroemer, G. The Hallmarks of Aging. *Cell* **2013**, *153*, 1194. [CrossRef]
26. Chen, F.; Liu, Y.; Wong, N.-K.; Xiao, J.; So, K.-F. Oxidative Stress in Stem Cell Aging. *Cell Transplant.* **2017**, *26*, 1483–1495. [CrossRef]
27. Zhao, K.; Chan, I.T.C.; Tse, E.H.Y.; Xie, Z.; Cheung, T.H.; Zeng, Y.A. Autophagy in Adult Stem Cell Homeostasis, Aging, and Disease Therapy. *Cell Regen.* **2025**, *14*, 14. [CrossRef]
28. Wei, Y.; Zheng, Z.; Zhang, Y.; Sun, J.; Xu, S.; Di, X.; Ding, X.; Ding, G. Regulation of Mesenchymal Stem Cell Differentiation by Autophagy. *Open Med.* **2024**, *19*, 20240968. [CrossRef]
29. Guan, J.L.; Simon, A.K.; Prescott, M.; Menendez, J.A.; Liu, F.; Wang, F.; Wang, C.; Wolvetang, E.; Vazquez-Martin, A.; Zhang, J. Autophagy in Stem Cells. *Autophagy* **2013**, *9*, 830–849. [CrossRef]
30. Holczer, M.; Hajdú, B.; Lőrincz, T.; Szarka, A.; Bánhegyi, G.; Kapuy, O. Fine-Tuning of AMPK-ULK1-MTORC1 Regulatory Triangle Is Crucial for Autophagy Oscillation. *Sci. Rep.* **2020**, *10*, 17803. [CrossRef]
31. Wu, F.; Chen, Z.; Liu, J.; Hou, Y. The Akt–MTOR Network at the Interface of Hematopoietic Stem Cell Homeostasis. *Exp. Hematol.* **2021**, *103*, 15–23. [CrossRef]
32. Magri, L.; Galli, R. MTOR Signaling in Neural Stem Cells: From Basic Biology to Disease. *Cell Mol. Life Sci.* **2013**, *70*, 2887–2898. [CrossRef]
33. Xiang, X.; Zhao, J.; Xu, G.; Li, Y.; Zhang, W. MTOR and the Differentiation of Mesenchymal Stem Cells. *Acta Biochim. Biophys. Sin.* **2011**, *43*, 501–510. [CrossRef]
34. Alhasan, B.A.; Gordeev, S.A.; Knyazeva, A.R.; Aleksandrova, K.V.; Margulis, B.A.; Guzhova, I.V.; Suvorova, I.I. The MTOR Pathway in Pluripotent Stem Cells: Lessons for Understanding Cancer Cell Dormancy. *Membranes* **2021**, *11*, 858. [CrossRef]
35. Fan, C.; Zhao, C.; Zhang, F.; Kesarwani, M.; Tu, Z.; Cai, X.; Davis, A.K.; Xu, L.; Hochstetler, C.L.; Chen, X.; et al. Adaptive Responses to MTOR Gene Targeting in Hematopoietic Stem Cells Reveal a Proliferative Mechanism Evasive to MTOR Inhibition. *Proc. Natl. Acad. Sci. USA* **2021**, *118*, e2020102118. [CrossRef]
36. Chang, N.C. Autophagy and Stem Cells: Self-Eating for Self-Renewal. *Front. Cell Dev. Biol.* **2020**, *8*, 138. [CrossRef]
37. Wang, C.; Haas, M.; Yeo, S.K.; Sebti, S.; Fernández, Á.F.; Zou, Z.; Levine, B.; Guan, J.L. Enhanced Autophagy in Becn1F121A/F121A Knockin Mice Counteracts Aging-Related Neural Stem Cell Exhaustion and Dysfunction. *Autophagy* **2022**, *18*, 409–422. [CrossRef]
38. He, Y.; Lu, H.; Zhao, Y. Development of an Autophagy Activator from Class III PI3K Complexes, Tat-BECN1 Peptide: Mechanisms and Applications. *Front. Cell Dev. Biol.* **2022**, *10*, 851166. [CrossRef]
39. Mizushima, N.; Ohsumi, Y.; Yoshimori, T. Autophagosome Formation in Mammalian Cells. *Cell Struct. Funct.* **2002**, *27*, 421–429. [CrossRef]
40. Cassidy, L.D.; Narita, M. Autophagy at the Intersection of Aging, Senescence, and Cancer. *Mol. Oncol.* **2022**, *16*, 3259–3275. [CrossRef]
41. Liu, Y.; Shi, L.; Chen, Y.; Luo, S.; Chen, Y.; Chen, H.; Lan, W.; Lu, X.; Cao, Z.; Ye, Z.; et al. Autophagy Regulates the Maturation of Hematopoietic Precursors in the Embryo. *Nat. Commun.* **2024**, *15*, 2255. [CrossRef]
42. Nitta, A.; Hori, K.; Tanida, I.; Igarashi, A.; Deyama, Y.; Ueno, T.; Kominami, E.; Sugai, M.; Aoki, K. Blocking LC3 Lipidation and ATG12 Conjugation Reactions by ATG7 Mutant Protein Containing C572S. *Biochem. Biophys. Res. Commun.* **2019**, *508*, 521–526. [CrossRef]
43. Liu, J.; Xiao, Y.; Cao, L.; Lu, S.; Zhang, S.; Yang, R.; Wang, Y.; Zhang, N.; Yu, Y.; Wang, X.; et al. Insights on E1-like Enzyme ATG7: Functional Regulation and Relationships with Aging-Related Diseases. *Commun. Biol.* **2024**, *7*, 382. [CrossRef]

44. Zhou, J.; He, H.; Zhang, J.J.; Liu, X.; Yao, W.; Li, C.; Xu, T.; Yin, S.Y.; Wu, D.Y.; Dou, C.L.; et al. ATG7-Mediated Autophagy Facilitates Embryonic Stem Cell Exit from Naive Pluripotency and Marks Commitment to Differentiation. *Autophagy* **2022**, *18*, 2946–2968. [CrossRef]
45. Shen, Y.; Li, T.; Sun, C.; Cheng, X.; Chen, Z.; Wang, G.; Yang, X. Atg7 Autophagy-Independent Role on Governing Neural Stem Cell Fate Could Be Potentially Applied for Regenerative Medicine. *Cell Death Differ.* **2024**, *31*, 1375–1388. [CrossRef]
46. Joshi, A.; Kundu, M. Mitophagy in Hematopoietic Stem Cells: The Case for Exploration. *Autophagy* **2013**, *9*, 1737–1749. [CrossRef]
47. Narendra, D.P.; Youle, R.J. The Role of PINK1-Parkin in Mitochondrial Quality Control. *Nat. Cell Biol.* **2024**, *26*, 1639–1651. [CrossRef]
48. Liu, K.; Li, X.; Li, Z.; Cao, J.; Li, X.; Xu, Y.; Liu, L.; Zhao, T. Evaluating Mitophagy in Embryonic Stem Cells by Using Fluorescence-Based Imaging. *Front. Cell Dev. Biol.* **2022**, *10*, 910464. [CrossRef]
49. Lin, Q.; Chen, J.; Gu, L.; Dan, X.; Zhang, C.; Yang, Y. New Insights into Mitophagy and Stem Cells. *Stem Cell Res. Ther.* **2021**, *12*, 452. [CrossRef]
50. Lampert, M.A.; Orogo, A.M.; Najor, R.H.; Hammerling, B.C.; Leon, L.J.; Wang, B.J.; Kim, T.; Sussman, M.A.; Gustafsson, Å.B. BNIP3L/NIX and FUNDC1-Mediated Mitophagy Is Required for Mitochondrial Network Remodeling during Cardiac Progenitor Cell Differentiation. *Autophagy* **2019**, *15*, 1182–1198. [CrossRef]
51. Settembre, C.; Di Malta, C.; Polito, V.A.; Arencibia, M.G.; Vetrini, F.; Erdin, S.; Erdin, S.U.; Huynh, T.; Medina, D.; Colella, P.; et al. TFEB Links Autophagy to Lysosomal Biogenesis. *Science* **2011**, *332*, 1429–1433. [CrossRef]
52. Audesse, A.J.; Dhakal, S.; Hassell, L.A.; Gardell, Z.; Nemtsova, Y.; Webb, A.E. FOXO3 Directly Regulates an Autophagy Network to Functionally Regulate Proteostasis in Adult Neural Stem Cells. *PLoS Genet.* **2019**, *15*, e1008097. [CrossRef]
53. Gómez-Puerto, M.C.; Verhagen, L.P.; Braat, A.K.; Lam, E.W.F.; Coffer, P.J.; Lorenowicz, M.J. Activation of Autophagy by FOXO3 Regulates Redox Homeostasis during Osteogenic Differentiation. *Autophagy* **2016**, *12*, 1804–1816. [CrossRef]
54. Warr, M.R.; Binnewies, M.; Flach, J.; Reynaud, D.; Garg, T.; Malhotra, R.; Debnath, J.; Passegué, E. FOXO3A Directs a Protective Autophagy Program in Haematopoietic Stem Cells. *Nature* **2013**, *494*, 323–327. [CrossRef]
55. Tan, A.; Prasad, R.; Jho, E.H. TFEB Regulates Pluripotency Transcriptional Network in Mouse Embryonic Stem Cells Independent of Autophagy-Lysosomal Biogenesis. *Cell Death Dis.* **2021**, *12*, 343. [CrossRef]
56. García-Prat, L.; Kaufmann, K.B.; Schneiter, F.; Voisin, V.; Murison, A.; Chen, J.; Chan-Seng-Yue, M.; Gan, O.I.; McLeod, J.L.; Smith, S.A.; et al. TFEB-Mediated Endolysosomal Activity Controls Human Hematopoietic Stem Cell Fate. *Cell Stem Cell* **2021**, *28*, 1838–1850.e10. [CrossRef]
57. Balzano, F.; Campesi, I.; Cruciani, S.; Garroni, G.; Bellu, E.; Giudici, S.D.; Angius, A.; Oggiano, A.; Rallo, V.; Capobianco, G.; et al. Epigenetics, Stem Cells, and Autophagy: Exploring a Path Involving MiRNA. *Int. J. Mol. Sci.* **2019**, *20*, 5091. [CrossRef]
58. Yang, L.; Wang, H.; Shen, Q.; Feng, L.; Jin, H. Long Non-Coding RNAs Involved in Autophagy Regulation. *Cell Death Dis.* **2017**, *8*, e3073. [CrossRef]
59. Wang, W.; Wang, Y.; Duan, C.; Tian, W.; Gao, L. LncRNA NEAT1-206 Regulates Autophagy of Human Umbilical Cord Mesenchymal Stem Cells through the WNT5A/Ca^{2+} Signaling Pathway under Senescence Stress. *Noncoding RNA Res.* **2025**, *11*, 234–248. [CrossRef]
60. Vitale, E.; Perveen, S.; Rossin, D.; Lo Iacono, M.; Rastaldo, R.; Giachino, C. Role of Chaperone-Mediated Autophagy in Ageing Biology and Rejuvenation of Stem Cells. *Front. Cell Dev. Biol.* **2022**, *10*, 912470. [CrossRef]
61. Lim, S.H.Y.; Hansen, M.; Kumsta, C. Molecular Mechanisms of Autophagy Decline during Aging. *Cells* **2024**, *13*, 1364. [CrossRef]
62. García-Prat, L.; Martínez-Vicente, M.; Perdiguero, E.; Ortet, L.; Rodríguez-Ubreva, J.; Rebollo, E.; Ruiz-Bonilla, V.; Gutarra, S.; Ballestar, E.; Serrano, A.L.; et al. Autophagy Maintains Stemness by Preventing Senescence. *Nature* **2016**, *529*, 37–42. [CrossRef]
63. Tang, A.H.; Rando, T.A. Induction of Autophagy Supports the Bioenergetic Demands of Quiescent Muscle Stem Cell Activation. *EMBO J.* **2014**, *33*, 2782–2797. [CrossRef]
64. Rastaldo, R.; Vitale, E.; Giachino, C. Dual Role of Autophagy in Regulation of Mesenchymal Stem Cell Senescence. *Front. Cell Dev. Biol.* **2020**, *8*, 276. [CrossRef]
65. Ma, W.; Lu, Y.; Jin, X.; Lin, N.; Zhang, L.; Song, Y. Targeting Selective Autophagy and beyond: From Underlying Mechanisms to Potential Therapies. *J. Adv. Res.* **2024**, *65*, 297–327. [CrossRef]
66. Chong, C.M.; Ke, M.; Tan, Y.; Huang, Z.; Zhang, K.; Ai, N.; Ge, W.; Qin, D.; Lu, J.H.; Su, H. Presenilin 1 Deficiency Suppresses Autophagy in Human Neural Stem Cells through Reducing γ-Secretase-Independent ERK/CREB Signaling. *Cell Death Dis.* **2018**, *9*, 879. [CrossRef]
67. Balnis, J.; Jackson, E.L.; Drake, L.A.; Singer, D.V.; Bossardi Ramos, R.; Singer, H.A.; Jaitovich, A. Rapamycin Improves Satellite Cells' Autophagy and Muscle Regeneration during Hypercapnia. *JCI Insight* **2025**, *10*, e182842. [CrossRef]
68. Li, Z.-H.; Wang, Y.-L.; Wang, H.-J.; Wu, J.-H.; Tan, Y.-Z. Rapamycin-Preactivated Autophagy Enhances Survival and Differentiation of Mesenchymal Stem Cells After Transplantation into Infarcted Myocardium. *Stem Cell Rev. Rep.* **2020**, *16*, 344–356. [CrossRef]
69. Ceccariglia, S.; Cargnoni, A.; Silini, A.R.; Parolini, O. Autophagy: A Potential Key Contributor to the Therapeutic Action of Mesenchymal Stem Cells. *Autophagy* **2020**, *16*, 28–37. [CrossRef]

70. Thannickal, V.J.; Fanburg, B.L. Reactive Oxygen Species in Cell Signaling. *Am. J. Physiol. Lung Cell Mol. Physiol.* **2000**, *279*, L1005–L1028. [CrossRef]
71. Juan, C.A.; de la Lastra, J.M.P.; Plou, F.J.; Pérez-Lebeña, E. The Chemistry of Reactive Oxygen Species (ROS) Revisited: Outlining Their Role in Biological Macromolecules (DNA, Lipids and Proteins) and Induced Pathologies. *Int. J. Mol. Sci.* **2021**, *22*, 4642. [CrossRef]
72. Boldogh, I.R.; Pon, L.A. Mitochondria on the Move. *Trends Cell Biol.* **2007**, *17*, 502–510. [CrossRef]
73. Urao, N.; Ushio-Fukai, M. Redox Regulation of Stem/Progenitor Cells and Bone Marrow Niche. *Free Radic. Biol. Med.* **2013**, *54*, 26–39. [CrossRef]
74. Tahara, E.B.; Navarete, F.D.T.; Kowaltowski, A.J. Tissue-, Substrate-, and Site-Specific Characteristics of Mitochondrial Reactive Oxygen Species Generation. *Free Radic. Biol. Med.* **2009**, *46*, 1283–1297. [CrossRef]
75. Murphy, M.P. How Mitochondria Produce Reactive Oxygen Species. *Biochem. J.* **2009**, *417*, 1–13. [CrossRef]
76. Bedard, K.; Krause, K.H. The NOX Family of ROS-Generating NADPH Oxidases: Physiology and Pathophysiology. *Physiol. Rev.* **2007**, *87*, 245–313. [CrossRef]
77. Maraldi, T.; Angeloni, C.; Prata, C.; Hrelia, S. NADPH Oxidases: Redox Regulators of Stem Cell Fate and Function. *Antioxidants* **2021**, *10*, 973. [CrossRef]
78. Ushio-Fukai, M. Compartmentalization of Redox Signaling through NaDPH Oxidase-Derived ROS. *Antioxid. Redox Signal.* **2009**, *11*, 1289–1299. [CrossRef]
79. Finkel, T.; Holbrook, N.J. Oxidants, Oxidative Stress and the Biology of Ageing. *Nature* **2000**, *408*, 239–247. [CrossRef]
80. Stavely, R.; Nurgali, K. The Emerging Antioxidant Paradigm of Mesenchymal Stem Cell Therapy. *Stem Cells Transl. Med.* **2020**, *9*, 985–1006. [CrossRef]
81. Kasper, G.; Mao, L.; Geissler, S.; Draycheva, A.; Trippens, J.; Kühnisch, J.; Tschirschmann, M.; Kaspar, K.; Perka, C.; Duda, G.N.; et al. Insights into Mesenchymal Stem Cell Aging: Involvement of Antioxidant Defense and Actin Cytoskeleton. *Stem Cells* **2009**, *27*, 1288–1297. [CrossRef]
82. Jang, Y.Y.; Sharkis, S.J. A Low Level of Reactive Oxygen Species Selects for Primitive Hematopoietic Stem Cells That May Reside in the Low-Oxygenic Niche. *Blood* **2007**, *110*, 3056–3063. [CrossRef]
83. Ludin, A.; Gur-Cohen, S.; Golan, K.; Kaufmann, K.B.; Itkin, T.; Medaglia, C.; Lu, X.J.; Ledergor, G.; Kollet, O.; Lapidot, T. Reactive Oxygen Species Regulate Hematopoietic Stem Cell Self-Renewal, Migration and Development, as Well as Their Bone Marrow Microenvironment. *Antioxid. Redox Signal.* **2014**, *21*, 1605–1619. [CrossRef]
84. Wilson, A.; Laurenti, E.; Oser, G.; van der Wath, R.C.; Blanco-Bose, W.; Jaworski, M.; Offner, S.; Dunant, C.F.; Eshkind, L.; Bockamp, E.; et al. Hematopoietic Stem Cells Reversibly Switch from Dormancy to Self-Renewal during Homeostasis and Repair. *Cell* **2008**, *135*, 1118–1129. [CrossRef]
85. Ito, K.; Hirao, A.; Arai, F.; Matsuoka, S.; Takubo, K.; Hamaguchi, I.; Nomiyama, K.; Hosokawa, K.; Sakurada, K.; Nakagata, N.; et al. Regulation of Oxidative Stress by ATM Is Required for Self-Renewal of Haematopoietic Stem Cells. *Nature* **2004**, *431*, 997–1002. [CrossRef]
86. Jing, Q.; Zhou, C.; Zhang, J.; Zhang, P.; Wu, Y.; Zhou, J.; Tong, X.; Li, Y.; Du, J.; Wang, Y. Role of Reactive Oxygen Species in Myelodysplastic Syndromes. *Cell Mol. Biol. Lett.* **2024**, *29*, 53. [CrossRef]
87. Valle-Prieto, A.; Conget, P.A. Human Mesenchymal Stem Cells Efficiently Manage Oxidative Stress. *Stem Cells Dev.* **2010**, *19*, 1885–1893. [CrossRef]
88. Gorbunov, N.V.; Garrison, B.R.; McDaniel, D.P.; Zhai, M.; Liao, P.J.; Nurmemet, D.; Kiang, J.G. Adaptive Redox Response of Mesenchymal Stromal Cells to Stimulation with Lipopolysaccharide Inflammagen: Mechanisms of Remodeling of Tissue Barriers in Sepsis. *Oxid. Med. Cell Longev.* **2013**, *2013*, 139–148. [CrossRef]
89. Liu, T.; Ma, X.; Ouyang, T.; Chen, H.; Lin, J.; Liu, J.; Xiao, Y.; Yu, J.; Huang, Y. SIRT1 Reverses Senescence via Enhancing Autophagy and Attenuates Oxidative Stress-Induced Apoptosis through Promoting P53 Degradation. *Int. J. Biol. Macromol.* **2018**, *117*, 225–234. [CrossRef]
90. Pan, H.; Guan, D.; Liu, X.; Li, J.; Wang, L.; Wu, J.; Zhou, J.; Zhang, W.; Ren, R.; Zhang, W.; et al. SIRT6 Safeguards Human Mesenchymal Stem Cells from Oxidative Stress by Coactivating NRF2. *Cell Res.* **2016**, *26*, 190–205. [CrossRef]
91. Kobayashi, C.I.; Suda, T. Regulation of Reactive Oxygen Species in Stem Cells and Cancer Stem Cells. *J. Cell Physiol.* **2012**, *227*, 421–430. [CrossRef] [PubMed]
92. Pervaiz, S.; Taneja, R.; Ghaffari, S. Oxidative Stress Regulation of Stem and Progenitor Cells. *Antioxid. Redox Signal.* **2009**, *11*, 2777–2789. [CrossRef] [PubMed]
93. Le Belle, J.E.; Orozco, N.M.; Paucar, A.A.; Saxe, J.P.; Mottahedeh, J.; Pyle, A.D.; Wu, H.; Kornblum, H.I. Proliferative Neural Stem Cells Have High Endogenous ROS Levels That Regulate Self-Renewal and Neurogenesis in a PI3K/Akt-Dependant Manner. *Cell Stem Cell* **2011**, *8*, 59–71. [CrossRef] [PubMed]
94. Juntilla, M.M.; Patil, V.D.; Calamito, M.; Joshi, R.P.; Birnbaum, M.J.; Koretzky, G.A. AKT1 and AKT2 Maintain Hematopoietic Stem Cell Function by Regulating Reactive Oxygen Species. *Blood* **2010**, *115*, 4030–4038. [CrossRef] [PubMed]

95. Borodkina, A.; Shatrova, A.; Abushik, P.; Nikolsky, N.; Burova, E. Interaction between ROS Dependent DNA Damage, Mitochondria and P38 MAPK Underlies Senescence of Human Adult Stem Cells. *Aging* **2014**, *6*, 481–495. [CrossRef]
96. Burova, E.; Borodkina, A.; Shatrova, A.; Nikolsky, N. Sublethal Oxidative Stress Induces the Premature Senescence of Human Mesenchymal Stem Cells Derived from Endometrium. *Oxid. Med. Cell Longev.* **2013**, *2013*, 474931. [CrossRef]
97. Dai, X.; Yan, X.; Wintergerst, K.A.; Cai, L.; Keller, B.B.; Tan, Y. Nrf2: Redox and Metabolic Regulator of Stem Cell State and Function. *Trends Mol. Med.* **2020**, *26*, 185–200. [CrossRef]
98. Kim, J.H.; Song, S.Y.; Park, S.G.; Song, S.U.; Xia, Y.; Sung, J.H. Primary Involvement of NADPH Oxidase 4 in Hypoxia-Induced Generation of Reactive Oxygen Species in Adipose-Derived Stem Cells. *Stem Cells Dev.* **2012**, *21*, 2212–2221. [CrossRef]
99. Li, S.Y.; Deng, Y.B.; Feng, J.Q.; Ye, W.B. Oxidative Preconditioning Promotes Bone Marrow Mesenchymal Stem Cells Migration and Prevents Apoptosis. *Cell Biol. Int.* **2009**, *33*, 411–418. [CrossRef]
100. Busletta, C.; Novo, E.; Valfrè Di Bonzo, L.; Povero, D.; Paternostro, C.; Ievolella, M.; Mareschi, K.; Ferrero, I.; Cannito, S.; Compagnone, A.; et al. Dissection of the Biphasic Nature of Hypoxia-Induced Motogenic Action in Bone Marrow-Derived Human Mesenchymal Stem Cells. *Stem Cells* **2011**, *29*, 952–963. [CrossRef]
101. Rodríguez-Carballo, E.; Gámez, B.; Ventura, F. P38 MAPK Signaling in Osteoblast Differentiation. *Front. Cell Dev. Biol.* **2016**, *4*, 40. [CrossRef] [PubMed]
102. Ji, A.R.; Ku, S.Y.; Cho, M.S.; Kim, Y.Y.; Kim, Y.J.; Oh, S.K.; Kim, S.H.; Moon, S.Y.; Choi, Y.M. Reactive Oxygen Species Enhance Differentiation of Human Embryonic Stem Cells into Mesendodermal Lineage. *Exp. Mol. Med.* **2010**, *42*, 175–186. [CrossRef] [PubMed]
103. Moliner, A.; Enfors, P.; Ibáñez, C.F.; Andäng, M. Mouse Embryonic Stem Cell-Derived Spheres with Distinct Neurogenic Potentials. *Stem Cells Dev.* **2008**, *17*, 233–243. [CrossRef] [PubMed]
104. Tsatmali, M.; Walcott, E.C.; Makarenkova, H.; Crossin, K.L. Reactive Oxygen Species Modulate the Differentiation of Neurons in Clonal Cortical Cultures. *Mol. Cell Neurosci.* **2006**, *33*, 345–357. [CrossRef]
105. Sart, S.; Song, L.; Li, Y. Controlling Redox Status for Stem Cell Survival, Expansion, and Differentiation. *Oxid. Med. Cell Longev.* **2015**, *2015*, 105135. [CrossRef]
106. Spitkovsky, D.; Sasse, P.; Kolossov, E.; Böttinger, C.; Fleischmann, B.K.; Hescheler, J.; Wiesner, R.J. Activity of Complex III of the Mitochondrial Electron Transport Chain Is Essential for Early Heart Muscle Cell Differentiation. *FASEB J.* **2004**, *18*, 1300–1302. [CrossRef]
107. Chung, S.; Dzeja, P.P.; Faustino, R.S.; Perez-Terzic, C.; Behfar, A.; Terzic, A. Mitochondrial Oxidative Metabolism Is Required for the Cardiac Differentiation of Stem Cells. *Nat. Clin. Pract. Cardiovasc. Med.* **2007**, *4* (Suppl. S1), S60–S67. [CrossRef]
108. Chung, S.; Dzeja, P.P.; Faustino, R.S.; Terzic, A. Developmental Restructuring of the Creatine Kinase System Integrates Mitochondrial Energetics with Stem Cell Cardiogenesis. *Ann. N. Y. Acad. Sci.* **2008**, *1147*, 254–263. [CrossRef]
109. Zhou, D.; Shao, L.; Spitz, D.R. Reactive Oxygen Species in Normal and Tumor Stem Cells. *Adv. Cancer Res.* **2014**, *122*, 1–67. [CrossRef]
110. Bartesaghi, S.; Graziano, V.; Galavotti, S.; Henriquez, N.V.; Betts, J.; Saxena, J.; Deli, A.; Karlsson, A.; Martins, L.M.; Capasso, M.; et al. Inhibition of Oxidative Metabolism Leads to P53 Genetic Inactivation and Transformation in Neural Stem Cells. *Proc. Natl. Acad. Sci. USA* **2015**, *112*, 1059–1064. [CrossRef]
111. Marin Navarro, A.; Pronk, R.J.; van der Geest, A.T.; Oliynyk, G.; Nordgren, A.; Arsenian-Henriksson, M.; Falk, A.; Wilhelm, M. P53 Controls Genomic Stability and Temporal Differentiation of Human Neural Stem Cells and Affects Neural Organization in Human Brain Organoids. *Cell Death Dis.* **2020**, *11*, 52. [CrossRef] [PubMed]
112. Huang, M.; Wu, Q.; Jiang, Z.H. Epigenetic Alterations under Oxidative Stress in Stem Cells. *Oxid. Med. Cell Longev.* **2022**, *2022*, 6439097. [CrossRef] [PubMed]
113. Berniakovich, I.; Laricchia-Robbio, L.; Belmonte, J.C.I. N-Acetylcysteine Protects Induced Pluripotent Stem Cells from In Vitro Stress: Impact on Differentiation Outcome. *Int. J. Dev. Biol.* **2012**, *56*, 729–735. [CrossRef] [PubMed]
114. Meng, Z.; Liu, J.; Feng, Z.; Guo, S.; Wang, M.; Wang, Z.; Li, Z.; Li, H.; Sui, L. N-Acetylcysteine Regulates Dental Follicle Stem Cell Osteogenesis and Alveolar Bone Repair via ROS Scavenging. *Stem Cell Res. Ther.* **2022**, *13*, 466. [CrossRef]
115. Asgari, R.; Mehran, Y.Z.; Weber, H.M.; Weber, M.; Golestanha, S.A.; Hosseini Kazerouni, S.M.; Panahi, F.; Mohammadi, P.; Mansouri, K. Management of Oxidative Stress for Cell Therapy through Combinational Approaches of Stem Cells, Antioxidants, and Photobiomodulation. *Eur. J. Pharm. Sci.* **2024**, *196*, 106715. [CrossRef]
116. Li, C.J.; Sun, L.Y.; Pang, C.Y. Synergistic Protection of N-Acetylcysteine and Ascorbic Acid 2-Phosphate on Human Mesenchymal Stem Cells against Mitoptosis, Necroptosis and Apoptosis. *Sci. Rep.* **2015**, *5*, 9819. [CrossRef]
117. Rodriguez, S.; Wang, L.; Mumaw, C.; Srour, E.F.; Lo Celso, C.; Nakayama, K.I.; Carlesso, N. The SKP2 E3 Ligase Regulates Basal Homeostasis and Stress-Induced Regeneration of HSCs. *Blood* **2011**, *117*, 6509–6519. [CrossRef]
118. Zeng, W.; Xiao, J.; Zheng, G.; Xing, F.; Tipoe, G.L.; Wang, X.; He, C.; Chen, Z.Y.; Liu, Y. Antioxidant Treatment Enhances Human Mesenchymal Stem Cell Anti-Stress Ability and Therapeutic Efficacy in an Acute Liver Failure Model. *Sci. Rep.* **2015**, *5*, 11100. [CrossRef]

119. Cai, J.; Yu, X.; Zhang, B.; Zhang, H.; Fang, Y.; Liu, S.; Liu, T.; Ding, X. Atorvastatin Improves Survival of Implanted Stem Cells in a Rat Model of Renal Ischemia-Reperfusion Injury. *Am. J. Nephrol.* **2014**, *39*, 466–475. [CrossRef]
120. Song, L.; Yang, Y.J.; Dong, Q.T.; Qian, H.Y.; Gao, R.L.; Qiao, S.B.; Shen, R.; He, Z.X.; Lu, M.J.; Zhao, S.H.; et al. Atorvastatin Enhance Efficacy of Mesenchymal Stem Cells Treatment for Swine Myocardial Infarction via Activation of Nitric Oxide Synthase. *PLoS ONE* **2013**, *8*, e65702. [CrossRef]
121. Shyh-Chang, N.; Ng, H.H. The Metabolic Programming of Stem Cells. *Genes. Dev.* **2017**, *31*, 336–346. [CrossRef] [PubMed]
122. Ito, K.; Suda, T. Metabolic Requirements for the Maintenance of Self-Renewing Stem Cells. *Nat. Rev. Mol. Cell Biol.* **2014**, *15*, 243–256. [CrossRef] [PubMed]
123. Zheng, X.; Boyer, L.; Jin, M.; Mertens, J.; Kim, Y.; Ma, L.; Ma, L.; Hamm, M.; Gage, F.H.; Hunter, T. Metabolic Reprogramming during Neuronal Differentiation from Aerobic Glycolysis to Neuronal Oxidative Phosphorylation. *Elife* **2016**, *5*, e13374. [CrossRef] [PubMed]
124. Rojas-Ríos, P.; Chartier, A.; Enjolras, C.; Cremaschi, J.; Garret, C.; Boughlita, A.; Ramat, A.; Simonelig, M. PiRNAs Are Regulators of Metabolic Reprogramming in Stem Cells. *Nat. Commun.* **2024**, *15*, 8405. [CrossRef]
125. Dodson, M.; Anandhan, A.; Zhang, D.D.; Madhavan, L. An NRF2 Perspective on Stem Cells and Ageing. *Front. Aging* **2021**, *2*, 690686. [CrossRef]
126. Kim, S.U.; Park, Y.H.; Kim, J.M.; Sun, H.N.; Song, I.S.; Huang, S.M.; Lee, S.H.; Chae, J.I.; Hong, S.; Sik Choi, S.; et al. Dominant Role of Peroxiredoxin/JNK Axis in Stemness Regulation during Neurogenesis from Embryonic Stem Cells. *Stem Cells* **2014**, *32*, 998–1011. [CrossRef]
127. Park, K.R.; Yun, H.M.; Yeo, I.J.; Cho, S.; Hong, J.T.; Jeong, Y.S. Peroxiredoxin 6 Inhibits Osteogenic Differentiation and Bone Formation Through Human Dental Pulp Stem Cells and Induces Delayed Bone Development. *Antioxid. Redox Signal.* **2019**, *30*, 1969–1982. [CrossRef]
128. Scadden, D.T. The Stem-Cell Niche as an Entity of Action. *Nature* **2006**, *441*, 1075–1079. [CrossRef]
129. Di Mattia, M.; Mauro, A.; Citeroni, M.R.; Dufrusine, B.; Peserico, A.; Russo, V.; Berardinelli, P.; Dainese, E.; Cimini, A.; Barboni, B. Insight into Hypoxia Stemness Control. *Cells* **2021**, *10*, 2161. [CrossRef]
130. Li, X.; Jiang, O.; Wang, S. Molecular Mechanisms of Cellular Metabolic Homeostasis in Stem Cells. *Int. J. Oral. Sci.* **2023**, *15*, 52. [CrossRef]
131. Chen, C.; Tang, Q.; Zhang, Y.; Yu, M.; Jing, W.; Tian, W. Physioxia: A More Effective Approach for Culturing Human Adipose-Derived Stem Cells for Cell Transplantation. *Stem Cell Res. Ther.* **2018**, *9*, 148. [CrossRef] [PubMed]
132. Yako, H.; Niimi, N.; Kato, A.; Takaku, S.; Tatsumi, Y.; Nishito, Y.; Kato, K.; Sango, K. Role of Pyruvate in Maintaining Cell Viability and Energy Production under High-Glucose Conditions. *Sci. Rep.* **2021**, *11*, 18910. [CrossRef] [PubMed]
133. Song, C.; Xu, F.; Ren, Z.; Zhang, Y.; Meng, Y.; Yang, Y.; Lingadahalli, S.; Cheung, E.; Li, G.; Liu, W.; et al. Elevated Exogenous Pyruvate Potentiates Mesodermal Differentiation through Metabolic Modulation and AMPK/MTOR Pathway in Human Embryonic Stem Cells. *Stem Cell Rep.* **2019**, *13*, 338–351. [CrossRef] [PubMed]
134. Yi, Y.; Lan, X.; Li, Y.; Yan, C.; Lv, J.; Zhang, T.; Jiang, W. Fatty Acid Synthesis and Oxidation Regulate Human Endoderm Differentiation by Mediating SMAD3 Nuclear Localization via Acetylation. *Dev. Cell* **2023**, *58*, 1670–1687.e4. [CrossRef]
135. Cao, Z.; Xie, Y.; Yu, L.; Li, Y. Hepatocyte Growth Factor (HGF) and Stem Cell Factor (SCF) Maintained the Stemness of Human Bone Marrow Mesenchymal Stem Cells (HBMSCs) during Long-Term Expansion by Preserving Mitochondrial Function via the PI3K/AKT, ERK1/2, and STAT3 Signaling Pathways. *Stem Cell Res. Ther.* **2020**, *11*, 329. [CrossRef]
136. Wang, Z.; Wang, L.; Jiang, R.; Li, C.; Chen, X.; Xiao, H.; Hou, J.; Hu, L.; Huang, C.; Wang, Y. Ginsenoside Rg1 Prevents Bone Marrow Mesenchymal Stem Cell Senescence via NRF2 and PI3K/Akt Signaling. *Free Radic. Biol. Med.* **2021**, *174*, 182–194. [CrossRef]
137. Ning, B.; Hang, S.; Zhang, W.; Mao, C.; Li, D. An Update on the Bridging Factors Connecting Autophagy and Nrf2 Antioxidant Pathway. *Front. Cell Dev. Biol.* **2023**, *11*, 1232241. [CrossRef]
138. Chang, K.C.; Liu, P.F.; Chang, C.H.; Lin, Y.C.; Chen, Y.J.; Shu, C.W. The Interplay of Autophagy and Oxidative Stress in the Pathogenesis and Therapy of Retinal Degenerative Diseases. *Cell Biosci.* **2022**, *12*, 1. [CrossRef]
139. Narendra, D.; Tanaka, A.; Suen, D.F.; Youle, R.J. Parkin Is Recruited Selectively to Impaired Mitochondria and Promotes Their Autophagy. *J. Cell Biol.* **2008**, *183*, 795–803. [CrossRef]
140. Cairns, G.; Thumiah-Mootoo, M.; Burelle, Y.; Khacho, M. Mitophagy: A New Player in Stem Cell Biology. *Biology* **2020**, *9*, 481. [CrossRef]
141. Kondoh, H.; Lleonart, M.E.; Nakashima, Y.; Yokode, M.; Tanaka, M.; Bernard, D.; Gil, J.; Beach, D. A High Glycolytic Flux Supports the Proliferative Potential of Murine Embryonic Stem Cells. *Antioxid. Redox Signal.* **2007**, *9*, 293–299. [CrossRef] [PubMed]
142. Liu, K.; Zhao, Q.; Liu, P.; Cao, J.; Gong, J.; Wang, C.; Wang, W.; Li, X.; Sun, H.; Zhang, C.; et al. ATG3-Dependent Autophagy Mediates Mitochondrial Homeostasis in Pluripotency Acquirement and Maintenance. *Autophagy* **2016**, *12*, 2000–2008. [CrossRef]

143. Vazquez-Martin, A.; Van den Haute, C.; Cufí, S.; Corominas-Faja, B.; Cuyàs, E.; Lopez-Bonet, E.; Rodriguez-Gallego, E.; Fernández-Arroyo, S.; Joven, J.; Baekelandt, V.; et al. Mitophagy-Driven Mitochondrial Rejuvenation Regulates Stem Cell Fate. *Aging* **2016**, *8*, 1330–1352. [CrossRef] [PubMed]
144. Xiang, G.; Yang, L.; Long, Q.; Chen, K.; Tang, H.; Wu, Y.; Liu, Z.; Zhou, Y.; Qi, J.; Zheng, L.; et al. BNIP3L-Dependent Mitophagy Accounts for Mitochondrial Clearance during 3 Factors-Induced Somatic Cell Reprogramming. *Autophagy* **2017**, *13*, 1543–1555. [CrossRef] [PubMed]
145. Cairns, G.; Thumiah-Mootoo, M.; Abbasi, M.R.; Gourlay, M.; Racine, J.; Larionov, N.; Prola, A.; Khacho, M.; Burelle, Y. PINK1 Deficiency Alters Muscle Stem Cell Fate Decision and Muscle Regenerative Capacity. *Stem Cell Rep.* **2024**, *19*, 673–688. [CrossRef]
146. Murakami, K.; Kurotaki, D.; Kawase, W.; Soma, S.; Fukuchi, Y.; Kunimoto, H.; Yoshimi, R.; Koide, S.; Oshima, M.; Hishiki, T.; et al. OGT Regulates Hematopoietic Stem Cell Maintenance via PINK1-Dependent Mitophagy. *Cell Rep.* **2021**, *34*, 108579. [CrossRef]
147. Ma, Q. Role of Nrf2 in Oxidative Stress and Toxicity. *Annu. Rev. Pharmacol. Toxicol.* **2013**, *53*, 401–426. [CrossRef]
148. Jin, H.; Zhang, L.; He, J.; Wu, M.; Jia, L.; Guo, J. Role of FOXO3a Transcription Factor in the Regulation of Liver Oxidative Injury. *Antioxidants* **2022**, *11*, 2478. [CrossRef]
149. Zhou, J.; Liao, W.; Yang, J.; Ma, K.; Li, X.; Wang, Y.; Wang, D.; Wang, L.; Zhang, Y.; Yin, Y.; et al. FOXO3 Induces FOXO1-Dependent Autophagy by Activating the AKT1 Signaling Pathway. *Autophagy* **2012**, *8*, 1712–1723. [CrossRef]
150. Lee, D.H.; Park, J.S.; Lee, Y.S.; Han, J.; Lee, D.K.; Kwon, S.W.; Han, D.H.; Lee, Y.H.; Bae, S.H. SQSTM1/P62 Activates NFE2L2/NRF2 via ULK1-Mediated Autophagic KEAP1 Degradation and Protects Mouse Liver from Lipotoxicity. *Autophagy* **2020**, *16*, 1949–1973. [CrossRef]
151. Bigarella, C.L.; Li, J.; Rimmelé, P.; Liang, R.; Sobol, R.W.; Ghaffari, S. FOXO3 Transcription Factor Is Essential for Protecting Hematopoietic Stem and Progenitor Cells from Oxidative DNA Damage. *J. Biol. Chem.* **2017**, *292*, 3005–3015. [CrossRef] [PubMed]
152. Tothova, Z.; Kollipara, R.; Huntly, B.J.; Lee, B.H.; Castrillon, D.H.; Cullen, D.E.; McDowell, E.P.; Lazo-Kallanian, S.; Williams, I.R.; Sears, C.; et al. FoxOs Are Critical Mediators of Hematopoietic Stem Cell Resistance to Physiologic Oxidative Stress. *Cell* **2007**, *128*, 325–339. [CrossRef] [PubMed]
153. Yalcin, S.; Luciano, J.P.; Zhang, X.; Vercherat, C.; Taneja, R.; Ghaffari, S. Foxo3 Modulation of ATM and Oxidative Stress Mediates Distinct Functions in the Regulation of Hematopoietic Stem and Progenitor Cell Fate. *Blood* **2007**, *110*, 1272. [CrossRef]
154. Mohammadzadeh, M.; Halabian, R.; Gharehbaghian, A.; Amirizadeh, N.; Jahanian-Najafabadi, A.; Roushandeh, A.M.; Roudkenar, M.H. Nrf-2 Overexpression in Mesenchymal Stem Cells Reduces Oxidative Stress-Induced Apoptosis and Cytotoxicity. *Cell Stress. Chaperones* **2012**, *17*, 553–565. [CrossRef]
155. Liu, P.; Cao, B.; Zhou, Y.; Zhang, H.; Wang, C. Human Umbilical Cord-Derived Mesenchymal Stem Cells Alleviate Oxidative Stress-Induced Islet Impairment via the Nrf2/HO-1 Axis. *J. Mol. Cell Biol.* **2023**, *15*, mjad035. [CrossRef]
156. Hammad, M.; Raftari, M.; Cesário, R.; Salma, R.; Godoy, P.; Emami, S.N.; Haghdoost, S. Roles of Oxidative Stress and Nrf2 Signaling in Pathogenic and Non-Pathogenic Cells: A Possible General Mechanism of Resistance to Therapy. *Antioxidants* **2023**, *12*, 1371. [CrossRef]
157. Jiang, L.L.; Liu, L. Effect of Metformin on Stem Cells: Molecular Mechanism and Clinical Prospect. *World J. Stem Cells* **2020**, *12*, 1455–1473. [CrossRef]
158. Cekuc, M.S.; Ergul, Y.S.; Pius, A.K.; Meagan, M.; Shinohara, I.; Murayama, M.; Susuki, Y.; Ma, C.; Morita, M.; Chow, S.K.H.; et al. Metformin Modulates Cell Oxidative Stress to Mitigate Corticosteroid-Induced Suppression of Osteogenesis in a 3D Model. *J. Inflamm. Res.* **2024**, *17*, 10383–10396. [CrossRef]
159. Zhang, Q.; Yang, Y.J.; Wang, H.; Dong, Q.T.; Wang, T.J.; Qian, H.Y.; Xu, H. Autophagy Activation: A Novel Mechanism of Atorvastatin to Protect Mesenchymal Stem Cells from Hypoxia and Serum Deprivation via AMP-Activated Protein Kinase/Mammalian Target of Rapamycin Pathway. *Stem Cells Dev.* **2012**, *21*, 1321–1332. [CrossRef]
160. Gorabi, A.M.; Kiaie, N.; Pirro, M.; Bianconi, V.; Jamialahmadi, T.; Sahebkar, A. Effects of Statins on the Biological Features of Mesenchymal Stem Cells and Therapeutic Implications. *Heart Fail. Rev.* **2021**, *26*, 1259–1272. [CrossRef]
161. Li, X.-H.; Qian, S.-D.; Chen, D.; Li, Z.-Z.; Chen, K.-Y.; Pan, Y.-P.; Lv, X.-H.; Jia, R.-Q.; Yu, X.-F. A New Mechanism in Steroid-Induced Osteonecrosis of the Femoral Head and the Protective Role of Simvastatin. *Exp. Cell Res.* **2025**, *446*, 114471. [CrossRef] [PubMed]
162. Yu, X.H.; Xu, X.M.; Zhang, S.X. Low-Dose Dexamethasone Promotes Osteoblast Viability by Activating Autophagy via the SGK1/FOXO3a Signaling Pathway. *Cell Biol. Int.* **2023**, *47*, 669–678. [CrossRef] [PubMed]
163. Zhong, C.; Xu, H.; Chen, J.; Cai, W.; Zhou, J.; Peng, H. Human Umbilical Cord Mesenchymal Stem Cells Prevent Steroid-Induced Avascular Necrosis of the Femoral Head by Modulating Cellular Autophagy. *Biomedicines* **2024**, *12*, 2817. [CrossRef] [PubMed]
164. Eldien, H.S.; Mostafa, N.A.; Sayed, D.; Mansor, S.G.; Elewa, F.M.; Meligy, F.Y. Resveratrol Antiaging Impact on Bone Marrow-Derived Mesenchymal Stem Cells in A Duration-Dependent Manner. *Egypt. J. Histol.* **2023**, *46*, 335–354. [CrossRef]
165. Hu, C.; Li, L. The Application of Resveratrol to Mesenchymal Stromal Cell-Based Regenerative Medicine. *Stem Cell Res. Ther.* **2019**, *10*, 307. [CrossRef]
166. Suvorova, I.I.; Knyazeva, A.R.; Petukhov, A.V.; Aksenov, N.D.; Pospelov, V.A. Resveratrol Enhances Pluripotency of Mouse Embryonic Stem Cells by Activating AMPK/Ulk1 Pathway. *Cell Death Discov.* **2019**, *5*, 61. [CrossRef]

167. Fu, J.; Zhao, S.D.; Liu, H.J.; Yuan, Q.H.; Liu, S.M.; Zhang, Y.M.; Ling, E.A.; Hao, A.J. Melatonin Promotes Proliferation and Differentiation of Neural Stem Cells Subjected to Hypoxia In Vitro. *J. Pineal Res.* **2011**, *51*, 104–112. [CrossRef]
168. Song, J.; Kang, S.M.; Lee, K.M.; Lee, J.E. The Protective Effect of Melatonin on Neural Stem Cell against LPS-Induced Inflammation. *Biomed. Res. Int.* **2015**, *2015*, 854359. [CrossRef]
169. Gong, X.; Ivanov, V.N.; Hei, T.K. 2,3,5,6-Tetramethylpyrazine (TMP) down-Regulated Arsenic-Induced Heme Oxygenase-1 and ARS2 Expression by Inhibiting Nrf2, NF-KB, AP-1 and MAPK Pathways in Human Proximal Tubular Cells. *Arch. Toxicol.* **2016**, *90*, 2187–2200. [CrossRef]
170. Ma, W.; He, F.; Ding, F.; Zhang, L.; Huang, Q.; Bi, C.; Wang, X.; Hua, B.; Yang, F.; Yuan, Y.; et al. Pre-Treatment with Melatonin Enhances Therapeutic Efficacy of Cardiac Progenitor Cells for Myocardial Infarction. *Cell. Physiol. Biochem.* **2018**, *47*, 1287–1298. [CrossRef]
171. Yoo, Y.M.; Han, T.Y.; Kim, H.S. Melatonin Suppresses Autophagy Induced by Clinostat in Preosteoblast MC3T3-E1 Cells. *Int. J. Mol. Sci.* **2016**, *17*, 526. [CrossRef] [PubMed]
172. Wang, F.W.; Wang, Z.; Zhang, Y.M.; Du, Z.X.; Zhang, X.L.; Liu, Q.; Guo, Y.J.; Li, X.G.; Hao, A.J. Protective Effect of Melatonin on Bone Marrow Mesenchymal Stem Cells against Hydrogen Peroxide-Induced Apoptosis In Vitro. *J. Cell Biochem.* **2013**, *114*, 2346–2355. [CrossRef] [PubMed]
173. Liu, C.; Zhou, W.; Li, Z.; Ren, J.; Li, X.; Li, S.; Liu, Q.; Song, F.; Hao, A.; Wang, F. Melatonin Protects Neural Stem Cells Against Tri-Ortho-Cresyl Phosphate-Induced Autophagy. *Front. Mol. Neurosci.* **2020**, *13*, 25. [CrossRef] [PubMed]
174. Tang, Y.; Jacobi, A.; Vater, C.; Zou, L.; Zou, X.; Stiehler, M. Icariin Promotes Angiogenic Differentiation and Prevents Oxidative Stress-Induced Autophagy in Endothelial Progenitor Cells. *Stem Cells* **2015**, *33*, 1863–1877. [CrossRef]
175. Yao, X.; Jing, X.; Guo, J.; Sun, K.; Deng, Y.; Zhang, Y.; Guo, F.; Ye, Y. Icariin Protects Bone Marrow Mesenchymal Stem Cells against Iron Overload Induced Dysfunction through Mitochondrial Fusion and Fission, PI3K/Akt/MTOR and MAPK Pathways. *Front. Pharmacol.* **2019**, *10*, 163. [CrossRef]
176. Liu, D.; Tang, W.; Zhang, H.; Huang, H.; Zhang, Z.; Tang, D.; Jiao, F. Icariin Protects Rabbit BMSCs against OGD-Induced Apoptosis by Inhibiting ERs-Mediated Autophagy via MAPK Signaling Pathway. *Life Sci.* **2020**, *253*, 117730. [CrossRef]
177. Li, W.; Huang, Y.; Fan, L.; Yangzom, D.; Zhang, K.; Shen, L.; Cao, S.; Gu, C.; Yu, S. Curcumin Liposomes Alleviate Senescence of Bone Marrow Mesenchymal Stem Cells by Activating Mitophagy. *Sci. Rep.* **2024**, *14*, 31291. [CrossRef]
178. Ruan, Y.; Luo, H.; Tang, J.; Ji, M.; Yu, D.; Yu, Q.; Cao, Z.; Mai, Y.; Zhang, B.; Chen, Y.; et al. Curcumin Inhibits Oxidative Stress and Autophagy in C17.2 Neural Stem Cell through ERK1/2 Signaling Pathways. *Aging Med.* **2024**, *7*, 559–570. [CrossRef]
179. Jiang, E.; Chen, X.; Bi, Y.; Pan, C.; Li, X.; Lan, X. Curcumin Inhibits Oxidative Stress and Apoptosis Induced by H_2O_2 in Bovine Adipose-Derived Stem Cells (BADSCs). *Animals* **2024**, *14*, 3421. [CrossRef]
180. Chen, C.; Liu, Y.; Liu, Y.; Zheng, P. MTOR Regulation and Therapeutic Rejuvenation of Aging Hematopoietic Stem Cells. *Sci. Signal.* **2009**, *2*, ra75. [CrossRef]
181. Rimmelé, P.; Lofek-Czubek, S.; Ghaffari, S. Resveratrol Increases the Bone Marrow Hematopoietic Stem and Progenitor Cell Capacity. *Am. J. Hematol.* **2014**, *89*, E235–E238. [CrossRef] [PubMed]
182. Fujino, T.; Asada, S.; Goyama, S.; Kitamura, T. Mechanisms Involved in Hematopoietic Stem Cell Aging. *Cell Mol. Life Sci.* **2022**, *79*, 473. [CrossRef] [PubMed]
183. Shaban, S.; El-Husseny, M.W.A.; Abushouk, A.I.; Salem, A.M.A.; Mamdouh, M.; Abdel-Daim, M.M. Effects of Antioxidant Supplements on the Survival and Differentiation of Stem Cells. *Oxid. Med. Cell Longev.* **2017**, *2017*, 5032102. [CrossRef] [PubMed]
184. Moustafa, E.M.; Moawed, F.S.M.; Abdel-Hamid, G.R. Icariin Promote Stem Cells Regeneration and Repair Acinar Cells in L-Arginine/Radiation-Inducing Chronic Pancreatitis in Rats. *Dose-Response* **2020**, *18*, 1559325820970810. [CrossRef]
185. Bai, L.; Liu, Y.; Zhang, X.; Chen, P.; Hang, R.; Xiao, Y.; Wang, J.; Liu, C. Osteoporosis Remission via an Anti-Inflammaging Effect by Icariin Activated Autophagy. *Biomaterials* **2023**, *297*, 122125. [CrossRef]
186. Wang, S.; Long, H.; Hou, L.; Feng, B.; Ma, Z.; Wu, Y.; Zeng, Y.; Cai, J.; Zhang, D.W.; Zhao, G. The Mitophagy Pathway and Its Implications in Human Diseases. *Signal Transduct. Target. Ther.* **2023**, *8*, 304. [CrossRef]

antioxidants

MDPI

Article

Luteolin Alleviates Cadmium-Induced Kidney Injury by Inhibiting Oxidative DNA Damage and Repairing Autophagic Flux Blockade in Chickens

Kanglei Zhang [1,2,3,†], Jiahui Li [1,2,3,†], Wenxuan Dong [4,†], Qing Huang [1,2,3], Xueru Wang [1,2,3], Kai Deng [1,2,3], Waseem Ali [1,2,3], Ruilong Song [1,2,3], Hui Zou [1,2,3], Di Ran [5,6], Gang Liu [1,2,3,7,*] and Zongping Liu [1,2,3,*]

1 College of Veterinary Medicine, Yangzhou University, Yangzhou 225009, China; dz120200021@stu.yzu.edu.cn (K.Z.); mz120211583@stu.yzu.edu.cn (J.L.); mx120221013@stu.yzu.edu.cn (Q.H.); dx120220199@stu.yzu.edu.cn (X.W.); mz120211581@stu.yzu.edu.cn (K.D.); 008301@yzu.edu.cn (W.A.); rlsong@yzu.edu.cn (R.S.); zouhui@yzu.edu.cn (H.Z.)

2 Jiangsu Co-Innovation Center for Prevention and Control of Important Animal Infectious Diseases and Zoonoses, Yangzhou 225009, China

3 Joint International Research Laboratory of Agriculture and Agri-Product Safety, The Ministry of Education of China, Yangzhou University, Yangzhou 225009, China

4 College of Veterinary Medicine, Qingdao Agricultural University, Qingdao 266000, China; dx120190152@stu.yzu.edu.cn

5 College of Veterinary Medicine, Southwest University, Chongqing 400715, China; diran@uic.edu

6 College of Medicine, University of Illinois at Chicago, Chicago, IL 60607, USA

7 Department of Pathology and Laboratory Medicine, Tulane University School of Medicine, New Orleans, LA 70112, USA

* Correspondence: gangliu@yzu.edu.cn (G.L.); liuzongping@yzu.edu.cn (Z.L.)

† These authors contributed equally to this work.

Abstract: Chickens are a major source of meat and eggs in human food and have significant economic value. Cadmium (Cd) is a common environmental pollutant that can contaminate feed and drinking water, leading to kidney injury in livestock and poultry, primarily by inducing the generation of free radicals. It is necessary to develop potential medicines to prevent and treat Cd-induced nephrotoxicity in poultry. Luteolin (Lut) is a natural flavonoid compound mainly extracted from peanut shells and has a variety of biological functions to defend against oxidative damage. In this study, we aimed to demonstrate whether Lut can alleviate kidney injury under Cd exposure and elucidate the underlying molecular mechanisms. Renal histopathology and cell morphology were observed. The indicators of renal function, oxidative stress, DNA damage and repair, NAD^+ content, SIRT1 activity, and autophagy were analyzed. In vitro data showed that Cd exposure increased ROS levels and induced oxidative DNA damage and repair, as indicated by increased 8-OHdG content, increased γ-H2AX protein expression, and the over-activation of the DNA repair enzyme PARP-1. Cd exposure decreased NAD^+ content and SIRT1 activity and increased LC3 II, ATG5, and particularly p62 protein expression. In addition, Cd-induced oxidative DNA damage resulted in PARP-1 over-activation, reduced SIRT1 activity, and autophagic flux blockade, as evidenced by reactive oxygen species scavenger NAC application. The inhibition of PARP-1 activation with the pharmacological inhibitor PJ34 restored NAD^+ content and SIRT1 activity. The activation of SIRT1 with the pharmacological activator RSV reversed Cd-induced autophagic flux blockade and cell injury. In vivo data demonstrated that Cd treatment caused the microstructural disruption of renal tissues, reduced creatinine, and urea nitrogen clearance, raised MDA content, and decreased the activities or contents of antioxidants (GSH, T-SOD, CAT, and T-AOC). Cd treatment caused oxidative DNA damage and PARP-1 activation, decreased NAD^+ content, decreased SIRT1 activity, and impaired autophagic flux. Notably, the dietary Lut supplement observably alleviated these alterations in chicken kidney tissues induced by Cd. In conclusion, the dietary Lut supplement alleviated Cd-induced chicken kidney injury through its potent antioxidant properties by relieving the oxidative DNA damage-activated PARP-1-mediated reduction in SIRT1 activity and repairing autophagic flux blockade.

Keywords: cadmium; luteolin; PARP-1; SIRT1; autophagic flux

1. Introduction

Cadmium (Cd) is a widely distributed environmental pollutant that seriously threatens global health and has attracted widespread attention from society. Cd is mainly released into the environment through human activities, such as mineral mining, metal smelting, fertilizer production, and waste disposal [1]. More seriously, the accumulation of Cd in water, soil, and sediments is still increasing [2,3]. The absorbed Cd accumulates in the body due to its low excretion rate and long biological half-life, eventually causing damage to various organs and tissues [4,5]. The kidney plays an important role in metabolic waste excretion and is also the primary target organ of Cd toxicity [6]. Renal tubular epithelial cells (RTECs) are very sensitive to Cd exposure. It has been reported that Cd-induced RTEC damage is irreversible, and continuous exposure to Cd can increase the risk of developing whole kidney damage [6]. Studies showed that Cd could cause kidney injury through various mechanisms, such as oxidative stress, apoptosis, autophagy, and inflammatory response [7–9]. However, the underlying mechanisms of Cd-induced kidney toxicity in chickens are not fully understood.

Oxidative stress is the key mechanism of Cd toxicity, which can oxidize biomolecules such as DNA to lose their biological function. As a DNA damage response protein, poly (ADP-ribose) polymerase 1 (PARP-1) is reported in all kinds of eukaryotic cells. It is activated during DNA damage reparation and maintains genome integrity [10]. Notably, PARP-1 activity requires consuming a large amount of nicotinamide adenine dinucleotide (NAD^+). Studies have shown that PARP-1 plays a dual role in pro-survival or pro-death based on varying degrees of DNA damage [11,12]. Silent mating-type information regulation 2 homolog-1 (SIRT1) is a vital deacetylase that regulates inflammation, aging, mitochondrial biogenesis, and autophagy [13,14]. Like PARP-1, SIRT1 activity is strictly dependent on NAD^+ levels. It has been reported that the excessive activation of PARP-1 causes massive NAD^+ depletion, leading to decreased SIRT1 activity [15]. Conversely, SIRT1 inhibits PARP-1 activity via deacetylation and protects mouse hearts from PARP-1-mediated cell death [16]. However, the role of SIRT1 or PARP-1 and their crosstalk in Cd-induced chicken kidney injury is still unclear.

Autophagy is an evolutionarily conserved metabolic process that degrades cellular components for recycling through lysosomes. Autophagy is considered as a protective response to changes in the microenvironment caused by various stimuli. However, defective or excessive autophagy contributes to the occurrence and development of multiple diseases [17–19]. SIRT1 plays an essential role in the transcription of autophagy-related genes and maintains autophagic flux [20,21]. Other studies have reported that SIRT1-regulated autophagy is associated with PARP-1 activation [22,23]. In addition, SIRT1 is degraded via the autophagic pathway to maintain its homeostasis [24]. Whether SIRT1 protects kidney injury induced by Cd in chickens by regulating autophagy deserves further study.

Luteolin (Lut) is a natural flavonoid compound, and peanut shell is one of the important extraction sources. It plays a key role in the antioxidation, anti-inflammation, and regulation of autophagy and thus benefits both human and animal health [25,26]. Many studies have found that Lut effectively ameliorates heavy metal-induced pathological lesions in various organs by enhancing antioxidant enzyme activities and reversing mitochondrial dysfunction [27–29]. Moreover, Lut inhibits PARP-1 activation and apoptosis induced by a mixture of heavy metals via reducing reactive oxide species (ROS) levels [30]. Recent studies have reported that the hepatorenal protective effects of Lut involve the activation of SIRT1 and the repair of impaired autophagic flux [31–33]. However, whether Lut can mitigate Cd-induced oxidative damage in chicken kidneys and its underlying mechanisms remain unknown.

In the present study, we aim to clarify the crosstalk between PARP-1 and SIRT1 and their roles in the regulation of autophagy in kidney injury under Cd exposure in vitro. We further demonstrate whether Lut can alleviate Cd exposure-induced kidney injury in chickens and its underlying mechanism. This study identifies effective therapeutic targets and provides potential medicine options for preventing kidney injury in poultry.

2. Materials and Methods

2.1. Reagents and Chemicals

Lut was obtained from Yuanye Bio-Technology Co., Ltd. (YuanYe, Shanghai, China). Cadmium chloride ($CdCl_2$, 202908), anti-p62 (P0067), anti-LC3 (L7543), and N-Acetyl-L-cysteine (NAC, 30498) were purchased from Sigma-Aldrich (Sigma, St. Louis, MO, USA). The PARP-1 inhibitor PJ34 (HY-13688A) and the SIRT1 activator resveratrol (RSV, HY-16561) were purchased from MedChemexpress CO., Ltd. (MCE, Shanghai, China). Anti-Beclin-1 (3495S), anti-β-actin (4970L), and anti-ATG5 (12994S) were purchased from (CST, Danvers, MA, USA). Anti-PARP-1(13371-1-AP) and anti-SIRT1 (13161-1-AP) were obtained from Wuhan Sanying Biotechnology Co., Ltd. (Proteintech, Wuhan, China). Anti-ac-H4K16 (ab109463) and anti-γ-H2AX (ab81299) were purchased from Abcam Trading Co., Ltd. (Abcom, Cambridge, UK). The ROS detection kit (S0033S), the NAD^+/NADH assay kit (S0179), and the BCA protein assay kit (P0009, Beyotime, Shanghai, China) were purchased from Beyotime Biotech Inc. (Beyotime, Shanghai, China). The malondialdehyde (MDA) assay kit (A003-1-2), reduced glutathione (GSH) assay kit (A006-2-1), total antioxidant capacity assay kit (T-AOC, A015-2-1), total superoxide dismutase (T-SOD) assay kit (A001-1-2) and catalase (CAT) assay kit (A007-1-1) were purchased from Nanjing Jiancheng Bio-Engineering Institute Co., Ltd. (Nanjing, China). AffiniPure™ Goat Anti-Rabbit IgG (AB_2337913) and AffiniPure™ Goat Anti-Mouse IgG (AB_2338447) were obtained from Jackson ImmunoResearch Laboratories Inc. (Jackson, CST, MA, USA). Chicken 8-hydroxy-2-deoxyguanosine (8-OHdG) ELISA kit (ml059825) was obtained from Shanghai Enzyme-linked Biotechnology Co., Ltd. (mlbio, Shanghai, China).

2.2. Animals and Experimental Design

One-day-old suvian green shell layer chickens ($n = 60$) were purchased from Yangzhou Xianglong Livestock Development Co., Ltd. (Yangzhou, Jiangsu, China). The average body weight was (83.62 ± 2.20 g). All chickens were reared at a constant temperature and humidity in a well-ventilated animal house. Balanced commercial feed and tap water were provided to the experimental chickens ad libitum. All animal care procedures and protocols employed in this study were approved by the Animal Care and Ethics Committee of Yangzhou University (Approved No. SYXK [Su] 2017-0044). The dosage of 50 mg/L $CdCl_2$ was chosen based on the previous studies but with slight modifications [34,35]. Previous studies have shown that the oral administration of 100 to 200 mg/kg Lut can alleviate heart and kidney injury in rats [36,37]. Our preliminary experiment found that oral treatment with 100, 150, and 200 mg/kg doses for 7 days had no effect on the growth and behavioral performance of chickens. Therefore, a moderate dose of 150 mg/kg was chosen to explore the protective effect of Lut on Cd-induced kidney injury in chickens. After 7 days of pre-feeding, the chickens were randomly and equally divided into 4 groups, with 15 chickens in each group. The chickens were grouped and treated as follows: the control/untreated group (were fed with basal diet continuously for the whole period), the Cd group (were pre-fed with basal diet for the first 7 days, and continued to be fed with basal diet supplemented with $CdCl_2$ for 1 month from the 8th day), the Cd + Lut group (were pre-fed with basal diet supplemented with Lut for the first 7 days and continued to be fed basal diet supplemented with $CdCl_2$ and Lut for 1 month from the 8th day), and the Lut group (were fed with basal diet supplemented with Lut continuously for the whole period). Both $CdCl_2$ and Lut were fed to the chickens by mixing material through the addition of drinking water. The total time period of the experimental trial was 37 days. After the completion of the experimental trial, all chickens were euthanized and dissected to collect the kidneys immediately, which were subsequently stored with neutral tissue and an electron microscope fixative or in an −80 °C ultra-low temperature freezer.

2.3. Extraction, Culture and Treatment of Chicken RTECs

The chicken RTECs were isolated from suvian green shell layer chicken embryos by gauze filtration and collagenase digestion combined with differential centrifugation. The 9 to 12-day-old chicken embryos were sterilized and placed on a sterile operating table. Kidney tissue was isolated and then digested using collagenase. The digestion was terminated using a complete culture medium, followed by filtration using gauze and subsequent differential centrifugation to harvest RTECs. Finally, the resuspended cells were seeded in appropriate cell culture dishes according to experimental requirements.

The isolated chicken RTECs were cultured in a cell incubator (37 °C; 5% CO_2) until the confluence rate reached about 60% before subsequent treatment. Cell experiments were grouped and treated as follows: (1) treatment with different concentrations of Cd was divided into 3 or 4 groups at 0 or 1.25, 2.5, and 5 μM $CdCl_2$ for 12 h, respectively; (2) NAC and Cd treatment were divided into the following 4 groups: control/untreated group (ultrapure water), Cd group (ultrapure water + 5 μM $CdCl_2$), Cd + NAC group (NAC pretreatment for 1 h, followed by NAC and $CdCl_2$ co-treatment for 12 h), and NAC group (200 μM NAC); (3) PJ34 and Cd treatment were divided into the following 4 groups: control/untreated group (DMSO), Cd group (MDSO + 5 μM $CdCl_2$), Cd + PJ34 group (pretreatment of PJ34 for 1 h, followed by PJ34 and $CdCl_2$ co-treatment for 12 h), and PJ34 group (10 μM PJ34); (4) RSV and Cd treatment were divided into the following 4 groups: control/untreated group (DMSO), Cd group (DMSO + 5 μM $CdCl_2$), Cd + RSV group (RSV pretreatment for 1 h, followed by RSV and $CdCl_2$ co-treatment for 12 h), RSV group (10 μM RSV).

2.4. Observation of Histopathology and Ultrastructure

The histopathological observation of renal tissues using hematoxylin and eosin (H&E) staining was performed as previously described in our studies [38]. Fresh renal cortex was isolated and immediately fixed in a neutral tissue fixative and subsequently dehydrated in alcohol, clear in xylene, and embedded in paraffin wax. The embedded tissues were sliced into sections of about 5–8 μm in thickness, flattened on a slide, and dried in an incubator. Tissue sections were deparaffinized in different concentrations of alcohol (75–100%) and stained with H&E staining. The prepared sections were observed under the bright field of a phase-contrast microscope (Leica, Wetzlar, Germany).

Ultrastructure observation was described in our previous studies [38]. Briefly, kidney tissues were fixed in 2.5% glutaraldehyde, washed overnight with a buffer, fixed in osmium tetroxide (2%), dehydrated in ethanol and propylene oxide, embedded, sectioned, and then stained with lead citrate combined with uranyl acetate. Finally, the prepared sections were visualized by transmission electron microscopy (TEM) (HT7700; Hitachi, Tokyo, Japan).

2.5. Detection of Biochemical Parameters

Blood was collected by exsanguinating the jugular vein of the chicken, which was placed at 37 °C for 30 min, followed by centrifugation at 2500 rpm for 10 min to separate the serum. The levels of creatinine (CREA), glucose (Glu), and uric acid (UA), which were related to renal function, were detected using an AU5800 automatic biochemical analyzer (Beckman Coulter, Brea, CA, USA).

2.6. Determination of Metal Concentrations

Renal tissue samples were placed in an oven for 48–72 h to ensure the dehydration of the samples. The dried kidney tissue was weighed and subsequently completely digested with nitric acid using a microwave digester (Intertek, London, UK). The digested solution was adjusted to the same volume. The relevant metal element content was determined using a flame atomic absorption spectrophotometer (FAAS) (PerkinElmer, Waltham, MA,

USA). The final statistical results were expressed as the ratio of the weight of the element (μg) to the weight of the dried kidney tissue (g).

2.7. Measurement of ROS and Oxidative Stress Indexes

The activities of CAT and T-SOD, the content of GSH and MDA, and T-AOC were measured using commercially available kits. The specific procedure was referred to in the previous study [38]. The protein concentration of the samples was determined using the BCA protein assay kit to normalize the MDA content as well as the content or activity of the above-mentioned antioxidants.

For cellular ROS detection, chicken RTECs were incubated using a DCFH-DA working solution for 20 min in a 37 °C incubator and subsequently digested with trypsin and centrifuged. After cells were resuspended and washed in a serum-free culture medium, ROS levels were analyzed using flow cytometry (BD, Franklin Lakes, NJ, USA). DCF fluorescence intensities were analyzed using FlowJo 7.6.1 software (BD, Franklin Lakes, NJ, USA).

2.8. Detection of NAD^+ and NADH Contents

The tissue or cell homogenate was centrifuged at 12,000× *g* in a freezing centrifuge to separate the supernatant, which was the sample to be tested. In total, 50 to 100 μL of the sample was treated at 60 °C for 30 min to decompose NAD^+ (for the detection of NADH), whereas the remaining sample was left untreated (for the detection of total NAD^+ and NADH). In total, 20 μL of the above two groups of samples was transferred to a 96-well plate, and blank wells and standard wells (NAD^+ standard solution) were set up simultaneously and then incubated with an alcohol dehydrogenase solution at 37 °C for 10 min in the dark. The chromogenic solution was added, and incubation continued for 30 min. The absorbance value was detected using a spectrophotometer at 450 nm, and the NAD^+ and NADH contents were calculated according to the standard curve. In addition, the protein concentration of each sample was determined using the BCA protein assay kit to normalize the NAD^+ or NADH content.

2.9. Determination of 8-OHdG Content

Homogenates of cells and tissues were transferred to ELISA-specific slats. The horseradish peroxidase-labeled assay antigen was added to each well and incubated at 37 °C for 60 min. After washing, a mixture of substrates A and B were supplemented and incubated at 37 °C for 15 min. The termination solution was subsequently added, and the absorbance value was detected using a spectrophotometer at 450 nm. 8-OHdG content was calculated from standard curves, and protein concentrations were used to normalize 8-OHdG content.

2.10. Immunohistochemistry (IHC)

Paraffin-embedded tissue sections were deparaffinized in xylene and then hydrated in a gradient of absolute ethanol and ultrapure water. Tissue sections were processed with citrate buffer for antigen repair for 30 min, treated with 3% hydrogen peroxide for 15 min, blocked with goat serum, incubated overnight with the LC3 antibody at 4 °C, applied a secondary antibody at room temperature for 2 h, before subsequently staining with DAB. Sections treated above continued to be counterstained with hematoxylin, differentiated in 1% hydrochloric ethanol, and dehydrated in ethanol and xylene. Finally, visualization was performed using a phase-contrast microscope.

2.11. TdT-Mediated dUTP Nick-End Labeling (TUNEL) Staining

In brief, tissue sections were deparaffinized with xylene, hydrated with gradient alcohol, washed with PBS, and then permeabilized with Proteinase K for 10–30 min at room temperature. This section was reacted for 1 h at 37 °C in a wet box using the TUNEL reaction mix, followed by three washes with PBS. Sections were incubated with Streptavidin labeled HRP for 30 min, followed by three washes with PBS. Sections were reacted with the DAB mixture for 10 min, then counterstained with hematoxylin, dehydrated with gradient alcohol, and cleared with xylene. Finally, the sections were observed using a phase-contrast microscope.

2.12. Western Blotting Analysis

Cell and renal tissue protein samples were extracted using the RIPA lysates buffer (20101ES60, NCM, Suzhou, China), and protein concentrations were normalized using the BCA protein assay kit. Samples were added with the SDS buffer and boiled for 8–15 min to denature the proteins. Protein samples were separated in 8–12% SDS-PAGE gel by electrophoresis and subsequently transferred to the 0.22 or 0.45 μm PVDF membrane (Merck Millipore, Darmstadt, HE, GER). Membranes were blocked with 5% nonfat milk, incubated with primary antibody at 4 °C overnight, and incubated with secondary antibody for 1–2 h at room temperature. Finally, Western blotting images were visualized using an enhanced chemiluminescence reagent (NCM, Suzhou, China) via the Tanon imaging system. Image J 1.42q software (NIH, Bethesda, MD, USA) was utilized to analyze protein expression, and the β-actin was used to normalize the protein expression.

2.13. Statistical Analysis

The results were analyzed using software IBM SPSS Statistics 19 statistical software (IBM, Armonk, NY, USA). Dates with normal distribution were presented with the mean ± standard error of the mean (SEM). One-way analysis of variance was used for comparison between the groups, and the least significant difference (LSD) was used for post hoc analysis. $p < 0.05$ was considered statistically significant. Graphs were drafted using GraphPad Prism 6 software (San Diego, CA, USA).

3. Results

3.1. Cd-Induced Oxidative DNA Damage, PARP-1 Over-Activation, Decreased SIRT1 Activity, and Autophagic Flux Blockade in Chicken RTECs

Chicken RTECs were treated with different concentrations of Cd for 12 h to study the underlying mechanisms of Cd on renal tubular epithelial cell injury. Bright-field observation showed that the cells were standard ovoid-shaped with high cell confluency in the control group, but low cell confluency and more shrinking cells were observed after Cd exposure (Figure 1A). The flow cytometry results showed that the level of ROS increased significantly ($p < 0.01$) in a concentration-dependent manner after Cd exposure (Figure 1B). 8-OHdG and γ-H2AX are widely recognized biomarkers of oxidative DNA damage. As shown in Figure 1C–E, compared with the control group, the 8-OHdG content and the protein expression of γ-H2AX and PARP-1 were observably increased after Cd treatment ($p < 0.05$ or $p < 0.01$). In addition, Cd exposure significantly decreased the NAD^+ content and the ratio of NAD^+/NADH ($p < 0.05$ or $p < 0.01$) (Figure 1F,G). Cd exposure dramatically decreased the protein expression of SIRT1 ($p < 0.01$) and increased the protein expression of ac-H4K16 ($p < 0.05$ or $p < 0.01$), respectively (Figure 1H,I). Furthermore, Cd exposure remarkably increased LC3 II, ATG5, and p62 protein expression in particular ($p < 0.05$ or $p < 0.01$) (Figure 1J). These results indicate that Cd caused oxidative DNA damage, PARP-1 over-activation, SIRT1 activity reduction, and autophagic flux blockade in chicken RTECs.

3.2. Alleviating Oxidative Stress Attenuated Cd-Induced PARP-1 Over-Activation, SIRT1 Inhibition, and Autophagic Flux Blocking in Chicken RTECs

NAC, a recognized potent ROS scavenger, is often used to determine whether oxidative stress is involved in risk factor-induced biotoxicity. The effects of oxidative stress on Cd-induced renal tubular epithelial cell injury were investigated by pretreatment with NAC and subsequent co-treatment with Cd for 12 h. NAC treatment improved the morphological abnormalities and low cell confluency induced by Cd (Figure 2A). Compared with the Cd-treated group, NAC treatment significantly decreased ($p < 0.01$) the ROS level (Figure 2B). We further investigated the effect of NAC on DNA damage and the autophagic flux blockade caused by Cd. NAC treatment observably reduced the 8-OHdG content ($p < 0.01$) and the protein expression of γ-H2AX and PARP-1 ($p < 0.05$ or $p < 0.01$) (Figure 2C–E). The NAC treatment dramatically reversed the reduction in NAD^+ content ($p < 0.01$) and the NAD^+/NADH ratio ($p < 0.01$) induced by Cd exposure (Figure 2F,G). Western blotting analysis showed that NAC treatment significantly increased SIRT1 protein expression ($p < 0.01$) and decreased ac-H4K16 protein expression ($p < 0.05$) (Figure 2H,I). Furthermore, NAC treatment observably reduced LC3 II and ATG5 protein expression ($p < 0.05$ or $p < 0.01$) (Figure 2J,K). Notably, NAC significantly decreased the Cd-induced increase of p62 protein expression ($p < 0.01$) (Figure 2J,K). These results suggest that the mitigation of oxidative stress using the antioxidant NAC effectively alleviated Cd-induced oxidative DNA damage, PARP-1 over-activation, and autophagic flux blockade in chicken RTECs.

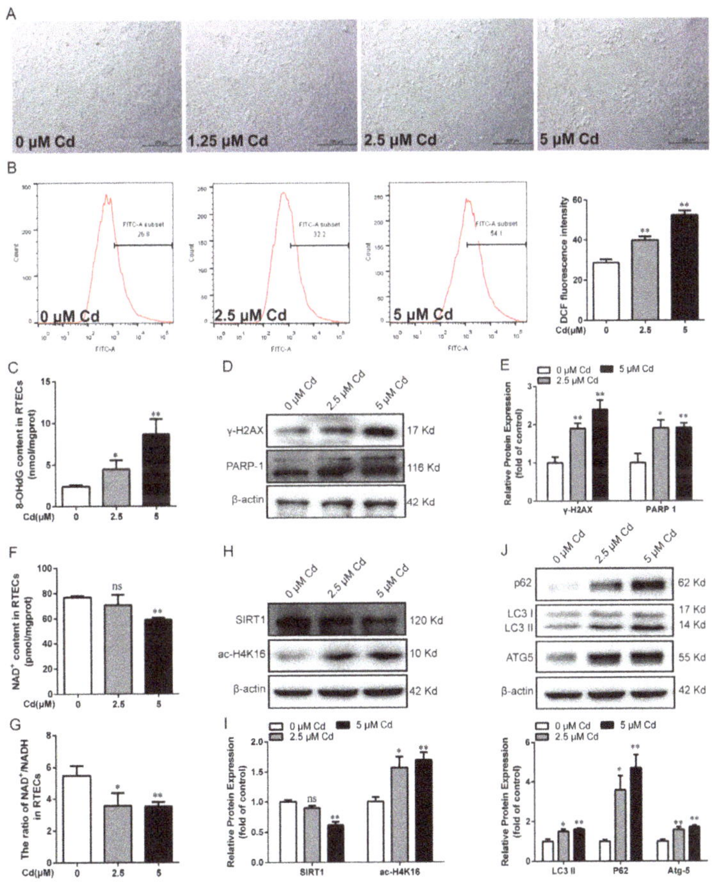

Figure 1. Effect of Cd on oxidative DNA damage, SIRT1 activity, and autophagy in chicken RTECs. (**A**) Cell morphology was observed by bright field under a phase-contrast microscope; scale bar: 200 μm. (**B**) The ROS content was detected by flow cytometry using DCFH-DA fluorescent probe staining. (**C**) The content of 8-OHdG was detected by ELISA. (**D**,**E**) Western blotting images and quantitative analysis of γ-H2AX and PARP-1 proteins. (**F**,**G**) Determination of NAD^+ content and NAD^+/NADH ratio using commercial kits. (**H**,**I**) Western blotting images and quantitative analysis of SIRT1 and ac-H4K16 proteins. (**J**) Western blotting images and quantitative analysis of autophagy-related proteins p62, LC3 II, and ATG5. Each experiment was duplicated at least three times. (ns: $p \geq 0.05$; *: $p < 0.05$, **: $p < 0.01$).

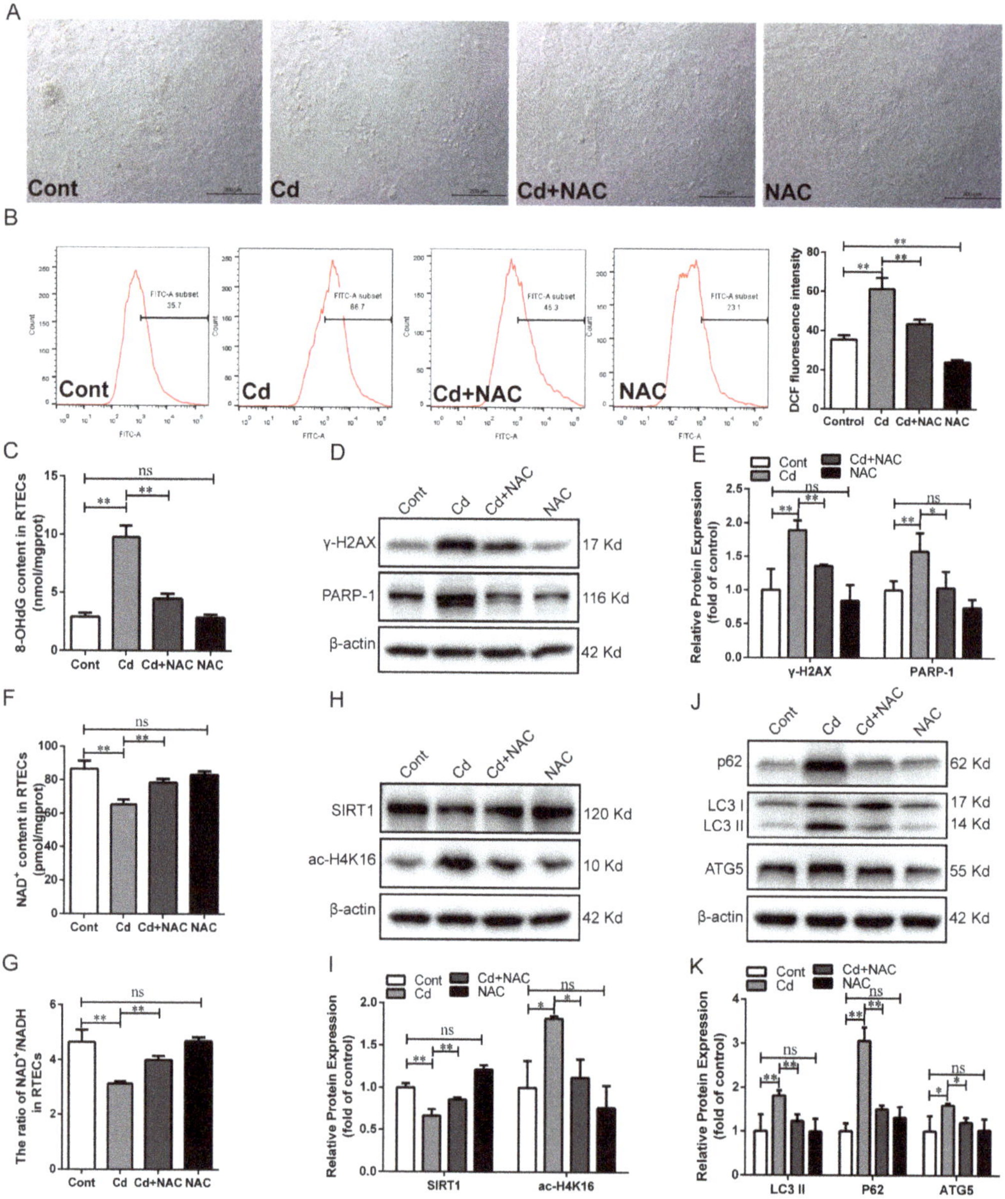

Figure 2. Effect of NAC on Cd-induced oxidative DNA damage, SIRT1 inhibition, and autophagic flux blockade in chicken RTECs. (**A**) Cell morphology was observed by bright field under a phase-contrast microscope; scale bar: 200 μm. (**B**) The ROS content was detected by flow cytometry using DCFH-DA fluorescent probe staining. (**C**) The content of 8-OHdG was detected by ELISA. (**D**,**E**) Western blotting images and quantitative analysis of γ-H2AX and PARP-1 proteins. (**F**,**G**) NAD^+ content and $NAD^+/NADH$ ratio in cells. (**H**,**I**) Western blotting images and quantitative analysis of SIRT1 and ac-H4K16 proteins. (**J**,**K**) Western blotting images and quantitative analysis of autophagy-related proteins p62, LC3 II, and ATG5. Each experiment was duplicated at least three times. (ns: $p \geq 0.05$; *: $p < 0.05$, **: $p < 0.01$).

3.3. Inhibition of PARP-1 Restored SIRT1 Activity and Autophagic Flux in Chicken RTECs

Next, chicken RTECs were pretreated with the PARP-1 inhibitor PJ34 followed by co-treatment with Cd for 12 h to study the effect of PARP-1 on SIRT1 activity and autophagic flux. The result showed that PJ34 treatment noticeably alleviated the cell morphological changes and reduced cell confluency compared with the Cd-treated group (Figure 3A). PJ34 treatment significantly weakened ROS accumulation ($p < 0.05$), inhibited PARP-1 protein over-activation ($p < 0.01$), and reduced γ-H2AX protein expression ($p < 0.01$) (Figure 3B,E,F). The reduction in NAD^+ content and the $NAD^+/NADH$ ratio, decreased SIRT1 protein, and increased ac-H4K16 protein induced by Cd was remarkably reversed by PJ34 treatment ($p < 0.05$ or $p < 0.01$) (Figure 3C,D,G,H). Furthermore, PJ34 treatment increased the expression of the LC3 II and ATG5 proteins but decreased the expression of the p62 protein ($p < 0.05$) (Figure 3I,J).

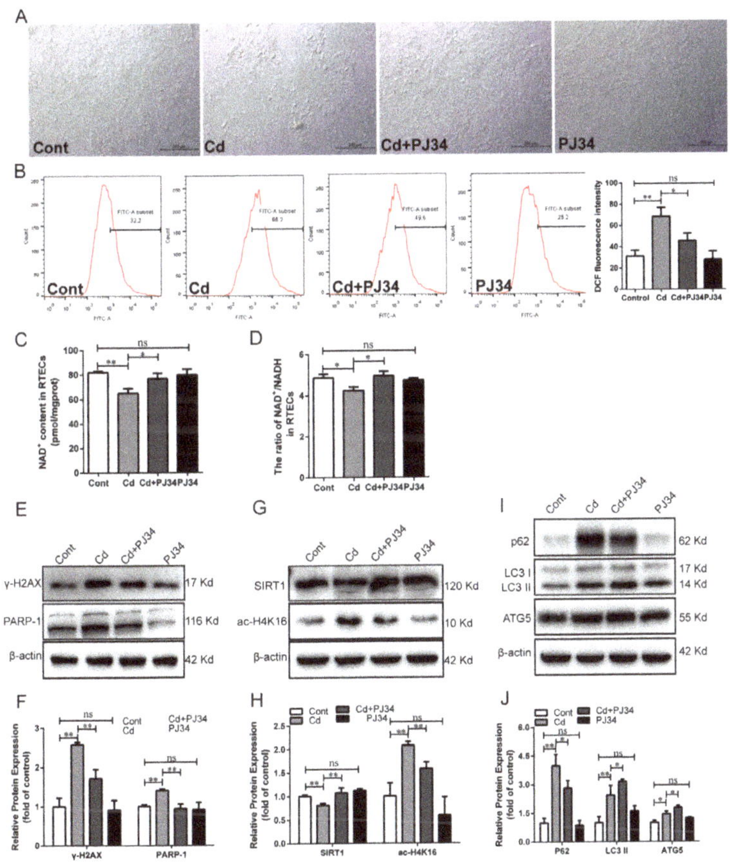

Figure 3. Effect of PARP-1 inhibition with PJ34 on Cd-induced SIRT1 activity reduction and autophagic flux blockade in chicken RTECs. (**A**) Bright-field observation of cell morphology under a phase-contrast microscope; scale bar: 200 μm. (**B**) The ROS content was detected by flow cytometry using DCFH-DA fluorescent probe staining. (**C**,**D**) NAD^+ content and $NAD^+/NADH$ ratio in cells. (**E**,**F**) Western blotting images and quantitative analysis of γ-H2AX and PARP-1 proteins. (**G**,**H**) Western blotting images and quantitative analysis of SIRT1 and ac-H4K16 proteins. (**I**,**J**) Western blotting images and quantitative analysis of autophagy-related proteins p62 and LC3 II. Each experiment was duplicated at least three times. (ns: $p \geq 0.05$; *: $p < 0.05$, **: $p < 0.01$).

In addition, chicken RTECs were pretreated with the SIRT1 activator RSV followed by co-treatment with Cd for 12 h to explore the regulatory role of SIRT1 on autophagy. Compared with the Cd-treated group, RSV significantly increased LC3 II protein expression ($p < 0.05$) but significantly reduced p62 protein expression ($p < 0.01$) (Figure 4A,B). Unsurprisingly, RSV treatment significantly reduced the ROS and 8-OHdG content ($p < 0.05$), as well as alleviating morphological changes (Figure 4C–E). These results indicated that the inhibition of PARP-1 restored SIRT1 activity reduction and the autophagic flux blockade caused by Cd in chicken RTECs.

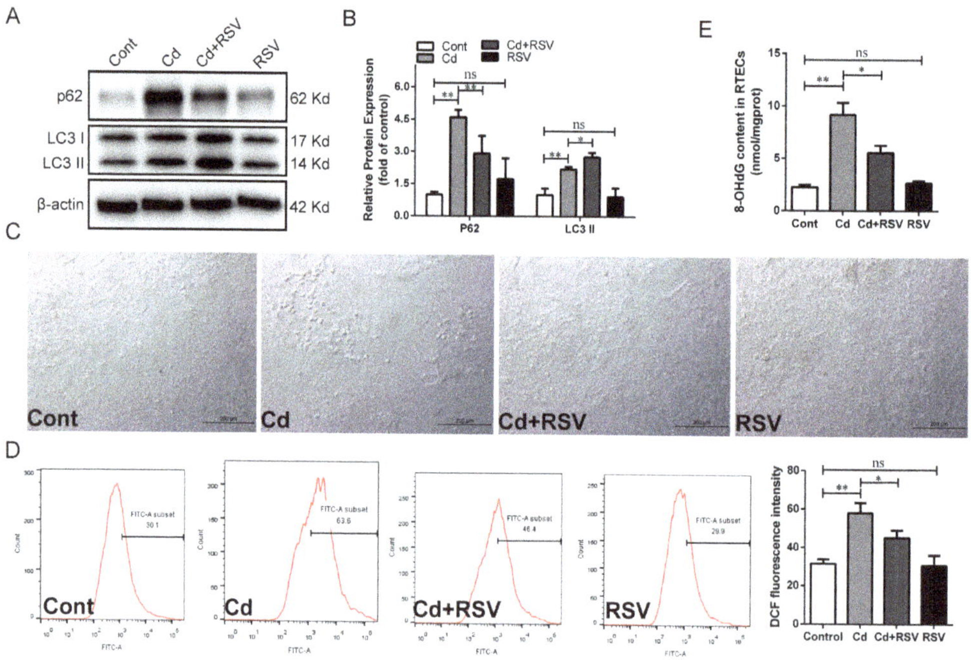

Figure 4. Effect of activating SIRT1 using RSV on Cd-induced autophagic flux blockade in chicken RTECs. (**A**,**B**) Western blotting images and quantitative analysis of autophagy-related proteins p62 and LC3 II. (**C**) Cell morphology was observed by bright field under a phase-contrast microscope; scale bar: 200 μm. (**D**) The ROS content was detected by flow cytometry using DCFH-DA fluorescent probe staining. (**E**) The content of 8-OHdG was detected by ELISA. Each experiment was duplicated at least three times. (ns: $p \geq 0.05$; *: $p < 0.05$, **: $p < 0.01$).

3.4. Lut Alleviates Cd-Induced Kidney Injury

We explored the protective effect of Lut against Cd-induced renal injury. The results showed that Cd content in renal tissues and serum significantly increased ($p < 0.01$) after Cd exposure but did not change considerably ($p > 0.05$) in the Cd + Lut-treated group (Figure 5A and Figure S1A). Cd exposure significantly reduced body weight ($p < 0.05$) compared to the control group, while the Lut supplement significantly alleviated the body weight loss caused by Cd ($p < 0.05$) (Figure 5B). However, Cd or Lut treatment had no significant effect on kidney weight ($p > 0.05$) (Figure 5C). Cd exposure significantly increased the kidney coefficient ($p < 0.05$), whereas the Lut supplement had a lower kidney coefficient than the Cd-treated group ($p < 0.05$) (Figure 5D). The histopathological evaluation by H&E staining showed that Cd exposure caused the irregular arrangement of renal tubular cells, swelling, and vacuolization of epithelial cells (Black arrows). However, the Lut supplement significantly alleviated Cd-induced tissue lesions (Figure 5E). Moreover, serum biochemical results showed that CREA, UA, and Glu levels increased dramatically ($p < 0.05$) after Cd exposure and were clearly reversed ($p < 0.05$ or $p < 0.01$) in the Cd + Lut-treated group (Figure 5F–H). These results suggest that the Lut supplement considerably ameliorated Cd-induced kidney injury mainly by repairing the renal structure and maintaining normal renal function.

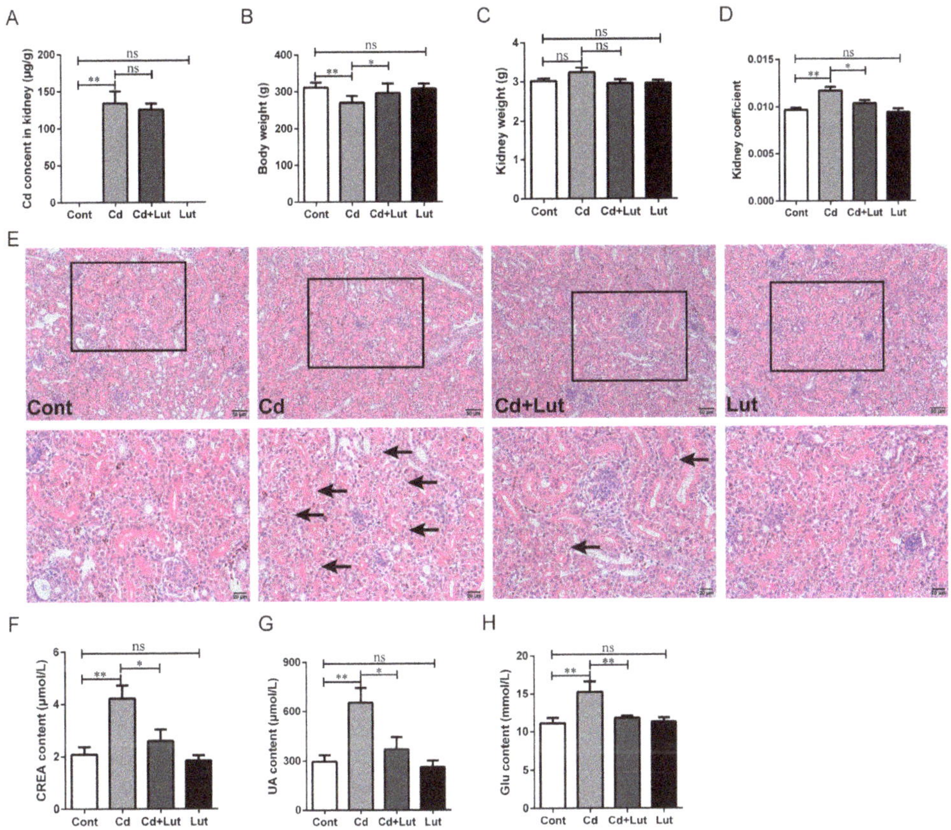

Figure 5. Effect of Lut and/or Cd on renal histopathology and renal function. (**A**) The Cd content in renal tissue was detected by FAAS. Statistical analysis of (**B**) body weight, (**C**) kidney weight, and (**D**) kidney coefficient. (**E**) Renal histopathological observation using H&E staining; scale bar (The black arrow indicates the abnormal morphology of the renal tubular, which is characterized by irregular arrangement of renal tubular cells, swelling and vacuolation of the epithelial cells). 50 μm or 20 μm. The contents of (**F**) CREA, (**G**) UA, and (**H**) Glu in serum were detected by an automatic biochemical analyzer. Each experiment was duplicated at least three times. (ns: $p \geq 0.05$; *: $p < 0.05$, **: $p < 0.01$).

3.5. Lut Alleviates Cd-Induced Oxidative Stress

We explored whether the Lut supplement could alleviate Cd-induced oxidative stress in renal tissue. The TEM result showed an irregular arrangement of mitochondrial cristae, even fragmentation or loss, and outer membrane disruption in the Cd-treated group. The Lut supplement significantly alleviated the disruption of the ultrastructure of mitochondria (Figure 6A). The MDA content and antioxidant indicator were measured to assess oxidative stress status in the kidneys. As shown in Figure 6B, compared with the Cd-treated group, the Lut supplement noticeably decreased renal MDA accumulation ($p < 0.01$) and GSH elevation ($p < 0.05$), and observably improved the activity of T-SOD, T-AOC, and

CAT ($p < 0.05$) (Figure 6C–F). Trace element results showed that Cd exposure significantly increased the contents of zinc (Zn) and copper (Cu) compared with the control group ($p < 0.01$). The Lut supplement considerably reduced Cd-induced increases in the Zn content but did not affect the Cu content ($p < 0.05$ or $p > 0.05$) (Figure 6G,H). However, no significant difference showed in iron (Fe) and selenium (Se) content among the groups ($p > 0.05$) (Figure 6I,J). These results suggest that the Lut supplement remarkably ameliorated renal oxidative stress under Cd exposure by reducing the accumulation of MDA and enhancing the activity of antioxidant enzymes.

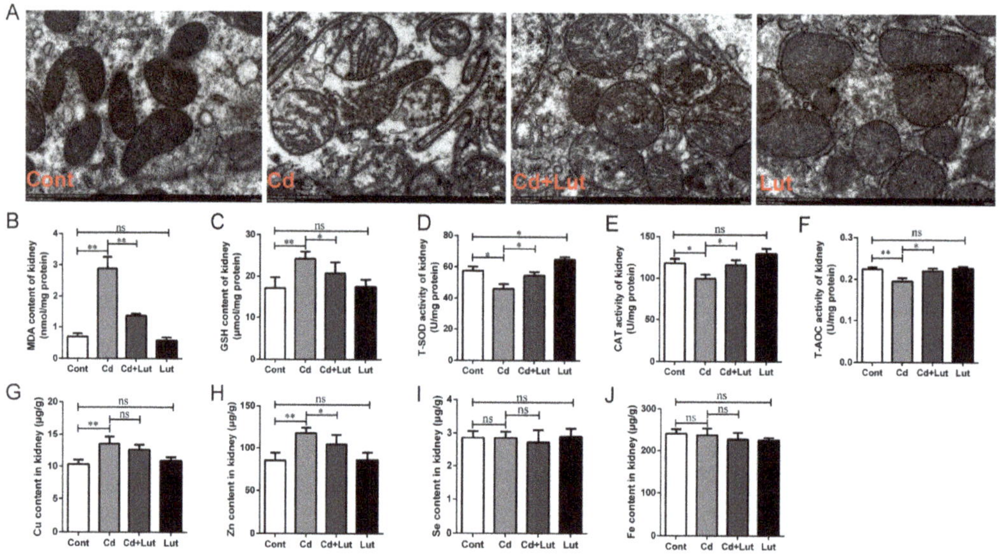

Figure 6. Effects of Lut and/or Cd on oxidative stress in chicken kidneys. (**A**) TEM observed mitochondrial ultrastructure; scale bar: 500 nm. (**B**) MDA content, (**C**) GSH content, (**D**) T-SOD activity, (**E**) CAT activity, and (**F**) T-AOC in renal tissues. The contents of (**G**) Cu, (**H**) Zn, (**I**) Se, and (**J**) Fe in renal tissues were measured by FAAS. Each experiment was duplicated at least three times. (ns: $p \geq 0.05$; *: $p < 0.05$, **: $p < 0.01$).

3.6. Lut Attenuates Cd-Induced DNA Damage and PARP-1 Activation

We studied the effects of Lut supplement and/or Cd exposure on DNA damage and PARP-1 activation. As shown in Figure 7A, the morphology of the nucleus was regularly round, and the nuclear membrane was intact in the control group, while the nuclear morphology was deformed in the Cd-treated group. The Lut supplement significantly alleviated the abnormal nuclear morphology caused by Cd. The number of TUNEL-positive cells was dramatically increased after Cd exposure and significantly decreased in the Cd + Lut-treated group (Figure 7B). As shown in Figure 7C–E, the Lut supplement significantly reduced the increases in 8-OHdG ($p < 0.01$), γ-H2AX ($p < 0.05$), and PARP-1 ($p < 0.05$) induced by Cd. These results demonstrate that Lut significantly alleviates Cd-induced DNA oxidative damage and PARP-1 activation in chicken kidney tissue.

3.7. Lut Restores Cd-Induced SIRT1 Inactivity and Autophagic Flux Blockade

We explored the effects of the Lut supplement and/or Cd exposure on SIRT1 activity and autophagy in the kidney. As shown in Figure 8A,B, Cd exposure significantly decreased the NAD^+ content ($p < 0.05$) and the ratio of $NAD^+/NADH$ ($p < 0.05$), which were observably improved by the Lut supplement ($p < 0.05$). Cd exposure greatly reduced the SIRT1 protein level ($p < 0.05$) but increased the ac-H4K16 protein expression ($p < 0.01$), and these changes were reversed considerably ($p < 0.05$) by the Lut supplement (Figure 8C,D).

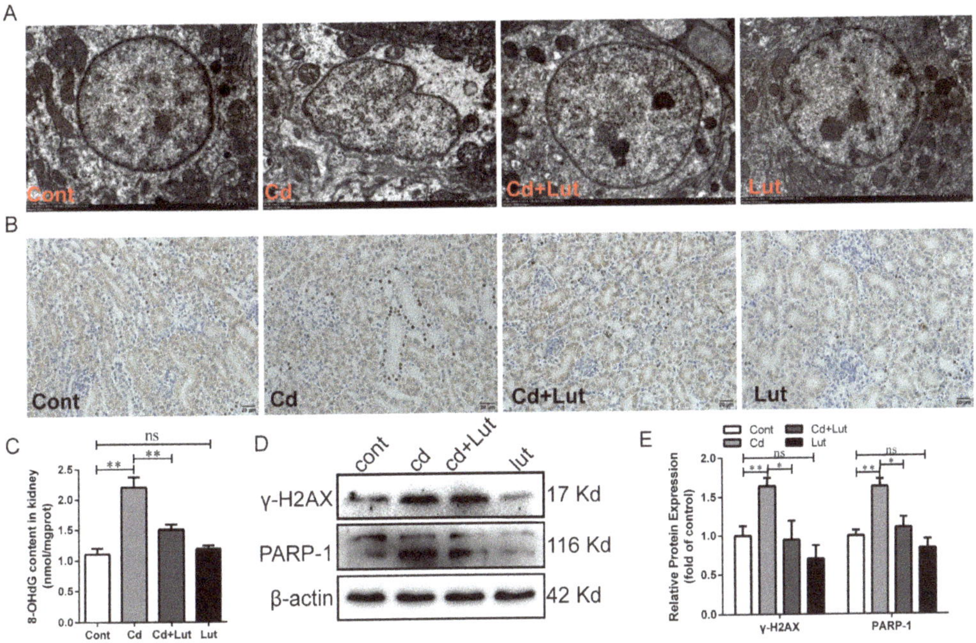

Figure 7. Effect of Lut and/or Cd on oxidative DNA damage and repair in chicken kidneys. (**A**) TEM observed nuclear morphology; scale bar: 1.0 μm. (**B**) DNA damage level detected by TUNEL staining; scale bar: 20 μm. (**C**) The content of 8-OHdG was detected by ELISA. (**D**,**E**) Western blotting images and quantitative analysis of γ-H2AX and PARP-1 proteins. Each experiment was duplicated at least three times. (ns: $p \geq 0.05$; *: $p < 0.05$, **: $p < 0.01$).

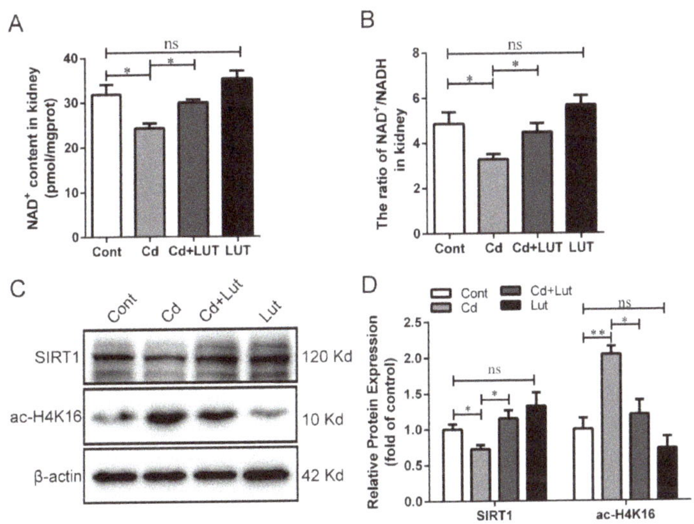

Figure 8. Effect of Lut and/or Cd on SIRT1 activity in chicken kidneys. (**A**) NAD^+ content and (**B**) NAD^+/NADH ratio in kidney tissues. (**C**,**D**) Western blotting images and quantitative analysis of SIRT1 and ac-H4K16. Each experiment was duplicated at least three times. (ns: $p \geq 0.05$; *: $p < 0.05$, **: $p < 0.01$).

Next, the TEM results show that the Lut supplement reduced the number of autophagosomes or autophagic vesicles elevated by Cd (Figure 9A). The IHC results showed that Cd exposure significantly increased LC3 protein expression, while this increase was weakened by the Lut supplement (Figure 9B). In addition, Western blotting analysis confirmed that the protein expression levels of p62, LC3 II, ATG5, and Beclin-1 were significantly increased ($p < 0.01$) after Cd exposure, while they were decreased considerably ($p < 0.05$ or $p < 0.01$) by the Lut supplement (Figure 9C,D). These results illustrate that the Lut supplement repaired the SIRT1 inactivity and autophagic flux blockade induced by Cd in chicken kidney tissue.

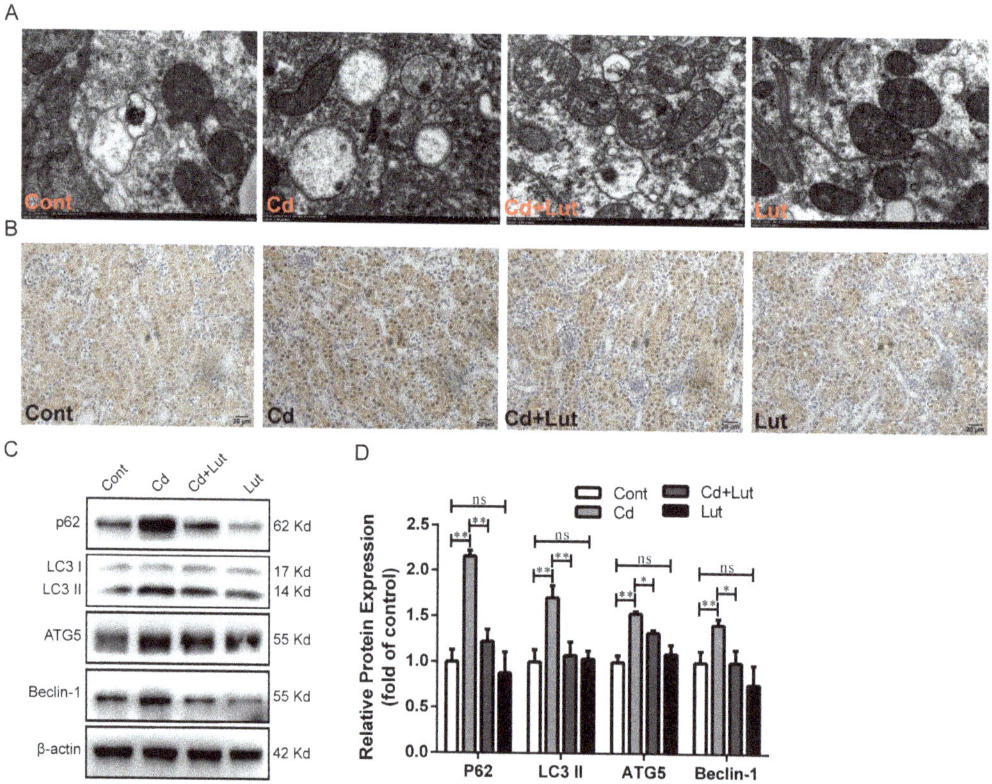

Figure 9. Effect of Lut and/or Cd on autophagy. (**A**) Observation of the number of autophagosomes or autolysosomes using TEM; scale bar: 500 nm. (**B**) LC3 protein expression was detected by the IHC; scale bar: 20 μm. (**C**,**D**) Western blotting and quantitative analysis of autophagy-related proteins p62, LC3 II, ATG5 and Beclin-1. Each experiment was duplicated at least three times. (ns: $p \geq 0.05$; *: $p < 0.05$, **: $p < 0.01$).

4. Discussion

Cd is a widely distributed environmental and occupational pollutant that has adverse effects on human and animal health and has been a global public health problem. Cd exposure is closely related to the development of various kidney diseases, including diabetes, interstitial renal fibrosis, glomerulosclerosis, and even renal cell carcinoma [39]. The exploration of effective therapeutic interventions is necessary to treat Cd-induced nephrotoxicity in animals and humans. Recently, Lut, a natural flavonoid, attracted much attention due to its various pharmacological activities. Studies have reported that Lut could protect organs such as the kidneys and liver from damage caused by heavy metals or chemicals [32,33]. However, the therapeutic effects of Lut on Cd-induced kidney injury in chickens have not been fully studied. Therefore, our study aimed to explore the protective effect of Lut against Cd-induced nephrotoxicity and elucidate the underlying molecular mechanisms.

Numerous studies have demonstrated that Cd causes renal pathological changes in poultry [40–43]. Lut can effectively improve kidney injury induced by various stimuli [31,32,44]. In addition, Lut also plays a protective role in resisting heavy metal poisoning [45,46]. Similar to previous studies, our results demonstrated that Cd exposure caused structural and functional abnormalities in the kidney, and Lut could significantly alleviate these changes. Studies have found that Lut reduces the accumulation of heavy metals in organs by chelating or increasing the excretion of heavy metals, including lead or mercury in the urine thereby alleviating the damage to the kidney and testis in rats [27,31]. Our study found that Cd exposure noticeably increased Cd contents in serum and renal tissues. However, Lut did not change its levels in the kidneys and serum, suggesting that the renoprotective effect of Lut is independent of reducing renal Cd accumulation. In addition to its chelating ability, the protective effect of Lut against organ damage is closely related to its potent antioxidant properties [47–49]. More and more studies have confirmed that oxidative stress is a crucial mechanism of Cd-induced nephrotoxicity [50,51]. In addition, studies have reported how Cd exposure causes an increase in lipid peroxidation products, a reduction in antioxidant enzyme capacity, and severe oxidative kidney injury in poultry [34,42,43]. Similar to previous reports, we found that Cd exposure caused the disruption or loss of mitochondrial crista and disruption of the outer membrane, increasing the MDA content and reducing antioxidant capacity or activity. In vitro studies also found that Cd exposure could significantly destroy cell morphology and elevate ROS content. ROS scavenger NAC treatment significantly reduced the ROS content and alleviated the morphological changes induced by Cd in RTECs. Expectedly, Lut also considerably improved Cd-induced oxidative stress, as indicated by the repair of mitochondrial ultrastructure damage, enhancing antioxidant enzyme activity, and reducing MDA content. The dyshomeostasis of trace elements in the body can promote oxidative damage and contribute to Cd toxicity [52]. Trace elements, including Zn, Cu, and Fe, are essential for maintaining normal cell structure and function. Cd can displace Zn and Cu and reduce antioxidant capacity [53,54]. The exploration of Cd could increase Cu and Zn levels but decrease Fe levels in chicken kidneys [34]. We found that Cd exposure caused an increase in Cu and Zn contents, and the Lut supplement reduced Zn content but did not affect Cu content. However, the contents of Se and Fe in renal tissue in each treatment group did not change significantly. The invariableness in Fe content may be related to the transfer of stored Fe from the liver to the kidney after Cd exposure [55]. Cu/Zn is a metal prosthetic group of the antioxidant enzyme SOD, and the activity of Cu/Zn-SOD was further detected to better evaluate the protective effect of Lut on Cd-induced oxidative renal injury. Our results demonstrate that Cd exposure induces oxidative kidney injury, while Lut enhances the antioxidant capacity to alleviate Cd-induced nephrotoxicity.

Cd can induce oxidative DNA damage in rat kidneys and RTECs due to excess ROS production [12,56]. Recently, studies reported that Cd exposure causes oxidative stress in duck testes and broiler liver, which leads to DNA damage and the activation of autophagy or apoptosis [57,58]. Our study found that Cd caused nuclear deformation and an increase in the number of TUNEL-positive cells in renal tissues. In addition, Cd exposure increased 8-OHdG content and the γ-H2AX protein level, indicating that Cd exposure caused oxidative DNA damage in chicken kidneys. Not surprisingly, Lut reversed the oxidative DNA damage induced by Cd exposure in renal tissue due to its enhanced antioxidant capacity. It is reported that Lut has a protective effect on ROS-induced DNA damage, which is more pronounced than quercetin and kaempferol [59]. PARP-1 plays an important role in maintaining DNA repair and genome integrity. Notably, PARP-1 activation requires the consumption of NAD^+ [60]. Cd causes oxidative stress and DNA fragmentation accompanied by PARP-1 activation and apoptosis in mammals and poultry [11,61]. Similar to previous studies, we also found that Cd caused a decrease in PARP-1 protein expression, NAD^+ content, and the NAD^+/NADH ratio. NAC could significantly alleviate the oxidative DNA damage induced by Cd, reduce PARP-1 activation, and increase NAD^+ content and the $NAD^+/NADH$ ratio. Thus, DNA damage takes the primary responsibility for PARP-1 activation induced by Cd. Like NAC, Lut alleviated Cd-induced changes in PARP-1 protein expression and NAD^+ content. Studies have found that the over-activation of PARP-1 induced by high concentrations of Cd promotes cell death, and conversely, moderate PARP-1 activation ameliorates cell damage induced by low concentrations of Cd [12,62]. Our study found that the inhibition of PARP-1 activation using PJ34 alleviated Cd-induced cell damage, suggesting that Cd-induced PARP-1 over-activation is detrimental to cell survival. In addition, PJ34 also reduced the expression of the γ-H2AX protein, which may be related to the alleviation of the ROS level induced by Cd. So, Lut protects the kidney from Cd toxicity by reversing oxidative DNA damage and PARP-1 over-activation.

SIRT1 is a deacetylase essential in regulating oxidative stress, inflammation, and autophagy by modifying downstream target proteins. In particular, SIRT1 activity also depends on the NAD^+ content. The crosstalk between SIRT1 and PARP-1 and their roles in ultimate cell fate determination has rarely been investigated. One study indicated that the activation of PARP-1 reduces SIRT1 activity, which may involve a large amount of NAD^+ consumption [63]. The inhibition of PARP-1 increases NAD^+ content and SIRT1 activity [64,65]. However, SIRT1 can inhibit PAPR-1 activity by its deacetylation [16]. Studies have found that the SIRT1 protein was reduced in the Cd-induced rat poisoning model [56,66,67]. Cd exposure also decreases chicken renal tissues' *SIRT1* and *SIRT3* gene expressions [34]. As expected, Cd exposure reduced the expression of the SIRT1 protein and increased the expression of its target protein ac-H4K16 both in vivo and in vitro. The Lut supplement reversed the changes in SIRT1 and ac-H4K16 proteins induced by Cd. Similarly, the results of NAC treatment were consistent with the Lut supplement. To further elucidate the role of PARP-1 activation on SIRT1 in Cd-induced chicken kidney injury, the inhibition of PARP-1 using PJ34 significantly upregulated the Cd-induced reduction in the NAD^+ content and $NAD^+/NADH$ ratio and increased the reduction in the SIRT1 protein. Our results demonstrate that Lut restores SIRT1 activity by inhibiting the over-activation of PARP-1 induced by Cd.

Autophagy is a metabolic process that relies on lysosomes to degrade and reuse cellular components. Autophagy is closely related to Cd-induced nephrotoxicity in poultry. Cd upregulates the protein expression of LC3 II, ATG5, and Beclin-1 and reduces the expression level of the autophagy adaptor protein p62 in duck kidneys [68,69]. Recent reports have shown that Cd causes autophagic flux blockade and lipid droplet accumulation, leading to liver injury in ducks [70]. In our study, Cd exposure increased the autophagosome number in chicken kidney tissues. Meanwhile, Cd increased the protein expression of LC3 II, ATG5, or Beclin-1, as well as p62 in vitro and in vivo. ATG5 and Beclin-1 proteins are responsible for forming an autophagic isolation membrane [71]. Studies have found that Cd impairs autophagic flux by interfering with the degradation function of lysosomes and blocking the fusion of autophagosomes and lysosomes, manifesting as autophagosome accumulation and the increase in p62 protein expression [72]. Our results suggest that Cd impaired autophagic flux without affecting autophagosome formation, which resulted in the accumulation of a large number of autophagosomes. Consistent with our findings, Cd leads to autophagosome accumulation-dependent apoptosis in neuronal cells by activating AKT-mediated autophagic flux blockade [17,73]. A similar mechanism has been reported in cisplatin-induced nephrotoxicity [74]. It is necessary to further elucidate the role of autophagy in Cd-induced kidney injury in chickens by regulating autophagy using autophagy modulators, such as the activator rapamycin or the inhibitor 3-MA. In addition, further studies are also needed to clarify the underlying mechanisms of Cd-induced autophagic flux blockade in chicken kidneys. Notably, Lut significantly reversed Cd-induced autophagy-related protein expression and autophagosome accumulation. Similarly, NAC treatment downregulated the expression of autophagy-related proteins induced by Cd. Thus, the regulation of autophagy by Lut may be related to its antioxidant activity. In addition, it has been reported that competitive NAD$^+$ depletion due to PARP-1 activation induced by DNA damage causes decreased autophagy, which is mediated by SIRT1 inactivation [22,75]. Moreover, the inhibition of PARP-1 further increased the protein expression of ATG5 and LC3 II and decreased p62 protein expression. It has been reported that activation of SIRT1 enhances autophagic flux in vivo, thereby protecting osteoporosis or alleviating hepatic steatosis [76,77]. We found that SIRT1 activation using RSV attenuated cell damage inhibited ROS production, increased LC3 II protein expression, and decreased p62 expression, indicating that Lut ameliorates autophagic flux blockade through PAPR-1 inhibition and SIRT1 activation to alleviate kidney injury in chickens.

5. Conclusions

Cd induces oxidative DNA damage and the over-activation of PARP-1, resulting in reduced SIRT1 activity and the blockade of autophagic flux in chicken kidney tissues and RTECs. The dietary supplementation of Lut protects the chicken kidney against Cd nephrotoxicity by repairing autophagic flux blockade via ameliorating oxidative DNA damage-dependent PARP-1 over-activation and SIRT1 activity reduction.

Supplementary Materials: The following supporting information can be downloaded at: https://www.mdpi.com/article/10.3390/antiox13050525/s1, Figure S1. Effect of Lut and/or Cd on serum Cd content. (A) Detection of serum Cd content by FAAS. Each experiment was duplicated at least three times. (ns: $p \geq 0.05$; *: $p < 0.05$, **: $p < 0.01$).

Author Contributions: Conceptualization, K.Z., J.L. and W.D.; Data curation, K.Z. and J.L.; Formal analysis, W.D., Q.H., X.W., K.D. and W.A.; Funding acquisition, G.L. and Z.L.; Investigation, K.Z. and J.L.; Methodology, K.Z. and J.L.; Project administration, R.S., H.Z., D.R., G.L. and Z.L.; Software, W.D., Q.H. and X.W.; Supervision, R.S., H.Z., D.R., G.L. and Z.L.; Validation, W.D. and X.W.; Visualization, Q.H. and W.A.; Writing—original draft, K.Z.; Writing—review and editing, G.L. and Z.L. All authors have read and agreed to the published version of the manuscript.

Funding: This research was funded by the National Key R&D Program of China (No. 2023YFD1801100), the National Natural Science Foundation of China (Nos. 32072933, 32072923 and 32273086), 111 Project D18007, a Project Funded by Priority Academic Program Development of Jiangsu Higher Education Institutions (PAPD) and the Postdoctoral Research Funding of Yangzhou University (Nos. 137070430). Ethics Approval and Consent to Participate: Every procedure and protocol involving animals were permitted by the Yangzhou University Comparative Medical Center (Jiangsu Province, China). The study was based on the Guide to Moral Control and Supervision in Animal Conservation and Use.

Institutional Review Board Statement: The animal study protocol was approved by the Animal Ethics Committee of Yangzhou University (protocol code: SYXK [Su] 2017-0044).

Informed Consent Statement: Not applicable.

Data Availability Statement: The datasets used and/or analyzed during the current study are available from the corresponding author on reasonable request.

Acknowledgments: The English language of this study was improved by native English speaker Roshan Riaz (Institution: Department of Animal Nutrition and Nutritional Diseases, Faculty of Veterinary Medicine, Kafkas University, Kars, Türkiye; E-mail: roshan.riaz@kafkas.edu.tr). We are very grateful to Roshan Riaz for making great improvements to the English language.

Conflicts of Interest: The authors declare that they have no known competing financial interests or personal relationships that could have appeared to influence the work reported in this paper.

References

1. Genchi, G.; Sinicropi, M.; Lauria, G.; Carocci, A.; Catalano, A. The Effects of Cadmium Toxicity. *Int. J. Environ. Res. Public Health* **2020**, *17*, 3782. [CrossRef]
2. Hu, B.; Shao, S.; Ni, H.; Fu, Z.; Hu, L.; Zhou, Y.; Min, X.; She, S.; Chen, S.; Huang, M.; et al. Current status, spatial features, health risks, and potential driving factors of soil heavy metal pollution in China at province level. *Environ. Pollut.* **2020**, *266*, 114961. [CrossRef]
3. Huang, Y.; Wang, L.; Wang, W.; Li, T.; He, Z.; Yang, X. Current status of agricultural soil pollution by heavy metals in China: A meta-analysis. *Sci. Total Environ.* **2019**, *651*, 3034–3042. [CrossRef]
4. Satarug, S.; Garrett, S.H.; Sens, M.A.; Sens, D.A. Cadmium, environmental exposure, and health outcomes. *Environ. Health Perspect.* **2010**, *118*, 182–190. [CrossRef]
5. Nordberg, G. Historical perspectives on cadmium toxicology. *Toxicol. Appl. Pharmacol.* **2009**, *238*, 192–200. [CrossRef]
6. Yan, L.; Allen, D. Cadmium-Induced Kidney Injury: Oxidative Damage as a Unifying Mechanism. *Biomolecules* **2021**, *11*, 1575. [CrossRef]
7. Zhao, Y.; Li, Z.; Zhang, D.; Wang, Z.; Wang, L. Quercetin alleviates Cadmium-induced autophagy inhibition via TFEB-dependent lysosomal restoration in primary proximal tubular cells. *Ecotoxicol. Environ. Saf.* **2021**, *208*, 111743. [CrossRef]
8. Yi, L.; Shang, X.J.; Lv, L.; Wang, Y.; Zhang, J.; Quan, C.; Shi, Y.; Liu, Y.; Zhang, L. Cadmium-induced apoptosis of Leydig cells is mediated by excessive mitochondrial fission and inhibition of mitophagy. *Cell Death Dis.* **2022**, *13*, 928. [CrossRef]
9. Liu, L.; Zhao, L.; Liu, Y.; Yu, X.; Qiao, X. Rutin Ameliorates Cadmium-Induced Necroptosis in the Chicken Liver via Inhibiting Oxidative Stress and MAPK/NF-κB Pathway. *Biol. Trace Elem. Res.* **2022**, *200*, 1799–1810. [CrossRef] [PubMed]
10. Pascal, J. The comings and goings of PARP-1 in response to DNA damage. *DNA Repair* **2018**, *71*, 177–182. [CrossRef] [PubMed]
11. Zhou, J.; Zeng, L.; Zhang, Y.; Wang, M.; Li, Y.; Jia, Y.; Wu, L.; Su, P. Cadmium exposure induces pyroptosis in testicular tissue by increasing oxidative stress and activating the AIM2 inflammasome pathway. *Sci. Total Environ.* **2022**, *847*, 157500. [CrossRef]
12. Luo, T.; Yu, Q.; Zou, H.; Zhao, H.; Gu, J.; Yuan, Y.; Zhu, J.; Bian, J.; Liu, Z. Role of poly (ADP-ribose) polymerase-1 in cadmium-induced cellular DNA damage and cell cycle arrest in rat renal tubular epithelial cell line NRK-52E. *Environ. Pollut.* **2020**, *261*, 114149. [CrossRef]
13. Morigi, M.; Perico, L.; Benigni, A. Sirtuins in Renal Health and Disease. *J. Am. Soc. Nephrol.* **2018**, *29*, 1799–1809. [CrossRef]
14. Lin, S.; Xing, H.; Zang, T.; Ruan, X.; Wo, L.; He, M. Sirtuins in mitochondrial stress: Indispensable helpers behind the scenes. *Ageing Res. Rev.* **2018**, *44*, 22–32. [CrossRef]
15. Chen, Q.; Cui, K.; Zhao, Z.; Xu, X.; Liu, Y.; Shen, Y.; Chen, F.; Mai, K.; Ai, Q. LPS stimulation stabilizes HIF-1α by enhancing HIF-1α acetylation via the PARP1-SIRT1 and ACLY-Tip60 pathways in macrophages. *FASEB J. Off. Publ. Fed. Am. Soc. Exp. Biol.* **2022**, *36*, e22418. [CrossRef]
16. Rajamohan, S.; Pillai, V.; Gupta, M.; Sundaresan, N.; Birukov, K.; Samant, S.; Hottiger, M.; Gupta, M. SIRT1 promotes cell survival under stress by deacetylation-dependent deactivation of poly(ADP-ribose) polymerase 1. *Mol. Cell. Biol.* **2009**, *29*, 4116–4129. [CrossRef]
17. Zhang, H.; Dong, X.; Zhao, R.; Zhang, R.; Xu, C.; Wang, X.; Liu, C.; Hu, X.; Huang, S.; Chen, L. Cadmium results in accumulation of autophagosomes-dependent apoptosis through activating Akt-impaired autophagic flux in neuronal cells. *Cell. Signal.* **2019**, *55*, 26–39. [CrossRef]
18. Kaushal, G.; Shah, S. Autophagy in acute kidney injury. *Kidney Int.* **2016**, *89*, 779–791. [CrossRef]
19. Pi, H.; Li, M.; Zou, L.; Yang, M.; Deng, P.; Fan, T.; Liu, M.; Tian, L.; Tu, M.; Xie, J.; et al. AKT inhibition-mediated dephosphorylation of TFE3 promotes overactive autophagy independent of MTORC1 in cadmium-exposed bone mesenchymal stem cells. *Autophagy* **2019**, *15*, 565–582. [CrossRef] [PubMed]
20. Shen, Q.; Shi, Y.; Liu, J.; Su, H.; Huang, J.; Zhang, Y.; Peng, C.; Zhou, T.; Sun, Q.; Wan, W.; et al. Acetylation of STX17 (syntaxin 17) controls autophagosome maturation. *Autophagy* **2020**, *17*, 1157–1169. [CrossRef] [PubMed]
21. Ou, X.; Lee, M.; Huang, X.; Messina-Graham, S.; Broxmeyer, H. SIRT1 positively regulates autophagy and mitochondria function in embryonic stem cells under oxidative stress. *Stem Cells* **2014**, *32*, 1183–1194. [CrossRef]
22. Zhang, Y.; Huang, W.; Zheng, Z.; Wang, W.; Yuan, Y.; Hong, Q.; Lin, J.; Li, X.; Meng, Y. Cigarette smoke-inactivated SIRT1 promotes autophagy-dependent senescence of alveolar epithelial type 2 cells to induce pulmonary fibrosis. *Free Radic. Biol. Med.* **2021**, *166*, 116–127. [CrossRef]
23. Fang, E.; Scheibye-Knudsen, M.; Brace, L.; Kassahun, H.; SenGupta, T.; Nilsen, H.; Mitchell, J.; Croteau, D.; Bohr, V. Defective mitophagy in XPA via PARP-1 hyperactivation and NAD(+)/SIRT1 reduction. *Cell* **2014**, *157*, 882–896. [CrossRef]
24. Wang, L.; Xu, C.; Johansen, T.; Berger, S.; Dou, Z. SIRT1—A new mammalian substrate of nuclear autophagy. *Autophagy* **2021**, *17*, 593–595. [CrossRef]
25. Nabavi, S.; Braidy, N.; Gortzi, O.; Sobarzo-Sanchez, E.; Daglia, M.; Skalicka-Woźniak, K.; Nabavi, S. Luteolin as an anti-inflammatory and neuroprotective agent: A brief review. *Brain Res. Bull.* **2015**, *119*, 1–11. [CrossRef]
26. Xu, H.; Yu, W.; Sun, S.; Li, C.; Zhang, Y.; Ren, J. Luteolin Attenuates Doxorubicin-Induced Cardiotoxicity Through Promoting Mitochondrial Autophagy. *Front. Physiol.* **2020**, *11*, 113. [CrossRef]
27. Al-Megrin, W.; Alomar, S.; Alkhuriji, A.; Metwally, D.; Mohamed, S.; Kassab, R.; Abdel Moneim, A.; El-Khadragy, M. Luteolin protects against testicular injury induced by lead acetate by activating the Nrf2/HO-1 pathway. *IUBMB Life* **2020**, *72*, 1787–1798. [CrossRef]

28. Tan, X.; Liu, B.; Lu, J.; Li, S.; Baiyun, R.; Lv, Y.; Lu, Q.; Zhang, Z. Dietary luteolin protects against HgCl-induced renal injury via activation of Nrf2-mediated signaling in rat. *J. Inorg. Biochem.* **2018**, *179*, 24–31. [CrossRef]
29. Domitrović, R.; Cvijanović, O.; Pugel, E.; Zagorac, G.; Mahmutefendić, H.; Škoda, M. Luteolin ameliorates cisplatin-induced nephrotoxicity in mice through inhibition of platinum accumulation, inflammation and apoptosis in the kidney. *Toxicology* **2013**, *310*, 115–123. [CrossRef]
30. Wang, Y.; Su, H.; Song, X.; Fiati Kenston, S.; Zhao, J.; Gu, Y. Luteolin inhibits multi-heavy metal mixture-induced HL7702 cell apoptosis through downregulation of ROS-activated mitochondrial pathway. *Int. J. Mol. Med.* **2018**, *41*, 233–241. [CrossRef]
31. Xu, X.; Yu, Z.; Han, B.; Li, S.; Sun, Y.; Du, Y.; Wang, Z.; Gao, D.; Zhang, Z. Luteolin alleviates inorganic mercury-induced kidney injury via activation of the AMPK/mTOR autophagy pathway. *J. Inorg. Biochem.* **2021**, *224*, 111583. [CrossRef]
32. Li, F.; Wei, R.; Huang, M.; Chen, J.; Li, P.; Ma, Y.; Chen, X. Luteolin can ameliorate renal interstitial fibrosis-induced renal anaemia through the SIRT1/FOXO3 pathway. *Food Funct.* **2022**, *13*, 11896–11914. [CrossRef]
33. Huang, C.; Chen, H.; Lo, C.; Wang, Y.; Li, C.; Liu, K.; Lii, C. Luteolin ameliorates palmitate-induced lipotoxicity in hepatocytes by mediating endoplasmic reticulum stress and autophagy. *Food Chem. Toxicol. Int. J. Publ. Br. Ind. Biol. Res. Assoc.* **2023**, *171*, 113554. [CrossRef]
34. Ge, J.; Zhang, C.; Sun, Y.; Zhang, Q.; Lv, M.; Guo, K.; Li, J. Cadmium exposure triggers mitochondrial dysfunction and oxidative stress in chicken (*Gallus gallus*) kidney via mitochondrial UPR inhibition and Nrf2-mediated antioxidant defense activation. *Sci. Total Environ.* **2019**, *689*, 1160–1171. [CrossRef]
35. Shi, Q.; Jin, X.; Fan, R.; Xing, M.; Guo, J.; Zhang, Z.; Zhang, J.; Xu, S. Cadmium-mediated miR-30a-GRP78 leads to JNK-dependent autophagy in chicken kidney. *Chemosphere* **2019**, *215*, 710–715. [CrossRef]
36. Oyagbemi, A.; Adejumobi, O.; Ajibade, T.; Asenuga, E.; Afolabi, J.; Ogunpolu, B.; Falayi, O.; Hassan, F.; Nabofa, E.; Olutayo Omobowale, T.; et al. Luteolin Attenuates Glycerol-Induced Acute Renal Failure and Cardiac Complications through Modulation of Kim-1/NF-κB/Nrf2 Signaling Pathways. *J. Diet. Suppl.* **2021**, *18*, 543–565. [CrossRef]
37. Oyagbemi, A.; Omobowale, T.; Ola-Davies, O.; Asenuga, E.; Ajibade, T.; Adejumobi, O.; Afolabi, J.; Ogunpolu, B.; Falayi, O.; Saba, A.; et al. Luteolin-mediated Kim-1/NF-kB/Nrf2 signaling pathways protects sodium fluoride-induced hypertension and cardiovascular complications. *BioFactors* **2018**, *44*, 518–531. [CrossRef]
38. Zhang, K.; Dong, W.; Li, J.; Gong, Z.; Liu, W.; He, S.; Zou, H.; Song, R.; Liu, G.; Liu, Z. Honokiol Antagonizes Cadmium-Induced Nephrotoxicity in Quail by Alleviating Autophagy Dysfunction, Apoptosis and Mitochondrial UPR Inhibition with Its Antioxidant Properties. *Life* **2022**, *12*, 1574. [CrossRef]
39. Satarug, S.; Vesey, D.; Gobe, G. Kidney Cadmium Toxicity, Diabetes and High Blood Pressure: The Perfect Storm. *Tohoku J. Exp. Med.* **2017**, *241*, 65–87. [CrossRef]
40. Zhuang, J.; Nie, G.; Yang, F.; Dai, X.; Cao, H.; Xing, C.; Hu, G.; Zhang, C. Cadmium induces cytotoxicity through oxidative stress-mediated apoptosis pathway in duck renal tubular epithelial cells. *Toxicol. Vitr. Int. J. Publ. Assoc. BIBRA* **2019**, *61*, 104625. [CrossRef]
41. Shi, L.; Cao, H.; Luo, J.; Liu, P.; Wang, T.; Hu, G.; Zhang, C. Effects of molybdenum and cadmium on the oxidative damage and kidney apoptosis in Duck. *Ecotoxicol. Environ. Saf.* **2017**, *145*, 24–31. [CrossRef]
42. Liu, L.; Yang, B.; Cheng, Y.; Lin, H. Ameliorative Effects of Selenium on Cadmium-Induced Oxidative Stress and Endoplasmic Reticulum Stress in the Chicken Kidney. *Biol. Trace Elem. Res.* **2015**, *167*, 308–319. [CrossRef]
43. Li, X.; Ge, M.; Zhu, W.; Wang, P.; Wang, J.; Tai, T.; Wang, Y.; Sun, J.; Shi, G. Protective Effects of Astilbin Against Cadmium-Induced Apoptosis in Chicken Kidneys via Endoplasmic Reticulum Stress Signaling Pathway. *Biol. Trace Elem. Res.* **2022**, *200*, 4430–4443. [CrossRef]
44. Hong, X.; Zhao, X.; Wang, G.; Zhang, Z.; Pei, H.; Liu, Z. Luteolin Treatment Protects against Renal Ischemia-Reperfusion Injury in Rats. *Mediat. Inflamm.* **2017**, *2017*, 9783893. [CrossRef]
45. Chu, N.; Zhang, X.; Chen, S.; Zhen, Q.; Wang, Y. Luteolin has a significant protective effect against cadmium-induced injury in lung epithelial Beas-2B cells. *Nan Fang Yi Ke Da Xue Xue Bao = J. South. Med. Univ.* **2021**, *41*, 729–735.
46. Al-Megrin, W.; Alkhuriji, A.; Yousef, A.; Metwally, D.; Habotta, O.; Kassab, R.; Abdel Moneim, A.; El-Khadragy, M. Antagonistic Efficacy of Luteolin against Lead Acetate Exposure-Associated with Hepatotoxicity is Mediated via Antioxidant, Anti-Inflammatory, and Anti-Apoptotic Activities. *Antioxidants* **2019**, *9*, 10. [CrossRef]
47. Owumi, S.; Lewu, D.; Arunsi, U.; Oyelere, A. Luteolin attenuates doxorubicin-induced derangements of liver and kidney by reducing oxidative and inflammatory stress to suppress apoptosis. *Hum. Exp. Toxicol.* **2021**, *40*, 1656–1672. [CrossRef]
48. Liu, M.; Cheng, C.; Li, X.; Zhou, S.; Hua, J.; Huang, J.; Li, Y.; Yang, K.; Zhang, P.; Zhang, Y.; et al. Luteolin alleviates ochratoxin A induced oxidative stress by regulating Nrf2 and HIF-1α pathways in NRK-52E rat kidney cells. *Food Chem. Toxicol. Int. J. Publ. Br. Ind. Biol. Res. Assoc.* **2020**, *141*, 111436. [CrossRef]
49. De Leo, E.; Elmonem, M.; Berlingerio, S.; Berquez, M.; Festa, B.; Raso, R.; Bellomo, F.; Starborg, T.; Janssen, M.; Abbaszadeh, Z.; et al. Cell-Based Phenotypic Drug Screening Identifies Luteolin as Candidate Therapeutic for Nephropathic Cystinosis. *J. Am. Soc. Nephrol.* **2020**, *31*, 1522–1537. [CrossRef]
50. Gobe, G.; Crane, D. Mitochondria, reactive oxygen species and cadmium toxicity in the kidney. *Toxicol. Lett.* **2010**, *198*, 49–55. [CrossRef]

51. Pavón, N.; Buelna-Chontal, M.; Macías-López, A.; Correa, F.; Uribe-Álvarez, C.; Hernández-Esquivel, L.; Chávez, E. On the oxidative damage by cadmium to kidney mitochondrial functions. *Biochem. Cell Biol. = Biochim. Biol. Cell.* **2019**, *97*, 187–192. [CrossRef] [PubMed]
52. Bhattacharya, S. Protective Role of the Essential Trace Elements in the Obviation of Cadmium Toxicity: Glimpses of Mechanisms. *Biol. Trace Elem. Res.* **2022**, *200*, 2239–2246. [CrossRef] [PubMed]
53. Zhu, Q.; Li, W.; Zheng, J. Life-cycle exposure to cadmium induced compensatory responses towards oxidative stress in the liver of female zebrafish. *Chemosphere* **2018**, *210*, 949–957. [CrossRef]
54. Taylor, C. Zinc, the pancreas, and diabetes: Insights from rodent studies and future directions. *Biometals Int. J. Role Met. Ions Biol. Biochem. Med.* **2005**, *18*, 305–312. [CrossRef] [PubMed]
55. Zhang, D.; Gao, J.; Zhang, K.; Liu, X.; Li, J. Effects of chronic cadmium poisoning on Zn, Cu, Fe, Ca, and metallothionein in liver and kidney of rats. *Biol. Trace Elem. Res.* **2012**, *149*, 57–63. [CrossRef] [PubMed]
56. Dong, W.; Zhang, K.; Gong, Z.; Luo, T.; Li, J.; Wang, X.; Zou, H.; Song, R.; Zhu, J.; Ma, Y.; et al. N-acetylcysteine delayed cadmium-induced chronic kidney injury by activating the sirtuin 1-P53 signaling pathway. *Chem. Biol. Interact.* **2023**, *369*, 110299. [CrossRef] [PubMed]
57. Pu, W.; Chu, X.; Guo, H.; Huang, G.; Cui, T.; Huang, B.; Dai, X.; Zhang, C. The activated ATM/AMPK/mTOR axis promotes autophagy in response to oxidative stress-mediated DNA damage co-induced by molybdenum and cadmium in duck testes. *Environ. Pollut.* **2023**, *316*, 120574. [CrossRef] [PubMed]
58. Yu, C.; Yang, C.; Song, X.; Li, J.; Peng, H.; Qiu, M.; Yang, L.; Du, H.; Jiang, X.; Liu, Y. Long Non-coding RNA Expression Profile in Broiler Liver with Cadmium-Induced Oxidative Damage. *Biol. Trace Elem. Res.* **2021**, *199*, 3053–3061. [CrossRef]
59. Jomova, K.; Hudecova, L.; Lauro, P.; Simunková, M.; Barbierikova, Z.; Malcek, M.; Alwasel, S.; Alhazza, I.; Rhodes, C.; Valko, M. The effect of Luteolin on DNA damage mediated by a copper catalyzed Fenton reaction. *J. Inorg. Biochem.* **2022**, *226*, 111635. [CrossRef]
60. Hurtado-Bagès, S.; Knobloch, G.; Ladurner, A.; Buschbeck, M. The taming of PARP1 and its impact on NAD metabolism. *Mol. Metab.* **2020**, *38*, 100950. [CrossRef]
61. Wang, M.; Wang, Y.; Wang, S.; Hou, L.; Cui, Z.; Li, Q.; Huang, H. Selenium alleviates cadmium-induced oxidative stress, endoplasmic reticulum stress and programmed necrosis in chicken testes. *Sci. Total Environ.* **2023**, *863*, 160601. [CrossRef] [PubMed]
62. Luo, T.; Yuan, Y.; Yu, Q.; Liu, G.; Long, M.; Zhang, K.; Bian, J.; Gu, J.; Zou, H.; Wang, Y.; et al. PARP-1 overexpression contributes to Cadmium-induced death in rat proximal tubular cells via parthanatos and the MAPK signalling pathway. *Sci. Rep.* **2017**, *7*, 4331. [CrossRef] [PubMed]
63. Pang, J.; Gong, H.; Xi, C.; Fan, W.; Dai, Y.; Zhang, T. Poly(ADP-ribose) polymerase 1 is involved in glucose toxicity through SIRT1 modulation in HepG2 hepatocytes. *J. Cell. Biochem.* **2011**, *112*, 299–306. [CrossRef] [PubMed]
64. Bai, P.; Cantó, C.; Oudart, H.; Brunyánszki, A.; Cen, Y.; Thomas, C.; Yamamoto, H.; Huber, A.; Kiss, B.; Houtkooper, R.; et al. PARP-1 inhibition increases mitochondrial metabolism through SIRT1 activation. *Cell Metab.* **2011**, *13*, 461–468. [CrossRef] [PubMed]
65. Waldman, M.; Nudelman, V.; Shainberg, A.; Abraham, N.; Kornwoski, R.; Aravot, D.; Arad, M.; Hochhauser, E. PARP-1 inhibition protects the diabetic heart through activation of SIRT1-PGC-1α axis. *Exp. Cell Res.* **2018**, *373*, 112–118. [CrossRef] [PubMed]
66. Guo, P.; Pi, H.; Xu, S.; Zhang, L.; Li, Y.; Li, M.; Cao, Z.; Tian, L.; Xie, J.; Li, R.; et al. Melatonin Improves mitochondrial function by promoting MT1/SIRT1/PGC-1 alpha-dependent mitochondrial biogenesis in cadmium-induced hepatotoxicity in vitro. *Toxicol. Sci. Off. J. Soc. Toxicol.* **2014**, *142*, 182–195. [CrossRef]
67. Hao, R.; Ge, J.; Song, X.; Li, F.; Sun-Waterhouse, D.; Li, D. Cadmium induces ferroptosis and apoptosis by modulating miR-34a-5p/Sirt1axis in PC12 cells. *Environ. Toxicol.* **2022**, *37*, 41–51. [CrossRef]
68. Zhang, C.; Wang, X.; Pi, S.; Wei, Z.; Wang, C.; Yang, F.; Li, G.; Nie, G.; Hu, G. Cadmium and molybdenum co-exposure triggers autophagy via CYP450s/ROS pathway in duck renal tubular epithelial cells. *Sci. Total Environ.* **2021**, *759*, 143570. [CrossRef] [PubMed]
69. Zhang, C.; Hu, Z.; Hu, R.; Pi, S.; Wei, Z.; Wang, C.; Yang, F.; Xing, C.; Nie, G.; Hu, G. New insights into crosstalk between pyroptosis and autophagy co-induced by molybdenum and cadmium in duck renal tubular epithelial cells. *J. Hazard. Mater.* **2021**, *416*, 126138. [CrossRef]
70. Sun, J.; Bian, Y.; Ma, Y.; Ali, W.; Wang, T.; Yuan, Y.; Gu, J.; Bian, J.; Liu, Z.; Zou, H. Melatonin alleviates cadmium-induced nonalcoholic fatty liver disease in ducks by alleviating autophagic flow arrest via PPAR-α and reducing oxidative stress. *Poult. Sci.* **2023**, *102*, 102835. [CrossRef]
71. Parzych, K.; Klionsky, D. An overview of autophagy: Morphology, mechanism, and regulation. *Antioxid. Redox Signal.* **2014**, *20*, 460–473. [CrossRef] [PubMed]
72. Li, M.; Pi, H.; Yang, Z.; Reiter, R.; Xu, S.; Chen, X.; Chen, C.; Zhang, L.; Yang, M.; Li, Y.; et al. Melatonin antagonizes cadmium-induced neurotoxicity by activating the transcription factor EB-dependent autophagy-lysosome machinery in mouse neuroblastoma cells. *J. Pineal Res.* **2016**, *61*, 353–369. [CrossRef]
73. Wang, X.Y.; Yang, H.; Wang, M.G.; Yang, D.B.; Wang, Z.Y.; Wang, L. Trehalose protects against cadmium-induced cytotoxicity in primary rat proximal tubular cells via inhibiting apoptosis and restoring autophagic flux. *Cell Death Dis.* **2017**, *8*, e3099. [CrossRef] [PubMed]

74. Yang, H.; Gao, Y.; Fan, X.; Liu, X.; Peng, L.; Ci, X. Oridonin Sensitizes Cisplatin-Induced Apoptosis via AMPK/Akt/mTOR-Dependent Autophagosome Accumulation in A549 Cells. *Front. Oncol.* **2019**, *9*, 769. [CrossRef] [PubMed]
75. El-Kott, A.; Abd-Lateif, A.; Khalifa, H.; Morsy, K.; Ibrahim, E.; Bin-Jumah, M.; Abdel-Daim, M.; Aleya, L. Kaempferol protects against cadmium chloride-induced hippocampal damage and memory deficits by activation of silent information regulator 1 and inhibition of poly (ADP-Ribose) polymerase-1. *Sci. Total Environ.* **2020**, *728*, 138832. [CrossRef] [PubMed]
76. Yang, X.; Jiang, T.; Wang, Y.; Guo, L. The Role and Mechanism of SIRT1 in Resveratrol-regulated Osteoblast Autophagy in Osteoporosis Rats. *Sci. Rep.* **2019**, *9*, 18424. [CrossRef]
77. Song, Y.; Lee, Y.; Kim, J.; Ham, D.; Kang, E.; Cha, B.; Lee, H.; Lee, B. Metformin alleviates hepatosteatosis by restoring SIRT1-mediated autophagy induction via an AMP-activated protein kinase-independent pathway. *Autophagy* **2015**, *11*, 46–59. [CrossRef]

antioxidants

MDPI

Article

Antioxidative Sirt1 and the Keap1-Nrf2 Signaling Pathway Impair Inflammation and Positively Regulate Autophagy in Murine Mammary Epithelial Cells or Mammary Glands Infected with *Streptococcus uberis*

Sohrab Khan [1], Tian Wang [1], Eduardo R. Cobo [2], Bingchun Liang [1], Muhammad Asfandyar Khan [1], Maolin Xu [1], Weijie Qu [3], Jian Gao [1], Herman W. Barkema [2], John P. Kastelic [2], Gang Liu [1,*] and Bo Han [1,*]

[1] College of Veterinary Medicine, China Agricultural University, Beijing 100193, China; drsohrab@cau.edu.cn (S.K.); b20223050426@cau.edu.cn (T.W.); liangbingchun@cau.edu.cn (B.L.); asfand@cau.edu.cn (M.A.K.); xx0517@cau.edu.cn (M.X.); gaojian2016@cau.edu.cn (J.G.)

[2] Faculty of Veterinary Medicine, University of Calgary, Calgary, AB T2N 4N1, Canada; ecobo@ucalgary.ca (E.R.C.); barkema@ucalgary.ca (H.W.B.); jpkastel@ucalgary.ca (J.P.K.)

[3] College of Veterinary Medicine, Yunnan Agricultural University, Kunming 650201, China; wjqu@ynau.edu.cn

* Correspondence: gangliu@cau.edu.cn (G.L.); hanbo@cau.edu.cn (B.H.); Tel.: +86-10-6273-3801 (B.H.)

Abstract: *Streptococcus uberis* mastitis in cattle infects mammary epithelial cells. Although oxidative responses often remove intracellular microbes, *S. uberis* survives, but the mechanisms are not well understood. Herein, we aimed to elucidate antioxidative mechanisms during pathogenesis of *S. uberis* after isolation from clinical bovine mastitis milk samples. *S. uberis*'s in vitro pathomorphology, oxidative stress biological activities, transcription of antioxidative factors, inflammatory response cytokines, autophagosome and autophagy functions were evaluated, and in vivo *S. uberis* was injected into the fourth mammary gland nipple of each mouse to assess the infectiousness of *S. uberis* potential molecular mechanisms. The results showed that infection with *S. uberis* induced early oxidative stress and increased reactive oxygen species (ROS). However, over time, ROS concentrations decreased due to increased antioxidative activity, including total superoxide dismutase (T-SOD) and malondialdehyde (MDA) enzymes, plus transcription of antioxidative factors (Sirt1, Keap1, Nrf2, HO-1). Treatment with a ROS scavenger (N-acetyl cysteine, NAC) before infection with *S. uberis* reduced antioxidative responses and the inflammatory response, including the cytokines IL-6 and TNF-α, and the formation of the Atg5-LC3II/LC3I autophagosome. Synthesis of antioxidants determined autophagy functions, with Sirt1/Nrf2 activating autophagy in the presence of *S. uberis*. This study demonstrated the evasive mechanisms of *S. uberis* in mastitis, including suppressing inflammatory and ROS defenses by stimulating antioxidative pathways.

Keywords: bovine mastitis; *Streptococcus uberis*; antioxidative pathway; inflammation; autophagy; murine mammary glands; mMECs

1. Introduction

Mastitis is an inflammatory syndrome that can irreversibly damage the mammary glands of dairy cattle [1], causing substantial financial losses due to reductions in milk production and quality, plus premature culling [2,3]. Bovine mastitis is often caused by various environmental and bacterial agents, including *Streptococcus uberis* [4], the most frequently isolated pathogen causing subclinical mastitis in the United Kingdom, Ireland, Australia and New Zealand [5]. The damaging consequences of *S. uberis* infection include inflammatory and autophagy responses [6] regulated by antioxidative factors [7]. Autophagy is a defensive catabolic mechanism to remove damaged organelles and control bacterial infections [8]. "Autophagy flux" refers to the entirety of autophagosome production, its maturation, fusion with lysosomes and subsequent breakdown, with release of macromolecules into the cytosol. Autolysosomes and degradation are key functions of autophagy [9].

Production of reactive oxygen species (ROS) significantly increases during infection, aids pathogen removal and contributes to inflammatory signaling cascades [10]. Production of ROS is regulated by antioxidative factors, including silent information regulator 1 (Sirt1), which reduces oxidative stress by modulating superoxide dismutase (SOD) [11] and decreases malondialdehyde (MDA), an oxidative stress marker [12]. Sirt1 also affects signaling pathways associated with inflammation and autophagy [13]. Other antioxidant effectors are Kelch-like ECH-associated protein 1 (Keap1) and Nuclear factor erythroid 2-related factor 2 (Nrf2) [14]. Under physiological conditions, Keap1 regulates Nrf2 activity in the cytoplasm and is a principal protective sensor for oxidative stress [15]. However, under oxidative stress, Nrf2 separates from Keap1 protein, moves into the nucleus and joins with antioxidant response elements to promote the production of heme oxygenase-1 (HO-1) and SOD [16,17]. Expression of inflammatory markers (namely TNF-α/IL-6) and oxidative damage are reduced by activation of the Nrf2/HO-1 signaling pathway [18,19]. Therefore, Nrf2/HO-1 is an antioxidant signal that aims to reduce inflammation provoked by infection and oxidative stress [20]. Dissociation of Nrf2 from Keap1 activates autophagy by coupling the stress-inducible p62/SQSTM1 protein complex [21]. This multifunctional protein core has multiple domains, including a Keap1-interacting region (KIR) and an LC3-interacting region (LIR) [22]. The lipidation of microtubule-associated protein 1A/1B-light chain 3 to generate LC3II is critical in promoting autophagy [23]. The protein P62 interacts with LC3 in the autophagy–lysosome pathway and targets ubiquitinated substrate cargoes for destruction [24]. Furthermore, Atg5 promotes autophagosome elongation and requires conversion of LC3I to LC3II [25].

Microbial pathogens that infect host cells can be subjected to autophagy. In this process, LC3, which is widely distributed in the cytoplasm, connects to targeted substrates [26]. Furthermore, Atg4 cuts the C-terminal portion of LC3 into LC3-I that is then activated by Atg7 (an E1-like enzyme), passed to Atg3 (an E2-like enzyme) and changed into membrane-bound LC3II. Invading pathogens with polyubiquitination are typically identified by the autophagy receptor P62 that delivers the targeted substrate to LC3II-bound membranes and facilitates autophagosome formation. Attracting autophagy-related proteins to phagocytic vesicle assembly sites, e.g., Atg5, is important in phagophore synthesis, and requires a signal for autophagy [27]. The usual outcome is containment of intracellular infections or recycling of cytosolic substances [28].

We identified autophagy as a crucial component of epithelial cell defense against mastitis pathogens, with the involvement of HIF-1α, AMPKα/ULK1 and the PTEN/PI3K-Akt-mTOR pathway [29–31]. Furthermore, we also reported that *S. uberis* infection induced autophagy by decreasing synthesis of pro-inflammatory cytokines [32]. However, the mechanisms that connect the antioxidative pathway and autophagy during *S. uberis* infection remain unclear. Hence, we tested the hypothesis that silencing/activation of antioxidative pathway factors will bring changes in autophagy mechanism.

Our objective was to characterize pathogenesis of *S. uberis* mastitis and the role of the antioxidative pathway in the modulation of autophagy, using murine in vitro and in vivo models of mammary epithelial cells (mMECs) and mammary glands, respectively. Specifically, we addressed antioxidative factors (Sirt1, Keap1 and Nrf2), inflammatory factors (IL-6 and TNF-α) and autophagy marker proteins (Atg5 and LC3II/LC3I). We concluded that Sirt1 and Keap1-Nrf2 were involved in the activation of autophagy by reducing T-SOD and MDA activity along with significant reductions in inflammatory responses.

2. Materials and Methods

2.1. Statement of Ethics

This study was reviewed and approved by the Ethical Committee of the College of Veterinary Medicine, China Agricultural University (CAU), Beijing, China (Protocol

SYXK, 2016-0008). Furthermore, it was conducted according to standard ethical guidelines implemented at CAU.

2.2. *S. uberis* Isolation

Milk samples from dairy cows with clinical mastitis were obtained from dairy farms in northern Beijing, China, and *S. uberis* was isolated from those samples [32]. Isolates were identified on Todd–Hewitt Agar (THA), a solid medium containing 5% sheep blood, and cultured for 24 h at 37 °C prior to infecting mouse mammary glands and mMECs. Selection of *S. uberis* was based on colony characteristics on THA medium, followed by Gram staining, API 20 Strep system (bioMérieux, Lyon, France), Lancefield grouping, and validation by PCR sequencing (Sangon Biotech, Shanghai, China). Isolates were multiplied in Todd–Hewitt broth (THB) liquid medium for 14 h at 37 °C on an orbital shaker at 120 rpm, and stored in 25% glycerol stock solutions at −70 °C. For each challenge, a single loop inoculum of stock solution was added to liquid THB medium containing 2% fetal bovine serum (FBS; Hyclone, Logan, UT, USA) to generate an exponential growth phase (OD600 = 0.5 to 0.7) at 37 °C for infections [32].

2.3. Cell Culture and *S. uberis* Infection

Murine mammary epithelial HC11 cell line (mMECs) (Shanghai Cell Bioscience Inc., Shanghai, China) was used as an in vitro model for infectious mastitis. Cells were cultured in Dulbecco modified Eagle medium (DMEM) supplemented with 10% FBS plus penicillin and streptomycin (100 U/mL each) in T-25/T-75 cell culture flasks. Cells were incubated with 5% CO_2 at 37 °C and at 80% confluence were harvested by the addition of 2 mL trypsin until 70% cell movement was achieved. Then, cells were collected, centrifuged for 5 min at 1000× *g* and stock solutions prepared in 5% DMSO (dimethyl sulfoxide; Life Tein, LLC, South Plainfield, NJ, USA) for cryopreservation (~1×10^8 cells per cryovial) in liquid nitrogen [32]. Each batch of cells were used from 2–5 passages in a T-25 cell culture flask. For transfection and infection experiments, cells were transferred into 6-well plates (~1×10^3 cells per well) and incubated until the desired confluence. The mMECs were challenged with *S. uberis* at multiplicity of infection (MOI) 5:1, followed by incubation in 5% CO_2 at 37 °C and subsequently collected for various analyses.

2.4. Murine *S. uberis* Mastitis Model

Mice were housed at the Experimental Animal Center of China Agricultural University with ad libitum access to feed and drinking water and a 12 h light/dark photocycle. Studies were conducted with 20 female albino mice (20 to 23 gm body weight) at 1 wk post parturition and 1 h after separation from their pups. These mice were randomly allocated into five groups (n = 4 mice per group): Sham (Control group); *S. uberis* (*S. uberis* group); *S. uberis* + NAC (*S. uberis* + NAC group); *S. uberis* + Cambinol (*S. uberis* + siSirt1); and *S. uberis* + NK-252 (*S. uberis* + Nrf2 activator). In the *S. uberis* + NAC group, mice were pretreated with an intramammary injection of 300 mg/kg NAC at 3 h prior to *S. uberis* challenge. In *S. uberis* + siSirt1 and Nrf2 activator groups, 50 mg/kg Cambinol and 10 mg/kg NK-252, respectively, were injected 6 h prior to challenge. For *S. uberis* challenge, mice were anesthetized (Zoletil® 50, 0.05 mg/kg IM) and *S. uberis* (1×10^5 CFU/mL diluted in sterile saline, final volume of 100 µL) was injected intramammarily. All intramammary injections were performed with a micro-syringe and 26-gauge needle (using a stereomicroscope to visualize openings) into the 4th nipple (counting forward) of each mouse, after disinfection with 75% alcohol. At 6 h post-inoculation, all mice were euthanized and mammary gland tissues excised.

2.5. Determination of ROS Production

An assay kit for ROS (Beyotime Biotechnology, Shanghai, China) was used to measure intracellular ROS concentrations in mMECs seeded in a 6-well plate and challenged with *S. uberis* (MOI 5:1) at 80% confluence. Cells were washed thrice with PBS and incubated in 5% CO_2 at 37 °C for 30 min in the dark with 10 μM of DCFH-DA fluorescent probe in serum-free DMEM. Then, cells were washed three times with serum-free culture medium, followed by DAPI staining (5 min). Fluorescent signals of stimulated cells were observed with a laser scanning confocal microscope at wavelengths of 405 and 488 nm.

2.6. Transmission Electron Microscopy

The mMECs were grown in 6-well plates up to 80% confluence and then challenged by *S. uberis* (MOI 5:1). At 6, 9 and 12 h post infection, cells were digested (500 μL trypsin per well), centrifuged at 1000× *g* for 5 min, washed thrice with PBS and fixed with 2.5% glutaraldehyde for 2 h at room temperature. Cells were stained with 1% osmium tetroxide for 2 h at 4 °C, dried in an ethanol gradient series, and embedded in epoxy resin–acetone mixtures for 2 h. Samples were immersed in resin solution overnight at 37 °C and cut in ultrathin sections (100 nm), and visualized with a light microscope to ensure only a single slice was loaded on a copper grid. Samples were stained with 2% saturated uranyl acetate and treated with 50% ethanol and 3% lead citrate. Copper grid with samples were examined with a transmission electron microscope (TEM; H7650, Tokyo, Japan) at an accelerating voltage of 80 kV.

2.7. Western Blot Analysis

The mMECs were cultured in 6-well plates until 80% cell confluence and challenged by *S. uberis* (MOI 5:1). Various pretreatments were used. For example, mMECs were pretreated (1–6 h prior to *S. uberis* infection) with NAC (30 μM) to scavenge intracellular production of ROS, 40 μM Cambinol for Sirt1 inhibition, 10 μM NK-252 for Nrf2 activation or 10 μM ML385 for Nrf2 inhibition.

The mMECs were harvested using a cell scraper on an ice block, rinsed thrice with cold PBS and lysed with RIPA lysis buffer (Beyotime Biotechnology). Supernatants were obtained by centrifugation at 12,000 rpm for 15 min at 4 °C and total protein concentrations determined with a Bicinchoninic acid (BCA) kit (Beyotime Biotechnology).

Protein was loaded into gels (equal amounts in each lane) and β-actin was used as a loading control. After being separated by SDS-PAGE, proteins were transferred to a polyvinylidene difluoride (PVDF) membrane that was washed thrice and blocked with 5% skim milk in tris-buffered saline +0.1% Tween® 20 Detergent (TBST) for 2 h at room temperature. Membranes were incubated overnight at 4 °C with the following primary antibodies: Sirt1 (Cell Signaling, #3931S; Danvers, MA, USA); Keap1 (Abcam, #ab227828; Cambridge, UK); Nrf2 (Proteintech, #16396-1-AP; Rosemont, IL, USA); HO-1 (Proteintech, #27282-1-AP; Rosemont, IL, USA); IL-6 (Invitrogen, #700480; Carlsbad, CA, USA); TNF-α (Proteintech, #17590-1-AP; Rosemont, IL, USA); Atg5 (Proteintech, #10181-2-AP; Rosemont, IL, USA); LC3 (Proteintech, #14600-1-AP; Rosemont, IL, USA); and β-actin (Proteintech #66009-1-Ig; Rosemont, IL, USA). Samples were incubated with secondary antibodies against rabbit or mouse IgG for 2 h at room temperature and signals developed by chemiluminescence using ECL reagents. ImageJ 1.49v software (http://imagej.nih.gov/ij, accessed on 18 December 2023, NIH, Bethesda, MD, USA) was used to assess band density.

2.8. T-SOD and MDA Activity

The mMECs were cultured overnight in 6-well plates and treated with NAC 1 h prior to *S. uberis* challenge (MOI 5:1). Total superoxide dismutase (T-SOD) and malondialdehyde (MDA) activity were measured at 6, 12 and 24 h post challenge. The T-SOD activity was measured using a T-SOD assay kit in a microplate reader (Beyotime Biotechnology), whereas MDA activity was evaluated with an MDA ELISA kit (Abcam, Shanghai, China). The same kits were used to determine the activities of T-SOD and MDA in murine mammary glands. Herein, tissues were collected, washed with PBS and stored at −20 °C. Then, tissues were transferred into a mortar with liquid nitrogen, ground to a powder, homogenized with 0.5% Triton X-100 and centrifuged at 14,000× *g* for 5 min at 4 °C to collect supernatants.

2.9. Labeling and Tracking Lysosomes

Lysosomes or mature autophagosomes were detected with Lyso-Tracker Red fluorescent probe (Beyotime Biotechnology). Lyso-Tracker Red penetrates mMECs and detects lysosomes or mature autophagosomes in an acidified environment [33]. In these experiments, mMECs were seeded in 6-well plates with coverslips and challenged with *S. uberis* at 80% confluence. Cells were washed thrice with ultra-sterilized PBS and incubated in 5% CO_2 at 37 °C for 30 min with 50 nM Lyso-Tracker Red in cell culture medium for lysosome red staining. The Lyso-Tracker Red was removed by three washes with PBS and nuclei stained with DAPI for 5 min. Fluorescent signals were observed under a laser scanning confocal microscope at wavelengths of 405, 488 and 561 nm.

2.10. Cell Transfection and Confocal Microscopy

Autophagy was monitored using Ad-GFP-LC3 and Ad-mCherry-GFP-LC3B (Beyotime Biotechnology), adenoviruses that express GFP-LC3 and mCherry-GFP-LC3B fusion proteins, respectively [34]. For transfection, mMECs were cultured in 6-well plates with coverslips and incubated for 12 h with 5% CO_2 at 37 °C. Then, Ad-GFP-LC3B and Ad-mCherry-GFP-LC3B were transfected into cells at 40% confluence in DMEM with 10% FBS, followed by a 24 h incubation. The mMECs were pretreated with Cambinol for Sirt1 inhibition and challenged with *S. uberis* (MOI 5:1) for 12 h. Cells were washed thrice with PBS and cell nuclei were stained with DAPI (10–20 µL per coverslip) for 5 min. After washes with ultra-sterilized PBS, anti-fluorescence quenching sealing solution (8 µL) was added to a clear glass slide. Then, coverslips were inverted on the glass slides and examined with a laser scanning confocal microscope. In an autophagy state, mMECs transfected with Ad-mCherry-GFP-LC3B overexpressed mRFP/mCherry-GFP tandem. Wavelengths of 405, 488 and 561 nm were used for imaging.

2.11. Immunofluorescence

The mMECs were cultured in 6-well plates with glass coverslips and incubated overnight at 37 °C with 5% CO_2 and pretreated (6 h) with a Nrf2 activator or inhibitor before being challenged with *S. uberis* (MOI 5:1) for 6 h. Cells were thrice washed with PBS and fixed with 4% paraformaldehyde for 20 min, followed by permeabilization with 0.25% Triton X-100 in PBS for 15 min. Cells were treated with 3% bovine serum at room temperature for 30 min and incubated with Nrf2 primary antibody overnight at 4 °C. After three PBS washes, cells were incubated with goat anti-rabbit IgG (H + L) tagged with Alexa Fluor 488 for 1 h at room temperature. Cell nuclei were stained with DAPI for 5 min and washed 3 times with PBS. Glass coverslips were inverted on clean glass slides and observed with a laser scanning confocal microscope (Olympus-FV3000, Olympus, Tokyo, Japan) at wavelengths of 405 and 488 nm, with images captured and analyzed with ImageJ software.

2.12. Hematoxylin and Eosin Staining of Murine Mammary Gland Tissues

Post *S. uberis* challenge and treatments, mammary gland tissues were excised, dehydrated and fixed in 4% paraformaldehyde for 20 min. Tissues were embedded in paraffin, sectioned (5 µm), treated with xylene for 5 min, and then exposed to 70, 80, 90 and 100% ethanol (10 s in each concentration). Slides were stained with hematoxylin (Beyotime Biotechnology) for 5 min, cleared with tap water for 10 min, rinsed with distilled water and stained with eosin (Beyotime Biotechnology) for 2 min. Slides were washed twice with 70% ethanol. Imaging was performed in a set of randomly chosen fields with an optical microscope (Olympus, Tokyo, Japan) at 100× magnification.

2.13. Statistical Analyses

The results of three independent experiments are presented as means ± standard deviation (SD). Data were analyzed by Student's *t*-test or one-way ANOVA, with Bonferroni correction for multiple comparisons using IBM SPSS statistics 29.0.10 software (https:

//www.ibm.com; Armonk, NY, USA). $p < 0.05$ and $p < 0.01$ were considered significant and highly significant, respectively.

3. Results

3.1. *S. uberis* Enhanced ROS Production and Autophagy Induction in mMECs

Oxidative stress in *S. uberis*-infected mMECs was gauged by intracellular ROS concentrations until 24 h post *S. uberis* challenge. Dichlorofluorescein diacetate (DCFH-DA) relative fluorescence emissions (as a measure of ROS concentrations) were higher at 3 to 9 h, but decreased by 12 and 24 h post *S. uberis* (Figure 1A). Infection with *S. uberis* induced autophagy and autolysosome formation in mMECs, as observed by transmission electron microscopy (TEM) (Figure 1B). Moreover, infected mMECs had mitochondrial vacuolization, autophagosome and lysosome formation and fusion at 12 h post challenge, whereas *S. uberis* were located intracellularly at 6 and 9 h post challenge.

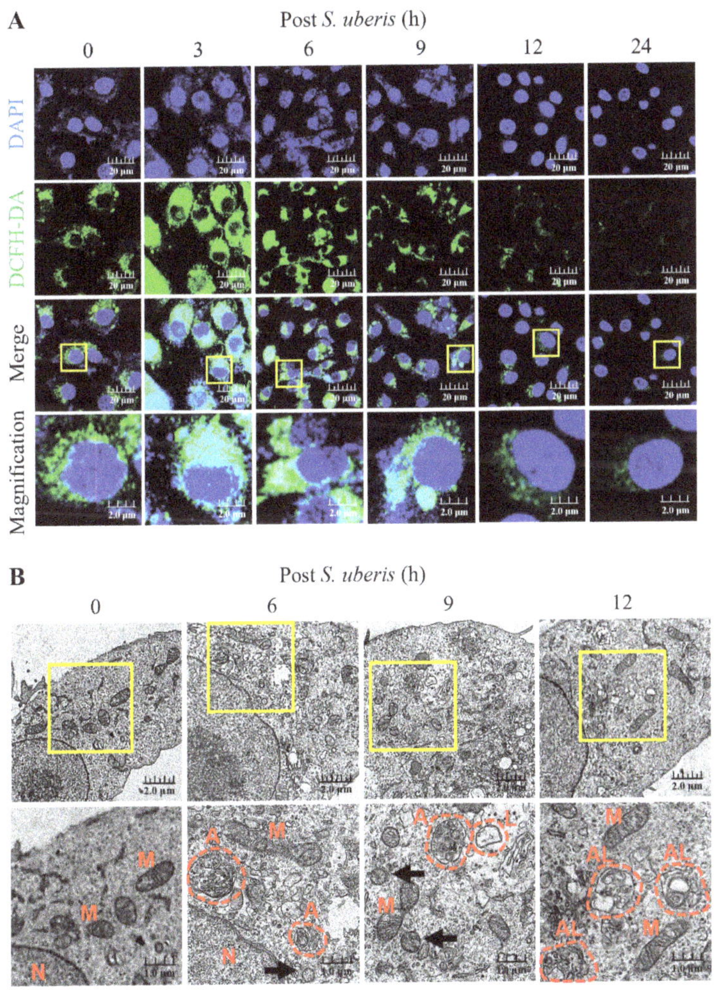

Figure 1. Infecting mMECs with *S. uberis* enhanced intracellular accumulation of ROS and induced autophagy. (**A**) The mMECs were challenged with *S. uberis* and ROS production was determined by

measuring the intensity of green fluorescence generated by DCFH-DA and captured with a confocal laser scanning microscope. (**B**) Autophagy induction was confirmed based on morphological and subcellular (TEM) images. Note the nuclei (N), mitochondria (M), autophagosomes (A), lysosomes (L), autolysosome (AL) and *S. uberis* (black arrowheads). Scale bar = 1.0 μm. Magnified figure It comes from the yellow box.

3.2. *S. uberis* Induced Antioxidative, Inflammatory and Autophagy Markers

Expressions of antioxidative Sirt1, Keap1 and Nrf2 were upregulated ($p < 0.01$) in mMECs at 3 to 9 h after *S. uberis* challenge (Figure 2A). Expressions of inflammatory cytokines IL-6 and TNF-α were decreased ($p < 0.01$) at 3 to 9 h, whereas autophagy LC3II/LC3I markers were increased ($p < 0.01$) at 6 to 12 h (Figure 2B). Expression levels of inflammatory cytokines had declined at 3 to 9 hpi (autophagy progression; Supplementary Figure S1).

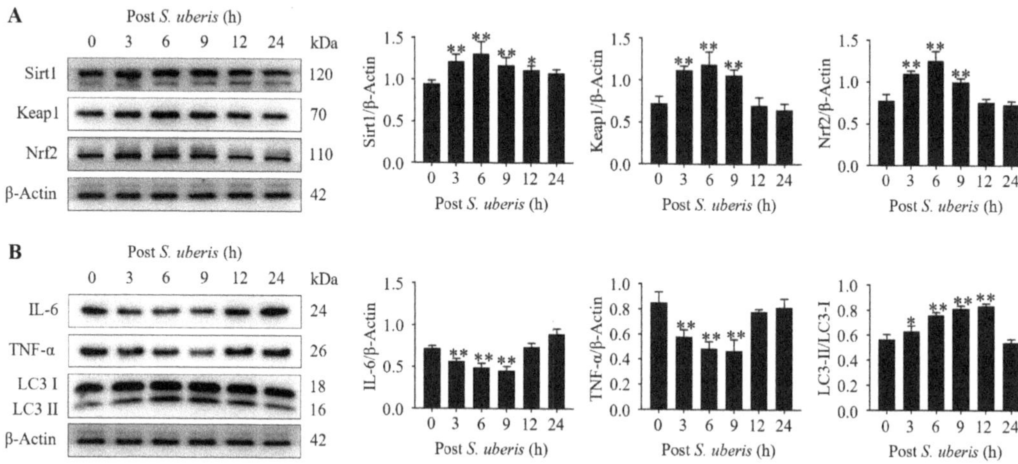

Figure 2. Infecting mMECs with *S. uberis* induced antioxidant and autophagy marker proteins and reduced inflammatory cytokines. (**A**) Western blot analyses of antioxidative Sirt1, Keap1 and Nrf2 isolated from *S. uberis*-challenged mMECs. Proteins were collected up to 24 h post challenge. (**B**) Inflammatory IL-6 and TNF-α, and autophagy of LC3II/LC3I, were also analyzed following *S. uberis* challenge. Mean and standard deviation (three independent experiments) of proteins (quantified with ImageJ 1.49v, http://imagej.nih.gov/ij, accessed on 18 December 2023). * $p < 0.05$, ** $p < 0.01$ (compared to the Sham).

3.3. NAC Pretreatment Mitigated Antioxidative Pathway Elements in *S. uberis*-Challenged mMECs

Antioxidative factors Sirt1, Nrf2 and HO-1 increased at 3 and 12 h post *S. uberis* challenge, but were reduced in NAC-pretreated cells (Figure 3A). Specifically, Sirt1 and Nrf2 expression increased ($p < 0.01$) at 3 h post challenge but it was comparatively lower at 12 h, whereas HO-1 was higher ($p < 0.01$) at 12 versus 3 h post challenge (Supplementary Figure S2). Expressions of Sirt1 were upregulated (not significantly), whereas Keap1 and Nrf2 were upregulated ($p < 0.01$) in *S. uberis*-challenged mMECs at 3 h post challenge; however, these responses were abrogated by Sirt1 inhibition in either transfected cells or those pretreated with Cambinol (Figure 3B). Cambinol/siSirt1 also decreased Keap1 and Nrf2 expression in either the presence or absence of *S. uberis* (Figure 9A).

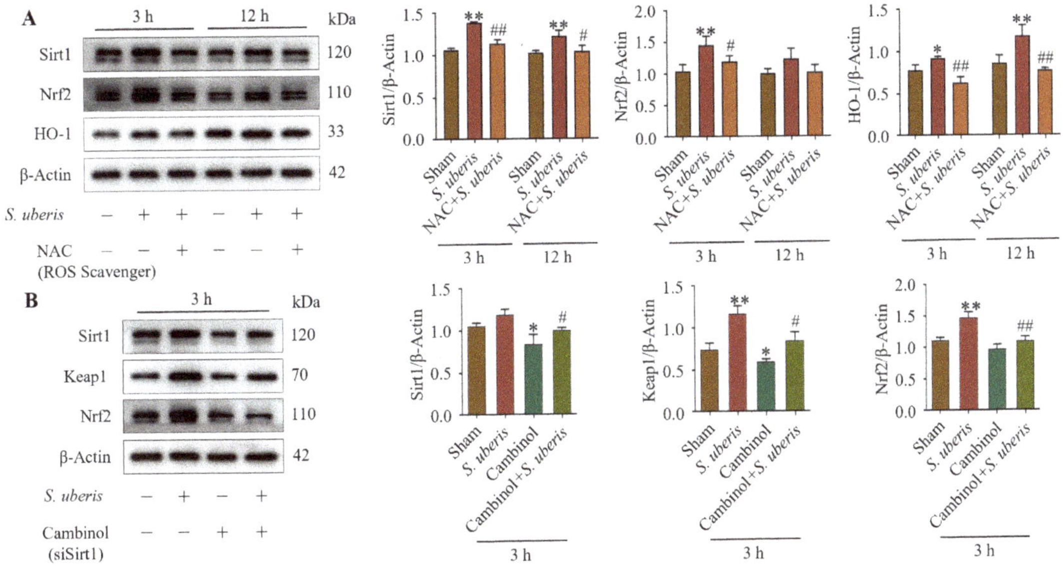

Figure 3. NAC pretreatment in *S. uberis*-challenged mMECs mitigated antioxidative responses. (**A**) Levels of Sirt1, Nrf2 and HO-1 in mMECs pretreated with 30 μM NAC and 1 h later challenged with *S. uberis*. (**B**) Levels of Sirt1, Keap1 and Nrf2 in mMECs pretreated with 40 μM Cambinol (siSirt1) and 6 h later challenged with *S. uberis*. Data were derived from assessments of Western blots and are mean ± SD of three independent trials. * $p < 0.05$ and ** $p < 0.01$ (compared to the Sham); # $p < 0.05$ and ## $p < 0.01$ (compared to the *S. uberis* group).

3.4. NAC Treatment Attenuated Inflammation and Cellular Damage in S. uberis-Challenged mMECs/Murine Mammary Glands via Reduced Oxidative Stress

S. uberis-challenged mMECs pretreated with NAC showed reduced oxidative stress. Although Nrf2, HO-1, IL-6 and TNF-α expression increased ($p < 0.01$) at 12 and 24 h post *S. uberis* challenge (Figure 4A), these levels were lesser in mMECs pretreated with NAC (Supplementary Figure S3). Activity of T-SOD in the *S. uberis*-challenged group was lower at 12 h ($p < 0.01$) and 24 h ($p < 0.05$) than at 6 h post *S. uberis* challenge (Figure 4B). Total SOD increased ($p < 0.05$) in the NAC + *S. uberis* group compared to the *S. uberis* group, but MDA activity was higher ($p < 0.05$) at 6 h post *S. uberis* compared to 12 or 24 h (Figure 4). In cells pretreated with NAC + *S. uberis*, MDA activity was progressively reduced at 6, 12 and 24 h.

3.5. NAC Treatment Attenuated Autophagy Mechanism in S. uberis-Challenged mMECs

Pretreatment with NAC in the presence of *S. uberis* impaired autophagy and antioxidative Keap1 at 12 and 24 h post challenge. Levels of Keap1, Atg5 and LC3II/LC3I were upregulated ($p < 0.01$) in *S. uberis*-challenged groups (Figure 5A); these levels peaked at 12 h compared to 24 h post *S. uberis* in cells pretreated with NAC (Supplementary Figure S4). Increased Lyso-Tracker red fluorescence ($p < 0.01$), indicative of autophagy, was observed in *S. uberis*-challenged mMECs (Figure 5B). Red fluorescence intensity increased from 0 to 6 and 12 h post challenge, but had subsequently decreased by 24 h.

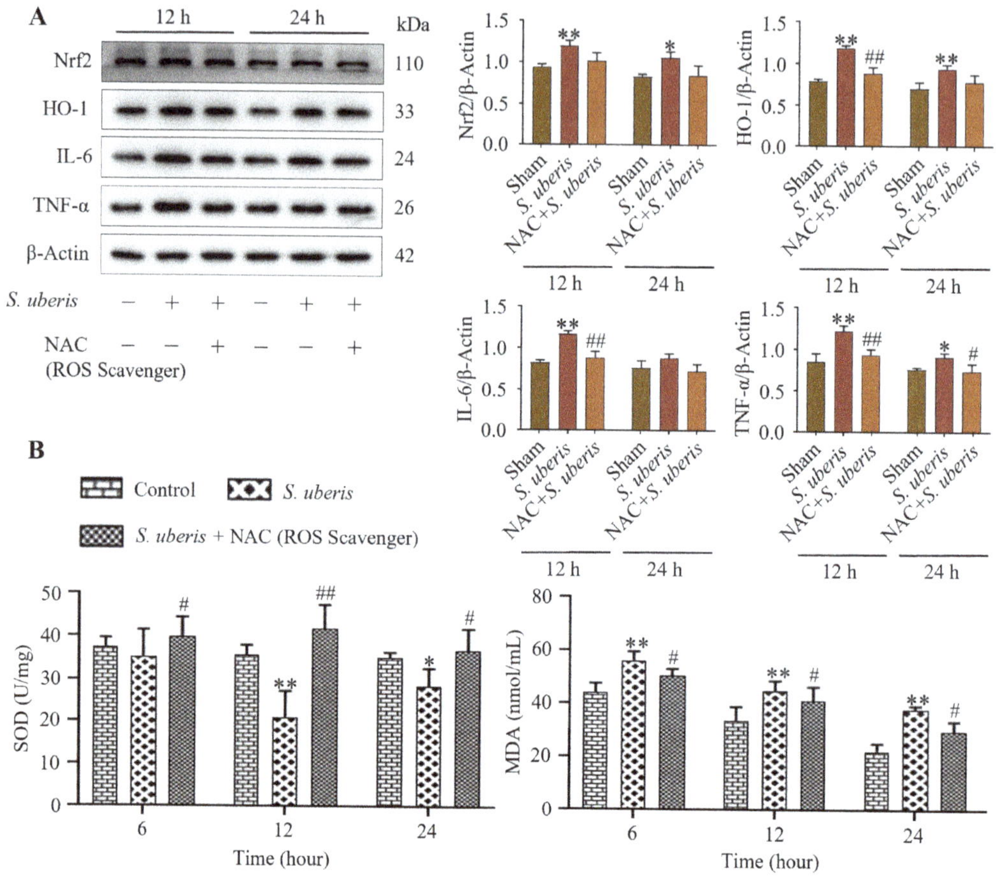

Figure 4. Pretreatment with NAC attenuated inflammatory and cellular damage in *S. uberis*-challenged mMECs and mammary glands by reducing oxidative stress. (**A**) Antioxidative Nrf2 and HO-1 and inflammatory IL-6 and TNF-α were determined in mMECs pretreated with NAC (30 μM) and 1 h later challenged with *S. uberis*. (**B**) Levels of total SOD and MDA activities at 6, 12 and 24 h post *S. uberis* challenge and pretreatment with NAC. Data represent mean ± SD of three independent experiments. * $p < 0.05$ and ** $p < 0.01$ (compared to the Sham); # $p < 0.05$ and ## $p < 0.01$ (compared to the *S. uberis* group).

3.6. Inhibition of Antioxidative Sirt1 Impaired Autophagy in mMECs by Inducing Inflammation

Concentrations of HO-1, IL-6, TNF-α and Atg5 were upregulated ($p < 0.05$) in mMECs challenged by *S. uberis*, but concentrations were reduced in mMECs pretreated with Sirt1 inhibitor (Cambinol) before *S. uberis* challenge (Figure 6A). In response to siSirt1 treatment, expressions of IL-6 increased numerically along with increases ($p < 0.05$) in TNF-α markers (Supplementary Figure S5). Autophagy dynamics changed in response to Cambinol. Vector Ad-mCherry-GFP-LC3B co-localized in autophagosomes in *S. uberis*-challenged cells (Figure 6B), but in Cambinol + *S. uberis* cells, the red fluorescence turned into yellow puncta ($p < 0.01$) due to a green GFP-LC3B co-localization in a non-acidic environment, indicative of autophagy inhibition.

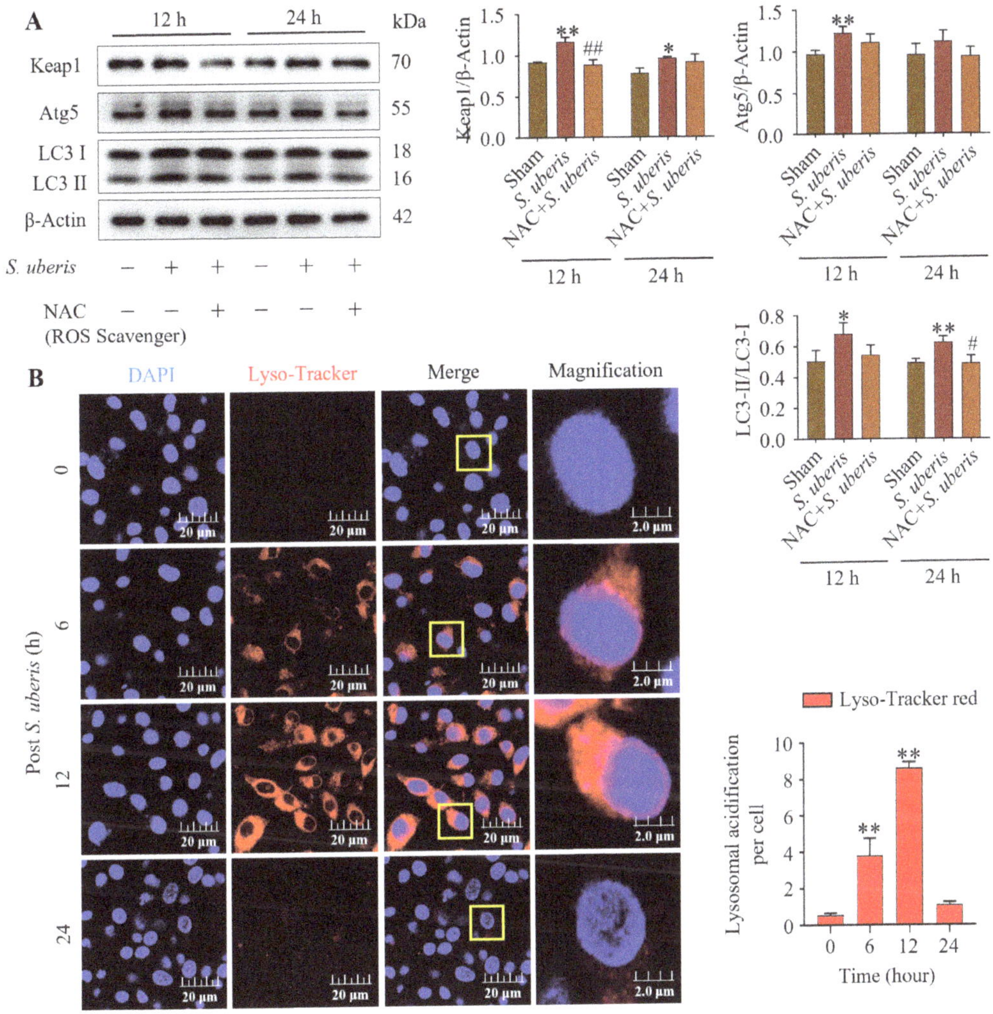

Figure 5. NAC treatment alleviated autophagy in *S. uberis*-challenged mMECs. (**A**) Protein concentrations of Keap1, Atg5 and LC3II/LC3I in mMECs pretreated with NAC (30 μM) 1 h prior to *S. uberis* challenge. (**B**) Formation of acidified lysosomes was quantified by measuring red fluorescence intensity. In total, 30 cells were selected for each group and 10 cells per sample with three repeats were quantified for statistical analyses. Data are representative means of three independent experiments. * $p < 0.05$ and ** $p < 0.01$ (compared to the Sham); # $p < 0.05$ and ## $p < 0.01$ (compared to the *S. uberis* group). Magnified figure It comes from the yellow box.

3.7. Antioxidative Nrf2 Activation Induced Autophagy by Alleviating Inflammatory Responses

At 12 and 24 hpi, concentrations of antioxidants Nrf2, HO-1, inflammatory IL-6, TNF-α and autophagy LC3II/LC3I markers were evaluated in the presence of NK-252 (Nrf2 activator) to identify the effects of the antioxidative pathway on inflammation and autophagy mechanisms. The mMECs infected with *S. uberis* expressed increased ($p < 0.01$) concentrations of Nrf2, HO-1, IL-6, and TNF-α and increased LC3II/LC3I markers compared to the Sham (Figure 7A). However, IL-6 and TNF-α had decreased ($p < 0.01$) at 12 hpi with NK-252 + infection compared to infection of *S. uberis* (Supplementary Figure S6). Additionally, green fluorescence in the *S. uberis* + NK-252 group had stronger intensity ($p < 0.01$)

than mMECs infected with *S. uberis* or non-infected mMECs (Sham) (Figure 7B), indicating Nrf2 activation at 6 hpi.

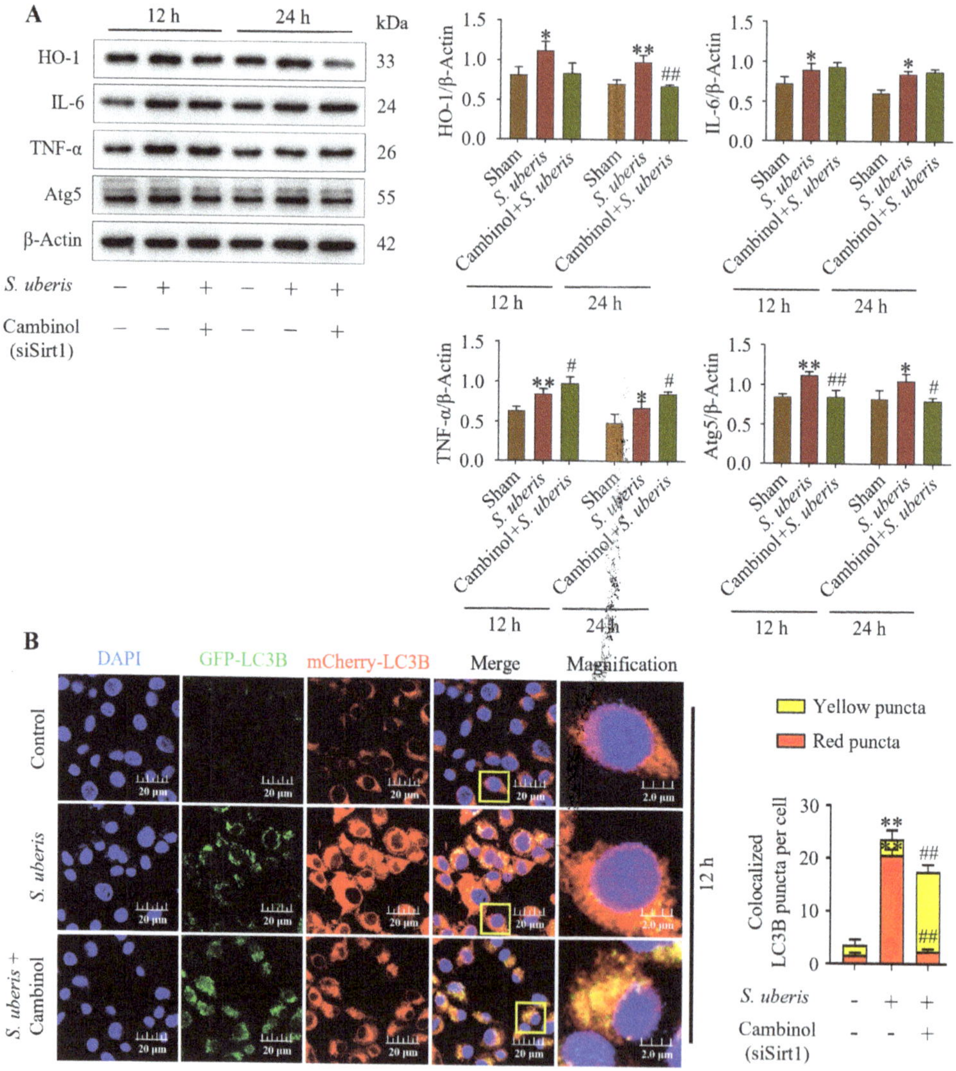

Figure 6. Silencing of Sirt1 in mMECs inhibited autophagy by inducing inflammation. (**A**) Protein expressions of HO-1, IL-6, TNF-α and Atg5 in mMECs pretreated with Cambinol (siSirt1) (40 μM) 6 h prior to *S. uberis* challenge. (**B**) Transfection of mMECs with Ad-mCherry-GFP-LC3B to determine autophagy inhibition in Cambinol treatment. Quantification of red, green and yellow fluorescence conducted by ImageJ 1.49v software with JaCoP plugin. Statistical data analyses were conducted on 10 cells per sample. Data represent mean ± SD of three independent experiments. * $p < 0.05$ and ** $p < 0.01$ (compared to the Sham); # $p < 0.05$ and ## $p < 0.01$ (compared to the *S. uberis* group). Magnified figure It comes from the yellow box.

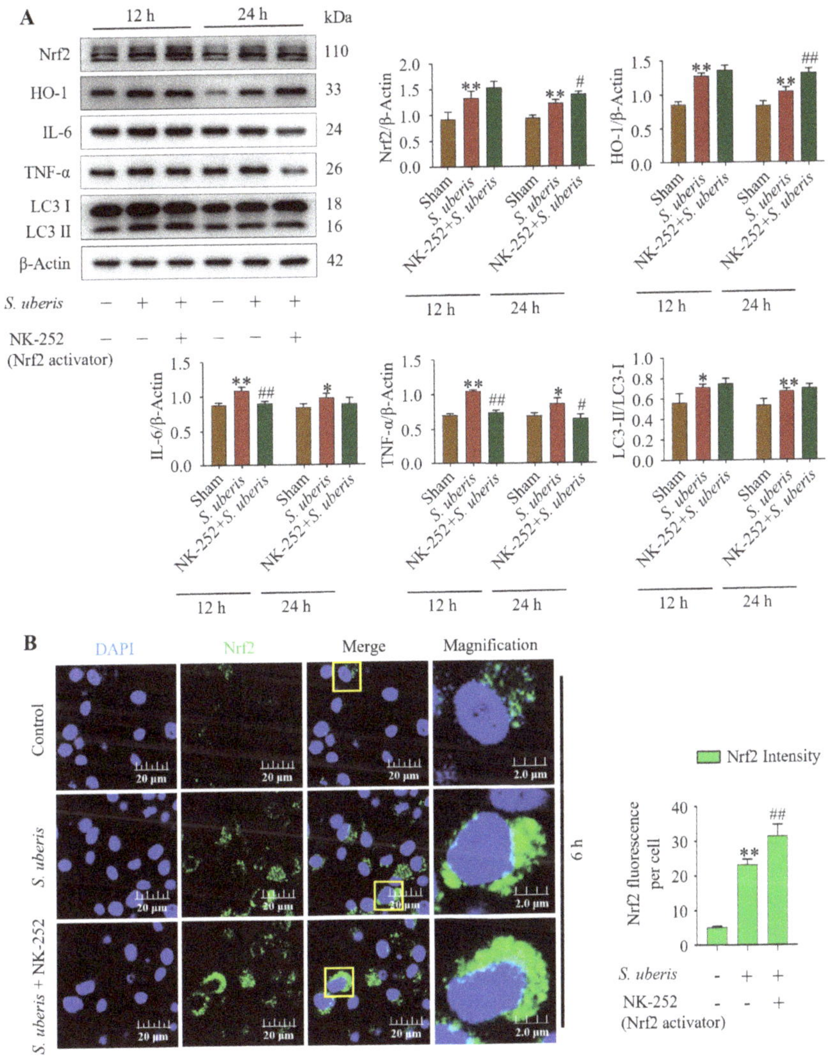

Figure 7. Activation of Nrf2 triggered autophagy by attenuating IL-6 and TNF-α. (**A**) Expression of Nrf2, HO-1, IL-6, TNF-α and LC3II/LC3I in mMECs pretreated with 10 μM of NK-252 (Nrf2 activator) 6 h prior to *S. uberis* challenge. (**B**) Nrf2 protein expressions in *S. uberis*-challenged mMECs analyzed by immunofluorescence assay. Nrf2 green fluorescence intensity was quantified using ImageJ software with JaCoP plugin. For statistical analyses, 10 cells were selected for each sample. The given data are representative of the mean of three independent experiments. * $p < 0.05$ and ** $p < 0.01$ (compared to the Sham); # $p < 0.05$ and ## $p < 0.01$ (compared to the *S. uberis* group). Magnified figure It comes from the yellow box.

3.8. Deactivation of Antioxidative Nrf2 Inhibited Autophagy by Increasing Inflammatory Responses

Infection with *S. uberis* induced ($p < 0.01$) Nrf2, HO-1, IL-6, TNF-α and Atg5 (Figure 8A). However, pretreatment with ML385 (Nrf2 inhibitor) followed by *S. uberis* challenge numerically decreased Nrf2, whereas HO-1 and Atg5 were reduced ($p < 0.01$) (Supplementary Figure S7). Concentrations of IL-6 increased ($p > 0.05$) and TNF-α was upregulated

($p < 0.01$) after Nrf2 inhibition, whereas HO-1 and autophagy Atg5 marker were downregulated ($p < 0.01$). Deactivation of Nrf2 in the presence of *S. uberis* was evident based on lower green fluorescence intensity ($p < 0.01$) in the ML385 + *S. uberis* group versus the *S. uberis* group (Figure 8B).

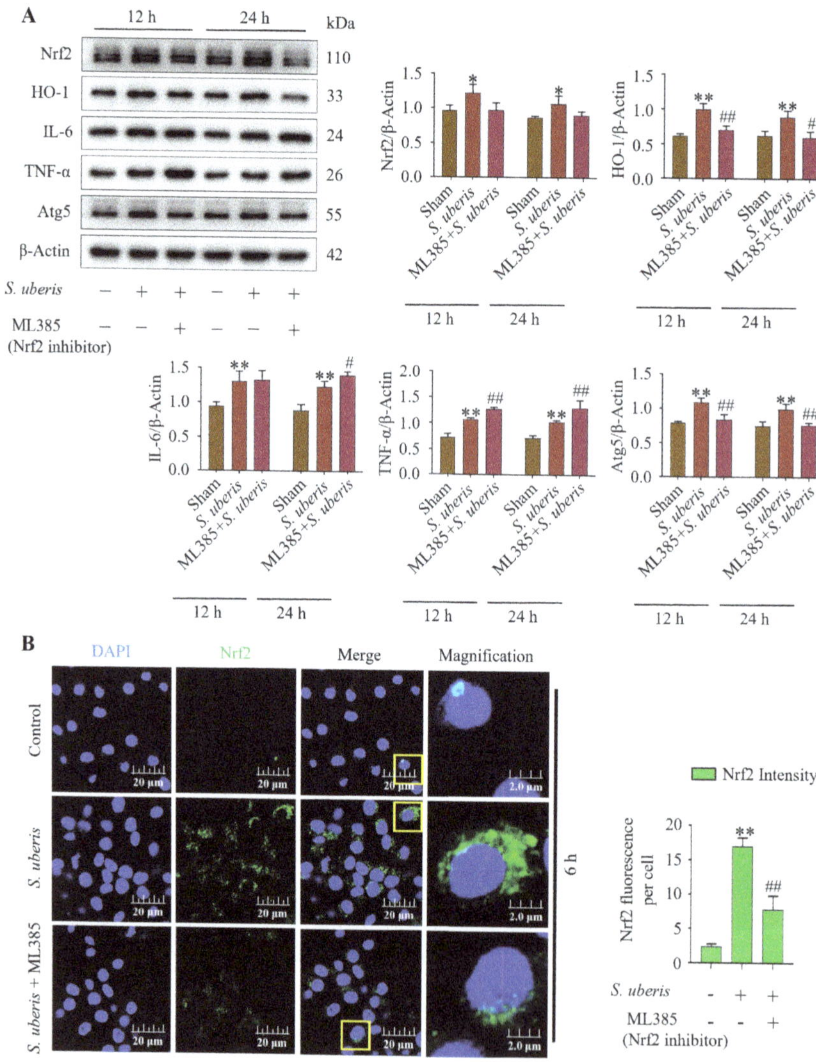

Figure 8. Suppression of antioxidative Nrf2 inhibited autophagy mechanism by increasing inflammation. (**A**) Nrf2 marker proteins were silenced by using 10 μM of ML385 in mMECs and Nrf2, HO-1, IL-6, TNF-α and Atg5 protein expression was analyzed at 12 and 24 h post *S. uberis* challenge. (**B**) Immunofluorescence confocal assay of Nrf2 in *S. uberis*-challenged mMECs. Quantitative image analysis of green Nrf2 intensity was conducted by ImageJ with JaCoP plugin in 10 cells/sample. Represented data are mean ± SD of three independent trials. * $p < 0.05$ and ** $p < 0.01$ (compared to the Sham); # $p < 0.05$ and ## $p < 0.01$ (compared to the *S. uberis* group). Magnified figure It comes from the yellow box.

3.9. Antioxidant Factors Were Increased in S. uberis-Challenged mMECs and Mammary Glands

Expression of Sirt1, Keap1, Nrf2, HO-1 and Atg5 was upregulated ($p < 0.01$) in *S. uberis*-challenged mMECs (Figure 9A). However, silencing of Sirt1 with Cambinol downregulated ($p < 0.05$) Sirt1, Keap1, Nrf2, HO-1 and Atg5 at 3 h, whereas inhibition of Nrf2 downregulated ($p < 0.05$) Nrf2, HO-1 and Atg5 at 6 h (Supplementary Figure S8). Therefore, Sirt1 and Keap1 preceded Nrf2 and HO-1 in the antioxidative pathway. In the murine model of mastitis, Sham mammary glands did not have sloughed mammary epithelial cells (Figure 9B). In contrast, mammary glands infected with *S. uberis* had damaged mammary epithelial cells, irrespective of Cambinol treatment. Compared to the *S. uberis* and Cambinol + *S. uberis* group, histopathological inflammatory changes were lower in the NAC + *S. uberis* and NK-252 + *S. uberis* groups.

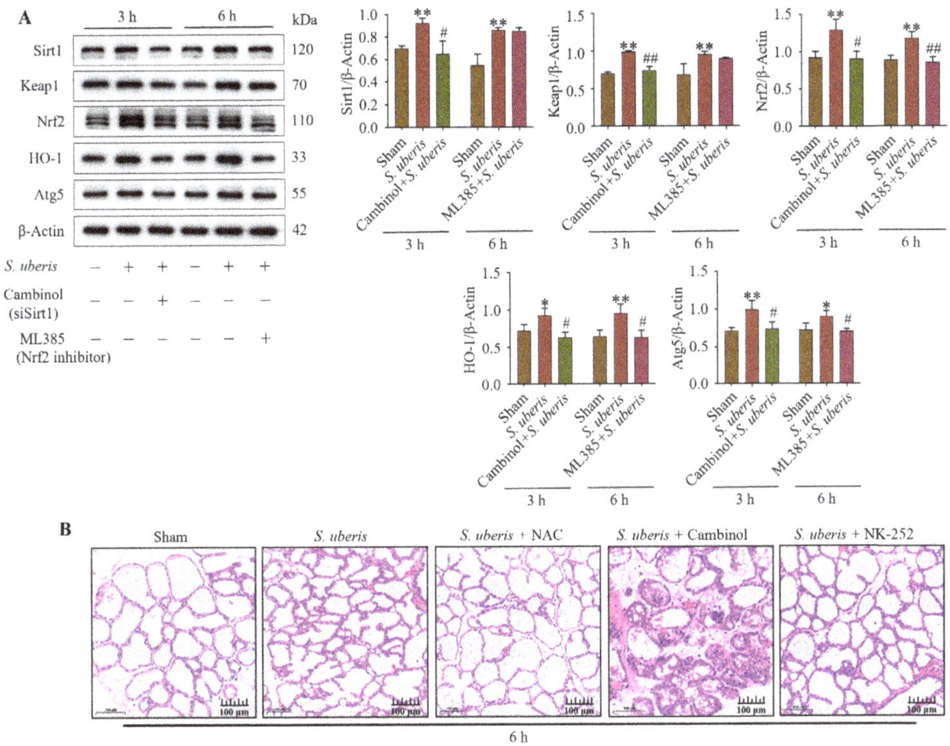

Figure 9. Mammary glands and mMECs activated antioxidative factors in response to oxidative stress provoked by *S. uberis*. (**A**) Expression of antioxidants Sirt1, Keap1, Nrf2, HO-1 and Atg5 in mMECs silenced in Sirt1 and Nrf2 previous to *S. uberis* at 3 h and 6 h challenge. (**B**) Mammary gland morphology after *S. uberis* challenge for 6 h in mice pretreated with NAC, Cambinol or NK-252. * $p < 0.05$ and ** $p < 0.01$ (compared to the Sham); # $p < 0.05$ and ## $p < 0.01$ (compared to the *S. uberis* group).

4. Discussion

As an important mediator of inflammation, *Streptococcus uberis* has been widely used to establish mastitis models in mice [35]. The mouse mastitis model established by injection of *S. uberis* was consistent with the clinical symptoms of cow mastitis [36]. The inflammatory factors TNF-α, IL-6 and IL-1β are closely associated with the response to bacterial *S. uberis* infection. *S. uberis* can stimulate inflammation cytokines, including IL-1β, TNF-α, IL-6 and IL-8, in bovine neutrophils, mammary epithelial cell and somatic milk cells models [37,38]. *S. uberis* is an important promoter in the NF-κB and MAPK inflammatory signaling pathways, which triggers inflammation in mammary epithelial cells [35]. Both TLR2 and TLR4 are involved in sensing *S. uberis* invasion. TLR2 is a principal receptor. The ability to stimulate TLR2 expression on the cell surface resulted in significant upregulation of both NF-κB and MAPK signaling pathways downstream [39]. In this study, murine mastitis models and mMECs were infected with *S. uberis* and the antioxidative, inflammatory and autophagy pathway elements were evaluated. We tested the hypothesis that silencing/activation of antioxidative pathway factors will bring changes in the autophagy mechanism. Whereas inflammatory changes and autophagy mechanisms were inversely correlated in our recent study [32], highlighting the role of Nrf2 in alleviating inflammation [40], this study examined the involvement of antioxidative pathways regulating autophagy. Key antioxidative elements, including Sirt1, Keap1, Nrf2 and HO-1 positively modulated the autophagy markers Atg5 and LC3II/LC3I and concurrently downregulated inflammatory IL-6 and TNF-α. Antioxidant SOD concentrations decreased, along with a reduction in MDA activity [41]. Thus, lower T-SOD and MDA activities reduced cellular damage due to oxidative stress in *S. uberis*-infected mammary glands, particularly epithelial cells. Furthermore, treatment with NAC attenuated morphological damage and reduced expressions of inflammatory markers but not autophagy, implying that oxidative stress and activation of the antioxidative pathway are key for inducing autophagy.

In response to oxidative stress at early stages of *S. uberis* infection, the antioxidative pathway was activated with increased key antioxidative regulatory factors (Sirt1, Keap1, Nrf2 and HO-1) [14,42]. Expression of inflammatory and autophagy markers also fluctuated with *S. uberis* infection. Therefore, the antioxidative pathway seemed to induce autophagy by modulating inflammatory responses. As inflammation and oxidative stress are directly associated, and excessive ROS activates numerous inflammatory mechanisms [43], we evaluated pathways associated with oxidative stress and mastitis. Inhibition of ROS with NAC prior to *S. uberis* infection reduced the need for antioxidative factors in mammary glands and mMECs. Furthermore, lower T-SOD and MDA activities also reduced oxidative stress damage. Thus, inflammatory IL-6 and TNF-α were downregulated, whereas autophagy Atg5 and LC3II/LC3I and the antioxidative Sirt1, Keap1, Nrf2 and HO-1 were increased.

In the present study, the antioxidative pathway was induced by *S. uberis* and counteracted oxidative stress in both mMECs and mastitis models. Sirt1 is the key element, as it reduced oxidative stress, whereas increases in Keap1, Nrf2 and HO-1 were dependent on Sirt1 marker proteins (indicating enhanced antioxidative activity) and suppressing inflammation. Nrf2 is a crucial regulator of cellular redox reactions [44] and a sensitive signal for scavenging ROS. Some pathogenic microbes enhance oxidative stress associated with expressions of the Nrf2/HO-1 pathway [45]. Similar outcomes following treatment with ML385 (Nrf2 inhibitor) and Cambinol (siSirt1) after *S. uberis* challenge implied that both Sirt1 and Nrf2 are antioxidative markers. Lack of suppression of Sirt1 and Keap1 with ML385 (Nrf2 inhibitor) indicated that Nrf2 and HO-1 are later components and led by Sirt1 and Keap1 antioxidative elements. Increases in the cytoprotective gene HO-1 after activation of Nrf2 would protect mMECs against oxidative damage [46], degrading heme to generate anti-inflammatory carbon monoxide (a vasodilatory gas) [47]. Moreover, downregulation of IL-6 and TNF-α with increased HO-1 due to activation of Nrf2 would promote autophagy.

Activation of the antioxidative pathway would stimulate autophagy by decreasing inflammation. IL-6 and TNF-α were downregulated during autophagy [32], along with increased expressions of antioxidative Sirt1, Keap1, Nrf2 and HO-1. Thus, inhibition of Nrf2 not only reduced antioxidant activity but also upregulated inflammatory IL-6 and TNF-α markers. Additionally, the antioxidative pathway had a positive and direct impact on autophagy. In fact, silencing Sirt1 impaired autophagy in the Ad-mCherry-GFP-LC3B transfection assay, with both GFP green and mCherry red fluorescence becoming yellow puncta [48].

We illustrated that *S. uberis* challenge indirectly induces autophagy in mMECs by targeting antioxidative Sirt1, Keap1, Nrf2 and Ho-1. Oxidative stress was increased, which also increased Sirt1 along with Keap1, Nrf2 and HO-1 as antioxidative mechanisms. Oxidative stress also dissociates Nrf2 from Keap1 protein, transfers Nrf2 to the nucleus, and induced expressions of HO-1. The increased antioxidative factors increase autophagous Atg5 and LC3II/LC3I by reducing inflammatory IL-6 and TNF-α. The inhibitory treatment of Sirt1 and Nrf2 have negative effects on autophagy induction, while Nrf2 activation enhanced autophagy activity. HO-1 increased the levels of total SOD and MDA contents against oxidative stress. Thus, autophagy inhibits oxidative stress and cellular damage in mastitis.

5. Conclusions

In conclusion, *S. uberis* infection induced oxidative stress in mouse mammary epithelial cells, which activated an antioxidative pathway that mitigated inflammatory responses and reduced cellular damage (Figure 10). Inflammation could thus be attenuated by the antioxidative pathway and autophagy mechanism.

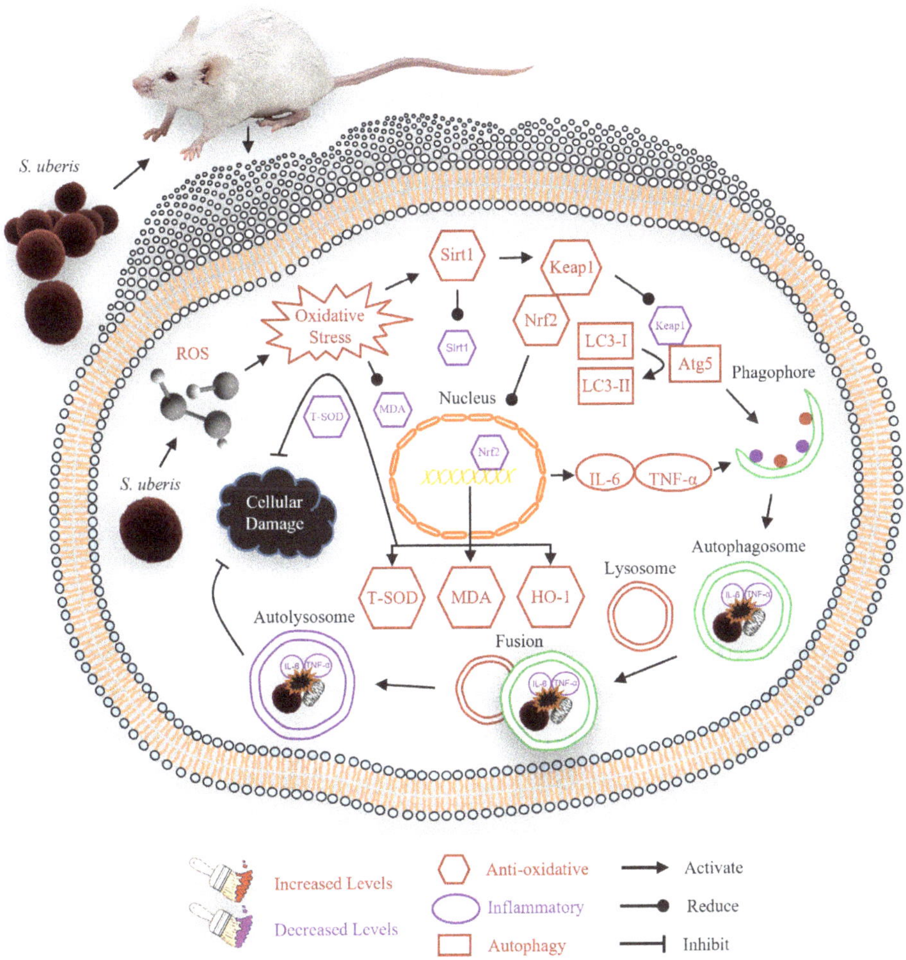

Figure 10. Theoretical scheme of antioxidative factors that regulate autophagy mechanism in mastitis.

Supplementary Materials: The following supporting information can be downloaded at: https://www.mdpi.com/article/10.3390/antiox13020171/s1. Figure S1: Original WB of *S. uberis*-infected mMECs induced antioxidant and autophagy marker proteins and reduced inflammatory cytokines; Figure S2: Original WB of NAC pretreatment in *S. uberis*-challenged mMECs mitigated antioxidative responses; Figure S3: Original WB of pretreatment with NAC attenuated inflammatory and cellular damage in *S. uberis*-challenged mMECs and mammary glands by reducing oxidative stress; Figure S4: Original WB of NAC treatment alleviated autophagy in *S. uberis*-challenged mMECs; Figure S5: Original WB of silencing of Sirt1 in mMECs inhibited autophagy by inducing inflammation; Figure S6: Original WB of activation of Nrf2 triggered autophagy by attenuating IL-6 and TNF-α; Figure S7: Original WB of suppression of antioxidative Nrf2 inhibited autophagy mechanism by increasing inflammation; Figure S8: Original WB of mammary glands and mMECs activated antioxidative factors in response to oxidative stress provoked by *S. uberis*.

Author Contributions: Conceptualization, B.H. and G.L.; methodology, S.K.; software, M.A.K. and M.X.; validation, T.W., M.X. and B.L.; formal analysis, S.K.; investigation, T.W. and M.X.; resources, J.G.; data curation, S.K., M.A.K. and M.X.; writing—original draft preparation, S.K., T.W., B.L., M.A.K., M.X., W.Q. and J.G.; writing—review and editing, E.R.C., H.W.B., J.P.K., G.L. and B.H.; visualization, S.K., T.W. and M.X.; supervision, B.H. and G.L.; project administration, B.H.; funding acquisition, B.H. All authors have read and agreed to the published version of the manuscript.

Funding: This work was supported in part by the National Natural Science Foundation of China (No. 32172928 and No. 31772813 to B.H.), the High-end Foreign Experts Recruitment Program (No. G2022108009L to B.H.).

Institutional Review Board Statement: This study was carried out according to the guidelines of the Declaration of Helsinki and was approved by the Animal Care Advisory Committee of College of Veterinary Medicine, China Agricultural University (CAU), Beijing, China (Protocol SYXK, 2016-0008). Furthermore, it was conducted according to standard ethical guidelines implemented at CAU.

Informed Consent Statement: Written informed consent has been obtained from the patient(s) to publish this paper.

Data Availability Statement: Data will be made available on request from the corresponding author.

Acknowledgments: The authors express their sincere appreciation to the Figdraw platform for providing drawing materials.

Conflicts of Interest: The authors declare no conflict of interest.

References

1. Majumder, S.; Eckersall, P.D.; George, S. Bovine mastitis: Examining factors contributing to treatment failure and prospects of nano-enabled antibacterial combination therapy. *ACS Agric. Sci. Technol.* **2023**, *7*, 562–582. [CrossRef]
2. Dalanezi, F.; Joaquim, S.; Guimarães, F.; Guerra, S.; Lopes, B.; Schmidt, E.; Cerri, R.; Langoni, H. Influence of pathogens causing clinical mastitis on reproductive variables of dairy cows. *J. Dairy Sci.* **2020**, *103*, 3648–3655. [CrossRef] [PubMed]
3. Heikkilä, A.M.; Liski, E.; Pyörälä, S.; Taponen, S. Pathogen-specific production losses in bovine mastitis. *J. Dairy Sci.* **2018**, *101*, 9493–9504. [CrossRef] [PubMed]
4. Wente, N.; Klocke, D.; Paduch, J.H.; Zhang, Y.; Tho Seeth, M.; Zoche-Golob, V.; Reinecke, F.; Mohr, E.; Krömker, V. Associations between *Streptococcus uberis* strains from the animal environment and clinical bovine mastitis cases. *J. Dairy Sci.* **2019**, *102*, 9360–9369. [CrossRef] [PubMed]
5. de Jong, E.; McCubbin, K.D.; Speksnijder, D.; Dufour, S.; Middleton, J.R.; Ruegg, P.L.; Lam, T.J.G.M.; Kelton, D.F. Invited review: Selective treatment of clinical mastitis in dairy cattle. *J. Dairy Sci.* **2023**, *106*, 3761–3778. [CrossRef] [PubMed]
6. Wang, Z.; Lan, R.; Xu, Y.; Zuo, J.; Han, X.; Phouthapane, V.; Luo, Z.; Miao, J. Taurine alleviates *Streptococcus uberis*-induced inflammation by activating autophagy in mammary epithelial cells. *Front. Immunol.* **2021**, *12*, 631113. [CrossRef] [PubMed]
7. Zhou, Y.; Lan, R.; Xu, Y.; Zhou, Y.; Lin, X.; Miao, J. Resveratrol alleviates oxidative stress caused by *Streptococcus uberis* infection via activating the Nrf2 signaling pathway. *Int. Immunopharmacol.* **2020**, *89*, 107076. [CrossRef] [PubMed]
8. Hu, W.; Chan, H.; Lu, L.; Wong, K.T.; Wong, S.H.; Li, M.X.; Xiao, Z.G.; Cho, C.H.; Gin, T.; Chan, M.T.V.; et al. Autophagy in intracellular bacterial infection. *Semin. Cell Dev. Biol.* **2020**, *101*, 41–50. [CrossRef]
9. Yu, L.; Chen, Y.; Tooze, S.A. Autophagy pathway: Cellular and molecular mechanisms. *Autophagy* **2018**, *14*, 207–215. [CrossRef]
10. Romeo, M.A.; Montani, M.S.G.; Benedetti, R.; Giambelli, L.; D'Aprile, R.; Gaeta, A.; Faggioni, A.; Cirone, M. The cross-talk between STAT1/STAT3 and ROS up-regulates PD-L1 and promotes the release of pro-inflammatory/immune suppressive cytokines in primary monocytes infected by HHV-6B. *Virus Res.* **2021**, *292*, 198231. [CrossRef]

11. Ren, Z.; He, H.; Zuo, Z.; Xu, Z.; Wei, Z.; Deng, J. The role of different SIRT1-mediated signaling pathways in toxic injury. *Cell. Mol. Biol. Lett.* **2019**, *24*, 1–10. [CrossRef] [PubMed]
12. Alshehri, A.; El-Kott, A.F.; Eleawa, S.; El-Gerbed, M.; Khalifa, H.; El-Kenawy, A.; Albadrani, G.M.; Abdel-Daim, M.M. Kaempferol protects against streptozotocin-induced diabetic cardiomyopathy in rats by a hypoglycemic effect and upregulating SIRT1. *J. Physiol. Pharmacol.* **2021**, *72*, 339–355.
13. Zhao, H.; Chen, S.; Gao, K.; Zhou, Z.; Wang, C.; Shen, Z.; Guo, Y.; Li, Z.; Wan, Z.; Liu, C.; et al. Resveratrol protects against spinal cord injury by activating autophagy and inhibiting apoptosis mediated by the SIRT1/AMPK signaling pathway. *Neuroscience* **2017**, *348*, 241–251. [CrossRef] [PubMed]
14. Huang, K.; Gao, X.; Wei, W. The crosstalk between Sirt1 and Keap1/Nrf2/ARE anti-oxidative pathway forms a positive feedback loop to inhibit FN and TGF-β1 expressions in rat glomerular mesangial cells. *Exp. Cell Res.* **2017**, *361*, 63–72. [CrossRef] [PubMed]
15. Baird, L.; Yamamoto, M. The molecular mechanisms regulating the KEAP1-NRF2 pathway. *Mol. Cell Biol.* **2020**, *40*, e00099-20. [CrossRef] [PubMed]
16. Mizunoe, Y.; Kobayashi, M.; Sudo, Y.; Watanabe, S.; Yasukawa, H.; Natori, D.; Hoshino, A.; Negishi, A.; Okita, N.; Komatsu, M.; et al. Trehalose protects against oxidative stress by regulating the Keap1–Nrf2 and autophagy pathways. *Redox Biol.* **2018**, *15*, 115–124. [CrossRef] [PubMed]
17. Shen, K.; Jia, Y.; Wang, X.; Zhang, J.; Liu, K.; Wang, J.; Cai, W.; Li, J.; Li, S.; Zhao, M.; et al. Exosomes from adipose-derived stem cells alleviate the inflammation and oxidative stress via regulating Nrf2/HO-1 axis in macrophages. *Free Radic. Biol. Med.* **2021**, *165*, 54–66. [CrossRef]
18. Chen, H.; Xie, K.; Chen, Y.; Wang, Y.; Wang, Y.; Lian, N.; Zhang, K.; Yu, Y. Nrf2/HO-1 signaling pathway participated in the protection of hydrogen sulfide on neuropathic pain in rats. *Int. Immunopharmacol.* **2019**, *75*, 105746. [CrossRef]
19. Jayasinghe, A.M.K.; Kirindage, K.G.I.S.; Fernando, I.P.S.; Han, E.J.; Oh, G.W.; Jung, W.K.; Ahn, G. Fucoidan isolated from sargassum confusum suppresses inflammatory responses and oxidative stress in TNF-α/IFN-γ-stimulated HaCaT keratinocytes by activating Nrf2/HO-1 signaling pathway. *Mar. Drugs* **2022**, *20*, 117. [CrossRef]
20. Shen, C.; Luo, Z.; Ma, S.; Yu, C.; Gao, Q.; Zhang, M.; Zhang, H.; Zhang, J.; Xu, W.; Yao, J.; et al. Microbe-derived antioxidants reduce lipopolysaccharide-induced inflammatory responses by activating the Nrf2 pathway to inhibit the ROS/NLRP3/IL-1β signaling pathway. *Int. J. Mol. Sci.* **2022**, *23*, 12477. [CrossRef]
21. Ichimura, Y.; Komatsu, M. Activation of p62/SQSTM1–Keap1–nuclear factor erythroid 2-related factor 2 pathway in cancer. *Front. Oncol.* **2018**, *8*, 210. [CrossRef] [PubMed]
22. Fan, X.; Huang, T.; Tong, Y.; Fan, Z.; Yang, Z.; Yang, D.; Mao, X.; Yang, M. p62 works as a hub modulation in the ageing process. *Ageing Res. Rev.* **2022**, *73*, 101538. [CrossRef] [PubMed]
23. Debnath, J.; Gammoh, N.; Ryan, K.M. Autophagy and autophagy-related pathways in cancer. *Nat. Rev. Mol. Cell Biol.* **2023**, *24*, 560–575. [CrossRef] [PubMed]
24. Xu, W.; Ocak, U.; Gao, L.; Tu, S.; Lenahan, C.J.; Zhang, J.; Shao, A. Selective autophagy as a therapeutic target for neurological diseases. *Cell. Mol. Life Sci.* **2021**, *78*, 1369–1392. [CrossRef] [PubMed]
25. Ding, X.; Zhu, C.; Wang, W.; Li, M.; Ma, C.; Gao, B. SIRT1 is a regulator of autophagy: Implications for the progression and treatment of myocardial ischemia-reperfusion. *Pharmacol. Res.* **2023**, *9*, 106957. [CrossRef] [PubMed]
26. Sudhakar, P.; Jacomin, A.C.; Hautefort, I.; Samavedam, S.; Fatemian, K.; Ari, E.; Gul, L.; Demeter, A.; Jones, E.; Korcsmaros, T.; et al. Targeted interplay between bacterial pathogens and host autophagy. *Autophagy* **2019**, *15*, 1620–1633. [CrossRef] [PubMed]
27. King, K.E.; Losier, T.T.; Russell, R.C. Regulation of autophagy enzymes by nutrient signaling. *Trends Biochem. Sci.* **2021**, *46*, 687–700. [CrossRef]
28. Galluzzi, L.; Bravo-San Pedro, J.M.; Levine, B.; Green, D.R.; Kroemer, G. Pharmacological modulation of autophagy: Therapeutic potential and persisting obstacles. *Nat. Rev. Drug Discov.* **2017**, *16*, 487–511. [CrossRef]
29. Zhao, W.; Xu, M.; Barkema, H.W.; Xie, X.; Lin, Y.; Khan, S.; Kastelic, J.P.; Wang, D.; Deng, Z.; Han, B. *Prototheca bovis* induces autophagy in bovine mammary epithelial cells via the HIF-1α and AMPKα/ULK1 pathway. *Front. Immunol.* **2022**, *13*, 934819. [CrossRef]
30. Xu, M.; Liu, Y.; Mayinuer, T.; Lin, Y.; Wang, Y.; Gao, J.; Wang, D.; Kastelic, J.P.; Han, B. *Mycoplasma bovis* inhibits autophagy in bovine mammary epithelial cells via a PTEN/PI3K-Akt-mTOR-dependent pathway. *Front. Microbiol.* **2022**, *13*, 2808. [CrossRef]
31. Liu, Y.; Deng, Z.; Xu, S.; Liu, G.; Lin, Y.; Khan, S.; Gao, J.; Qu, W.; Kastelic, J.P.; Han, B. *Mycoplasma bovis* subverts autophagy to promote intracellular replication in bovine mammary epithelial cells cultured in vitro. *Vet. Res.* **2021**, *52*, 130. [CrossRef] [PubMed]
32. Khan, S.; Yang, J.; Cobo, E.R.; Wang, Y.; Xu, M.; Wang, T.; Shi, Y.; Liu, G.; Han, B. *Streptococcus uberis* induced expressions of pro-inflammatory IL-6, TNF-α, and IFN-γ in bovine mammary epithelial cells associated with inhibited autophagy and autophagy flux formation. *Microb. Pathog.* **2023**, *183*, 106270. [CrossRef] [PubMed]
33. Ruan, L.; Bai, J.; Ji, X.; Zhao, W.; Dong, X. A series of meso amide BODIPY based lysosome-targeting fluorescent probe with high photostability and sensitivity. *Anal. Chim. Acta* **2022**, *1205*, 339771. [CrossRef] [PubMed]
34. Klionsky, D.J.; Abdel-Aziz, A.K.; Abdelfatah, S.; Abdellatif, M.; Abdoli, A.; Abel, S.; Abel, S.; Abeliovich, H.; Abildgaard, M.H.; Abudu, Y.P.; et al. Guidelines for the use and interpretation of assays for monitoring autophagy. *Autophagy* **2021**, *17*, 1–382. [CrossRef] [PubMed]

35. Zhou, G.; Zhang, W.; Wen, H.; Su, Q.; Hao, Z.; Liu, J.; Gao, Y.; Zhang, H.; Ge, B.; Tong, C.; et al. Esculetin improves murine mastitis induced by *Streptococcus* isolated from bovine mammary glands by inhibiting NF-κB and MAPK signaling pathways. *Microb. Pathog.* **2023**, *185*, 106393. [CrossRef] [PubMed]
36. Vander Elst, N.; Bellemans, J.; Lavigne, R.; Briers, Y.; Meyer, E. Endolysin NC5 improves early cloxacillin treatment in a mouse model of *Streptococcus uberis* mastitis. *Appl. Microbiol. Biotechnol.* **2024**, *108*, 118. [CrossRef] [PubMed]
37. Goto, S.; Mikami, O.; Nagasawa, Y.; Watanabe, A. Bovine neutrophils stimulated with *Streptococcus uberis* induce neutrophil extracellular traps and cause cytotoxicity, and transcriptional upregulation of inflammatory cytokine genes in bovine mammary epithelial cells. *J. Vet. Med. Sci.* **2023**, *ahead of print*. [CrossRef]
38. Wellnitz, O.; Berger, U.; Schaeren, W.; Bruckmaier, R. Mastitis severity induced by two Streptococcus uberis strains is reflected by the mammary immune response in vitro. *Schweiz Arch. Tierheilkd.* **2012**, *154*, 317–323. [CrossRef] [PubMed]
39. Li, B.; Xi, P.; Wang, Z.; Han, X.; Xu, Y.; Zhang, Y.; Miao, J. PI3K/Akt/mTOR signaling pathway participates in *Streptococcus uberis*-induced inflammation in mammary epithelial cells in concert with the classical TLRs/NF-κB pathway. *Vet. Microbiol.* **2018**, *227*, 103–111. [CrossRef]
40. Zhao, W.; Deng, Z.; Barkema, H.W.; Xu, M.; Gao, J.; Liu, G.; Lin, Y.; Kastelic, J.P.; Han, B. Nrf2 and NF-κB/NLRP3 inflammasome pathways are involved in *Prototheca bovis* infections of mouse mammary gland tissue and mammary epithelial cells. *Free Radic. Biol. Med.* **2022**, *184*, 148–157. [CrossRef]
41. Zalewska-Ziob, M.; Adamek, B.; Kasperczyk, J.; Romuk, E.; Hudziec, E.; Chwalińska, E.; Dobija-Kubica, K.; Rogoziński, P.; Bruliński, K. Activity of antioxidant enzymes in the tumor and adjacent noncancerous tissues of non-small-cell lung cancer. *Oxid. Med. Cell Longev.* **2019**, *31*, 2901840.
42. Pu, Q.; Guo, X.X.; Hu, J.J.; Li, A.L.; Li, G.G.; Li, X.Y. Nicotinamide mononucleotide increases cell viability and restores tight junctions in high-glucose-treated human corneal epithelial cells via the SIRT1/Nrf2/HO-1 pathway. *Biomed. Pharmacother.* **2022**, *147*, 112659. [CrossRef]
43. Zhao, M.; Wang, Y.; Li, L.; Liu, S.; Wang, C.; Yuan, Y.; Yang, G.; Chen, Y.; Cheng, J.; Lu, Y.; et al. Mitochondrial ROS promote mitochondrial dysfunction and inflammation in ischemic acute kidney injury by disrupting TFAM-mediated mtDNA maintenance. *Theranostics* **2021**, *11*, 1845–1863. [CrossRef] [PubMed]
44. Wei, W.; Ma, N.; Fan, X.; Yu, Q.; Ci, X. The role of Nrf2 in acute kidney injury: Novel molecular mechanisms and therapeutic approaches. *Free Radic. Biol. Med.* **2020**, *158*, 1–12. [CrossRef] [PubMed]
45. Molagoda, I.M.N.; Lee, K.T.; Choi, Y.H.; Kim, G.Y. Anthocyanins from Hibiscus syriacus L. inhibit oxidative stress-mediated apoptosis by activating the Nrf2/HO-1 signaling pathway. *Antioxidants* **2020**, *9*, 42. [CrossRef] [PubMed]
46. Xu, D.; Liu, J.; Ma, H.; Guo, W.; Wang, J.; Kan, X.; Li, Y.; Gong, Q.; Cao, Y.; Cheng, J.; et al. Schisandrin A protects against lipopolysaccharide-induced mastitis through activating Nrf2 signaling pathway and inducing autophagy. *Int. Immunopharmacol.* **2020**, *78*, 105983. [CrossRef] [PubMed]
47. Petsouki, E.; Cabrera, S.N.S.; Heiss, E.H. AMPK and NRF2: Interactive players in the same team for cellular homeostasis? *Free Radic. Biol. Med.* **2022**, *190*, 75–93. [CrossRef] [PubMed]
48. Ma, J.; Han, Z.; Jiao, R.; Yuan, G.; Ma, C.; Yan, X.; Meng, A. Irisin ameliorates PM2. 5-induced acute lung injury by regulation of autophagy through AMPK/mTOR pathway. *J. Inflamm. Res.* **2023**, *16*, 1045–1057. [CrossRef]

MDPI AG
Grosspeteranlage 5
4052 Basel
Switzerland
Tel.: +41 61 683 77 34

Antioxidants Editorial Office
E-mail: antioxidants@mdpi.com
www.mdpi.com/journal/antioxidants

www.ingramcontent.com/pod-product-compliance
Lightning Source LLC
Chambersburg PA
CBHW061825210926
51850CB00006B/808
9783725858231